SURGERY - PROCEDURES, COMPLICATIONS, AND RESULTS

ADVANCES IN EXPERIMENTAL SURGERY

VOLUME 2

Surgery - Procedures, Complications, and Results

Additional books in this series can be found on Nova's website under the Series tab.

Additional e-books in this series can be found on Nova's website under the e-Books tab.

SURGERY - PROCEDURES, COMPLICATIONS, AND RESULTS

ADVANCES IN EXPERIMENTAL SURGERY

VOLUME 2

HUIFANG CHEN
AND
PAULO N. MARTINS
EDITORS

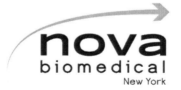

Copyright © 2018 by Nova Science Publishers, Inc.

All rights reserved. No part of this book may be reproduced, stored in a retrieval system or transmitted in any form or by any means: electronic, electrostatic, magnetic, tape, mechanical photocopying, recording or otherwise without the written permission of the Publisher.

We have partnered with Copyright Clearance Center to make it easy for you to obtain permissions to reuse content from this publication. Simply navigate to this publication's page on Nova's website and locate the "Get Permission" button below the title description. This button is linked directly to the title's permission page on copyright.com. Alternatively, you can visit copyright.com and search by title, ISBN, or ISSN.

For further questions about using the service on copyright.com, please contact:
Copyright Clearance Center
Phone: +1-(978) 750-8400   Fax: +1-(978) 750-4470   E-mail: info@copyright.com.

NOTICE TO THE READER

The Publisher has taken reasonable care in the preparation of this book, but makes no expressed or implied warranty of any kind and assumes no responsibility for any errors or omissions. No liability is assumed for incidental or consequential damages in connection with or arising out of information contained in this book. The Publisher shall not be liable for any special, consequential, or exemplary damages resulting, in whole or in part, from the readers' use of, or reliance upon, this material. Any parts of this book based on government reports are so indicated and copyright is claimed for those parts to the extent applicable to compilations of such works.

Independent verification should be sought for any data, advice or recommendations contained in this book. In addition, no responsibility is assumed by the publisher for any injury and/or damage to persons or property arising from any methods, products, instructions, ideas or otherwise contained in this publication.

This publication is designed to provide accurate and authoritative information with regard to the subject matter covered herein. It is sold with the clear understanding that the Publisher is not engaged in rendering legal or any other professional services. If legal or any other expert assistance is required, the services of a competent person should be sought. FROM A DECLARATION OF PARTICIPANTS JOINTLY ADOPTED BY A COMMITTEE OF THE AMERICAN BAR ASSOCIATION AND A COMMITTEE OF PUBLISHERS.

Additional color graphics may be available in the e-book version of this book.

Library of Congress Cataloging-in-Publication Data

ISBN: 978-1-53612-773-7

Published by Nova Science Publishers, Inc. † New York

CONTENTS

Foreword vii
    Pierre Daloze

Preface ix
    Huifang Chen and Paulo N. Martins

Section I. General and Specific Experimental Surgeries Models 1

Chapter 1   Laparoscopic Experimental Surgery Models   3
    Natalie Bath, Demetrius Litwin and Paulo N. Martins

Chapter 2   Experimental Models of Sepsis   37
    Norbert Nemeth, Mihai Oltean and Bela Fulesdi

Chapter 3   Bariatric Experimental Surgery Models   73
    Osman Bilgin Gulcicek

Chapter 4   Animal Models of Heart Failure   81
    Mouer Wang

Chapter 5   Hepatopancreatobiliary Surgery Experimental Models   107
    Paulo N. Martins, Natalie Bath and Adel Bozorgzadeh

Section II. Other Experimental Models 157

Chapter 6   Animal Models of Acute Graft-Versus-Host and Host-Versus-Graft Responses and Disease   159
    Abraham Matar and Raimon Duran-Struuck

Chapter 7   Microfluidic Devices and Micro-Dissected Tissue to Predict Therapeutic Response in Patients with Prostate Cancer   183
    Robin Guay-Lord, Muhammad Abdul Lateef, Kayla Simeone, Benjamin Péant, Jennifer Kendall-Dupont, Anne-Marie Mes-Masson, Thomas Gervais and Fred Saad

Chapter 8	Of Mice and Rats: Animal Models for Use in Laparoscopy and Laparotomy with Human Ovarian Cancer Cell Line Intraperitoneal Xenografts *Philippe Sauthier, Anne-Marie Mes-Masson, Louise Champoux, Michèle Bally and Diane M. Provencher*	211

Section III. Advance Techniques in Experimental Surgery 227

Chapter 9	Organ Bioengineering through Decellularization and Recellularization Approaches *Maria Jaramillo and Basak E. Uygun*	229
Chapter 10	Wound Healing and Scarring *A. Samandar Dowlatshahi*	255
Chapter 11	Organ Preservation *Cheng Yang, Jiawei Li and Ruiming Rong*	269
Chapter 12	Machine Organ Preservation *Hazel L. Marecki, Isabel Brüggenwirth and Paulo N. Martins*	289
Chapter 13	Microcirculation *Norbert Nemeth and Andrea Szabo*	317
Chapter 14	Experimental Gene Therapy Using Naked DNA *Eiji Kobayashi*	359
Chapter 15	Robotic Surgery in Experimental Medicine *Sandra S. Y. Kim, David Ian Harriman and Christopher Nguan*	373

About the Editors	403
Index	405

FOREWORD

Pierre Daloze, CM, CQ, MD, FRCSC
Professor Emeritus,
Department of Surgery, University of Montreal, Canada

Experimental surgery is a key link for developments in clinical surgery, research and teaching. Throughout the history of medicine, many discoveries and techniques developed from experimental surgery. Most modern surgeons are now learning or improving their surgical techniques firstly via experimental surgery. Reviewing the 20th century surgical developing history, most clinical achievements were related to experimental surgery. Some were real landmarks, such as successful vascular sutures, opening the striking advances of vascular surgery and organ transplantation. In recent years, experimental surgery has achieved new advances, like laparoscopic and robotic surgery, tissue engineering and gene therapy, which are now applied in clinic and have saved many patients.

Both editors of this book, Drs. Huifang Chen and Paulo Martins as well as their colleagues have been contributing to experimental surgery at the University of Montreal, Canada and the University of Massachusetts, US. Their achievements in experimental surgical models in small and large animals, including nonhuman primates, have been applied in clinical trials.

It is my pleasure to write this foreword for this impressive book, *Advances in Experimental Surgery*, which Drs. Chen and Martins provide as a reference for surgeons, residents, surgical researchers, physicians, immunologists, veterinarians and nurses in surgery. I am sure these two volumes will provide an abundance of imperative information for these individuals and their patients.

PREFACE

Huifang Chen and Paulo N. Martins

Experimental surgery is an important link for developments in clinical surgery, research and teaching. Experimental surgery has been a part of the most important surgical discoveries in the past century. Since 1901, nine Nobel Prizes have been awarded to the pioneers who had remarkable achievements in basic or practical surgery. In recent years, experimental surgery has achieved new advances, like laparoscopic and robotic surgery, tissue engineering, and gene therapy which are widely applied in clinic surgery.

The present book covers wide experimental surgery in preclinical research models subdivided into two volumes. Volume I introduces basic surgical notions, techniques, and different surgical models involved in basic experimental surgery, and reviews the biomechanical models, ischemia/reperfusion injury models, repair and regeneration models, and organ and tissue transplantation models, respectively. Volume II introduces several specific experimental models such as laparoscopic and bariatric experimental surgical models. The second volume also introduces graft-versus-host diseases, and other experimental models. A review of the advances and development of recent techniques such as tissue engineering, organ preservation, wound healing and scarring, gene therapy and robotic surgery is included. This book documents the enormous volume of knowledge scientists have acquired in the field of experimental surgery.

The editors have invited experts from the United States, Canada, France, Germany, China, Japan, Korea, UK, Sweden, Netherlands, Hungary and Turkey to contribute 15 chapters in the fields of their expertise. This volume is a compilation of basic experimental surgery and updated advances of new developments in this field that will be invaluable to any experimental surgery lab.

The editors are grateful to Dr. Pierre Daloze for writing the foreword and reviewing these volumes. The editors also want to thank all of the authors for their contributions and the time they spent to make this book successful. We also appreciate Dr. Muhammad Zafarullah and Dr. Lijun Song for contributing their valuable time in proofreading the entirety of this book.

Dr. Huifang Chen, MD., PhD.
Professor of Surgery
Laboratory of Experimental Surgery, Research Center, CHUM
10th floor, R10. 480, University of Montreal
900 rue Saint Denis, Montreal, Quebec, Canada H2X 0A9
E. Mail: hui.fang.chen@umontreal.ca

Dr. Paulo N. Martins, MD., PhD, FAST, FACS
Department of Surgery
Division of Transplantation
UMass Memorial Medical Center
University of Massachusetts
Worcester, MA, USA
E. Mail: Paulo.martins@umassmemorial.org

SECTION I. GENERAL AND SPECIFIC EXPERIMENTAL SURGERIES MODELS

In: Advances in Experimental Surgery. Volume 2
Editors: Huifang Chen and Paulo N. Martins
ISBN: 978-1-53612-773-7
© 2018 Nova Science Publishers, Inc.

Chapter 1

LAPAROSCOPIC EXPERIMENTAL SURGERY MODELS

Natalie Bath MD[1], Demetrius Litwin MD and Paulo N. Martins MD, PhD [*]

[1]Department of Surgery, UMass Memorial Medical Center, University Campus, Worcester, MA
[2]Department of Surgery, Division of Organ Transplantation, UMass Memorial Medical Center, University Campus, Worcester, MA

ABSTRACT

Laparoscopy and minimally invasive surgery has continued to play an increasingly large role across all surgical fields including general surgery, gynecology, colorectal surgery, hepatobiliary surgery, and urology. By minimizing trauma to the abdominal wall, allowing faster recovery postoperatively, decreasing length of hospital stay, and improving cosmesis, laparoscopy has become the gold standard approach for many operations due to these improved outcomes. However, laparoscopic surgery demands its own unique set of surgical skills due to loss of tactile feedback, operating within a three-dimensional space as seen on a two-dimensional monitor, and the importance of recognizing spatial relationships. A learning curve is found to exist as one is further developing these skills. In order to further develop these skills prior to utilizing them in the operating room, live animal models and laparoscopic simulators have been developed. Live animal models including pigs, rabbits, and rats have been used for training, and it has been found that *in vivo* models appear to most closely resemble operating on patients; therefore, animal models are the ideal training model to be used in laparoscopic surgery training. As laparoscopy continues to become more popular throughout surgery, it also continues to evolve in order to further reduce the invasiveness of surgery as seen in robotic surgery, single incision laparoscopic surgery (SILS), and natural orifice translumenal endoscopic surgery (NOTES). These surgical techniques are the future of laparoscopic surgery and as their use becomes more widespread, training on experimental models specific to these methods will become even more important in order to optimize surgical outcomes for patients.

---

[*] Corresponding author: Paulo N. Martins, MD, PhD, Department of Surgery, Division of Organ Transplantation, 55 Lake Avenue North, Worcester, MA 01655, Tel: 508-334-2023,
Email: paulo.martins@umassmemorial.org.

Keywords: laparoscopic surgery, experimental laparoscopy, learning curve, animal models, laparoscopic simulator, future laparoscopy

ABBREVIATIONS

dVSS	de Vinci Skills Simulator
FLS	Fundamentals of Laparoscopic Surgery
MISTVR	Minimally Invasive Surgery Trainer Virtual Reality
NOTES	Natural orifice translumenal endoscopic surgery
OSATS	Objective Structured Assessment of Technical Skill
SEP	Sim-Surgery Educational Plateform
SILS	Single Incision Laparoscopic Surgery
TAPP	Transabdominal Preperitonal Practice
TEP	Totally Extraperitonal
VR	Virtual Reality

IMPORTANCE OF LAPAROSCOPIC TRAINING

Laparoscopic surgery requires a unique and at times more complex skill set than open surgery. In order to further develop these skills prior to utilizing them in the operating room, live animal models and laparoscopic simulators have been developed. Live animal models including pigs, rabbits, and rats have been used for training, and it has been found that *in vivo* models appear to most closely resemble operating on a live patient.

Laparoscopic surgery traces its roots to the early twentieth century when pioneers such as Dimitri Ott, Georg Kelling, and Hans Christian Jacobeus first began using laparoscopy as a diagnostic technique (Vecchio 2000). However, it was not until the early 1980s that a paradigm shift was made in the field of laparoscopy when laparoscopic procedures evolved from an invasive diagnostic tool to an efficient instrument for surgical treatment (Buia 2015). Over the last thirty years, laparoscopy has played an increasingly more predominant role across all surgical sub-specialties. As procedures become more complex and technically challenging, a need for additional robust laparoscopic skills training has been created. With ongoing improvements in surgical training, imaging, tools and instruments, laparoscopic surgery has been able to be safely used in innumerable fields. Additionally, experimental laparoscopic surgery helps to create a path for continuing evolution and new roles for laparoscopy to play in the future.

Laparoscopy has multiple advantages over open surgery such as minimizing trauma to the abdominal wall, which ultimately results in faster recovery, reduced hospital stay, and faster return to normal activity. As a result, laparoscopy has become the gold standard for many procedures despite lack of randomized controlled trials. Moreover, laparoscopy has been able to be used for oncological surgeries without providing inferior oncological results when compared to open surgery (Buia 2015).

Open appendectomy has been performed since the late 1800s with laparoscopic appendectomy gaining popularity during the 1980s. Meta-analyses comparing the two procedures have indicated that while operating times were increased with open appendectomies, there was found to be shorter hospital stay, less postoperative pain, faster recovery, and lower complication rates found in the laparoscopic appendectomy group. Meta-analysis of randomized controlled trials comparing laparoscopic to open appendectomy have found that although operative time was shorter for the open procedure, laparoscopic surgery was associated with earlier consumption of liquid and solid diet, shorter hospital stay, decreased use of oral and parenteral analgesics, and decreased wound infection amongst several other advantages (Li 2010; Ohtani 2012).

Similar to appendectomy, open cholecystectomy initially was the gold standard for treatment of symptomatic cholelithiasis for over one hundred years. However, with the gaining prevalence of minimally invasive techniques, laparoscopic cholecystectomy gained prominence in the 1980s and allowed a greater liberalization of indications for surgery (Antoniou 2014). Meta-analyses comparing these two approaches have showed that while no significant differences were found between these approaches with regards to mortality, complication rates, and operative time, laparoscopic cholecystectomy is associated with significantly shorter hospital stay and quicker overall recovery (Keus 2006).

The benefits of laparoscopy can also be extended to anti-reflux and adrenal surgery. Open Nissen fundoplication during which the gastric fundus is wrapped around the distal esophagus has been used in treatment for moderate to severe gastroesophageal reflux disease since the 1950s, but the laparoscopic technique was not introduced until 1991 by Dallemagne (Memon 2015). It was hypothesized that the benefits of laparoscopic surgery including less post-operative pain, faster recovery time, improved cosmesis, and reduced rate of wound infection could also be conferred to laparoscopic anti-reflux surgery. However, initial studies demonstrated complications including esophageal and gastric perforation, paraesophageal herniation and wrap migration into the chest (Peters 2009). As experience with laparoscopic anti-reflux surgery has increased in addition to improved surgical techniques and training, the laparoscopic approach has proved to be a safe and effective alternative to an open technique in that laparoscopy allows a faster recovery, reduced risk of complications, and similar treatment outcomes between groups.

Despite the fact that minimally invasive surgery has facilitated improved surgical outcomes amongst various specialties, there are drawbacks to laparoscopy over open surgery. Work hour restrictions for residents, cost of operating room time, and increased learning curve for laparoscopic training creates the need for surgical trainees to acquire a large part of these skills outside of the operating room and in a more efficient manner (Roberts 2006; Trehan 2015; Alaker 2016). Furthermore, laparoscopic surgery requires a unique and at times more complex skill set than open surgery, which furthers the need for training facilities outside of the operating room in order for these skills to be further developed without putting the patient's safety at risk (Alaker 2016). In order to fill the need for additional training outside the operating room, surgical simulation has emerged as an opportunity to instruct surgical trainees on how to safely develop laparoscopic skills away from the time and financial constraints of the operating room. These simulators allow the issues of patient safety and risk management concerns to be addressed more efficiently and effectively while also helping trainees acquire skills needed to perform complex procedures before utilizing these skills on live patients (Roberts 2006).

LAPAROSCOPIC SURGERY LEARNING CURVE

Laparoscopy has continued to evolve over the last two decades, and this evolution has allowed it to gain a larger presence amongst many fields ranging from bariatric surgery to colorectal surgery to urology. As laparoscopic surgery has become increasingly more widespread as the method of choice for many procedures, this increased exposure has allowed surgeons across specialties to apply basic laparoscopic skills to more technically demanding surgeries. For both the novice and expert laparoscopic surgeon, a learning curve exists when learning how to perform basic and advanced tasks, respectively. Specific to laparoscopic surgery, laparoscopy requires a new, different skill set than what is required by open surgery. Laparoscopy can prove to be difficult to learn and is very different from open surgery due to loss of tactile perception, using a two-dimensional video screen to work within a three-dimensional space, spatial relationships, developing ambidextrous skills, and the fulcrum effect (Grantcharov 2009; Greco 2010; Buckley 2014). Due to these added challenges, a steeper learning curve exists within laparoscopic surgery when compared to open surgery, and it is during this phase that an increased incidence of serious complications may occur (Grantcharov 2009). As a result, it is imperative that trainees complete adequate training prior to operating on patients. In order to facilitate the teaching and assessment of trainees' fundamental knowledge and technical skills in laparoscopy, The Fundamentals of Laparoscopic Surgery (FLS) program was developed. The FLS curriculum consists of five simulation stations, which aim to teach and assess basic laparoscopic surgery skills: peg transfer, precision cutting, loop ligation, and suturing with extracorporeal and intracorporeal knot tying (Zendejas 2016). The FLS curriculum, which originally evolved from the McGill Inanimate System for Training and Evaluation of Laparoscopic Skills (MISTELS), also consists of web-based didactics, hands-on skills training and a written exam. Both the Society of American Gastrointestinal and Endoscopic Surgeons (SAGES) and the American College of Surgeons (ACS) have endorsed the FLS training program, which is now a prerequisite for board eligibility in general surgery. The FLS program has been found to be effective in regards to training; however, fewer studies exist which further explore the validity of the assessment component of FLS (Fried 2004).

Acquisition of skill in both laparoscopic and open surgery by trainees has been described in the literature as a "learning curve". The learning curve can be defined as the observation that repetitive performance of motor skills results in improvement over time. This improvement is most notable early on with sequentially smaller improvements as the number of repetitions increase (Feldman 2009). The learning curve can be divided into three main parameters: the starting point, the learning rate, and learning plateau. The starting point is the skill level at which performance begins. It is at the starting point and early portion of the curve that higher incidence of complications, increased rates of conversion to laparoscopic to open, and longer operating times are seen to be experienced. The learning rate is the slope along the curve which is measured by how quickly a level of performance is reached, and the learning plateau is the plateau or asymptote level at which performance flattens and no longer improves (Cook 2007). When applied to surgical skills, learning curves vary between surgeons and are influenced by multiple factors including a surgeon's innate ability, previous experience, motivation, available technology, task complexity, case-mix and operative findings, and other members of the surgical team (Cook 2004; Sachdeva 2007). In applications to surgery, identifying where a trainee's skill level is located on their own learning curve can help to predict whether or not the trainee's skills will continue to improve. Traditionally, learning curves have been statistically analyzed by dividing the curve into halves or thirds with subsequent comparison of outcomes between earlier and later time periods. Although this approach may be useful for quantifying improvements over a period of time, it does not describe the underlying curve itself and does not allow for precise estimation of where the curve flattens and at what level this occurs. Furthermore, it does not allow for the estimation of individual skill differences between surgeons (Feldman 2009). By fitting an inverse curve to the performance curve of trainees, the learning curve effect can be estimated including the starting point, speed of learning, and plateau. Although not calculated on a regular basis amongst trainees, this technique may have a role in laparoscopic simulation when comparing groups of trainees who have been exposed to different educational interventions (Feldman 2009).

Although it has been shown that laparoscopic simulation helps trainees progress along the learning curve, some trainees possess an aptitude for laparoscopic skills which others may lack. This innate ability may allow for others to progress more quickly along the learning curve, and conversely, a lack of ability may prevent others from achieving adequate laparoscopic skills. In a study which examined this hypothesis, two groups of medical students with disparate innate ability were selected. Innate ability was defined as exceptional visuospatial ability, depth perception and psychomotor ability as measured by validated tests. Each group was tested on a laparoscopic skill trainer until they achieved proficiency in performing a laparoscopic appendectomy. The mean number of attempts to complete the procedure for the more skilled group was six attempts versus fourteen in the less skilled group. Furthermore, three participants in the less skilled group did not reach proficiency after eighteen attempts. This study demonstrated that high innate ability is directly related to a faster learning curve in achieving proficiency for a laparoscopic task (Buckley 2012).

Aptitude testing can further be applied to more difficult laparoscopic skills such as laparoscopic suturing and intracorporeal knot tying. As indicated in previously mentioned studies, aptitude can be used to predict the rate at which a trainee is able to become proficient at basic skills. In turn, one's aptitude can also be used to predict how quickly one is able to achieve proficiency at more complex laparoscopic procedures. Students in the high aptitude group were found to have higher visual spatial, perceptual and psychomotor ability than those in the low aptitude group. After didactic teaching on how to perform laparoscopic suturing, students in each group were asked to perform this task. Figure 1.1 compares path length, economy of movement, and time scores between surgical novices with low or high aptitude. Group A achieved proficiency faster than group B. In the low-aptitude group, 30% achieved proficiency after a mean attempt of fourteen while 40% demonstrated improvement but did not achieve proficiency over the course of sixteen attempts; 30% failed to progress altogether and were unable to progress along the learning curve as seen in Figure 1.1B. Group A achieved proficiency in a shorter amount of time in both economy of movement and time scores as shown in Figure 1.3C and 1.1E, respectively. Figures 1.1D and 1.1F demonstrate the results seen in group B: 30% reached proficiency, 40% showed improvement but did not reach proficiency, and 30% failed to progress. Figure 1.1 demonstrates the mean number of attempts to achieve proficiency. For group A the average was seven (range, 4–10) in comparison to group B who required on average fourteen attempts (range, 10–16). In group B, 30% failed to progress and dropped out of the study. From this study, it can be concluded that distinct learning curves based on innate ability also exist for technically more challenging tasks such as laparoscopic suturing. A significant proportion of those with lower aptitude were unable to achieve proficiency, which brings up the question of whether or not aptitude should be used to select surgical trainees. However, these tasks were performed in a simulated environment; therefore, it is unclear whether or not these skills would be transferrable to the operating room (Buckley 2014).

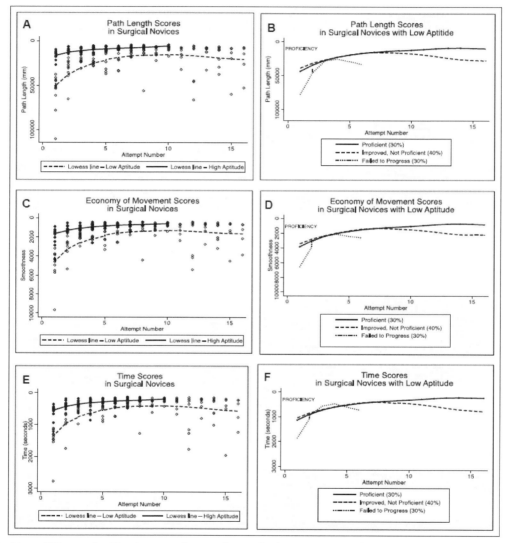

Buckley, C.E., et al., *The impact of aptitude on the learning curve for laparoscopic suturing.* The American Journal of Surgery, 2014. 207(2): p. 263−270.

Figure 1.1. (A) Comparison of path length scores in surgical novices and (B) path length scores for all attempts in those with low aptitude. (C) Comparison of economy of movement scores in surgical novices and (D) economy of movement scores for all attempts in those with low aptitude.
(E) Comparison of time scores in surgical novices and (F) time scores for all attempts in those with low aptitude.

Although it has been established that separate learning curves exist for those with and without an innate aptitude for laparoscopy, it is important to further delineate what makes this distinction between groups and whether or not this discrepancy is surmountable. Visual-spatial ability is thought to play a large role in achieving proficiency in both open and laparoscopic procedures. A group of thirty-seven surgical residents were asked to complete six tests in order to assess visual-spatial ability. After these tests were completed, residents were then asked to complete a Z-plasty procedure. This procedure consists of one or more Z-shaped incisions being made with the diagonals forming one straight line and two triangular sections, which is used for cosmetic reasons or can be functional in order to elongate and relax scars. Residents with higher visual-spatial scores performed better in the Z-plasty procedure in comparison to those with lower scores. However, after additional practice, residents with lower scores were also able to achieve competency (Wanzel 2002). This finding suggests that despite the fact that learning curves differed between the groups, additional practice and feedback may be able to make up for the innate differences between groups. In a separate study that examined visual-spatial ability and manual dexterity among dental students, surgical residents, and staff surgeons, it was found that higher visual-spatial ability scores were associated with a more skilled performance among surgical novices. However, superior visual-spatial ability among the more advanced trainees and experts was not found to correlate with superior performance on procedures. Therefore, these findings suggest that although aptitude testing may not be able to be used to predict who will perform well in a surgical career; however, it may be able to predict who would likely benefit from additional surgical training prior to entering the operating room (Wanzel 2003).

As previously stated, it has been established that laparoscopic procedures are associated with a learning phase during which there is an increased prevalence of serious complications. The learning curve for laparoscopic procedures is typically based on the time to procedure completion and the number of complications; however, multiple factors play a role in complications in the operating room in addition to surgeon experience such as the entire team involved in patient care at that time. In addition to describing time to proficiency, learning curve patterns may potentially also be used to identify surgical trainees who will be unable to achieve proficiency despite additional training (Grantcharov 2004). A virtual-reality trainer was used to measure the following parameters which have previously been validated in studies: time to complete task, number of errors, and economy of motion score (Taffinder 1998). Figure 1.2 shows the four learning curves that were identified: surgeons who (1) demonstrated proficiency from the beginning of the learning session (5.4%); (2) advanced with practice and achieved predefined expert criteria between two and nine repetitions (70.3%); (3) slow and steady acquisition of skills but unable to achieve proficiency level within ten repetitions (16.2%); and (4) underperformed from the beginning and showed no tendency to skills improvement (8.1%) (Grantcharov 2009; Kramp 2016). Trainees in the first group demonstrated impressive innate ability, potentially indicating a strong future in minimally invasive surgery; whereas those in the fourth group not only did not demonstrate any aptitude for laparoscopic surgery at the beginning, but they also failed to show any progression towards achieving proficiency. Although the role of surgeon involves skills such as communication and strong clinical judgment, technical skills play a large role. Therefore, one's performance on laparoscopic trainers should not be viewed in isolation; however, technical performance should be taken into consideration in order to help determine one's success in pursuing a surgical career (Grantcharov 2009).

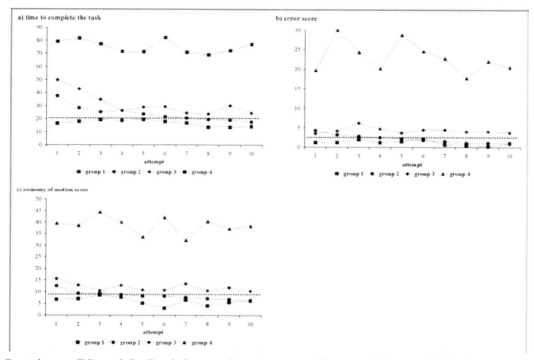

Grantcharov, T.P. and P. Funch-Jensen, Can everyone achieve proficiency with the laparoscopic technique? Learning curve patterns in technical skills acquisition. *The American Journal of Surgery*, 2009. 197(4): p. 447–449.

Figure 1.2. Learning curves. Time to perform the task. (a) Error scores. (b) Economy-of-motion scores. (c) Dotted line indicates the proficiency level for each parameter.

In addition to visual-spatial ability, several other cognitive abilities can be assessed in order to more completely understand one's aptitude in laparoscopy. A cognitive aptitude test may be used to assess trainees prior to laparoscopic simulator training. Ultimately, a surgeon's cognitive aptitude is related to the learning curve for minimally invasive surgery and the possibility of success in achieving proficiency (Luursema 2010; Luursema 2012). Spatial memory describes the ability to record information about one's environment and its spatial orientation. It can be viewed as an indicator of one's ability to learn the procedural aspects of tasks. Spatial memory is also related to the early learning phase of basic laparoscopic tasks (Luursema 2010). Perceptual speed is the ability to quickly identify a given shape or dissimilar shape from a number of alternatives. It is related to efficiency of movement in early learning, and it is also related to the associative phase of learning, which indicates that part of laparoscopic tasks might become automated during training. The fourth element of cognitive ability is reasoning ability. Increases in perceptual speed, a skill crucial due to the time critical nature of laparoscopic surgery, are found to be related to improved laparoscopic performance. The fourth element, reasoning ability, was found to be related to early learning of laparoscopic procedures. Reasoning ability was found to be less of an influence as skill level increased (Keehner 2006).

Since laparoscopic surgery requires a different mental skill set, it should be expected that the cognitive abilities of visual-spatial ability, spatial memory, perceptual speed, and reasoning ability should predict the learning curve for basic tasks on a laparoscopic simulator. Laparoscopic surgery requires each of these skills; therefore trainees who perform exceedingly well on cognitive aptitude tests are expected to show high levels of performance in the following areas: (1) number of practice sessions in order to achieve proficiency; (2) time to task completion; (3) damage to surrounding tissue; (4) efficiency of movement on basic laparoscopic simulator tasks. Despite these expectations, cognitive aptitude was found to neither be related to total number of sessions required to achieve proficiency in a task, nor did it predict learning rate during training. Participants with lower cognitive aptitude scores were not found to require more practice sessions to reach proficiency in comparison to those with higher scores. Although trainees became quicker and more efficient in performing basic laparoscopic tasks on a simulator, damage to surrounding tissue remained constant. Cognitive aptitude did not affect the amount of tissue damage that was found. Although learning rates for trainees with discrepancies between their cognitive aptitude scores were similar, trainees with higher levels of cognitive aptitude were found to consistently outperform those with lower levels. Overall, there was no effect of cognitive aptitude on the learning curve across multiple sessions (Groenier 2014).

All four aspects of cognitive aptitude were associated with higher efficiency of movement. Visual-spatial and reasoning ability were associated with less time to complete a given task. The role of cognitive aptitude did change, however, when the influence of a cognitive ability was corrected for the effect of the other cognitive abilities. Perceptual speed remained positively associated with efficiency of movement; spatial memory and perceptual speed were associated with the amount of tissue damage.

ANIMAL MODELS OF LAPAROSCOPIC SURGERY TRAINING

Operating skills can be acquired via three methods, all of which have benefits and drawbacks. The first method involves the use of bench models, for which benefits include lower cost, ready availability, and reuse of materials (Martin 1997). Basic laparoscopy skills may be learned and further honed on trainer boxes or with virtual reality models, but as the trainee becomes more skilled, the need for more challenging and life-like models is required for skills to be further developed. As a result, animal models have become a popular way to simulate procedures in the operating room. The porcine model is the most commonly used model due to the pig's anatomical and physiological similarities to humans (Kobayashi 2012). The second method involves practicing of skills in the animal laboratory. The animal model represents an important step in the training process due to the fact that the direct step from the pelvic trainer model to the operating room may be too difficult for a trainee. The animal model also allows trainees to gain confidence in trocar use and positioning (Piechaud 2006). Although this method is expensive and also presents the issue of limited resources and funding, the use of animals very closely simulates operating on actual patients. The cadaver as a model also offers a very effective way to gain an understanding of anatomy through a laparoscopic view. Cadavers also provide macroscopic anatomy and improved spatial perception of anatomy. However, cadavers present certain disadvantages due to the fact that they do not bleed, the visual field is also clear, and no hemostasis can be done (Piechaud 2006). The third method takes place in the operating room under the supervision of a preceptor where trainees can gain real life experience. The drawback to this method is that this can potentially be a dangerous situation in which trainees are further developing their skills on real patients. Training in the operating room is also limited by the fact that time and financial constraints limit the ability for trainees to perfect their skills here.

As more complex procedures are now being performed with laparoscopy in addition to shortened residency work hours, the need for intensive, efficient laparoscopy training is necessary for novices. This training can be conducted in a safe, controlled, and standardized environment within a simulation center; however, limited access to training centers does not always make this training possible. In order to provide additional training to general surgeons and graduating surgical residents, intensive training programs have been developed throughout the country as an alternative to simulation centers. Most intensive training programs are set up at locations throughout the country where general surgeons, residents, and fellows can travel to in order to complete an intensive training program over the course of several days. Intensive training programs may consist of lectures, laparoscopic videos, and practical training either on animal training models or laparoscopic trainers. Skill improvement is assessed using objective structured assessment of technical skill (OSATS). Most participants are found to have an improvement in their overall performance after finishing these courses (Castillo 2015).

For those that have access to simulation centers at their local institutions, there are numerous methods that can be used for preclinical training including virtual reality, box trainer simulators, operations on cadavers, or animal models. Although virtual reality or box trainer simulators have been used successfully by beginning trainees to acquire skills, they may be too simple and do not correlate closely enough to the actual procedure in the operating room. Therefore, human cadaveric and animal models have been introduced for more real-to-life training. Animal models have been found to be the ideal model due their realistic anatomy and surgical workflow similar to humans. Animal models are also ideal because they allow pathological findings such as cholelithiasis and inflammatory findings to be present, which is not possible in virtual reality or cadaveric models. Animal models are needed for two purposes. First, they allow new, minimally invasive procedures to be evaluated for their feasibility and effectiveness in comparison to standard techniques. Secondly, animal models provide training that most accurately resembles operating on real patients; therefore, it may also be used for training of both conventional and new methods of laparoscopic surgery (Ryska 2016). Due to both of these considerations, animal models are used throughout multiple surgical sub-specialties for preclinical training.

Hepatobiliary Surgery

Training in laparoscopic hepatobiliary surgery with animal models has not gained large traction internationally due in part to its level of difficulty; however, success has been found when using the porcine model for training. Several differences exist between human and porcine liver anatomy, which can present a challenge to new trainees, but with the appropriate amount of preoperative preparation, the porcine model can offer a very realistic training model for laparoscopic liver surgery (Figures 1.3–6) (Martins 2013). Bovine and porcine livers are most frequently used due to their similarity to human livers in terms of size and density. These animals are also farm animals that are readily available and relatively inexpensive (Ong 2013).

The porcine liver has three hepatic ducts (left, right and middle) and join to form the common hepatic duct at the hepatic porta. The cystic duct is relatively long prior to joining the common hepatic duct, which also makes the porcine model a good model for laparoscopic cholecystectomy. The hepatic vein and inferior vena cava (IVC) confluence is intraparenchymal in pigs, which makes this dissection more challenging than in humans. The IVC and intraparenchymal hepatic veins have extremely thin walls and the nearby diaphragm is easily damaged. Although external morphology of the porcine liver differs from the human liver, the segmental anatomy in regards to its vascularity and biliary tree is very similar to the human liver. Novice trainees were able to successfully perform Pringle maneuvers, left lateral segmentectomy and division of the liver ligaments. With appropriate preparation, the porcine model appears to be an adequate model for laparoscopic hepatobiliary surgery (Komorowski 2015). In other studies, laparoscopic left hepatectomy was successfully completed using a four-portal technique without the use of specialized instruments such as a LigaSure device, which further helps to decrease operative cost as seen in Figures 1.5, 1.6, 1.7, 1.8, and 1.9. This procedure offers a safe, feasible technique for laparoscopic left hepatectomy in pigs, which could additionally serve as a useful model for investigating liver disease, regeneration and offer preclinical information in order to improve hepatobiliary surgical procedures (Zhang 2014). Dogs have also been used in animal models to help surgeons further develop technical skills necessary to perform laparoscopic common bile duct exploration. Previously it has been difficult to find a suitable animal model that possesses a bile duct diameter large enough to accommodate a fiber optic choledochoscope required for stone extraction. The dog model has been found to be an effective and reliable model, which will allow surgeons to not only further hone skills but to also develop new techniques in laparoscopic bile duct exploration (Crist 1994).

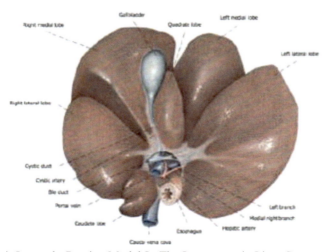

Komorowski Andrzej, L., et al., Porcine Model In The Laparoscopic Liver Surgery Training, in *Polish Journal of Surgery*. 2015. p. 425.

Figure 1.3. Caudoventral view of the visceral aspect of an isolated swine liver. © 2015 Andrzej L. Komorowski et al., published by De Gruyter Open. This chapter is distributed under the terms of the Creative Commons Attribution 4.0 Public License. (CC BY 4.0). Figure was not altered.

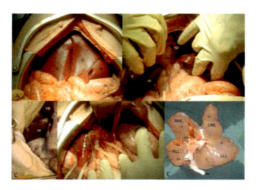

Figure 1.4. View of pig liver. Figure courtesy of Dr. Paulo Martins, MD PhD.

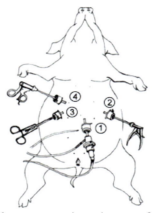

Zhang, H., et al., Laparoscopic left hepatectomy in swine: a safe and feasible technique. *Journal of Veterinary Science*, 2014. **15**(3): p. 417–422.

Figure 1.5. Portal locations. Portal 1 (laparoscope) was located 2–3 cm below the umbilicus along the ventral midline (portal 1 was shifted 2–3 cm to the left male pigs). Portals 2 and 3 were 3–5 cm cranial to portal 1 and 8-10 cm to the left and right of the ventral midline, respectively. Portal 4 was 3–5 cm cranial to portal 3 and 8–10 cm to the left of the ventral midline. These portals were used to introduce various laparoscopic instruments.

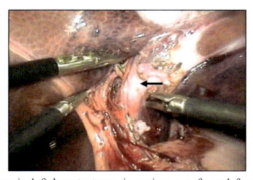

Zhang, H., et al., Laparoscopic left hepatectomy in swine: a safe and feasible technique. *Journal of Veterinary Science*, 2014. 15(3): p. 417–422.

Figure 1.6. Intraoperative view. The left branches of the portal vein (arrow) were dissected and then clamped with medium titanium clips before cutting.

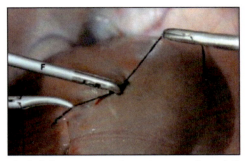

Zhang, H., et al., Laparoscopic left hepatectomy in swine: a safe and feasible technique. *Journal of Veterinary Science*, 2014. 15(3): p. 417−422.

Figure 1.7. Simulated intraoperative view. A knot was tied between the ends of the snipped sutures with the aid of needle-holding forceps (F).

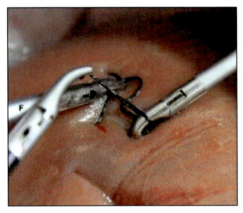

Zhang, H., et al., Laparoscopic left hepatectomy in swine: a safe and feasible technique. *Journal of Veterinary Science*, 2014. 15(3): p. 417−422.

Figure 1.8. Simulated intraoperative view. A knot was tied with the aid of needle-holding forceps (F) inserted from the third trocar.

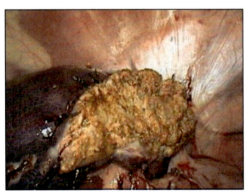

Zhang, H., et al., Laparoscopic left hepatectomy in swine: a safe and feasible technique. *Journal of Veterinary Science*, 2014. 15(3): p. 417−422.

Figure 1.9. Intraoperative view. The raw area observed immediately after liver resection.

Colorectal Surgery

Laparoscopy has been prevalent in colorectal surgery for many years at this point in time. New advances are being made within this sub-specialty with techniques such as natural orifice translumenal endoscopic surgery (NOTES). NOTES is an emerging technique that combines both endoscopic and laparoscopic approaches and uses natural body orifices as an entry site to the peritoneal cavity. This technique has already been applied to cholecystectomy and appendectomy but a purely NOTES technique has yet to be implemented in colorectal surgery. Hybrid techniques combining NOTES and laparoscopic techniques have yielded promising results in colorectal procedures such as colon resections. In order to further investigate this method, an experimental model using sheep was employed. Sheep were used to perform excision of the left colon using a transvaginal approach, which was chosen due to the similarity of external genital organs to female human genitals. Additionally, sheep share with humans a similar position of the left colon within the abdominal cavity. The totally transvaginal approach appears to be feasible in an animal model; however, application to the human population should be used with caution due to the technically challenging nature of the procedure and lack of long-term outcomes in the human patient population (Alba 2012). In addition to sheep models, porcine and rat models have also been used in colorectal surgery in order to further investigate sealing techniques of colorectal anastomoses in both *ex vivo* and *in vivo* models (Holmer 2011). Porcine models were used to evaluate the feasibility, safety, and efficacy of using a LigaSure device for dividing and sealing rectal stump during colorectal anastomosis creation versus a conventional stapler. The LigaSure device was found to be feasible in this experimental model but is less reliable than a stapler leading to a significantly greater fail rate (Sánchez-De Pedro 2014).

Urology

Laparoscopy has gained increased importance in urology over the last twenty years, which has led to the development of laparoscopic reconstructive procedures such as pyeloplasty, pelvic floor reconstruction, and radical prostatectomy. Training models include dry-lab, *ex vivo* animal models, and live animal models to be used for laparoscopic, robotic and endourologic training (Soria 2010; Aydin 2016). On porcine models, trainees are able to perform laparoscopic nephrectomy, ureteropelvic anastomosis, and suturing an incision on the bladder. Video trainers remain important in urologic laparoscopy training, but porcine laparoscopy has gained increased importance. Laparoscopic training on porcine models confers the benefits of training on animal models in general including haptic feedback, handling vitalized tissues that respond and bleed, and an overall similarity to real operative procedures; however, pig genitourinary anatomy is not identical to that of the human, which presents some limitations to this model. The pig has no retroperitoneal fat. The kidneys are adherent to the posterior abdominal wall and covered by a thin layer of peritoneum, which makes retroperitoneal dissection training difficult. Additionally, the ureter is thick and fatty with a narrow lumen. These anatomical limitations of the porcine model make human cadavers a popular alternative in urologic laparoscopic training (Katz 2003).

BARIATRIC SURGERY

Obesity continues to be a growing problem in the United States with an estimated 15.8 million adults qualifying for bariatric surgery (Ponce). Bariatric surgery techniques target weight loss through restriction, malabsorption, or a mix of both. The two most popular weight loss surgeries currently being performed are vertical sleeve gastrectomy (restrictive) and Roux-en-Y gastric bypass (mixed). Within laparoscopic and bariatric surgery, there has been a tendency for large laboratory animals such as pigs to be used. Bariatric experimental surgery on animals is useful for developing and perfecting techniques. Animal experimentation in bariatric surgery can also be used to study the relationship between metabolism and surgery in order to find improvements in treatment in the co-morbidities associated with morbid obesity. Lastly, research in this area can also focus on manipulating intake via central and vagal control (Del Castillo Dejardin 2004). Although it is now an abandoned malabsorptive technique, the jejunoileal bypass was previously the most studied bariatric surgical technique. Genetically-determined Zucker-type obese rats were used for the first time in bariatric research. From this research, subsequent studies of hormonal mechanisms responsible for weight loss and resolution of co-morbidities such as type 2 diabetes took place (Polyzogopoulou 2003). Current studies are aimed at further investigating the relationship between metabolism and surgery, specifically with gastric bypass in Zucker-type obese rats. This animal research looks at peptide hormones such as ghrelin, which regulates food intake and therefore plays a role in weight loss. In addition to Zucker-type obese rats, dogs and pigs have been used with the restrictive and mixed techniques with the goal of improving techniques for laparoscopy. Gastric persistalsis in reduction of intake is also being studied in rats, dogs, pigs, and rabbits in order to discover new options for patients in bariatric surgery. In order to draw meaningful conclusions, it is important to use obese animals in this area of research (Del Castillo Dejardin 2004).

GENERAL SURGERY

Inguinal hernia repair is one of the most frequently performed surgical procedures with over 800,000 hernia repairs performed annually in the USA. Despite the common nature of this procedure, key problems still exist following repair including complications secondary to invasive fixation of mesh, poor quality of tissue ingrowth induced by the mesh, and early mesh migration to and penetration into neighboring organs after implantation (Scheidbach 2004; Panaro 2015). Porcine animal models have been used for laparoscopic training purposes for hernia repairs for quite some time, but this animal model is further being utilized in order to compare surgical approaches and type of mesh used in hernia repairs. Polypropylene mesh is a common mesh used in millions of hernia repair operations, but variations in the type of polypropylene mesh used in repair result in a difference in their biocompatibility and handling characteristics during surgery. Porcine models may be used to further characterize these differences between mesh including shrinkage, chronic inflammatory reaction, and mesh incorporation into the surrounding tissue (Scheidbach 2004). Studies have also been done using the porcine model in order to further investigate various approaches to hernia repair including NOTES technique, totally extraperitoneal (TEP) and transabdominal preperitoneal (TAPP) (Dhumane 2013). Although this area of research may not purely focus on laparoscopic training, the results of such studies have a direct impact on the future standard of care in inguinal hernia repairs in patients.

PEDIATRIC SURGERY

Laparoscopic training outside of the operating room is of particular importance in pediatric surgery due to the increasingly complicated surgeries that are now being performed laparoscopically; however, the number of pediatric patients requiring these complicated procedures is usually small, which makes training outside of the operating room of the utmost importance in order to reduce complications and operating error. The porcine model is the most widely used animal model in laparoscopic training in fields such as adult minimally invasive surgery, colorectal, urologic and gynecological surgery. Despite this fact, very few studies have described the role of animal models for laparoscopic training in the pediatric population. Although the pig can be used in pediatric surgery training, the rabbit model could be helpful for pediatric surgery training due to its smaller size, which is comparable to the operative field encountered when operating on neonates and small children (Kirlum 2005). The piglet also poorly simulates the pediatric population due to its larger size weighing between 20 and 40 kg. In comparison, a rabbit that weighs 3–4 kg will have an abdominal cavity that measures approximately 15 cm long, 10 cm wide, and 8 cm high, which mimics the dimensions of the abdominal cavity in a newborn baby. Rabbits have been found to be good surgical models for repair of inguinal hernia and hiatal hernia due to their patent inguinal ring with retractile or intraabdominal testes and naturally gaping diaphragmatic hiatus, respectively. In contrast, it is difficult to mobilize the esophagus or perform cholecystectomy in the pig model due to its huge, multi-lobulated liver (Esposito 2016). Laparoscopic nephrectomy can also be challenging to perform in the porcine model due to the difficult access to the kidneys caused by large, distended bowel loops. Nephrectomy is more straight-forward in the rabbit model due to the anterior location of the kidneys and scant intraabdominal and perineal fat (Molinas 2004). Other laparoscopic procedures can be performed additionally including intestinal anastomosis, splenectomy, and congenital diaphragmatic hernia repair. In an analysis of trainees' performances on rabbit versus porcine models, it was found that surgeons had higher performance scores and statistically shorter operative times for advanced procedures in the rabbit model. Overall, the rabbit model appears to provide a viable approach to technical training in basic and advanced laparoscopic procedures (Esposito 2016).

ALTERNATIVES TO ANIMAL SURGERY IN LAPAROSCOPIC SURGERY

Due to high costs, regulatory constraints, opposed public opinion, and complex logistics (maintenance, anesthesia) associated with animal experiments, other alternatives for training have been proposed. Simulation-based training allows trainees to further hone their laparoscopic skills in a safe, non-threatening environment prior to entering the operating room. The repetition of tasks and simulated procedures has been shown to reduce the risk of adverse surgical events and further decrease operating time (Hyltander 2002). Although training that occurs in the OR, on cadaver, and animal models may be a better method than simulation training, it appears that skills acquired in a simulation setting are transferable to the OR such as laparoscopic suturing and knot tying skills (Sutherland 2006; Al-Kadi 2013; Zendejas 2013). Simulation-based training can lead to demonstrable benefits of surgical skills in the operating room, and it is an effective way to teach laparoscopic surgery skills, increase translation of laparoscopic skills to the OR, and increase patient safety (Vanderbilt 2015). Numerous laparoscopic training tools exist, each of which have their own benefits and drawbacks.

A box trainer is a simple box that uses a camera, screen, light source and instruments. It incorporates conventional laparoscopic equipment in order to perform basic skills. It can be used for training on animal parts in addition to synthetic inanimate models. Complex task trainers are hybrid models that provide visual, audio and touch cues and use integrated hardware in order to replicate a clinical setting. They may also be composed of a partial component of a simulator or body part such as an arm or a leg. Video trainers are more sophisticated box trainers that have embedded motion sensors and recorders which measure distance and direction moved in order to calculate economy of movement. Table 1.1 lists the different types of training tools and their individual capabilities (Vanderbilt 2015; Alaker 2016).

In addition to physical box trainers and video trainers, virtual reality plays an increasingly large role in laparoscopic training; multiple modalities that utilize virtual reality for laparoscopic simulation training exist. Virtual reality uses screen-based computer software and hardware similar to that used in laparo-endoscopic surgery. Virtual reality (VR) can further be broken down into low-fidelity and high-fidelity groups. Low fidelity VR simulators use computer-training programs that provide an abstract environment to teach basic laparo-endoscopic skills whereas high-fidelity uses motorized instruments in order to provide haptic feedback and more closely resembles live tissue. Minimally Invasive Surgical Trainer – Virtual Reality (MIST VR), a part-task virtual reality laparoscopic simulator, not only simulates surgical tasks and operations but is also able to provide an objective assessment of psychomotor skills by the operator. It will then generate an overall score, taking into consideration errors committed and time taken to complete six different tasks. When assessing surgical novices and practicing surgeons, experienced surgeons scored consistently and significantly better than their counterparts in all tasks, suggesting that the simulator is measuring surgically relevant parameters. Therefore, MIST-VR appears to be a validated tool in objectively assessing laparoscopic skills (Chaudhry 1999). In a systematic review and meta-analysis comparing virtual reality to other simulation models, it was found that virtual reality simulation was significantly more effective than video trainers and at least as good as box trainers in laparoscopic simulation training (Nagendran 2013; Alaker 2016). Moreover, virtual reality training appears to be a superior training method in comparison to standard laparoscopic training in the operating room (Gurusamy 2009; Al-Kadi 2012; Larsen 2012; Willaert 2013).

Virtual or box trainer simulators have been shown to be effective at the beginning of training; however, fresh-frozen cadavers are another method of providing laparoscopic training that more closely resembles operating on patients. Cadavers provide full haptic and tactile feedback, which is vital in laparoscopic simulation and is unfortunately difficult to incorporate into virtual systems (Buckley 2014). They can also be stored at a low temperature for an indefinite amount of time (Sharma 2012). In comparison of cost, an initial fee is incurred to purchase with a small added cost for maintenance for simulators whereas cadaver bodies are typically donated free of charge; however, high cost is associated with maintenance of a cadaver laboratory and cremation of used bodies. Other drawbacks to use of cadavers for training

Table 1.1. Laparoscopic training tools, definitions, and procedures commonly used in surgery

Type of simulation	Definition	Camera Navigation	Clipping and cutting	Suturing and knot tying	Lifting and grasping	Dissection
Box Trainer	A box that incorporates conventional laparoscopic equipment to perform basic skills, is versatile, and enables training on animal parts and synthetic models	+	+	+	+	+
Task Trainer	A partial component of a simulator or simulation modality such as an arm, leg or torso		+	+		+
MIST-VR	Virtual reality simulator with six different tasks to simulate maneuvers performed during laparoscopic cholecystectomy in a computerized environment	+	+		+	+
LapMentor/ LapMentor II	Virtual reality simulator consisting of camera and two calibrated working instruments. Motion of the instruments is translated to a two-dimensional computer screen for student practices	+	+	+	+	+
LapSim	A computer-based simulator creating a virtual laparoscopic setting through a computer operating system, a video monitor, a laparoscopic interface containing two pistol-grip instruments, and a diathermy pedal without haptic feedback	+	+	+	+	+
EndoTower	EndoTower software consists of an angled telescope simulator composed of rotating camera and telescopic components.	+	+			

MISTELS/FLS trainer	McGill Inanimate System for Training and Evaluation of Laparoscopic Skills (MISTELS)- this inexpensive, portable, and flexible system allows students to practice in a virtual Endotrainer box		+	+	+	
SIMENDO VR	Computer software used to train eye-hand coordination skills by camera navigation and basic drills.	+		+	+	
URO Mentor	A hybrid simulator, consisting of a personal computer based system linked to a mannequin with real endoscopes. Cystoscopic and ureteroscopic procedures are performed using either flexible or semi rigid endoscopes	+	+		+	+
Da Vinci Skills Simulator	A portable simulator containing a variety of exercises and scenarios specifically designed to give users the opportunity to improve their proficiency with surgical controls.	+	+	+	+	+

Vanderbilt, A.A., et al., *Randomized Controlled Trials: A Systematic Review of Laparoscopic Surgery and Simulation-Based Training.* Global Journal of Health Science, 2015. **7**(2): p. 310–327. This is an open-access article distributed under the terms and conditions of the Creative Commons Attribution license (http://creativecommons.org/licenses/by/3.0/). Table was not altered

include limited availability, avital tissues, and inability to injure vasculature or other structures (Sharma 2012; Ryska 2016).

Robotic surgery continues to grow in popularity worldwide. Although it is a derivative of minimally invasive surgery, the skills required to perform robotic surgery are unique from those required in either open or laparoscopic surgery. There are currently four commercially available simulators: the da Vinci Skills simulator (dVSS), the Mimic dV-Trainer (dV-Trainer), the Robotic Surgical Simulator, and Sim-Surgery Educational Platform (SEP). All four trainers are able to assess robotic skill. Three of the four simulators (dVSS, dV-Trainer, RoSS) demonstrate the ability to improve basic robotic skills, with proficiency-based training being the most effective training style. The skills obtained on a VR training curriculum appear to be similar to those obtained through dry laboratory simulation (Bric 2016).

An alternative to virtual reality simulators and fresh frozen cadavers is the Open-source Heidelberg laparoscopy phantom (OpenHELP), which combines realistic anatomy and tissue properties with reusable simulation specimens. OpenHELP is based on a digital three-dimensional model obtained from a CT scan of a male body and uses a flexible torso, via an elastic abdominal wall, or rigid, with a plastic shell, filled with artificial organs made from silicon casts. Pneumoperitoneum could successfully be attained by both methods (Kenngott 2015). As NOTES become more prevalent, training models specific for this technique are needed. A new training model for the NOTES procedures was developed known as the endoscopic-laparoscopic interdisciplinary training entity (ELITE). This model is composed of a synthetic package with all the intrabdominal organs, including the greater omentum. The synthetic appendix is made from gelatin material, which allows for dissection with high-frequency tools. The ELITE training model appears to be well suited for the training of NOTES procedures (Gillen 2012).

In addition to *in vivo* training, pieces of animal tissues may also be removed from the animal specimen and be used to recreate the anatomic conditions of a specific procedure. When used for this purpose, the animal tissue is traditionally placed in a pelvic trainer or dry box in order to more closely simulate a specific laparoscopic surgery for the trainee. Animal tissue may also be placed in human body simulators in order to more closely imitate both human anatomy and realistic operating conditions by including real tissue that will allow tactile feedback and will respond when being manipulated. The advantages of using pieces of animal tissue include high availability, low cost, lack of need for anesthesia, and no animal maintenance (van Velthoven 2006).

LAPAROSCOPIC SURGERY IN SMALL ANIMAL MODELS

A wide variety of small animal models exist in order to provide a sophisticated training model for the advanced laparoscopic trainee. Each of these models not only have advantages and disadvantages, but they also possess characteristics which may make them better suited for certain surgical sub-specialties over other small animal models. Overall, the ideal training model should provide the skills required, be inexpensive, universally available, and anatomically and physiologically identical to the anesthetized patient. Mice, rats, rabbits, and guinea pigs are universally accepted and are bred for both surgical and medical research due to cheaper costs, easy handling and care, and a more favorable public opinion. Although primates such as monkeys and apes most closely represent humans physiologically and anatomically, the use of primates is limited only to special circumstances in which any other animal model would be deemed unreliable. Animal models are typically utilized for reproduction of the following systems for training purposes due to the relative ease of reproducing surgical conditions: musculoskeletal, genitourinary, integumentary, vascular, cardiothoracic, and digestive system (Hassan 2005).

Mice, despite being studied extensively and being ideal for immunologic or oncologic studies, are too small to be used in laparoscopic procedures. On the other hand, the larger animal model, the rat, has been previously used for laparoscopic training such as in transperitoneal laparoscopic research (Gutt 1998). The rat model is inexpensive and easily handled due to size. This model has previously been described as a model for retroperitoneal mini laparoscopic nephrectomy, but the rat can also be used universally throughout laparoscopic sub-specialties as a way for the trainee to acquire advanced laparoscopic skills and microsurgical suturing skills (Kaouk 2000). However, due to the limited workspace, the rat model requires the trainee to have already acquired the skills necessary to work with 3-mm instruments in a very small space.

In comparison to the rat model, the rabbit model is not only inexpensive but also provides a larger workspace, which makes it a more realistic model. This model has been used as an *in vivo* training model for laparoscopic skills such as knot-tying, suturing, and using cutting and coagulation modes for dissection (Molinas 2004). The rabbit model has been shown to be well-suited for the use as a new training tool that emphasizes the repetition of simple procedures due to its ability to easily monitor progress when comparing learning curves between experienced and inexperienced surgeons such as gynecologists and medical students, respectively. With additional practice, shorter operating times and fewer complications were noted. This small animal model is also being used in experimental settings to evaluate the oxidative stress production on a transplanted kidney during laparoscopy (Demirbas 2004). As previously discussed, the rabbit model provides a very realistic model for pediatric surgery training due to the small operative field similar to that seen in the pediatric population. Due to the potential risks of carbon dioxide pneumoperitoneum in the neonate and infant population, the concept of gasless laparoscopy was first developed in the rabbit model. In the gasless model, the animals were neither intubated nor mechanically ventilated. After incision was made and the peritoneum was entered, an abdominal wall elevator was inserted which provided excellent visualization of the abdominal cavity (Luks 1995).

At the Center for the Development of Advanced Medical Technology (CDAMTec) in Japan, both wild-type and genetically modified pigs are used as multi-purpose models for medical skill education, the development of therapeutic strategies, and innovations for new tools for endo- and laparoscopic procedures. Unlike dogs, few spontaneous disease models exist in pigs. Pigs also share similar immune systems with humans as seen in inbred pigs such as the Clawn minipig, which further allows genetically modified pigs to be used in experimental models for liver, intestine, kidney, pancreas, and lung transplantation (Kobayashi 2012). At the CDAMTec research center, three different types of pigs are used: domestic pigs, miniature pigs, and genetically modified miniature pigs as seen in Figures 1.10 and 1.11. Pigs may vary in size from 30 to 40 kg as young pigs to approximately 100 kg once at mature body weight. Domestic pigs are easily obtained and are inexpensive since they are well established as a food source. Miniature pigs are generally easier to handle; however, they are more expensive than domestic pigs due to their limited annual production for experimental use in Japan. A mature miniature pig weighs 40 to 50 kg, similar to the weight seen in immature domestic pigs. In order to use the pigs available more effectively, after they have been euthanized, their tissues can undergo "second use" after being donated to other researchers for additional experiments, which ultimately results in fewer total number of experimental animals needed for research and decreases the other resources that are set aside for the proper care and disposal of animals after being euthanized (Tanaka 2006).

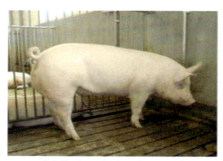

Kobayashi, E., et al., The pig as a model for translational research: overview of porcine animal models at Jichi Medical University. *Transplantation Research*, 2012. 1: p. 8–8.

Figure 1.10. Domestic pig used in experimental research. This is an Open Access article distributed under the terms of the Creative Commons Attribution License (http://creativecommons.org/licenses/by/2.0), which permits unrestricted use, distribution, and reproduction in any medium, provided the original work is properly cited.

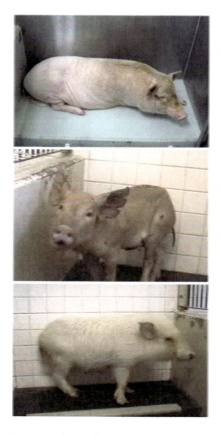

Figure 1.11. Miniature pigs used for experimental research. KCG pig (top), Mexican hairless pig (middle), Clawn pig (bottom). Kobayashi, E., et al., The pig as a model for translational research: overview of porcine animal models at Jichi Medical University. *Transplantation Research*, 2012. 1: p. 8–8. This is an Open Access article distributed under the terms of the Creative Commons Attribution License (http://creativecommons.org/licenses/by/2.0), which permits unrestricted use, distribution, and reproduction in any medium, provided the original work is properly cited. This figure was not altered.

Table 1.2. Advantages and disadvantages of *ex-vivo* and *in-vivo* models.

Models	Applications	Advantages	Disadvantages
Ex-vivo (non-perfused) models	• Compare the efficacy of different antenna configurations. • Trial of different energy settings	• Allow histological examination of whole lesion to study zones of tissue after thermal energy (i.e., ablation) applied • Inexpensive • Larger study sample size • Easy to manipulate during experiment • Does not require ethical approval/animal license	• Non-physiological • Homogenous parenchyma • Absence of respiratory excursion and motion of subject being studied • Lack of cooling effect secondary to tissue perfusion • Inability to study heat sink effect
In-vivo models	• Study of lesion evolution over time • Histological examination of lesion • Study of heat sink effect • Study of systemic responses to thermal energy applied • Study of effect of large volume thermal energy applied to tissues (in larger animals)	Small animals • Easier to handle • Cheaper • Ability to have larger sample size Large animals • Closer resemblance to human anatomy and physiology (for example, the liver)	Small animals • Small organ volume (i.e., liver) • Not suitable for the study of large volume thermal energy application (i.e., ablation) Large animals • Size and temperament poses challenges during anesthesia • Difficult vascular access in porcine models • Limited by strict ethic regulation • Small study sample size
Isolated perfused *ex-vivo* models	• Study of lesion evolution over time • Study of heat sink effect • Study of early inflammatory response	• Cheaper than *in-vivo* experiments • Does not require ethical approval • Greater control of perfusion characteristics (i.e., in liver, portal vein and hepatic arterial flows and pressures)	• Expensive • Expertise in animal handling and anesthesia is required • Duration of study is limited to the lifespan of the model • Absence of interacting organ systems • Inability to assess the impact of thermal energy on end organs • Perfusion circuit itself may activate some degree of systemic response

Ong, S. L., G. Gravante, M. S. Metcalfe and A. R. Dennison (2013). "History, ethics, advantages and limitations of experimental models for hepatic ablation." *World Journal of Gastroenterology : WJG* 19(2): 147-154.

LIMITATIONS OF ANIMAL MODELS

Animal models in laparoscopic training act as a great tool to help trainees improve their laparoscopic skills in a setting that closely resembles operating on patients. However, animal experimentation has several drawbacks including cost, availability, time required to provide adequate care to the animals both before and after operative intervention, and the ethical implications of using animals for medical experimentation. From a legal perspective, these experiments are likely to continue on animals until viable alternatives exist for testing prior to introduction of certain surgical procedures to the general public or until legislation allows the introduction of surgical treatment to the general public without first being tested on animals.

The Greeks described animal experimentation almost 2500 years ago when both Aristotle and Erasistratus performed studies on live animals (Singer 1922; Wilson 1959). Once general anesthesia emerged in the 1840s, this allowed unconscious animals to be studied, which led to a turning point in the medical and scientific communities' ability to use animal models in surgical experimentation. Animals can be used either as *ex vivo* or *in vivo* models. The major limitations of *ex vivo* models include absence of blood flow and vitalized tissues, which will respond to movement and maneuvers performed by the surgeon, and they also have limited lifespans during which valid data can be obtained. The absence of other interacting organs in *ex vivo* models may also affect the extent of systemic responses during experimentation. The use of living animals with *in vivo* studies requires specific laboratory facilities and research teams with expertise in anesthetizing and handling different species. The size of the animal also poses a barrier, for example when a larger animal such as a pig or cow needs to be anesthetized, moved, or examined post-operative (Hildebrand 2007; Ong 2013). The advantages and disadvantages of *ex vivo* and *in vivo* models for experimentation are compared in Table 1.2.

FUTURE OF LAPAROSCOPIC SURGERY

Laparoscopic surgery has evolved immensely from its initial use as a diagnostic procedure to the first laparoscopic cholecystectomy being performed in 1985 to its widespread use across all surgical subspecialties. Laparoscopy has further developed over the last thirty years in part due to the development of new instruments, which allows more complex operations to be performed. Laparoscopic camera equipment is now available in high-definition, with automatic focus and zoom, and three-dimensional images. Several different types of energy devices are now available including monopolar electrocautery scissors, ultrasonic coagulating shears, and electrothermal bipolar vessel sealers, which can be used for dissection and division of tissue, bowel, and vascular structures (Blackmore 2014). The development of new surgical instruments and imaging devices expands not only the type of surgery but also the surgical fields that are now able to use laparoscopy. In addition to these new contributions to the field, laparoscopy continues to evolve through different methods in which laparoscopic surgery can be performed including robotic surgery, single incision laparoscopic surgery (SILS), natural orifice translumenal endoscopic surgery (NOTES), and three-dimensional laparoscopy.

Robotic surgery was first seen in the field of urology and cardiac surgery with over 50,000 robotic prostatectomies being performed in 2007 in the USA alone. It was not used in colorectal surgery until 2002 (Blackmore 2014). Robotic surgery confers several advantages including high-definition three-dimensional visualization, increased freedom of movement, and minimization of tremor. These advantages provide for a more controlled, delicate dissection compared to laparoscopy. Several urologic procedures are now routinely being performed robotically including radical prostatectomy, transperitoneal and retroperitoneal partial nephrectomy, radical nephrectomy with caval thrombectomy, and pyeloplasty (Rogers 2008; Abaza 2011; Patel 2013; Stepanian 2016). Studies have indicated that robotic-assisted partial nephrectomy is associated with excellent outcomes in terms of perioperative complications and functional results when performed by experienced surgeons. Robotic surgery could potentially also be applied to removal of complex tumors (Novara). Robotic technology has also been extended to liver surgery and represents an accepted alternative to open and laparoscopic techniques in certain cases. Robotic liver surgery allows precise dissection and microsuturing in narrow operative fields, and with this technology, there is greater potential for more major resections and difficult segmentectomies to be performed through minimally invasive methods. Current data suggests that robotic liver resections have at the very least similar perioperative and postoperative outcomes while conferring the general benefits of minimally invasive surgery. Advantages of minimally invasive robotic surgery appear to be able to be applied additionally to right hepatectomy for living liver donors including faster post-operative recovery. Similar early allograft dysfunction, complications, and one-year recipient liver function were found between the open and robotic groups (Chen 2016). The technology used in robotic surgery also helps integrate and facilitate newer technologies such as near-infrared fluorescence (Giulianotti 2016). However, there are limitations to robotic surgery, which include higher associated costs and the need for specialized training for the primary surgeon, secondary surgeon, and OR nurses.

The next step to decrease the invasiveness and improve cosmesis of laparoscopic surgery is to decrease the size and number of incisions made as seen in single incision laparoscopic surgery (SILS). Through this technique, all instruments are introduced into the body cavity through a single access port. As laparoscopy has resulted in decreased trauma to the abdominal wall, improved pain control, and quicker recovery post-operatively, single-site incision surgery has further capitalized on these advantages of minimally invasive surgery by decreasing the number of incisions made. However, SILS requires a skill set and has ergonomic demands, which cannot directly be adapted from laparoscopic surgery. Therefore, in order to avoid higher complication rates as seen in both early laparoscopic cases and now initial SILS cases, evidence- and competency-based SILS curriculum should be instituted.

The first reported SILS cholecystectomy was performed in 1995 with new applications to other fields such as appendectomies and complex bariatric procedures. As was seen in the early days of laparoscopic surgery, increased complication rates at the advent of SILS makes it clear that appropriate training should occur before utilizing this technique on patients. The Laparoendoscopic Single-site Surgery Consortium for Assessment and Research (LESSCAR) set out a 2009 whitepaper, which addresses some of the issues regarding appropriate training for new techniques. LESSCAR recommends a stepwise format for training with a progression from inanimate models to animal procedures to supervised human SILS cases. These are the same principles that can be applied to laparoscopic or robotic training. As seen in case studies that examine SILS outcomes, there exists a significant learning curve even for laparoscopic surgeons who adopt SILS as seen through greater operative time and increased conversion from single to multi-port laparoscopy. Skills required for SILS do not appear to be automatically conferred from laparoscopic surgery, which further makes it important that adequate, safe training is available in order to make surgeons proficient (Pucher 2013). Needlescopic cholecystectomy is an additional method, which further reduces traumatic stress during and after surgery and hastens full recovery. A meta-analysis comparing needlescopic versus laparoscopic cholecystectomy indicated that needlescopic is not only safe and effective procedure for management of gallstone disease, but it is superior to laparoscopy for less post-operative pain and better cosmetic results despite being associated with longer operative time and higher conversion rate.

Natural orifice translumenal endoscopic surgery (NOTES) has gained traction in the surgical community as a technique to further advance minimally invasive techniques towards being truly non-invasive (Figure 1.12). This method requires a flexible endoscope to be inserted via a natural orifice such as the mouth, anus, vagina or umbilicus in order to gain access to the abdominal cavity thereby without leaving a scar. NOTES has gained popularity as a method to perform cholecystectomy or appendectomy. NOTES is truly a non-invasive surgery since it eliminates external postoperative wounds and other advantages including reduction in trauma to the abdominal wall, decreased recovery time, decreased clinical costs, and improved overall cosmetic results (Spivak 1997; MacFadyen 2005; Richards 2005; Ponsky 2006). Initial clinical outcomes following transvaginal hybrid NOTES cholecystectomy indicate that this method appears to be safe when performed by appropriately trained surgeons and may result in a faster return to normal activities and decreased postoperative pain (Sodergren 2015).

As with any new operative technique, appropriate training and investigation into post-operative outcomes should be performed prior to routine use of the NOTES technique. Differences between laparoscopic and NOTES procedures are that the NOTES technique requires the surgeon to operate an endoscope and other instruments through a single access point, rather than three or four other ports as frequently used in laparoscopy. Many NOTES procedures are currently being performed via hybrid fashion in which both an endoscope and trans-abdominal instruments are used; however, there is still significant loss of traction and the in-line instrument approach using the instrument ports in the endoscope hand-piece remain unfamiliar to most surgeons. Additionally, there is no gastrointestinal lumen to support the endoscope; thus, the distal end of the endoscope is manipulated in the open abdominal cavity using the incision site, internal organs and gravitational force to navigate and position the endoscope and instruments. As a result, the middle section of the endoscope is prone to rolling and twisting in the abdomen. Similar to SILS, the skill set required to operate an endoscope and associated surgical instruments is unique and cannot be directly transferred from laparoscopic and endoscopic skills (Korzeniowski 2016). Virtual reality simulators have found to be effective training tools for other minimally invasive techniques; however, a virtual reality trainer specific to NOTES procedures is required in order to proceed with further training. As a result, the natural orifice virtual surgery (NOViSE) simulator was developed due to the lack of established curriculum for NOTES training. NOViSE is a first prototype whose main focus is teaching the endoscopic manipulation skills required for NOTES and includes integration of a force-feedback-enabled virtual reality simulator for NOTES training with a virtual flexible endoscope. NOViSE is currently only able to simulate trans-gastric hybrid cholecystectomy procedure using a flexible endoscope as seen in Figure 1.12. Promising initial results following its implementation as a training device indicate that may be able to contribute to surgical training and to improving technical skills for NOTES procedures without putting patients at risk (Korzeniowski 2016).

One of the challenges of laparoscopic surgery is that surgeons face the loss of depth perception and spatial orientation due to the fact that they are working in a three-dimensional (3D) space but being guided by two-dimensional (2D) images. This disadvantage leads to a high visual and cognitive load. Therefore, 3D imaging was developed as an alternative to conventional 2D imaging. 3D imaging was introduced as early as the 1990s; however, its use is still not standard at hospitals, which may be secondary to the degraded view of the operative field resulting from poor image resolution, the necessity to wear uncomfortable eyewear (which alone can lead to eye strain, headaches, dizziness, and physical discomfort), and high cost. However, as technology has further evolved and high-definition monitors are now available, these disadvantages may be minimized when using the newest technology (Sorensen 2016).

Laparoscopic Experimental Surgery Models

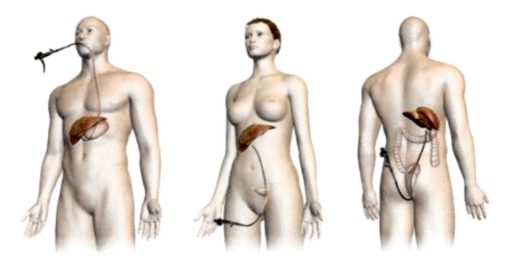

Korzeniowski, P., et al., *NOViSE: a virtual natural orifice transluminal endoscopic surgery simulator*. International Journal of Computer Assisted Radiology and Surgery, 2016: p. 1–13

Figure 1.12. NOTES approaches via trans-gastric (left), trans-vaginal (middle), and trans-rectal (right). This article is distributed under the terms of the Creative Commons Attribution 4.0 International License (http://creativecommons.org/licenses/by/4.0/), which permits unrestricted use, distribution, and reproduction in any medium, provided you give appropriate credit to the original author(s) and the source, provide a link to the Creative Commons license, and indicate if changes were made.

Overall, 3D laparoscopy appears to confer a reduction in performance time, is more affordable than robotic systems, and a reduction in errors is observed when compared to 2D technology. Most importantly, however, 3D laparoscopy allows improved depth perception, which is significant due to the fact that most common laparoscopic injuries occur due to visual misperceptions (Way 2003).

CONCLUSION

The prevalence of laparoscopy throughout surgery has increased exponentially over the past thirty years. As laparoscopy as a field has continued to grow, its applications are being applied to both new surgical procedures that previously were only being performed open, and an increasing number of surgical subspecialties are using laparoscopy. As a result, laparoscopic experimental surgery models have played a crucial role in surgical training, which ultimately impacts the diversity of surgical procedures that may be safely performed in patients. Animal models are the ideal training model to be used in laparoscopic surgery training because they confer the benefits of ideal haptic feedback, handling vitalized tissues that respond and bleed, and an overall similarity to real operative procedures. Animal experimental models have been crucial to the development of new techniques and procedures and for the training of surgeons in laparoscopic surgery. Due to its success, laparoscopy and other minimally invasive procedures have been applied to more complex surgeries in fields such as hepatobiliary, transplant, colorectal, and pediatric surgery. Laparoscopy and other minimally invasive techniques such as robotic surgery and NOTES require their own set of surgical skills, which makes it imperative that proper training is available prior to both novice surgeons using basic techniques and experienced surgeons using advanced or new techniques on patients. Laparoscopic trainers, virtual reality, cadavers, and *in vivo* animal models are all options for laparoscopic training with *in vivo* animal models providing the most real-to-life models for practice due to their anatomical and physiologic similarities to humans. As minimally invasive surgery continues to evolve from laparoscopy to robotic, single-incision laparoscopic surgery, and NOTES procedures, the need for additional animal training will be a necessity in order to ensure optimal outcomes for patients.

REFERENCES

Abaza, RR. Robotic surgery and minimally invasive management of renal tumors with vena caval extension. *Current opinion in urology*, 2011, 21(2), 104–109.

Al-Kadi, AS; Donnon, T. Using simulation to improve the cognitive and psychomotor skills of novice students in advanced laparoscopic surgery: a meta-analysis. *Med. Teach.*, 2013, 35 Suppl 1, S47–55.

Al-Kadi, AS; Donnon, T; Oddone Paolucci, E; Mitchell, P; Debru, E; Church, N. The effect of simulation in improving students' performance in laparoscopic surgery: a meta-analysis. *Surg. Endosc.*, 2012, 26(11), 3215–3224.

Alaker, M; Wynn, GR; Arulampalam, T. Virtual reality training in laparoscopic surgery: A systematic review & meta-analysis. *Int. J. Surg.*, 2016, 29, 85–94.

Alba Mesa, F; Amaya Cortijo, A; Romero Fernandez, TM; Komorowski, AL; Sanchez Hurtado, MA; Sanchez Margallo, FM. Totally transvaginal resection of the descending colon in an experimental model. *Surgical Endoscopy*, 2012, 26(3), 877–881.

Antoniou, SA; Antoniou, GA; Koch, OO; Pointner, R; Granderath, FA. Meta-analysis of laparoscopic vs open cholecystectomy in elderly patients. *World Journal of Gastroenterology: WJG*, 2014, 20(46), 17626–17634.

Aydin, A; Raison, N; Khan, MS; Dasgupta, P; Ahmed, K. Simulation-based training and assessment in urological surgery. *Nat. Rev. Urol.*, 2016, 13(9), 503–519.

Blackmore, AE; Wong, MT; Tang, CL. Evolution of laparoscopy in colorectal surgery: an evidence-based review. *World J. Gastroenterol.*, 2014, 20(17), 4926–4933.

Bric, JD; Lumbard, DC; Frelich, MJ; Gould, JC. Current state of virtual reality simulation in robotic surgery training: a review. *Surgical Endoscopy*, 2016, 30(6), 2169–2178.

Buckley, CE; Kavanagh, DO; Nugent, E; Ryan, D; Traynor, OJ; Neary, PC. The impact of aptitude on the learning curve for laparoscopic suturing. *The American Journal of Surgery*, 2014, 207(2), 263–270.

Buckley, CE; Kavanagh, DO; Traynor, O; Neary, PC. Does aptitude matter? *Journal of the American College of Surgeons*, 2012, 215(3), S116.

Bui, A; Stockhausen, F; Hanisch, E. Laparoscopic surgery: A qualified systematic review. *World J. Methodol*, 2015, 5(4), 238–254.

Castillo, R; Buckel, E; León, F; Varas, J; Alvarado, J; Achurra, P; Aggarwal, R; Jarufe, N; Boza, C. Effectiveness of Learning Advanced Laparoscopic Skills in a Brief Intensive Laparoscopy Training Program. *Journal of Surgical Education*, 2015, 72(4), 648–653.

Chaudhr, A; Sutton, C; Wood, J; Stone, R; McCloy, R. Learning rate for laparoscopic surgical skills on MIST VR, a virtual reality simulator: quality of human-computer interface. *Annals of The Royal College of Surgeons of England*, 1999, 81(4), 281–286.

Chen, PD; Wu, CY; Hu, RH; Ho, CM; Lee, PH; Lai, HS; Lin, MT; Wu, YM. Robotic liver donor right hepatectomy – a pure, minimally invasive approach. *Liver Transplantation*, 2016, 22 (11), 1509–1518.

Cook, JA; Ramsay, CR; Fayers, P. Using the literature to quantify the learning curve: A case study. *International Journal of Technology Assessment in Health Care*, 2007, 23(2), 255–260.

Cook, JA; Ramsaya, CR; Fayers, P. Statistical evaluation of learning curve effects in surgical trials. *Clinical Trials*, 2004, 1(5), 421–427.

Crist, DW; Davoudi, MM; Parrino, PE; Gadacz, TR. An experimental model for laparoscopic common bile duct exploration. *Surg. Laparosc. Endosc.*, 1994, 4(5), 336–339.

Del Castillo Dejardin, D; Sabench Pereferrer, F; Hernandez Gonzale, M; Blanco Blasco, S; Abello Sala, M. The evolution of experimental surgery in the field of morbid obesity. *Obes. Surg.*, 2004, 14(9), 1263–1272.

Demirbas, M; Samli, M; Aksoy, Y; Guler, C; Kilinc, A; Dincel, C. Comparison of changes in tissue oxidative-stress markers in experimental model of open, laparoscopic, and retroperitoneoscopic donor nephrectomy. *Journal of endourology*, 2004, 18(1), 105–108.

Dhumane, P; Donatelli, G; Chung, H; Dallemagne, B; Marescaux, J. Feasibility of transumbilical flexible endoscopic preperitoneoscopy (FLEPP) and its utility for inguinal hernia repair: experimental animal study. *Surg. Innov.*, 2013, 20(1), 5–12.

Esposito, CC. Training Models in Pediatric Minimally Invasive Surgery: Rabbit Model Versus Porcine Model: A Comparative Study. *Journal of laparoendoscopic & advanced surgical techniques. Part A*, 2016, 26(1), 79–84.

Feldman, LS; Cao, J; Andalib, A; Fraser, S; Fried, GM. A method to characterize the learning curve for performance of a fundamental laparoscopic simulator task: Defining "learning plateau" and "learning rate". *Surgery*, 2009, 146(2), 381–386.

Fried, GM; Feldman, LS; Vassiliou, MC; Fraser, SA; Stanbridge, D; Ghitulescu, G; Andrew, CG. Proving the Value of Simulation in Laparoscopic Surgery. *Annals of Surgery*, 2004, 240(3), 518–528.

Gillen, S; Gröne, J; Knödgen, F; Wolf, P; Meyer, M; Friess, H; Buhr, HJ; Ritz, JP; Feussner, H; Lehmann, KS. Educational and training aspects of new surgical techniques, experience with the endoscopic–laparoscopic interdisciplinary training entity (ELITE) model in training for a natural orifice translumenal endoscopic surgery (NOTES) approach to appendectomy. *Surgical Endoscopy*, 2012, 26(8), 2376–2382.

Giulianotti, PC; Bianco, FM; Daskalaki, D; Gonzalez-Ciccarelli, LF; Kim, J; Benedetti, E. Robotic liver surgery: technical aspects and review of the literature. *Hepatobiliary Surgery and Nutrition*, 2016, 5(4), 311–321.

Grantcharov, TP; Funch-Jensen, P. Can everyone achieve proficiency with the laparoscopic technique? Learning curve patterns in technical skills acquisition. *The American Journal of Surgery*, 2009, 197(4), 447–449.

Grantcharov, TPTP. [*Evaluation of surgical competence*]. Ugeskrift for læger, 2004, 166(21), 2023–2025.

Greco, EFEF. Identifying and classifying problem areas in laparoscopic skills acquisition: can simulators help? *Academic medicine*, 2010, 85(10 suppl), S5–S8.

Groenier, M; Schraagen, JMC; Miedema, HAT; Broeders, IAJM. The role of cognitive abilities in laparoscopic simulator training. *Advances in Health Sciences Education*, 2014, 19(2), 203−217.

Gurusamy, KS; Aggarwal, R; Palanivelu, L; Davidson, BR. Virtual reality training for surgical trainees in laparoscopic surgery. *Cochrane Database Syst Rev*, 2009, (1), Cd006575.

Gutt, CNC. Standardized technique of laparoscopic surgery in the rat. *Digestive surgery*, 1998, 15(2), 135−139.

Hassan, A; Kadima, KB; Remi-adewumi, BD; Awasum, CA; Abubakar, MT. Animal models in surgical training, choice and ethics. *Nigerian journal of surgical research*, 2005, 7(3−4), 260−267.

Hildebrand, P; Kleemann, M; Roblick, U; Mirow, L; Bruch, HP; Bürk, C. Development of a perfused ex vivo tumor-mimic model for the training of laparoscopic radiofrequency ablation. *Surgical Endoscopy*, 2007, 21(10), 1745−1749.

Holmer, C; Winter, H; Kröger, M; Nagel, A; Jaenicke, A; Lauster, R; Kraft, M; Buhr, HJ; Ritz, JP. Bipolar radiofrequency-induced thermofusion of intestinal anastomoses—feasibility of a new anastomosis technique in porcine and rat colon. *Langenbeck's Archives of Surgery*, 2011, 396(4), 529−533.

Hyltander, A; Liljegren, E; Rhodin, PH; Lönroth, H. The transfer of basic skills learned in a laparoscopic simulator to the operating room. *Surgical Endoscopy And Other Interventional Techniques*, 2002, 16(9), 1324−1328.

Kaouk, JH; Gill, IS; Meraney, AM; Desai, MM; Carvalhal, EF; Fergany, AF; Sung, GT. Retroperitoneal minilaparoscopic nephrectomy in the rat model. *Urology*, 2000, 56(6), 1058−1062.

Katz, RR. Cadaveric versus porcine models in urological laparoscopic training. *Urologia internationalis*, 2003, 71(3), 310−315.

Keehner, M; Lippa, Y; Montello, DR; Tendick, F; Hegarty, M. Learning a spatial skill for surgery: How the contributions of abilities change with practice. *Applied cognitive psychology*, 2006, 20(4), 487−504.

Kenngott, HG; Wünscher, JJ; Wagner, M; Preukschas, A; Wekerle, AL; Neher, P; Suwelack, S; Speidel, S; Nickel, F; Oladokun, D; Maier-Hein, L; Dillmann, R; Meinzer, HP; Müller-Stich, BP. Open HELP (Heidelberg laparoscopy phantom): development of an open-source surgical evaluation and training tool. *Surgical Endoscopy*, 2015, 29(11), 3338−3347.

Keus, F; de Jong, J; Gooszen, HG; Laarhoven, CJ. Laparoscopic versus open cholecystectomy for patients with symptomatic cholecystolithiasis. *Cochrane Database of Systematic Reviews*, 2006, (4), CD006231

Kirlum, HJ; Heinrich, M; Tillo, N; Till, H. Advanced Paediatric Laparoscopic Surgery: Repetitive Training in a Rabbit Model Provides Superior Skills for Live Operations. *Eur. J. Pediatr. Surg.*, 2005, 15(03), 149−152.

Kobayashi, E; Hishikawa, S;Teratani, T; Lefor, AT. The pig as a model for translational research: overview of porcine animal models at Jichi Medical University. *Transplantation Research*, 2012, 1, 1−8.

Komorowski Andrzej, L; Mituś Jerzy, W; Hurtado Miguel Angel, S; Margallo Francisco Miguel, S. Porcine Model In The Laparoscopic Liver Surgery Training. *Polish Journal of Surgery*, 2015, 87, 425.

Korzeniowski, P; Barrow, A; Sodergren, MH; Hald, N; Bello, F. NOViSE: a virtual natural orifice transluminal endoscopic surgery simulator. *International Journal of Computer Assisted Radiology and Surgery*, 2016, 1–13.

Kramp, KH; van Det, MJ; Hoff, C; Veeger, NJ; ten Cate Hoedemaker, HO; Pierie, JP. The predictive value of aptitude assessment in laparoscopic surgery: a meta-analysis. *Med. Educ.*, 2016, 50(4), 409–427.

Larsen, CR; Oestergaard, J; Ottesen, BS; Soerensen, JL. The efficacy of virtual reality simulation training in laparoscopy: a systematic review of randomized trials. *Acta. Obstet. Gynecol. Scand.*, 2012, 91(9), 1015–1028.

Li, X; Zhang, J; Sang, L; Zhang, W; Chu, Z; Li, X; Liu, Y. Laparoscopic versus conventional appendectomy - a meta-analysis of randomized controlled trials. *BMC Gastroenterology*, 2010, 10(1), 1–8.

Luks, FI; Peers, KHE; Deprest, JA; Lerut, TE. Gasless laparoscopy in infants: The rabbit model. *Journal of Pediatric Surgery*, 1995, 30(8), 1206–1208.

Luursema, JM; Buzink, SN; Verwey, WB; Jakimowicz, JJ. Visuo-spatial ability in colonoscopy simulator training. *Advances in Health Sciences Education*, 2010, 15(5), 685–694.

Luursema, JM; Verwey, WB; Burie, R. Visuospatial ability factors and performance variables in laparoscopic simulator training. *Learning and Individual Differences*, 2012, 22(5), 632–638.

MacFadyen, BV; Cuschieri, A. Endoluminal surgery. *Surgical Endoscopy and Other Interventional Techniques*, 2005, 19(1), 1–3.

Martin, JA; Regehr, G; Reznick, R; Macrae, H; Murnaghan, J; Hutchison, C; Brown, M. Objective structured assessment of technical skill (OSATS) for surgical residents. *British Journal of Surgery*, 1997, 84(2), 273–278.

Martins, P; Markmann, JF; Hertl, M; (2013). Liver transplantation in the pig. *Experimental Organ Transplantation*. H. Chen and S. Quin, Nova Science Publishers, 271–296.

Memon, MA; Subramanya, MS; Hossain, MB; Yunus, RM; Khan, S; Memon, B. Laparoscopic Anterior Versus Posterior Fundoplication for Gastro-esophageal Reflux Disease: A Meta-analysis and Systematic Review. *World Journal of Surgery*, 2015, 39(4), 981–996.

Molinas, CR; Binda, MM; Mailova, K; Koninckx, PR. The rabbit nephrectomy model for training in laparoscopic surgery. *Human Reproduction*, 2004, 19(1), 185–190.

Nagendran, M; Gurusamy, KS; Aggarwal, R; Loizidou, M; Davidson, BR. Virtual reality training for surgical trainees in laparoscopic surgery. *Cochrane Database Syst. Rev.*, 2013, (8), Cd006575.

Novara, G; La Falce, S; Kungulli, A; Gandaglia, G; Ficarra, V; Mottrie, A. Robot-assisted partial nephrectomy. *International Journal of Surgery*, 2016, 36, 554–559.

Ohtani, H; Tamamori, Y; Arimoto, Y; Nishiguchi, Y; Maeda, K; Hirakawa, K. Meta-analysis of the Results of Randomized Controlled Trials that Compared Laparoscopic and Open Surgery for Acute Appendicitis. *Journal of Gastrointestinal Surgery*, 2012, 16(10), 1929–1939.

Ong, SL; Gravante, G; Metcalfe, MS; Dennison, AR. History, ethics, advantages and limitations of experimental models for hepatic ablation. *World Journal of Gastroenterology: WJG*, 2013, 19(2), 147–154.

Panaro, F; Matos-Azevedo, AM; Fatas, JA; Marin, J; Navarro, F; Zaragoza-Fernandez, C. Endoscopic and histological evaluations of a newly designed inguinal hernia mesh implant,

Experimental studies on porcine animal model and human cadaver. *Ann. Med. Surg. (Lond)*, 2015, 4(2), 172–178.

Patel, M; Porter, J. Robotic retroperitoneal partial nephrectomy. *World Journal of Urology*, 2013, 31(6), 1377–1382.

Peters, MJ; Mukhtar, A; Yunus, RM; Khan, S; Pappalardo, J; Memon, B; Memon, MA. Meta-Analysis of Randomized Clinical Trials Comparing Open and Laparoscopic Anti-Reflux Surgery. *Am. J. Gastroenterol.*, 2009, 104(6), 1548–1561.

Piechaud, PT; Pansadoro, A. Transfer of skills from the experimental model to the patients. *Curr. Urol. Rep.*, 2006, 7(2), 96–99.

Polyzogopoulou, EV; Kalfarentzos, F; Vagenakis, AG; Alexandrides, TK. Restoration of Euglycemia and Normal Acute Insulin Response to Glucose in Obese Subjects With Type 2 Diabetes Following Bariatric Surgery. *Diabetes*, 2003, 52(5), 1098–1103.

Ponce, J; DeMaria, EJ; Nguyen, NT; Hutter, M; Sudan, R; Morton, JM. American Society for Metabolic and Bariatric Surgery estimation of bariatric surgery procedures in 2015 and surgeon workforce in the United States. *Surgery for Obesity and Related Diseases*, 2016, 12(9), 1637–1639.

Ponsky, JL. Endoluminal surgery: past, present and future. *Surgical Endoscopy And Other Interventional Techniques*, 2006, 20(2), S500–S502.

Pucher, PH; Sodergren, MH; Singh, P; Darzi, A; Parakseva, P. Have we learned from lessons of the past? A systematic review of training for single incision laparoscopic surgery. *Surg. Endosc.*, 2013, 27(5), 1478–1484.

Richards, WO; Rattner, DW. Endoluminal and transluminal surgery: no longer if, but when. *Surgical Endoscopy And Other Interventional Techniques*, 2005, 19(4), 461–463.

Roberts, KE; Bell, RL; Duffy, AJ. Evolution of surgical skills training. *World J. Gastroenterol.*, 2006, 12(20), 3219–3224.

Rogers, CG; Singh, A; Blatt, AM; Linehan, WM; Pinto, PA. Robotic Partial Nephrectomy for Complex Renal Tumors, Surgical Technique. *European Urology*, 2008, 53(3), 514–523.

Ryska, O; Serclova, Z; Martinek, J; Dolezel, R; Kalvach, J; Juhas, S; Juhasova, J; Bunganic, B; Laszikova, E; Ryska, M. A new experimental model of calculous cholecystitis suitable for the evaluation and training of minimally invasive approaches to cholecystectomy. *Surgical Endoscopy*, 2016, 1–8.

Sachdeva, AK; Russell, TR. Safe Introduction of New Procedures and Emerging Technologies in Surgery: Education, Credentialing, and Privileging. *Surgical Oncology Clinics of North America*, 2007, 16(1), 101–114.

Sánchez-De Pedro, F; Moreno-Sanz, C; Morandeira-Rivas, A; Tenías-Burillo, JM; Alhambra-Rodríguez De Guzmán, C. Colorectal anastomosis facilitated by the use of the LigaSure® sealing device: comparative study in an animal model. *Surgical Endoscopy*, 2014, 28(2), 508–514.

Scheidbach, H; Tamme, C; Tannapfel, A; Lippert, H; Köckerling, F. *In vivo* studies comparing the biocompatibility of various polypropylene meshes and their handling properties during endoscopic total extraperitoneal (TEP) patchplasty: an experimental study in pigs. *Surgical Endoscopy And Other Interventional Techniques*, 2004, 18(2), 211–220.

Sharma, M; Horgan, A. Comparison of Fresh-Frozen Cadaver and High-Fidelity Virtual Reality Simulator as Methods of Laparoscopic Training. *World Journal of Surgery*, 2012, 36(8), 1732–1737.

Singer, CJ. *Greek biology and Greek medicine*. Oxford: Clarendon Press, 1922.

Sodergren, MH; Markar, S; Pucher, PH; Badran, IA; Jiao, LR; Darzi, A. Safety of transvaginal hybrid NOTES cholecystectomy: a systematic review and meta-analysis. *Surgical Endoscopy*, 2015, 29(8), 2077−2090.

Sorensen, SM; Savran, MM; Konge, L; Bjerrum, F. Three-dimensional versus two-dimensional vision in laparoscopy: a systematic review. *Surg. Endosc.*, 2016, 30(1), 11−23.

Soria, F; Delgado, MI; Rioja, LA; Blas, M; Pamplona, M; Duran, E; Uson, J; Sanchez, FM. Ureteral double-J wire stent effectiveness after endopyelotomy: an animal model study. *Urol. Int.*, 2010, 85(3), 314−319.

Spivak, H; Hunter, JG. Endoluminal surgery. *Surgical Endoscop.*, 1997, 11(4), 321−325.

Stepanian, S; Patel, M; Porter, J. Robot-assisted Laparoscopic Retroperitoneal Lymph Node Dissection for Testicular Cancer: Evolution of the Technique. *European Urology*, 2016, 70(4), 661−667.

Sutherland, LM; Middleton, PF; Anthony, A; Hamdorf, J; Cregan, P; Scott, D; Maddern, GJ. Surgical simulation: a systematic review. *Ann. Surg.*, 2006, 243(3), 291−300.

Taffinder, NN. Validation of virtual reality to teach and assess psychomotor skills in laparoscopic surgery: results from randomised controlled studies using the MIST VR laparoscopic simulator. *Studies in health technology and informatics*, 1998, 50, 124−130.

Tanaka, H; Kobayashi, E. Education and research using experimental pigs in a medical school. *Journal of Artificial Organs*, 2006, 9(3), 136−143.

Trehan, A; Barnett-Vanes, A; Carty, MJ; McCulloch, P; Maruthappu, M. The impact of feedback of intraoperative technical performance in surgery: a systematic review. *BMJ Open*, 2015, 5(6), e006759.

van Velthoven, RF; Hoffmann, P. Methods for laparoscopic training using animal models. *Current Urology Reports*, 2006, 7(2), 114−119.

Vanderbilt, AA; Grover, AC; Pastis, NJ; Feldman, M; Granados, DD; Murithi, LK; Mainous, AG. Randomized Controlled Trials: A Systematic Review of Laparoscopic Surgery and Simulation-Based Training. *Global Journal of Health Science*, 2015, 7(2), 310−327.

Vecchio, R; MacFayden, BV; Palazzo, F. History of laparoscopic surgery. *Panminerva. Med.*, 2000, 42(1), 87−90.

Wanzel, KR; Hamstra, SJ; Anastakis, DJ; Matsumoto, ED; Cusimano, MD. Effect of visual-spatial ability on learning of spatially-complex surgical skills. *The Lancet*, 2002, 359(9302), 230−231.

Wanzel, KR; Hamstra, SJ; Caminiti, MF; Anastakis, DJ; Grober, ED; Reznick, RK. Visual-spatial ability correlates with efficiency of hand motion and successful surgical performance. *Surgery*, 2003, 134(5), 750−757.

Way, LW; Stewart, L; Gantert, W; Liu, K; Lee, CM; Whang, K; Hunter, JG. Causes and Prevention of Laparoscopic Bile Duct Injuries: Analysis of 252 Cases From a Human Factors and Cognitive Psychology Perspective. *Annals of Surgery*, 2003, 237(4), 460−469.

Willaert, W; Van De Putte, D; Van Renterghem, K; Van Nieuwenhove, Y; Ceelen, W; Pattyn, P. Training models in laparoscopy: a systematic review comparing their effectiveness in learning surgical skills. *Acta. Chir. Belg.*, 2013, 113(2), 77−95.

Wilson, LGL. Erasistratus, Galen, and the pneuma. *Bulletin of the history of medicine*, 1959, 33, 293−314.

Zendejas, B; Brydges, R; Hamstra, SJ; Cook, DA. State of the evidence on simulation-based training for laparoscopic surgery: a systematic review. *Ann. Surg.*, 2013, 257(4), 586−593.

Zendejas, B; Ruparel, RK; Cook, DA. Validity evidence for the Fundamentals of Laparoscopic Surgery (FLS) program as an assessment tool: a systematic review. *Surg. Endosc.*, 2016, 30(2), 512–520.

Zhang, H; Liu, T; Wang, Y; Liu, HF; Zhang, JT; Wu, YS; Lei, L; Wang, HB. Laparoscopic left hepatectomy in swine: a safe and feasible technique. *Journal of Veterinary Science*, 2014, 15(3), 417–422.

In: Advances in Experimental Surgery. Volume 2
Editors: Huifang Chen and Paulo N. Martins
ISBN: 978-1-53612-773-7
© 2018 Nova Science Publishers, Inc.

Chapter 2

EXPERIMENTAL MODELS OF SEPSIS

Norbert Nemeth[1,], Mihai Oltean[2] and Bela Fulesdi[3]*

[1]Department of Operative Techniques and Surgical Research, Faculty of Medicine,
University of Debrecen, Debrecen, Hungary
[2]The Transplantation Institute, Sahlgrenska University Hospital, Gothenburg, Sweden
[3]Department of Anesthesiology and Intensive Care, Faculty of Medicine,
University of Debrecen, Debrecen, Hungary

ABSTRACT

Sepsis is a clinical syndrome manifesting as a complex systemic response to infection. In spite of significant developments in diagnostic, monitoring and intensive care, sepsis remains a major cause of morbidity and mortality as well as a significant economic burden. Despite inherent limitations, experimental models remain an essential tool for understanding the intricate mechanisms and pathways activated during sepsis and for developing new therapeutic approaches. However, most strategies proved as effective experimentally, have been disappointing in the clinical trials conducted so far. These unsatisfactory attempts in translating the treatment options to bedside may be attributed to the involvement of multiple mediators and pathways in sepsis with only few components being recognized and targeted but also to general or specific shortcomings of each animal model. Herein, we provide a brief overview of the pathophysiology of sepsis and concise descriptions of relevant experimental models including considerations for further refinements (i.e., animal age, gender and co-morbidities) that are further required to ensure an effective translation of the findings into the clinical setting.

Keywords: sepsis, animal models, clinical versus experimental sepsis

---

[*] Corresponding author; Norbert Nemeth M.D., Ph.D., Department of Operative Techniques and Surgical Research, Faculty of Medicine, University of Debrecen, 22 Moricz Zs. krt., H-4032 Debrecen, Hungary , Tel: +36 52 416 915, E-mail: nemeth@med.unideb.hu.

ABBREVIATIONS

ARDS	acute respiratory distress syndrome
AST	aspartate aminotransferase
ATP	adenosine triphosphate
CASP	colon ascendens stent peritonitis model
CLP	cecal ligation and puncture model
DIC	disseminated intravascular coagulation
EVLW	extra-vascular lung water
GCS	Glasgow Coma Scale
HR	heart rate
ICU	intensive care unit
IL	interleukin
LPS	lipopolysaccharide
MAP	mean arterial pressure
MODS	multiorgan dysfunction syndrome
MOF	multiple organ failure
NFκB	nuclear factor kappa B
NO	nitric oxide
NOD	nucleotide-binding oligomerization domain-like (receptor)
PEEP	positive end-expiratory pressure
PiCCO	Pulse index Continuous Cardiac Output monitoring device
SIRS	systemic inflammatory response syndrome
SOFA	sequential organ failure assessment (score)
TLR	toll-like receptor
TNF-α	tumor necrosis factor alpha

INTRODUCTION

The last decades witnessed a tremendous increase in the volume of research and number of publications on sepsis, both in clinical and experimental setting (Figure 2.1). Despite the advancement of the diagnostic and therapeutic possibilities and the accumulating evidence-based treatment options, sepsis remains a main cause of death in the intensive care units (ICU) of developed countries. According to a recent report, there have been 31.5 million cases of sepsis annually, among them 19.4 million severe cases, with potentially 5.3 million deaths occurring annually (Daniels 2011; Fleischmann 2016).

A better understanding of the pathophysiology of the sepsis and the development of novel therapeutical methods require a great deal of animal experimentation. Publications on animal sepsis have increased in logarithmic fashion in the past decades (Figure 2.1). Although rodents remain the most common species used, other species are also subjected to sepsis studies (Figure 2.2). Depending on the goals of each particular study and the peculiarities of various models and species, each existing model has different advantages but also result in several limitations and difficulties when extrapolating results into the clinical scenarios or trials (Fink 2001; Esmon 2004; Bara 2014; Kingsley 2016).

Planning and conducting a sepsis study on animals requires careful consideration of numerous essential aspects that may influence the results, conclusions and the as well as the reproducibility of the study. In this chapter we aimed to briefly overview the clinical problem, pathophysiology, the animal models, their advantages and limitations.

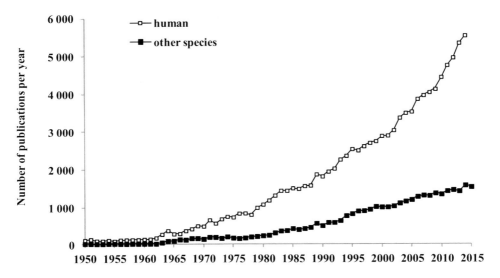

Figure 2.1. Number of publications per year on the human and animal sepsis (PubMed search, 12 November 2016).

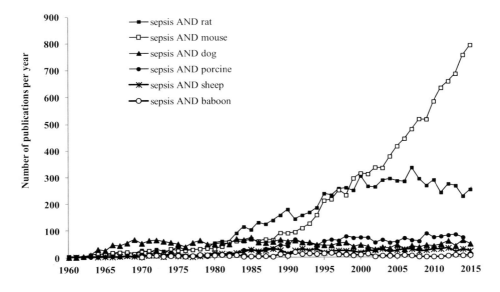

Figure 2.2. Number of publications per year on animal sepsis by species (PubMed search, 12 November 2016).

In the last decades, increasing number of papers has been published on sepsis, both in clinical and experimental settings (Figure 2.1).

To better understand the pathophysiology of sepsis and to develop therapeutic methods, experiments conducted on animals are still necessary. Publications on animal sepsis have increased significantly in the past decades (Figure 2.1). Although the most common species are rodents, other animals such as dog, pig, sheep and non-human primate are also used in sepsis studies in a significant number (Figure 2.2). However, the models are different; besides their advantages, animal models have several limitations and difficulties when extrapolating results. These issues have been discussed in the literature intensively in the last decades (Wichterman 1980; Fink 2001; Schulz 2002; Esmon 2004; Remick 2005; Rittirsch 2007; Chiavolini 2008; Poli-de-Figueiredo 2008; Dyson 2009; van der Poll 2012; Ward 2012; Ziaja 2012; Bara 2014; Chen 2014; Efron 2014; Fink 2014; Shrum 2014; Lilley 2015; Kingsley 2016; Lewis 2016). To plan and conduct a sepsis model using animals, there are numerous essential aspects to consider.

CLINICAL DEFINITIONS OF SEPSIS

It is noteworthy that the past three decades have seen various definitions for sepsis and severe sepsis. Initially, sepsis was defined as a clinical response arising from infection, independently from the cause of infection (bacterial, viral or fungal) (American College of Chest Physicians/Society of Critical Care Medicine Consensus Conference 1992). This initial definition also introduced the concept of systemic inflammatory response syndrome (SIRS).

It has been postulated that sepsis and SIRS have similar clinical appearance, although, major differences exist among the underlying causes (i.e., infections and non-infections causes such as, burns, trauma). At this stage, sepsis was defined based on simple clinical criteria such as: body temperature > 38°C or < 36°C; pulse rate > 90/minutes; breathing frequency > 20/minutes and/or pCO_2 < 30 mmHg; leukocyte count > 12 G/l or lower than 4 G/l along with more than 10% immature forms. For making the diagnosis of sepsis, two of the above listed parameters were necessary to be present. At that time, severe sepsis was defined as basic symptoms of sepsis plus organ dysfunctions, hypotension and hypoperfusion related to infection. Consequently, a very large number of patients were diagnosed as having sepsis based on these criteria.

The next attempt to revise this definition retained these clinically determined criteria, further stating that an expanded list of signs and symptoms of sepsis may better reflect the clinical response to infection, but also included several biochemical markers for use in septic patients (Table 2.1) (Levy 2003). In its very recent definition, sepsis is described as a *"life threatening organ dysfunction caused by a dysregulated host response to infection"* (Singer 2016).

The key points to be taken into account according to this newly developed definition are heterogeneity of the patients that is influenced by underlying co-morbidities, concurrent injuries (such as surgery), medications and source of infections. This statement differentiates sepsis from infection. Sepsis is an aberrant or dysregulated host response and the presence of organ dysfunction. Accordingly, the main definitions of the septic process are as follows:

Table 2.1. Diagnostic criteria for sepsis according to the 2001 definition (Levy 2003)

Infection
Documented or suspected *and* some of the following:
General parameters
Fever (core temperature >38.3°C)
Hypothermia (core temperature <36°C)
Heart rate >90 bpm or >2 SD above the normal value for age
Tachypnea: >30 bpm
Altered mental status
Significant edema or positive fluid balance (>20 ml/kg over 24 h)
Hyperglycemia (plasma glucose >110 mg/dl or 7.7 mM/l) in the absence of diabetes
Inflammatory parameters
Leukocytosis (white blood cell count >12,000/µl)
Leukopenia (white blood cell count <4,000/µl)
Normal white blood cell count with >10% immature forms
Plasma C reactive protein>2 SD above the normal value
Plasma procalcitonin >2 SD above the normal value
Hemodynamic parameters
Arterial hypotension (systolic blood pressure <90 mmHg, mean arterial pressure <70, or a systolic blood pressure decrease >40 mmHg in adults or <2 SD below normal for age)
Mixed venous oxygen saturation >70%
Cardiac index >3.5 l min^{-1} m
Organ dysfunction parameters
Arterial hypoxemia (PaO$_2$/FIO2 <300)
Acute oliguria (urine output <0.5 ml kg^{-1} h^{-1} or 45 mM/l for at least 2 h)
Creatinine increase ≥0.5 mg/dl
Coagulation abnormalities (international normalized ratio >1.5 or activated partial thromboplastin time >60 s)
Ileus (absent bowel sounds)
Thrombocytopenia (platelet count <100,000/µl)
Hyperbilirubinemia (plasma total bilirubin >4 mg/dl or 70 mmol/l)
Tissue perfusion parameters
Hyperlactatemia (>3 mmol/l)
Decreased capillary refill or mottling

- *Sepsis* is defined as life-threatening organ dysfunction caused by a dys-regulated host response to infection.
- *Organ dysfunction* can be identified as an acute change in total SOFA score >2 points consequent to the infection.
- *Septic shock* is a subset of sepsis in which underlying circulatory and cellular/metabolic abnormalities are profound enough to substantially increase mortality. Patients with septic shock can be identified with persisting hypotension requiring vasopressors to maintain MAP > 65 mmHg and having a serum lactate level, > 2 mmol/L (18 mg/dL) despite adequate volume resuscitation.

Table 2.2. The Sequential Organ Failure Assessment or Sepsis-related Organ Failure Assessment score (SOFA) score (Vincent 1996)

	0	1	2	3	4
Respiration					
PaO2/FiO2 (mmHg)	>400	<400	<300	<200 with respiratory support	<100 with respiratory support
Coagulation					
Platelets ($\times 10^3/\mu L$)	>150	<150	<100	<50	<20
Liver					
Bilirubin (μmol/L)	<1.2	1.2–1.9	2.0–5.9	6.0–11.9	>12
Cardiovascular					
	MAP >70 mmHg	MAP <70 mmHg	Dopamine < 5 or dobutamine any dose	Dopamine 5.1-15 or epinephrine <0.1 or norepinephrine < 0.1	Dopamine >15 or epinephrine >0.1 or norepinephrine >0.1
Central nervous system					
GCS	15	13–14	10–12	6–9	< 6
Renal					
Creatinine (μmol/L)	<110	110–170	171–299	300–440	> 440
Urine output (mL/D)				< 500	< 200

The main categories of Sequential Organ Failure Assessment Score (SOFA Score) are summarized in Table 2.2 (Vincent 1996).

A BRIEF OVERVIEW ON THE PATHOPHYSIOLOGY OF SEPSIS

In recent decades it has become clear that different pathogens exert their action by interacting with specific targets (represented by toll-like receptors) at the surface of various cell types. In case of non-infectious origin, SIRS is evoked through the activation of the nucleotide-binding oligomerization domain-like (NOD) receptors. Macrophages are key actors in the process as activation of their NF-κB by protein kinases results in the production of pro- and anti-inflammatory cytokines triggering the general inflammatory process (Figure 2.3). As it is demonstrated in the figure, the "cytokine storm" causes gradual changes at the level of capillary function and coagulation system. These complex changes determine the severity of SIRS and sepsis in their later course (Brides 2005; Remick 2007; Wynn 2010; Nduka 2011; Dellinger 2013; Semeraro 2015; Bhan 2016). In the view of this, in the following sections, we summarize the main pathophysiological alterations and their consequences in different organ systems.

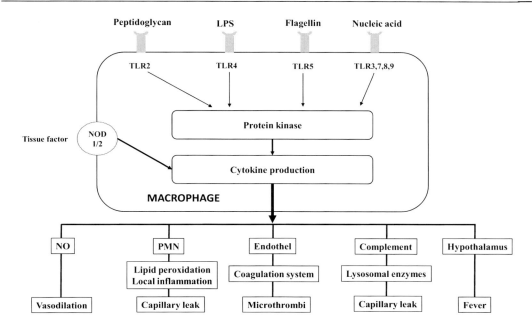

Figure 2.3. The involvement of macrophages in the septic process.

Causes of Capillary Dysfunction in Sepsis

The capillary network is responsible for the transport of oxygen and the main nutritional products to the tissues. Its function is influenced by the distribution of the capillary network in certain tissue, by the actual condition of the capillaries (dilated or constricted), by the inter-capillary distance and by hemorheological factors (Further details in Chapter 13).

Sepsis is currently considered as a microcirculatory disorder (Astiz 1995; Ince 2005, 2016; Trzeciak 2007, 2008; Tyagi 2009; Ostergaard 2015). The microcirculatory failure usually is generalized; however, it is often tested on the sublingual surface and/or on skin (Young 1995; Trzeciak 2007, 2008; Wester 2011; Kiss 2015). Factors leading to microcirculatory problems in sepsis are complex. Several mechanisms act on the pre-capillary, capillary and post-capillary regions of the microcirculation, as summarized in Table 2.3.

The mechanisms leading to deterioration of micro-rheological factors are dominantly non-specific. Red blood cell deformability can be impaired by (1) local metabolic and acid-base changes (pH, lactate concentration, oxygenation level, micro-environmental osmolarity); (2) decrease in ATP and consequent failure of active pump mechanisms, a condition that leads to alteration in surface to volume ratio; as well as by (3) reactive oxygen species (Baskurt 2007; Piagnerelli 2003; Nemeth 2012). Red blood cells can be damaged mechanically as well due to the presence of thrombi and micro-thrombi (DIC), or even by the associated mechanical trauma to blood during therapeutic efforts such as the direct removal of toxins from the bloodstream by high-volume hemofiltration (Kameneva 2007; Borthwick 2013).

Table 2.3. Events and factors leading to microcirculatory disturbances in sepsis (based on papers by Piagnerelli 2003; Spronk 2004; Lundy 2009)

Event, factor	Dominant site of the effect
vasodilatation and vasopressor hyporeactivity (vasoplegia)	arterioles
redistribution of organ blood flow, hemodynamic changes	
congestion, intravascular pooling	arterioles, venules
opening AV shunts	
endothelial cell activation, endothelial dysfunction	arterioles, capillaries, venules
hemorrhage	
decreased neutrophil deformability	
enhanced neutrophil aggregation	
impaired red blood cell deformability	
microthrombi, DIC	
increased plasma viscosity	
increased microvascular permeability	capillaries
edema formation	
neutrophil adhesion and aggregation	capillaries, venules

Enhanced red blood cell aggregation is a common observation in manifest sepsis. In most of the clinical and experimental studies, the developed sepsis and severe sepsis has been found with increased fibrinogen and plasma viscosity, impaired red blood cell deformability and markedly enhanced erythrocyte aggregation (Chien 1972; Baskurt 1997; Kirschenbaum 2000; Piagnerelli 2003; Pöschl 2003; Alt 2004; Sordia 2006; Moutzouri 2007; Reggiori 2009). The rise in fibrinogen concentration is one of the factors that lead to enhanced erythrocyte aggregation. Furthermore, free radical effects, ultrastructural alterations of the cell surface glycocalyx as well as cellular morphology changes might also influence red blood cell aggregation in its magnitude and kinetics (Baskurt 2007, 2012; Nemeth 2012). However, it has been also shown in a porcine model of fulminant sepsis that during the early phase of the process, the red blood cell aggregation might be decreased (Nemeth 2015, 2016), probably due to the early fibrinogen consumption (Asakura 2014; Semeraro 2015), the direct effect of NO and the bacteria themselves *(Escherichia coli)* on erythrocytes.

Deformability of neutrophils also decreases and their aggregation increases in severe sepsis and septic shock (Yodice 1997; Nishino 2005; Brown 2006). Adhered leukocytes affect local flow pattern and rigid cells may plug microcapillaries. Furthermore, altered blood rheology drives margination of the leukocytes: increased erythrocyte aggregation enhances axial flow, resulting in a widening cell deprived layer (Poiseuille-zone) in the vicinity of the endothelial surface, and so the flow pattern facilitates leukocyte tethering and margination (Nash 2008).

Capillary perfusion is usually described by the term 'capillary driving pressure' and by the actual condition of the pre- and post-capillary sphincters. Low volume state during sepsis may be attributed to 2 main factors: (1) Due to the peripheral vasodilation, a large amount of fluid is stored in the dilated vessels; and (2) due to capillary leak, a large amount of fluid may leave the intravascular compartment thus resulting in an interstitial fluid accumulation. Capillary leakage is also believed to be the consequence (at least in part) of the excessive NO production of the endothelium. From experimental observations, it is known that high levels of NO decreases the cyclic opening-closing function of the endothelial tight junctions and it is believed that this is a key factor in capillary leakage (Gomez-Jimenez 1995; Morel 2013). Additionally, activated leucocytes and complement enzymes may also damage capillary wall integrity.

Based on experimental observations, dominantly precapillary sphincters in gram-positive sepsis are dilated, while in case of gram-negative pathogens, this phenomenon occurs at the level of postcapillary sphincters. Thus, capillary perfusion itself is also influenced by the actual pathogen causing the septic process. Taking into account that capillary driving pressure is also influenced by systemic blood pressure, low systemic blood pressure that develops in severe sepsis, may result in a decreased capillary driving pressure. Due to local regulatory mechanisms, when driving pressure decreases, capillary sphincters get further dilated in order to enhance local blood flow. Unfortunately, as shown in Figure 2.3, coagulation system is also activated during the septic process leading to micro-thrombi formation and thus resulting in worsening of the local oxygen and nutritional transport.

Alterations in lymphatic flow also show a blend picture in sepsis. Endotoxaemia can be associated with an increase in thoracic duct lymph flow (Kutner 1967; Williemas 1973; Smith 1988). When the thoracic duct was ligated in a canine model of peritonitis sepsis, it had a negative effect on liver function and survival; bacterial count in peritoneal fluid, endotoxin level in portal vein, nitrite and AST level were significantly elevated (Guler 1999). In a porcine model, Lattuada and Hedenstierna (Lattuada 2006) found that during endotoxin sepsis (LPS infusion), the lymph flow from the abdomen increased. The flow was measured by ultrasonic probe placed around the thoracic duct. They have also observed that mechanical ventilation with high PEEP impedes lymphatic drainage and also cold increases the lymph production, while flow increased and lymphatic drainage of abdominal edema improved by spontaneous breathing (Lattuada 2006). Elias and co-workers in their ovine model found that endotoxin (i.v., 3.3 – 33 µg/kg) reduces lymphatic pump activity, contributing to the edema formation in sepsis (Elias 1987). Intrahepatic lymph stasis in endotoxaemia in rats can be caused by decreased pumping activity of extra- and intrahepatic large lymph vessels (Shibayama 1992). It has been showed in LPS-induced sepsis model in guinea pigs that there is an early increase in mesenteric lymph flow rate being mediated by vascular hyperpermeability and plasma albumin leakage (Nemoto 2011).

Microcirculatory and Mitochondrial Distress Syndrome

As described above, the excessive systemic reaction to the inflammatory insult finally leads to a critical imbalance of oxygen and nutritional products supply and demand. In the recent decade, it has been speculated that compensatory mechanisms in sepsis may be described as a 2-phase process. In the beginning, microvascular compensation dominates. During this phase, the decreased tissue perfusion and tissue hypoxia result in enhanced production of potent vasodilatory substances (mainly NO) (Gomez-Jimenez 1995). This reaction aims to increase the tissue perfusion. Whenever this compensation fails, in the second mitochondrial phase, cells are trying to turn into an "energy-saving mode" by decreasing their energy needs. The main actor in this process is again the overproduced NO. It passes easily through the cellular and mitochondrial membranes as oxygen and blocks cytochrome oxidase at complex IV. This compensatory mechanism however is a double-edged sword; although it decreases cellular energy need (and thus contributes to survival) but only until a certain limit: as a secondary consequence of complex IV block, reactive nitrogen species (most importantly peroxinitrites) are produced. Large amounts of reactive nitrogen species contribute to cell necrosis in severe, end-stage states of sepsis.

Multiple Organ Failure (MOF) in Sepsis

The continuum of sepsis is depicted in Figure 2.4. Based on the underlying pathophysiological mechanisms, different organs may be affected during the septic process (Albert 2004; Langenberg 2005; Remick 2007; Wynn 2010; Nduka 2011; Bhan 2016; Doi 2016).

- In the *cardiovascular system*, newly developing atrial fibrillation can be considered as early warning sign of developing sepsis. Beside this, decreased central venous and mean arterial blood pressures as well as a decreased peripheral vascular resistance are typical signs of septic cardiovascular affection. Cardiac contractility may eventually be higher in the early phase of sepsis, however, in the late phase of septic shock, cardiac contractility also decreases due to inappropriate oxygenation of the myocardium. Recent clinical observations suggest that PiCCO monitoring enables checking the cardiovascular consequences.
- *Pulmonary consequences:* Based on experimental and pathological observations, there is an inflammatory exudate accumulation within the alveoli. This exudate worsens the effectiveness of the alveolo-capillary gas exchange. It contributes to the washout of the surfactant, thus leading to alveolar collapse and atelectasis formation. Additionally capillary leak also affects the pulmonary capillaries and contributes to extravascular fluid accumulation within the lung. This extravascular lung water may lead to further compression of the alveoli (due to extraalveolar forces) and also leads to an increase of the alveolo-capillary distance that worsens gas exchange. The most sensitive parameter that describes the function of the alveolo-capillary gas exchanges is PaO_2/FiO_2 ratio. Extravascular lung water can be measured by PiCCO monitoring (EVLW).
- *Consciousness disturbances* of different severity are early signs of sepsis development. At early stages, sepsis causes confusions or delirious states. The correct terminology for the cerebral affection in sepsis is sepsis-associated encephalopathy. This is a multifactorially-determined functional disturbance that develops along with the progression of the septic process, leading to somnolence, or coma in late phases. Cerebral functions can be monitored by the GCS score and EEG.
- In early stages of systemic hypoperfusion, the urine output decreases and septic patients are prone to development of acute kidney injury. Along with the advancement of severe sepsis, oliguria may turn to anuria and serum creatinine progressively increases.

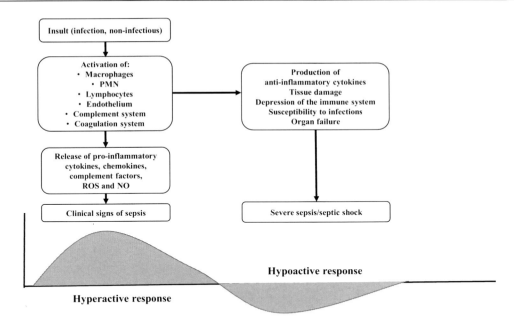

Figure 2.4. The continuum of sepsis.

- Hypoperfusion of the liver has different consequences: albumin and vitamin K-dependent coagulation factor production decreases. In severe cases where parenchymal damage is advanced, bilirubin increases (by canalicular damage and hepatocytolysis) (> 70 mmol/l) and icterus may develop.
- Severe hypoperfusion also affects gastrointestinal organs. As a consequence, bowel ischemia, ileus, pancreas apoplexy and acalculous cholecystitis may develop.

EXPERIMENTAL MODELS FOR STUDYING SEPSIS

According to Fink (2001), the 'ideal' animal sepsis model should be (1) capable of predicting both positive and negative results of a trial; (2) inexpensive; (3) reproducible (within and among laboratories); (4) humane and fully respecting the 3Rs; (5) able to provide a mortality endpoint; (6) characterized by hemodynamic, hematologic, and biochemical features similar to those observed in human sepsis (Fink 2001). Unfortunately there is no 'ideal' model known to date.

Experimental sepsis can be induced via generating toxemia by intravenous or intraperitoneal administration of live bacteria (pure or mixed cultures), inhalation, intrabronchial instillation, implantation or seeding into tissues or by disruption of the host-barriers (mechanically or by ischemia), or in combination. Behind these major approaches to develop sepsis models, there are numerous variations and sub-models that can be classified in the following main categories:

- endotoxin models
- bacteremia models

- peritonitis models
- pneumonia models
- meningitis models
- soft tissue infection models (abscess models)

Table 2.4 summarizes some major characteristics of these models. Each of these strategies reproduces one or several pathophysiological mechanisms activated during sepsis, yet the multitude of existing approaches indicate limitations of each model to mimic the clinical scenario. Many of the limitations depend on the species of animals or bacteria used while others depend on technical and conceptual details behind each model.

Not only the way of sepsis induction, but the choice of the animal species itself is also crucial. Table 2.5 gives a summary of various species in consideration of sepsis models (based on Fink 2001).

Following sections provide the technical description of the methods for inducing experimental sepsis as well as brief considerations on their advantages and limitations.

Endotoxin Models

Endotoxin is a lipoprotein-carbohydrate complex that can be found in the cell wall of all gram-negative bacteria. Endotoxins were originally isolated by André Boivin (Bactéries et Virus, Paris, Presses Universitaires de France, 1941).

The simplest way is to inject single bolus of LPS intravenously (as the most common way) or intraperitoneally. The pro-inflammatory processes occur suddenly and last briefly when endotoxicosis is induced by LPS injection (single bolus). Endotoxin can be administered via intraperitoneal injection as well (Laschke 2007). In case of infection, the inflammatory stimulus is much more obvious with gradual development and persisting longer. It has been shown that TNF-α concentration is much higher and showing a peak around 60–90 minutes after LPS injection (i.v. or i.p.) compared to a focal infection model (e.g., fecal peritonitis) (Eskandari 1992; Fink 2001). After endotoxin administration, plasma concentration of host response mediators such as TNF-α, IL-1, IL-6 and IL-10 rapidly increase as an acute and transient elevation. LPS binds to TLR-4 and so activates inflammatory pathways, including NF-κβ.

The sensitivity of various animal species to LPS and the physiologic and immunologic response to this stimulus is different. Humans are very sensitive to LPS; in volunteers 2–4 ng/kg LPS may produce obvious symptoms. In mice 1–25 ng/kg LPS is needed to generate septic symptoms. A very interesting study aimed at reaching a similar IL-6 response in mice and humans revealed that 2 ng of endotoxin administered intravenously in humans were enough to elicit the same IL-6 plasma levels as 500 ng given intraperitoneally to mice (Copeland 2005). Other species such as rabbit, pig and sheep are also sensitive to endotoxin, similarly to human. Interestingly, the rodents or even monkeys such as baboons are resistant to endotoxin. About 5 μg/kg LPS is lethal in sheep, 100 μg/kg is the LD_{80} in rabbits, while mice and baboons needs incomparably higher dose for lethality (LD_{70} dose is about 6 mg/kg in baboon; LD_{100} dose is about 20–80 mg/kg in the mouse) (Fink 2001). Overall, endotoxemia models are relatively far from the clinical sepsis scenario. Furthermore, the resistance of rodents to LPS also puts a serious limitation of extrapolating the results to the human (Kingsley 2016).

There are several techniques and materials for increasing the sensitivity of rodents to LPS such as D-galactosamine, a non-ionic polyoxyethylene-polypropylene copolymer (Pluronic F127), carageenan, berrylium phosphate, lead acetate or carbon tetrachloride. Administration of platelet-activating factor or heat-killed bacteria a week prior to LPS injection can also cause enhanced sensitivity (Katschinski 1992; Rabinovici 1993; Fink 2001; Gumenscheimer 2002).

Rittirsch and co-workers reported in their paper that the LPS endotoxemia differs from cecal ligation and puncture (CLP) model in rodents. After LPS infusion, the symptoms such as rapid hypothermia developed within a few hours, together with leukopenia followed by leukocytosis. The scenario is also characterized by an early increase and high transient levels of pro-inflammatory cytokines (IL-1β, TNF-α, IL-6) and the protective effect of anti-TNF-α is shown. In CLP model, the symptoms developed within 12–24 hours, leukocytosis or leukopenia was also present, whereas, the pro-inflammatory cytokines (IL-1β, TNF-α, IL-6, C5a) were expressed later at moderately high levels. Anti-LPS or anti-TNF-α were not protective (Rittirsch 2007).

Intravenous, intraperionoteal or intraarticular administration of zymosan (a polysaccharide cell wall component derived from *Saccharomyces cerevisiae*), producing a prolonged activation of the alternative complement pathway and generalized inflammation, is another example for endotoxaemia models, mostly in rodents (mouse, rat) and rabbit (Sharkey 1984; Volman 2005; Cash 2009; Guerra 2016; Hong 2016;).

Bacteremia Models

Intravenous administration of live *Escherichia coli* is used for studying sepsis since decades. The early studies used typically large animals (dogs, pigs, monkeys) (Guenter 1969; Cryer 1971; Hinshaw 1976; Wichterman 1980). Later, rodent usage has been also spread out widely. Contrary to the rapid bolus infusion, which results in rapid hypoglycemia and death, further models have been established to provide more time for the response reactions approaching closer to the clinical scenarios. Postel et al. developed a canine model in which the animals were continuously infused with *Pseudomonas aeruginosa* for 5 hours (10^6/ml/min for 2–5 hours or 4×10^7/ml/min for 5 hours), and observed the animals for 24 hours. This model provided more time for developing wider response reactions and for observation of kinetics (Postel 1975).

In sepsis models with bacterial infusion, the exact number of bacteria can be estimated only that might influence the reproducibility compared to the better standardized endotoxin infusion models (Fink 2001). The most commonly used bacteria are the gram-negative *Escherichia coli*. Other gram-positive bacteria, such as *Staphylococcus aureus*, *Staphylococcus epidermidis*, *Streptococcus pyogenes* or *Pseudomonas aeruginosa*, or fungi such as *Candida albicans* can be also used in various animal species (mouse, rat, rabbit, dog, pig, sheep, baboon).

PERITONITIS MODELS

The surgical models are particularly relevant models of sepsis since a significant number of sepsis cases are the result of intraabdominal leakage of intestinal content after abdominal surgery or perforated diverticulitis or appendicitis (Browne 1976; Wichterman 1980; Krisher 2001; Wryzykowski 2005; Catry 2016). These models generate a polymicrobial sepsis which closely resembles the clinical situation in terms of mechanism and clinical course. The peritonitis may be induced by perforating the bowel or by instillation of bacteria or fecal material in the peritoneal cavity.

Cecal Ligation and Puncture (CLP)

This simple and reproducible model has become a gold standard in sepsis research because of its relative technical simplicity and versatility (Wichterman 1980; Hubbard 2005; Dejager 2011; Toscano 2011; Schabbauer 2012; Siempos 2014). Nonetheless, ensuring reproducibility requires that a few important details should be carefully considered throughout the procedure including preoperative fasting of the animals to generate similar intestinal contents as well as consistency in several other technical details. In addition, short-acting methods of anesthesia (i.e., isoflurane inhalation) should be chosen in order to minimize prolonged anesthesia-induced cardiovascular alterations postoperatively (Hubbard 2005). Following midline incision, the cecum is identified and carefully exteriorized. Then, the cecum is ligated distal to the ileocecal valve and perforated using one or two needle punctures (Figure 2.5). Both the length of the ligated cecum (Singleton 2003) and the needle size (Ebong 1999; Otero-Anton 2001) can be used to influence the CLP outcome and give a lethal or nonlethal sepsis. For instance, two punctures created with an 18G needle result in 100% mortality in BALB/c mice, while the same procedure yields mortality rates of 50% or 0% when performed with 21G or 25G needles, respectively (Ebong 1999).

The cecum is gently compressed to expel a small amount of intestinal content through the perforation, thereafter is returned to the abdomen and the wound is closed in two layers. The cecum will become necrotic within 24 hours but it may ultimately be resected to remove the source of infection as part of the treatment strategy.

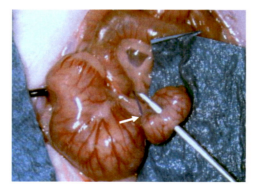

Figure 2.5. Cecal ligation and puncture (CLP) in anesthetized rat. White arrow shows the site of the ligature. The excluded cecum punctured through by a 19 G needle.

The postoperative care is a significant element of this particular experimental model as fluid resuscitation and antibiotic treatment may influence significantly both the pathophysiology and animal survival (Zanotti-Cavazzoni 2009). In the rat, this model induces a complex cardiovascular response with an early, hyperdynamic phase characterized by increased cardiac output, increased tissue perfusion and decreased peripheral resistance. This is followed by a late, hypodynamic phase characterized by reduced microvascular blood flow in various tissues and increased peripheral resistance (Yang 2002; Yang 1999). Results in mice and rats indicate that fluid resuscitation (typically isotonic saline as subcutaneous injection) and antibiotics may increase the 48 hour survival rate from 0 to around 20–40% (Hollenberg 2001) depending on type of fluid, volume and concentration (Zanotti-Cavazzoni 2009).

Colon Ascendens Stent Peritonitis (CASP)

The model of colon ascendens stent peritonitis (Zantl 1998) is more recent than the previously described CLP and has been introduced following numerous observations that animals undergoing cecal ligation and puncture often develop only localized peritonitis (Schabbauer 2012). The cecal perforations are spontaneously covered by the surrounding intestinal loops leading to abscess formation (Maier 2004). This in its turn may result in two different pathologic conditions not entirely comparable (diffuse peritonitis vs. large abscess) and with different response to various treatment alternatives.

The surgery is preceded by the preparation of plastic venous catheters of variable sizes. In the rat model, the survival rate is strictly dependent on the diameter of the implanted stent and a stent diameter of 14G leads to 100% mortality whereas smaller stent diameters generates sublethal models (16G stent leads to a 71% mortality whereas mortality is 53% when a 18G stent is used) (Lustig 2007). Similarly, approximately 70% of the mice expired within 48 hours when a 16G stent was used whereas the death rate dropped to 50% with an 18G stent (Maier 2004). After creating a marking at a distance of 3 mm from the tip, the catheter is circumferentially incised with a 1 mm scalpel beyond the marking sparing only a narrow bridge of plastic.

Inhalational anesthesia is advocated by the majority of the authors (ether, isoflurane, sevoflurane) (Lohner 2013; Islam 2016; Schöneborn 2016) due to the lower impact on the hemodynamics as well as the short postoperative recovery. The abdominal wall is opened through midline incision and the ascending colon is exposed using soft cotton earbuds. After adequate exposure of the ascending colon, the prepared catheter is inserted into the lumen of the ascending colon through the antimesenteric wall approximately 10 mm from the ileocecal valve and fixed with two stitches of non-absorbable suture (7/0) (Figure 2.6). Thereafter, the inner needle of the stent is removed and the stent is cut at the marked site. To verify the adequate intraluminal placement of the stent and the immediate initiation of the fecal leakage, stool is milked from the cecum into the ascending colon and the stent is filled until a small drop of stool appears at its end. The procedure is completed through abdominal wall closure in two layers and fluid resuscitation (Zantl 1998).

Bacterial Suspension Inoculation (Intraabdominal Abscess Models)

Classic models include the inoculation of defined bacterial isolates (e.g., *E. coli*, *B. fragilis*) mixed with barium sulfate and autoclaved rat fecal material, suspended and loaded into gelatin capsule and implanted intraperitoneally, or agar pellets containing bacteria, or suspension containing hemoglobin, mucin and bacteria *(E. coli)*, or impregnated fibrin clot (Onderdonk 1976; Wichterman 1980; Fink 2001; Kingsley 2016). Inoculation of autologous feces and other clinically-relevant model dominantly in pigs (for instance simulating the case of bowel anastomosis insufficiency), in which a definitive amount (e.g., 0.5 g/kg) of autologous feces is suspended in saline solution (e.g., 200 ml), incubated (e.g., for 6 hours at 38°C) and inoculated into the peritoneal cavity through drains, or via incision and/or Veres needle (Chvojka 2008; Zsikai 2012) (Table 2.6).

Interventions that Partly Destroy Barriers of Gastrointestinal Tract

Intestinal ischemia models. An example is the creation of an ischemic bowel loop results in severe diffuse peritonitis (Wichterman 1980). Hau and Simmons (1977) and which reported 90% mortality rate within 10 days after making a loop of terminal ileum ischemia in dogs. Simpler intestinal ischemia-reperfusion models with longer follow-up period, allowing time for development of symptoms, are also capable for mimicking abdominal sepsis.

Cholecystitis models. In the canine study of Perbellini and co-workers, *E. coli* was injected directly into the gall bladder after ligating the cystic artery. The ischemic and infected gall bladder showed similarities to clinically seen cholecystitis (Perbellini 1978; Wichterman 1980).

Pneumonia Models

In this simple and clinically relevant model type, *Streptocossus pneumoniae*, *Klebsiella pneumoniae*, *Pseudomonas aeruginosa* are the most common bacteria which are introduced via a tracheal route (tube in rodents, or even with bronchoscope in large animals), or via nasal route (Fink 2011; Kinglsey 2016).

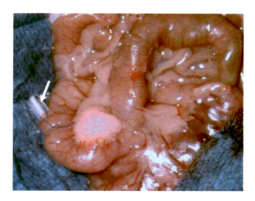

Figure 2.6. Colon ascendens stent peritonitis (CASP) in anesthetized rat. White arrow shows the fixed stent (size: 16 G).

Meningitis Models

Several murine models have been developed using intracerebral, intraperitoneal, intravenous, intranasal or intracisternal inoculation methods (Chiavolini 2008). In the latter category, a well-established model is inoculation by injecting 10 μL of bacterial suspension into the cisterna magna using a 32 G needle (Mook-Kanamori 2012; 2015).

Meningitis in rats can be produced by intranasal inoculation of *Haemophilus influenzae* in newborn rats, or in young adult animals by intraperitoneal inoculation (Smith 1984). *Streptococcus pneumoniae* is also used for meningitis models. Intraperitoneal route provokes hematogenous meningitis. The intranasal inoculation can act non-hematogenously as well along the olfactory nerves (Chiavolini 2008).

Soft Tissue Infection Models (Abscess Models)

Intramuscular abscess models. Hermreck and Thal (1969) described a model in which 5-cm wicks of umbilical tape were seeded with the dog's own feces and immersed into porcine mucin solution. These wicks then were embedded into the thigh (unilaterally) of the dog subcutaneously and intramuscularly. The animals were followed-up for a week.

Dermal abscess models. In 1964, Walker et al. published a rat model mimicking dermal abscess. *Pseudomonas aeruginosa*, isolated from a patient with septicemia after second and third degree burn injury, was used to seed subcutaneous tissues. On the dorsum, a 5×7 cm area was excised (~20% of the body surface), and the fascia in the base of the wound was seeded by the bacterial culture. The area then was covered with split-thickness (0.012 inch) skin autograft. In their study, a comparison was made with intraperitoneal and subcutaneous injection of the bacterial culture as well (Walker 1964).

Intramuscular, subdermal bacterial injections, subcutaneous pockets filled with gauze and injected bacteria, infected cotton suture are further examples for soft tissue infections models (Fink 2001).

EXTRAPOLATION OF THE RESULTS: EXPERIMENTAL VERSUS CLINICAL SEPSIS

The final goal of all medical research is and must be the benefit to the patient, by exploring and understanding the nature of various disorders and its pathophysiology mechanisms as well as developing preventive or therapeutic agents. In this process, animal studies are still necessary, since in the translational process, there must be a stage of *in vivo* study before any human application.

Unfortunately, numerous pharmacological agents which have been promising and effective in animal models, failed in large well-designed human clinical trials (e.g., methylprednisolone sodium succinate, IL1-RA, CDP571, BN 5021, BB-822, TCV-309, TAK-242, lenercept, tifacogin) (Fink 2014; Lakshmikanth 2016).

Practically speaking, all the experimental sepsis models fail to reproduce entirely the clinical scenario. This explains the relatively large number of models used to induce severe systemic infections and continuous search for a better mirror to the clinical situation. Accordingly, numerous authors have discussed the comparability of animal sepsis models and human sepsis (Wichterman 1980; Fink 2001; Esmon 2004; Rittirsch 2007; Nemzek 2008; Poli-de-Figueiredo 2008; Dyson 2009; Fink 2014; Lilley 2015).

In the clinical practice, the most frequent infection sites are the lung, the abdomen and urinary tract. Gram-positive and gram-negative infections show almost the same frequency, followed by fungi and parasites. The initial insult or infection activates the innate immune system bursting the pro-inflammatory cascades and mediators with SIRS as result. Anti-inflammatory factors appear as compensatory mechanism but any imbalance can cause further deterioration: exaggerated pro-inflammatory effect results in uncontrolled, excessive inflammatory response and consecutive effects; stronger anti-inflammatory steps may lead to immunosuppression (Rittirsch 2007).

Virtually all the experimental sepsis models in rodents fail to reproduce entirely the clinical scenario due to limitations related to design or the species used. Moreover, seemingly minor technical details (Ebong 1999; Singleton 2003) or the choice of the animals used in terms of age and gender impacts on the pathophysiology and the outcome (Turnbull 2003). Compared with humans, rodents are quite resistant to endotoxin, have a distinct hemodynamic profile, and limited blood volume (Copeland 2005). All these factors explain the relatively large number of models used to induce severe systemic infections and the ongoing search for refined designs to better mirror the clinical situation.

Microbiological Actors Causing Sepsis

In human sepsis, gram-positive bacteria and fungi act for causing sepsis in higher incidence than gram-negative organisms, however, in animal studies mostly gram-negative bacteria have been used (Poli de Figueiredo 2008).

Experimental Considerations Related to the Pathomechanism of Sepsis

In clinical scenario, usually there is a septic focus which intermittently or persistently scatters bacteria. Different ways of sepsis induction act differently, as it has been discussed previously and overviewed in Table 2.4.

The Time Factor (Follow-Up)

For development of sepsis, time is needed that differs according to the way of induction (Table 2.4). Endotoxemia and infusion of bacteria provide prompt effects, while infection site models obviously need more time to develop the response reactions and the septic symptoms. The choice of the model depends on the primary aim of the study itself.

Table 2.4. Summary of various septic models by its nature, origin, most commonly used species, advantages and disadvantages (based on papers by Fink 2001; Esmon 2004; Volman 2005; Rittirsch 2007; Poli de Figueiredo 2008; Engel 2011; Mai 2012; Fink 2014; Kingsley, 2016)

Sepsis origin	Model	Species	Characteristic hemodynamic response	Persistent inflammatory response	Cytokine response characteristics	Advantages	Disadvantages	Special notes
Toxemia	Endotoxin (LPS) administration	*Most commonly used:* mouse, rat *More rarely used:* rabbit, dog, pig, sheep, non-human primates	immediate early hypodynamic phase	no	Early rise of TNF-α, rapid transient increase	Easy model. LPS dosage is well-controllable. Innate immune system activation can be well studied. Well-suited to test the mechanism of inflammatory cascade activation and the efficacy of anti-inflammatory compounds.	Far from clinical scenario. Different sensitivity amongst the species (relatively endotoxin resistant species: rodents, cat, dog; sensitivity with enhanced response: rabbit, sheep, non-human primates). Dose dependency (concentration and way of administration)	Toxin can be given: i.v., i.a., i.p. LPS effect can be enhanced by administration of D-galactosamine, pluronic F 127, carageenan, lead acetate, beryllium phosphate, carbon tetrachloride, platelet-activating factor, co-administration of heat-killed bacteria (e.g., *P. acnes, C. parvum, M. bovis*), mostly in rodents.
	TLR agonist administration (i.v.)	rodents	Not specified.	no	Rapid immune activation and inflammation, elevation of IL-6 and IFN-β within 2 h	Technically easy model.	Nonspecific indicator of inflammation, short half-time of agents, immunological effects often controversial	Mostly TLR-9, TLR-7, TLR-3 agonists
	Administration of zymosan	rodents (most frequently rabbits), rarely in sheep	early drop in cardiac index and stroke volume index	no	Prolonged activation of the alternative complement pathway, generalized inflammation	Easy to perform. Can be used for studying sterile peritonitis, MODS and acute lung injury as well.	Early mortality rate is high.	Toxin can be given: i.v., i.a., i.p., intraarticularly. Acute inflammation peaking within few hours. Marked hypoxaemia, interstitial edema, pulmonary neutrophil sequestration.

Table 2.4. (Continued)

Sepsis origin	Model	Species	Characteristic hemodynamic response	Persistent inflammatory response	Cytokine response characteristics	Advantages	Disadvantages	Special notes
Bacteremia	Intravascular infusion of live bacteria	rodents, dog, pig, sheep, non-human primates	hypotensive shock	no	Rise of TNF-α and IL-1β, rapid transient increase	DIC presents.	Relatively far from clinical scenario.	Most commonly used bacteria: *E. coli* Others: *S. aureus, P. aeruginosa, S. pyogenes, S. epidermidis, C. albicans* Variations: Bolus (single or multiple), increasing concentration via infusion pump.
Peritonitis	cecal ligation and puncture (CLP)		hemodynamic and metabolic phases	yes	moderate increase	Clinically highly relevant.	Not specified.	-
	colon ascendens stent peritonitis (CASP)	most commonly rodents	prolonged hemodynamic instability	yes	steady, continuous systemic increase	Clinically highly relevant. Lethality is accompanied by MOF.	Not specified.	-
	polymicrobial peritoneal contamination and infection (PCI)		early hyperdynamic response	yes		Clinically highly relevant.	Not specified.	e.g., intraperitoneal injection of a human feces suspension
	implantation model (implanting fibrin clot impregnated with live bacteria)	rat dog, pig		yes	Similar to human sepsis.	Clinically highly relevant.	Not specified.	Most commonly used bacteria: *E. coli* Others: *B. fragilis* in combination with *E. coli*

Sepsis origin	Model	Species	Characteristic hemodynamic response	Persistent inflammatory response	Cytokine response characteristics	Advantages	Disadvantages	Special notes
	faecal peritonitis (inoculation of autologous faeces or faecal suspension)	pig	early hyperdynamic response	yes	Similar to human sepsis.	Clinically highly relevant.	Not specified.	-
Pneumonia	Direct administration of bacteria (S. pneumoniae, P. aeruginosa, K.pneumoniae) via trachea or nasal route	mouse, rat	absent	yes	Strain-specific (e.g., TNF-α decrease after S. pneumoniae infection)	Clinically relevant.	Not specified.	-
	Instillation of living bacteria into bronchi via bronchoscope	pig	Not specified.	yes	Not specified.	Clinically highly relevant.	Not specified.	-
Sof tissue infection	Injecting bacteria or implanting contaminated materials into soft tissue	rodents, dog	Not specified.	yes	Not specified.	Clinically relevant.	Not specified.	Intramuscular, subdermal bacterial injections, subcutaneous pockets filled with contaminated gauze or cotton suture
Meningitis	Inoculation of bacteria (intracerebral, intraperitoneal, intravenous, intranasal, intracisternal)	mostly rodents	Not specified.	yes	Strain-specific.	Clinically relevant.	Not specified.	Most commonly used bacteria: H. influenza, S. pneumoniae

Table 2.5. Summary of advantages and disadvantages of various animal species in sepsis studies (based on Fink 2001, with additions and modifications)

Species	Advantages	Disadvantages
mouse *(Mus musculus)*	inexpensive, inbred or transgenic strains available, immunological reagents widely available	repetitive blood sampling is difficult, problematic hemodynamic measurements – special instruments needed, moderately resistant to LPS
rat *(Rattus norvegicus)*	inexpensive, inbred, outbred or transgenic strains available, immunological reagents widely available, most hemodynamic measurements feasible, chronic instrumentation feasible, faecal flora shows certain similarities to that of human	very resistant to LPS
guinea pig *(Rattus norvegicus)*	inexpensive, various outbred strains available, immunological reagents available, most hemodynamic measurements feasible, chronic instrumentation feasible, very sensitive to LPS	gram-positive faecal flora, coprophagy (caecotrophia)
rabbit *(Oryctolagus cuniculus)*	inexpensive, most hemodynamic measurements feasible, chronic instrumentation feasible, very sensitive to LPS, septic acute lung injury reminiscent of human ARDS	gram-positive faecal flora, caecotrophia
sheep *(Ovies aries)*	relatively inexpensive for a large animal, faecal flora similar to that of human, well-suited for hemodynamic measurements, repetitive blood sampling and chronic instrumentation, septic acute lung injury reminiscent of human ARDS – so good for studying pulmonary pathophysiology, very sensitive to LPS, often are used in chronic, examples for unanesthetized models	chronic study is difficult
pig *(Sus scrofa domestica)*	relatively inexpensive, renal, cardiovascular and digestive anatomy and physiology as well as faecal flora close to human, well-suited for hemodynamic measurements and repetitive blood sampling, septic acute lung injury reminiscent of human ARDS, relatively sensitive to LPS	chronic study is difficult (acute or subacute models only)
cat *(Felis catus)*	well-suited for hemodynamic measurements and repetitive blood sampling, but not a typical species for sepsis study rather for research on central nervous system	heightened public concerns as companion animal
dog *(Canis familiaris)*	faecal flora similar to that of human, well-suited for hemodynamic measurements and repetitive blood sampling, chronic instrumentation feasible	heightened public concerns as companion animal, moderately resistant to LPS, relatively expensive, postal venous hypertension after endotoxic challenge
nonhuman primates, e.g., baboons *(Papio doguera, Papio anubis, Papio cynocephalus, etc.)*, cynomolgus macaque *(Macaca fascicularis)*, rhesus macaque *(Macaca mulatta)*	well-suited for hemodynamic measurements and repetitive blood sampling, antibodies against human proteins commonly cross-react, studies to closely replicate the human inflammatory response	heightened public concerns, very expensive, chronic instrumentation difficult, very resistant to LPS, potential zoonotic disease transmisison

Inter-Species Differences in Sensitivity and Immune Response

Several inter-species differences have been discussed in previous sub-sections. To list some other ones, it is interesting to mention that *Salmonella typhi* does not cause systemic infection in rodents, but causes typhoid fever in humans. *Salmonella typhimurium* causes systemic infection in rodents, but has low virulence in humans (Piper 1996; Poli de Figueiredo 2008).

The evolutionary adaptation and environmental factors have rendered rodents much less sensitive to bacterial products including endotoxin, as discussed previously. In addition to that, rodents usually react to endotoxemia differently than humans. Cecal ligation and puncture in the rat elicits a biphasic cardiovascular response. An early hyperdynamic phase is usually found during the first 6 hours, and it is characterized by increased cardiac output and tissue perfusion, increased oxygen delivery and oxygen consumption as well as decreased peripheral resistance (Wang 1996; Yang 1999). If inadequately resuscitated, these are replaced by a late, hypodynamic phase towards the end of the first 24 hours after the initiation of sepsis. This late phase is characterized by reduced microvascular blood flow in various tissues, decreased oxygen delivery and increased peripheral resistance. These changes are the key events leading to the development of MOF and ultimately to death. Besides a different cardiovascular response, the immunologic response in rodents differs from humans. A murine study reported similar outcome (mortality and morbidity) but significant differences in the kinetics of cytokine production Thus, TNF-α usually peaks at 1–2 hrs after endotoxin challenge in both rodents and humans but normalizes by 4 hrs and 2.5–10 hrs, respectively (Remick 2000).

Normovolemic septic patients typically present increased cardiac output, hypotension, decreased peripheral resistance and oliguria. In dogs, for instance, the endotoxemia is associated with hypotension but with increased peripheral resistance (Wichterman 1980; Kaszaki 1997). The differences between animal species in response to living bacteria infusion can be different. For instance, *E. coli* may cause either hypodynamic or hyperdynamic circulatory response (Fink, 2001).

Concerning species-specific differences, it is important to mention that pigs and sheep may express marked pulmonary hypertension and increased pulmonary endothelial permeability and other characteristics of acute lung injury after injection of endotoxin or gram-negative bacteria. The reason is that the pulmonary intravascular macrophages (PIM) are embedded within the endothelial liming of pulmonary arterioles (Traber 1978; Judges 1986; Fink 2001).

In a chronically instrumented pig model, Haberstroh and co-workers used a relatively low dose of viable *P. aeruginosa* for 84 hours. They found triphasic hemodynamic response: (1) pulmonary hypertension and decrease in cardiac output (0–12 hours), (2) normalization (12–60 hours), and (3) secondary rise in pulmonary arterial pressure, systemic artery hypotension and increased cardiac output (60–84 hours) (Haberstroh 1995; Fink 2001).

Table 2.6. Methodological summary of some selected recent sepsis studies in pigs with different sepsis induction methods and various anesthesia protocols and observation periods

Strain, Sex, Weight	Method of inducing sepsis	Protocol	Anesthesia, drugs, fluid administration	Other related interventions	Duration of observation	Reference
domestic outbred stock, either sex, 15 kg	LPS i.v.	Ultrapure *E. coli* LPS (strain 0111:B4) dissolved in sterile water. A total amount of 0.03 mg LPS/kg was infused intravenously over 30 min.	ketamine (20 mg/kg), atropine (0.4 mg) and azaperone 40 mg/ml (1.5 ml), i.m. isoflurane (end tidal cc: 1%), morphine, 50-100 mg pentobarbital i.v., 1 mkg/kg/h, i.v., mechanical ventillation (PEEP=5 cmH$_2$O, FiO$_2$=0.3), Ringer acetate, 8 ml/kg/h	preparation and cannulation of external jugular vein l.d., carotid artery l.d., pulmonary artery catheter,	6 hours	Thorgersen 2010
domestic outbred stock, either sex, 15 kg	living bacteria i.v.	Live *E. coli* (strain LE392; ATCC 33572) infused intravenously at an increasing rate: 3.75 × 10^7 bacteria/h from 0 to 60 min, 1.5 × 10^8 bacteria/h from 60 to 90 min, and 6.0 × 10^8 bacteria/h from 90 to 240 min		tracheostomy, urinary bladder catheter via skin incision	6 hours	Thorgersen 2010
domestic outbred stock, either sex, 25-35 kg	living bacteria i.v.	Live *E. coli* (strain LE392; ATCC 33572) 1.5x10^8/ml infused intravenously at an increasing rate. In low dose: total of 4x10^9 bacteria, increase from 4 ml/h after 60 min to 16 ml/h after 90 min, thereafter constant. In high dose: total of 16x10^9 bacteria, increase from 4 ml/h after 30 min to 16 ml/h after 60 min, to 64 ml/h after 90 min, thereafter constant.			3 hours	Castellheim 2008
domestic outbred stock, either sex, 25-35 kg	living bacteria into the bronchus	Live *E. coli* (strain LE392; ATCC 33572) 20 ml of 1.5x10^9/ml suspension instilled into each main bronchus via a flexible bronchoscope			5 hours	Castellheim 2008
domestic outbred stock, females, 16-18 kg	living bacteria i.v.	*Escherichia coli* suspension (2.5x10^5/ml; strain: ATCC 25922,) infused intravenously at an increasing rate: 2 ml in the first 30 min, then 4 ml in 30 min and afterwards 16 ml/h for 2 hours. A total of 9.5×10^6 *E. coli* within 3 hours	Induction: i.m. 15 mg/kg ketamin and 1 mg/kg xylazin, maintenance i.m., pressure support mechanical ventilation (Pa O$_2$: 100–130 mmHg, PaCO$_2$: 35–45 mmHg).	preparation and cannulation of external jugular vein l.s. (thermodilution sensors, pressure monitoring, blood sampling, fluid and anesthetic drug intake), femoral artery l.s. (thermodilution sensors, pressure monitoring, blood sampling) (tracheostomy inferior (assisted ventilation)	8 hours	Nemeth 2015

Strain, Sex, Weight	Method of inducing sepsis	Protocol	Anesthesia, drugs, fluid administration	Other related interventions	Duration of observation	Reference
domestic outbred stock, either sex, 27–35 kg	faecal peritonitis (autologous faeces inoculation)	0.5 g/kg of autologous faeces suspended in 200 ml saline was inoculated into the peritoneal cavity through drains.	Induction: i.v. 0.5 mg atropine, 1 to 2 mg/kg propofol 2% and 2 mg/kg ketamine. Mechanically ventilation (PEEP=10 cmH$_2$O, FiO$_2$=0.4, tidal volume: 10 ml/kg) Surgical anaesthesia: intravenous 5-10 mg/kg/hour thiopental and 5-15 µg/kg/hour fentanyl. Pancuronium (4 to 6 mg/kg/hour), infusion of Plasma Lyte solution (7–15 ml/kg/hour), 20% glucose to maintain blood glucose levels between 4.5 and 7 mmol/l.	central venous and pulmonary artery catherers, external jugular vein and femoral artery cannulation. Midline laparotomy, drainage, urinary bladder catheterization via epicystostomy.	22 hours (after 8 hours of stabilization)	Chvojka 2008
Vietnamese minipig, either sex, 24 ± 3 kg	faecal peritonitis (autologous faeces inoculation)	0.5 g/kg of autologous faeces suspended in 200 ml saline was incubated for 6 hours at 38 °C, then the suspension was intraperitoneally inoculated via a small incision above the umbilical scar and through a Veres-needle.	Anesthesia for sepsis induction: i.m. 20 mg/kg ketamin and 2 mg/kg xylazin, then 6 mg/kg/h i.v. propofol. After the induction process, animals were sedated and analgesic was used (4 mg/kg ketamin, 0.6 mg/kg nalbuphin). 15 hours later the animals were re-anaesthetized for invasive monitoring. Ringer-lactate 15 ml/kg/h, Voluvel 6% 130 kDa/0.4 5 ml/kg/h, and in case of need: 0.015 µg/kg/h i.v.	Unilateral preparation and cannulation of external jugular vein (pressure monitoring, sampling, infusion). Endotracheal intubation. Unilateral preparation and cannulation of femoral artery and vein (thermodilution sensors, pressure monitoring). Urinary bladder catheterization via inguinal incision.	24 hours (measurements started 15 hours after sepsis induction)	Zsikai 2012

Effect of Age, Gender, and Co-Morbidities

Age is an important issue both in clinical and experimental scenarios (Watters 2001; Starr 2014). In most of the experimental models, the animals are usually young adults and healthy animals, without co-morbidities. Agent is a toxin or a defined type of micro-organism. The treatment protocol (if any) is standardized and initiated soon after the onset of sepsis. The animals are usually anesthetized. Coprophagy is common.

In humans, sepsis often is seen at extreme ages (neonates or elderly), the origin is more often an infection site usually not recognized or frequently, the infection is polymicrobial. The treatment is initiated usually late (hours or days) after the start of infection and frequently the antibiotics are ineffective and are very different between cases. The presence of the co-morbidities is increasingly common (atherosclerosis, hypertension, diabetes mellitus, cancer, etc.) (Esmon 2004).

Gender differences have been also observed. Receptors for sex hormones have been identified on various immune cells, suggesting direct effects of these hormones on immune function (Albertsmeier 2014).

There are models with immunosuppressed host and so-called sequential challenge models. Co-morbidities can be induced by acute ethanol ingestion, CCl_4-induced cirrhosis, hemorrhagic shock, trauma, splenectomy, thermal injury, etc., mostly in rodents (Fink 2001).

Anesthesia, Drugs, Resuscitation

The clinical management of septic animals versus septic patients is a very important point of view, such as volume therapy, electrolytes, antibiotics, ventilation, etc. These protocols in experiments have unquestionable importance (Naumann 2015). Table 2.6 summarizes methodological details of some selected porcine sepsis models, which include the sepsis induction, the instrumentation, the anesthesia, drugs, resuscitation protocols as well as the follow-up periods are different.

CONCLUSION

Unfortunately, sepsis remains a severe clinical challenge with numerous unsolved problems. Animal models are both useful and necessary to explore the pathophysiology and develop effective therapeutic strategies. Nonetheless, besides their advantages, the experimental models of sepsis have numerous limitations that need to be considered when translating the experimental findings into clinical trials.

Some of the main factors have to be taken into consideration when planning, conducting and evaluating experimental sepsis models:

- the method of sepsis induction
- the agent (type of toxin or microorganism)
- choice of animal species

- species-specific characteristics in immune response sensitivity, in physiological and even anatomical features
- age and gender of the animals
- effect of anesthesia, drugs, fluid intake, resuscitation
- co-morbidities (absence or presence)
- duration of the follow-up (observation period)

In general it can be also concluded that small animal models (e.g., mouse, rat) are useful to test certain pathophysiological pathways and for developing/testing drugs, while large animal models (e.g., pig, non-human primate) may provide a better scenario for testing novel treatment strategies being closer to the clinical practice by size, physiology and opportunities for intervention.

REFERENCES

Albert, M; Losser, MR; Hayon, D; Faivre, V; Payen, D. Systemic and renal macro- and microcirculatory responses to arginine vasopressin in endotoxic rabbits. *Crit. Care Med.*, 2004, 32(9), 1891–1898.

Albertsmeier, M; Pratschke, S; Chaudry, I; Angele, MK. Gender-specific effects on immune response and cardiac function after trauma hemorrhage and sepsis. *Viszeralmedizin.*, 2014, 30(2), 91–96.

Alt, E; Amann-Vesti, BR; Madl, C; Funk, G; Koppensteiner, R. Platelet aggregation and blood rheology in severe sepsis/septic shock: relation to the Sepsis-related Organ Failure Assessment (SOFA) score. *Clin. Hemorheol. Microcirc.*, 2004, 30(2), 107–115.

American College of Chest Physicians/Society of Critical Care Medicine Consensus Conference: definitions for sepsis and organ failure and guidelines for the use of innovative therapies in sepsis. *Crit. Care Med.*, 1992, 20(6), 864–874.

Asakura, H. Classifying types of disseminated intravascular coagulation: clinical and animal models. *J. Int. Care*, 2014, 2(1), 20–26.

Astiz, ME; DeGent, GE; Lin, RY; Rackow, EC. Microvascular function and rheologic changes in hyperdynamic sepsis. *Crit. Care Med.*, 1995, 23(2), 265–271.

Bara, M; Joffe, AR. The ethical dimension in published animal research in critical care: the public face of science. *Crit. Care.*, 2014, 18(1), R15–R21.

Baskurt, OK; Neu, B; Meiselman, HJ. *Red Blood Cell Aggregation.* Boca Raton: CRC Press, 2012.

Baskurt, OK; Temiz, A; Meiselman, HJ. Red blood cell aggregation in experimental sepsis. *J. Lab. Clin. Med.*, 1997, 130(2), 183–190.

Baskurt, OK. Mechanisms of blood rheology alterations. In: Baskurt OK, Hardeman MR, Rampling MW, Meiselman HJ, editors. *Handbook of Hemorheology and Hemodynamics.* Amsterdam: IOS Press, 2007. pp. 170–190.

Bhan, C; Dipankar, P; Chakraborty, P; Sarangi, PP. Role of cellular events in the pathophysiology of sepsis. *Inflamm. Res,.* 2016, 65(11), 853–868.

Borthwick, EM; Hill, C; Rabindranath, KS; Maxwell, AP; McAuley, DF; Blackwood, B. High-volume haemofiltration for sepsis. *Cochrane Database Syst. Rev.*, 1, 2013, CD008075.

Bridges, EJ; Dukes, S. Cardiovascular aspects of septic shock: pathophysiology, monitoring, and treatment. *Crit. Care Nurse.*, 2005, 25(2), 14–40.

Brown, KA; Brain, SD; Pearson, JD; Edgeworth, JD; Lewis, SM; Treacher, DF. Neutrophils in development of multiple organ failure in sepsis. *The Lancet*, 2006, 368(9530), 157–169.

Browne, MK; Leslie, GB. Animal models of peritonitis. *Surg. Gynecol. Obstet.*, 1976, 143(5), 738–740.

Cash, JL; White, GE; Greaves, DR. Chapter 17. Zymosan-induced peritonitis as a simple experimental system for the study of inflammation. *Methods in Enzymology (Chemokines, Part B)*, 2009, 461, 379–396.

Castellheim, A; Thorgersen, EB; Hellerud, BC; Pharo, A; Johansen, HT; Brosstad, F; Gaustad, P; Brun, H; Fosse, E; Tonnessen, TI; Nielsen, EW; Mollnes, TE. New biomarkers in an acute model of live Escherichia coli-induced sepsis in pigs. *Scand. J. Immunol.*, 2008, 68(1), 75–84.

Catry, J; Brouquet, A; Peschaud, F; Vychnevskaia, K; Abdalla, S; Malafosse, R; Lambert, B; Costaglioli, B; Benoist, S; Penna, C. Sigmoid resection with primary anastomosis and ileostomy versus laparoscopic lavage in purulent peritonitis from perforated diverticulitis: outcome analysis in a prospective cohort of 40 consecutive patients. *Int. J. Colorectal. Dis.*, 2016, 31(10), 1693–1699.

Chen, P; Stanojcic, M; Jeschke, MG. Differences between murine and human sepsis. *Surg. Clin. North. Am.*, 2014, 94(6), 1135–1149.

Chiavolini, D; Pozzi, G; Ricci, S. Animal models of Streptococcus pneumoniae disease. *Clin. Microbiol. Rev.*, 2008, 21(4), 666–685.

Chien, S; Usami, S; Dellenback, J; Magazinovic, V. Blood rheology after hemorrhage and endotoxin. *Adv. Exp. Med. Biol.*, 1972, 33, 75–93.

Chvojka, J; Sykora, R; Krouzecky, A; Radej, J; Varnerova, V; Karvunidis, T; Hes, O; Novak, I; Radermacher, P; Matejovic, M. Renal haemodynamic, microcirculatory, metabolic and histopathological responses to peritonitis-induced septic shock in pigs. *Crit. Care.*, 2008, 12(6), R164. http://ccforum.biomedcentral.com/articles/10.1186/cc7164.

Copeland, S; Warren, HS; Lowry, SF; Calvano, SE; Remick, D. Acute inflammatory response to endotoxin in mice and humans. *Clin. Diagn. Lab. Immunol.*, 2005, 12(1), 60–67.

Cryer, PE; Herman, CM; Sode, J. Carbohydrate metabolism in the baboon subjected to gram-negative (*E. coli*) septicemia. I. Hyperglycemia with depressed plasma insulin concentrations. *Ann. Surg.*, 1971, 174(1), 91–100.

Daniels, R. Surviving the first hours in sepsis: getting the basics right (an intensivist's perspective). *J. Antimicrob. Chemother.*, 2011, 66(Suppl 2), 11–13.

Dejager, L; Pinheiro, I; Dejonckheere, E; Libert, C. Cecal ligation and puncture: the gold standard model for polymicrobial sepsis? *Trends Microbiol.*, 2011, 19(4), 198–208.

Dellinger, RP; Levy, MM; Rhodes, A; Annane, D; Gerlach, H; Opal, SM; Sevransky, JE; Sprung, CL; Douglas, IS; Jaeschke, R; Osborn, TM; Nunnally, ME; Townsend, SR; Reinhart, K; Kleinpell, RM; Angus, DC; Deutschman, CS; Machado, FR; Rubenfeld, GD; Webb, SA; Beale, RJ; Vincent, JL; Moreno, R. Surviving Sepsis Campaign Guidelines Committee including the Pediatric Subgroup. Surviving sepsis campaign: international guidelines for management of severe sepsis and septic shock: 2012. *Crit. Care Med.*, 2013, 41(2), 580–637.

Doi, K. Role of kidney injury in sepsis. *J. Int. Care*, 2016, 4, 17–22.

Dyson, A; Singer, M. Animal models of sepsis: why does preclinical efficacy fail to translate to the clinical setting? *Crit. Care Med.*, 2009, 37(1 Suppl), S30–S37.

Ebong, S; Call, D; Nemzek, J; Bolgos, G; Newcomb, D; Remick, D. Immunopathologic alterations in murine models of sepsis of increasing severity. *Infect. Immun.*, 1999, 67(12), 6603–6610.

Efron, PA; Mohr, AM; Moore, FA; Moldawer, LL. The future of murine sepsis and trauma research models. *J. Leukoc. Biol.*, 2015, 98(6), 945–952.

Elias, RM; Johnston, MG; Hayashi, A; Nelson, W. Decreased lymphatic pumping after intravenous endotoxin administration in sheep. *Am. J. Physiol.*, 1987, 253(6 Pt 2), H1349–H1357.

Engel, AL; Holt, GE; Lu, H. The pharmacokinetics of Toll-like receptor agonists and the impact on the immune system. *Expert Rev. Clin. Pharmacol.*, 2011, 4(2), 275–289.

Eskandari, MK; Bolgos, G; Miller, C; Nguyen, DT; DeForge, LE; Remick, DG. Anti-tumor necrosis factor antibody therapy fails to prevent lethality after cecal ligation and puncture or endotoxemia. *J. Immunol.*, 1992, 148(), 2724–2730.

Esmon, CT. Why do animal models (sometimes) fail to mimic human sepsis? *Crit. Care Med.*, 2004, 32(5 Suppl), S219–S222.

Fink, MP. Animal models of sepsis and the multiple organ dysfunction syndrome. In: Souba WW, Wilmore DW, editors. *Surgical Research*. Amsterdam: Elsevier Academic Press, 2001, pp. 875–891.

Fink, MP. Animal models of sepsis. *Virulence*, 2014, 5(1), 143–153.

Fleischmann, C; Scherag, A; Adhikari, NK; Hartog, CS; Tsaganos, T; Schlattmann, P; Angus, DC; Reinhart, K. International Forum of Acute Care Trialists. Assessment of Global Incidence and Mortality of Hospital-treated Sepsis. Current Estimates and Limitations. *Am. J. Respir. Crit. Care Med.*, 2016, 193(3), 259–272.

Franks, Z; Carlisle, M; Rondina, MT. Current challenges in understanding immune cell functions during septic syndromes. *BMC Immunology*, 2015, 16, 11–16.

Gomez-Jimenez, J; Salgado, A; Mourelle, M; Martin, MC; Segura, RM; Peracaula, R; Moncada, S. L-arginine: nitric oxide pathway in endotoxemia and human septic shock. *Crit. Care Med.*, 1995, 23(2), 253-258.

Guenter, CA; Fiorica, V; Hinshaw, LB. Cardiorespiratory and metabolic responses to liver *E. coli* and endotoxin in the monkey. *J. Appl. Physiol.*, 1969, 26(6), 780–786.

Guerra, GC; de Menezes, MS; de Araújo, AA; de Araújo Júnior, RF; de Medeiros, CA. Olmesartan prevented intra-articular inflammation induced by zymosan in rats. *Biol. Pharm. Bull.*, 2016, 39(11), 1793–1801.

Guler, O; Ugras, S; Aydin, M; Dilek, FH; Dilek, ON; Karaayvaz, M. The effect of lymphatic blockage on the amount of endotoxin in portal circulation, nitric oxide synthesis, and the liver in dogs with peritonitis. *Surg. Today*, 1999, 29(8), 735–740.

Gumenscheimer, M; Mitov, I; Galanos, C; Freudenberg, MA. Beneficial or deleterious effects of a preexisting hypersensitivity to bacterial components on the course and outcome of infection. *Infect. Immun.*, 2002, 70(10), 5596–5603.

Haberstroh, J; Breuer, H; Lücke, I; Massarrat, K; Früh, R; Mand, U; Hagerdorn, L; von Specht, BU. Effect of recombinant human granulocyte colony-stimulating factor on hemodynamic and cytokine response in a porcine model of *Pseudomonas* sepsis. *Shock*, 1995, 4(3), 216–224.

Hau, T; Simmons, RL. Animal models of peritonitis. *Surg. Gynecol. Obstet.*, 1977, 144(5), 755–756.

Hermreck, AS; Thal, AP. Mechanisms for the high circulatory requirements in sepsis and septic shock. *Ann. Surg.*, 1969, 170(4), 677–695.

Hinshaw, LB; Beller, BK; Archer, LT; Benjamin, B. Hypoglycemic response of blood to live *Escherichia coli* organisms and endotoxin. *J. Surg. Res.*, 1976, 21(3), 141–150.

Hollenberg, SM; Dumasius, A; Easington, C; Colilla, SA; Neumann, A; Parrillo, JE. Characterization of a hyperdynamic murine model of resuscitated sepsis using echocardiography. *Am. J. Respir. Crit. Care Med.*, 2001, 164(5), 891–895.

Hong, Y; Sun, LI; Sun, R; Chen, H; Yu, Y; Xie, K. Combination therapy of molecular hydrogen and hyperoxia improves survival rate and organ damage in a zymosan-induced generalized inflammation model. *Exp. Ther. Med.*, 2016, 11(6), 2590–2596.

Hubbard, WJ; Choudhry, M; Schwacha, MG; Kerby, JD; Rue, LW; 3rd. Bland, KI; Chaudry, IH. Cecal ligation and puncture. *Shock.*, 2005, 24(Suppl 1), 52–57.

Ince, C; Mik, EG. Microcirculatory and mitochondrial hypoxia in sepsis, shock, and resuscitation. *J. Appl. Physiol.*, 2016, 120(2), 226–235.

Ince, C. The microcirculation is the motor of sepsis. *Crit. Care.*, 2005, 9(Suppl 4), S13–S19.

Islam, S; Jarosch, S; Zhou, J; Parquet Mdel, C; Toguri, JT; Colp, P; Holbein, BE; Lehmann, C. Anti-inflammatory and anti-bacterial effects of iron chelation in experimental sepsis. *J. Surg. Res.*, 2016, 200(1), 266–273.

Judges, D; Sharkey, P; Cheung, H; Craig, I; Driedger, AA; Sibbald, WJ; Finley, R. Pulmonary microvascular fluid flux in a large animal model of sepsis: evidence for increased pulmonary endothelial permeability accompanying surgically induced peritonitis in sheep. *Surgery*, 1986, 99(2), 222–234.

Kameneva, MV; Antaki, JF. Mechanical trauma to blood. In: Baskurt OK, Hardeman MR, Rampling MW, Meiselman HJ, editors. *Handbook of Hemorheology and Hemodynamics.* Amsterdam: IOS Press, 2007, pp. 206–227.

Kaszaki, J; Wolfrad, A; Boros, M; Baranyi, L; Okada, H; Nagy, S. Effects of antiendothelin treatment on the early hemodynamic changes in hyperdynamic endotoxemia. *Acta Chir. Hung.*, 1997, 36(1-4), 152–153.

Katschinski, T; Galanos, C; Coumbos, A; Freudenberg, MA. Gamma interferon mediates Proprionibacterium acnes-induced hypersensitivity to lipopolysaccharide. *Infect. Immun.*, 1992, 60(5), 1994–2001.

Kingsley, SM; Bhat, BV. Differential paradigms in animal models of sepsis. *Curr. Infect. Dis. Rep.*, 2016, 18(9), 26–36.

Kirschenbaum, LA; Aziz, M; Astiz, ME; Saha, DC; Rackow, EC. Influence of rheologic changes and platelet-neutrophil interactions on cell filtration in sepsis. *Am. J. Respir. Crit. Care Med.*, 2000, 161(5), 1602–1607.

Kiss, F; Molnar, L; Hajdu, E; Deak, A; Molnar, A; Berhes, M; Szabo, J; Nemeth, N; Fulesdi, B. Skin microcirculatory changes reflect early the circulatory deterioration in a fulminant sepsis model in the pig. *Acta Cir. Bras.*, 2015, 30(7), 470–477.

Klag, T; Cantara, G; Sechtem, U; Athanasiadis, A. Interleukin-6 kinetics can be useful for early treatment monitoring of severe bacterial sepsis and septic shock. *Infect Dis Rep.*, 2016, 8(1), 6213. http:// www.pagepress.org/journals/index.php/idr/ article/view/6213/ 5524

Krisher, SL; Browne, A; Dibbins, A; Tkacz, N; Curci, M. Intra-abdominal abscess after laparoscopic appendectomy for perforated appendicitis. *Arch. Surg.*, 2001, 136(4), 438–441.

Kutner, FR; Schwartz, SI; Adams, JT. The effect of adrenergic blockade on lymph flow in endotoxin shock. *Ann. Surg.*, 1967, 165(4), 518–527.

Lakshmikanth, CL; Jacob, SP; Chaithra, VH; de Castro-Faria-Neto, HC; Marathe, GK. Sepsis: in search of cure. *Inflamm. Res.*, 2016, 65(8), 587–602.

Langenberg, C; Bellomo, R; May, C; Wan, L; Egi, M; Morgera, S. 2005. Renal blood flow in sepsis. *Crit. Care.*, 9(4), R363–R374.

Laschke, MW; Menger, MD; Wang, Y; Lindell, G; Jeppsson, B; Thorlacius, H. Sepsis-associated cholestasis is critically dependent on P-selectin-dependent leukocyte recruitment in mice. *Am. J. Physiol. Gastrointest. Liver Physiol.*, 2007, 292(5), G1396–G1402.

Lattuada, M; Hedenstierna, G. Abdominal lymph flow in an endotoxin sepsis model: influence of spontaneous breathing and mechanical ventilation. *Crit. Care Med.*, 2006, 34(11), 2792–2798.

Levy, MM; Fink, MP; Marshall, JC; Abraham, E; Angus, D; Cook, D; Cohen, J; Opal, SM; Vincent, JL; Ramsay, G. International Sepsis Definitions Conference. 2001 SCCM/ESICM/ACCP/ATS/SIS International Sepsis Definitions Conference. *Intensive Care Med.*, 2003, 29(4), 530–538.

Lewis, AJ; Seymour, CW; Rosengart, MR. Current murine models of sepsis. *Surg. Infect. (Larchmt).*, 2016, 17(4), 385–393.

Lilley, E; Armstrong, R; Clark, N; Gray, P; Hawkins, P; Mason, K; López-Salesansky, N; Stark, AK; Jackson, SK; Thiemermann, C; Nandi, M. Refinement of animal models of sepsis and septic shock. *Shock*, 2015, 43(4), 304–316.

Lohner, R; Schwederski, M; Narath, C; Klein, J; Duerr, GD; Torno, A; Knuefermann, P; Hoeft, A; Baumgarten, G; Meyer, R; Boehm, O. Toll-like receptor 9 promotes cardiac inflammation and heart failure during polymicrobial sepsis. *Mediators Inflamm.*, 2013, 2013, 261049. https://www.hindawi.com/journals/mi/2013/261049/.

Lundy, DJ; Trzeciak, S. Microcirculatory dysfunction in sepsis. *Crit. Care Clin.*, 2009, 25(4), 721–731.

Lustig, MK; Bac, VH; Pavlovic, D; Maier, S; Gründling, M; Grisk, O; Wendt, M; Heidecke, CD; Lehmann, C. Colon ascendens stent peritonitis – a model of sepsis adopted to the rat: physiological, microcirculatory and laboratory changes. *Shock*, 2007, 28(1), 59–64.

Mai, S; Khan, M; Liaw, P; Fox-Robichaud, A. Experimental sepsis models. In: Azevedo L, editor. Sepsis - An ongoing and significant challenge. *InTech*, 2012. http://www.intechopen.com/ books/sepsis-an-ongoing-and-significant-challenge/experimental-sepsis-models.

Maier, S; Traeger, T; Entleutner, M; Westerholt, A; Kleist, B; Hüser, N; Holzmann, B; Stier, A; Pfeffer, K; Heidecke, CD. Cecal ligation and puncture versus colon ascendens stent peritonitis: two distinct animal models for polymicrobial sepsis. *Shock*, 2004, 21(6), 505–511.

Martins, GS. Sepsis, severe sepsis and septic shock: changes in incidence, pathogens and outcomes. *Expert Rev. Anti Infect. Ther.*, 2012, 10, 701–706.

Mook-Kanamori, B; Geldhoff, M; Troost, D; van der Poll, T; van de Beek, D. Characterization of a pneumococcal meningitis mouse model. *BMC Infect. Dis.*, 2012, 12, 71.

Mook-Kanamori, BB; Valls Serón, M; Geldhoff, M; Havik, SR; van der Ende, A; Baas, F; van der Poll, T; Meijers, JC; P Morgan, B; Brouwer, MC; van de Beek, D. Thrombin-activatable fibrinolysis inhibitor influences disease severity in humans and mice with pneumococcal meningitis. *J. Thromb. Haemost.*, 2015, 13(11), 2076–2086.

Morel, J; Li, JY; Eyenga, P; Meiller, A; Gustin, MP; Bricca, G; Molliex, S; Viale, JP. Early adverse changes in liver microvascular circulation during experimental septic shock are not linked to an absolute nitric oxide deficit. *Microvasc. Res.*, 2013, 90, 187–191.

Moutzouri, AG; Skoutelis, AT; Gogos, CA; Missirlis, YF; Athanassiou, GM. Red blood cell deformability in patients with sepsis: a marker for prognosis and monitoring of severity. *Clin. Hemorheol. Microcirc.*, 2007, 36(4), 291–299.

Nash, GB; Watts, T; Thornton, C; Barigou, M. Red cell aggregation as a factor influencing margination and adhesion of leukocytes and platelets. *Clin. Hemorheol. Microcirc.*, 2008, 39(1-4), 303–310.

Naumann, DN; Dretzke, J; Hutchings, S; Midwinter, MJ. Protocol for a systematic review of the impact of resuscitation fluids on the microcirculation after haemorrhagic shock in animal models. *Systematic Reviews*, 2015, 4, 135–141.

Nduka, OO; Parrillo, JE. The pathophysiology of septic shock. *Crit. Care Nurs. Clin. North Am.*, 2011, 23(1), 41–66.

Nemeth, N; Berhes, M; Kiss, F; Hajdu, E; Deak, A; Molnar, A; Szabo, J; Fulesdi, B. Early hemorheological changes in a porcine model of intravenously given E. coli induced fulminant sepsis. *Clin. Hemorheol. Microcirc.*, 2015, 61(3), 479–496.

Nemeth, N; Fulesdi, B. Concerning hemorheological disturbances in sepsis. De omnibus dubitandum est… *Series on Biomechanics*, 2016, 30(1), 20–26.

Nemeth, N; Miko, I; Furka, A; Kiss, F; Furka, I; Koller, A; Szilasi, M. Concerning the importance of changes in hemorheological parameters caused by acid-base and blood gas alterations in experimental surgical models. *Clin. Hemorheol. Microcirc.*, 2012, 51(1), 43–50.

Nemoto, K; Sato, H; Tanuma, K; Okamura, T. Mesenteric lymph flow in endotoxemic guinea pigs. *Lymphat. Res. Biol.*, 2011, 9(3), 129–134.

Nemzek, JA; Hugunin, KM; Opp, MR. Modeling sepsis in the laboratory: merging sound science with animal well-being. *Comp. Med.*, 2008, 58(2), 120–128.

Nishino, M; Tanaka, H; Ogura, H; Inoue, Y; Koh, T; Fujita, K; Sugimoto, H. Serial changes in leukocyte deformability and whole blood rheology in patients with sepsis or trauma. *J. Trauma*, 2005, 59(6), 1425–1431.

Onderdonk, AB; Bartlett, JG; Louie, T; Sullivan-Seigler, N; Gorbach, SL. Microbial synergy in experimental intra-abdominal abscess. *Infect. Immun.*, 1976, 13(1), 22–26.

Ostergaard, L; Granfeldt, A; Secher, N; Tietze, A; Iversen, NK; Jensen, MS; Andersen, KK; Nagenthiraja, K; Gutiérrez-Lizardi, P; Mouridsen, K; Jespersen, SN; Tonnesen, EK. Microcirculatory dysfunction and tissue oxygenation in critical illness. *Acta Anaesthesiol. Scand.*, 2015, 59, 1246–1259.

Otero-Anton, E; Gonzalez-Quintela, A; Lopez-Soto, A; Lopez-Ben, S; Llovo, J; Perez, LF. Cecal ligation and puncture as a model of sepsis in the rat: influence of the puncture size on mortality, bacteremia, endotoxemia and tumor necrosis factor alpha levels. *Eur. Surg. Res.*, 2001, 33(2), 77–79.

Perbellini, A; Shatney, CH; MacCarter, DJ; Lillehei, RC. A new model for the study of septic shock. *Surg. Gynecol. Obstet.*, 1978, 147(1), 68–74.

Piagnerelli, M; Boudjeltia, KZ; Vanhaeverbeek, M; Vincent, JL. Red blood cell rheology in sepsis. *Intensive Care Med.*, 2003, 29(7), 1052–1061.

Piper, RD; Cook, DJ; Bone, RC; Sibbald, WJ. Introducing critical appraisal to studies of animal models investigating novel therapies in sepsis. *Crit. Care Med.*, 1996, 24(12), 2059–2070.

Poli-de-Figueiredo, LF; Garrido, AG; Nakagawa, N; Sannomiya, P. Experimental models of sepsis and their clinical relevance. *Shock*, 2008, 30(Suppl 1), 53–59.

Pöschl, JMB; Leray, C; Ruef, P; Cazenave, JP; Lindekamp, O. Endotoxin binging to erythrocyte membrane and erythrocyte deformability in human sepsis and *in vitro*. *Crit. Care Med.*, 2003, 31(3), 924–928.

Postel, J; Schloerb, PR; Furtado, D. Pathophysiologic alterations during bacterial infusions for the study of bacteremic shock. *Surg. Gynecol. Obstet.*, 1975, 141(5), 683–692.

Rabinovici, R; Bugelski, PJ; Esser, KM; Hillegass, LM; Griswold, DE; Vernick, J; Feuerstein, G. Tumor necrosis factor-primed rats. *J. Pharmacol. Exp. Ther.*, 1993, 267(3), 1550–1557.

Reggiori, G; Occhipinti, G; De Gasperi, A; Vincent, JL; Piagnerelli, M. Early alterations of red blood cell rheology in critically ill patients. *Crit. Care Med.*, 2009, 37(12), 3041–3046.

Remick, DG; Newcomb, DE; Bolgos, GL; Call, DR. Comparison of the mortality and inflammatory response of two models of sepsis: lipopolysaccharide vs. cecal ligation and puncture. *Shock*, 2000, 13(2), 110–116.

Remick, DG; Ward, PA. Evaluation of endotoxin models for the study of sepsis. *Shock*, 2005, 24(Suppl 1), 7–11.

Remick, DG. Pathophysiology of sepsis. *Am. J. Pathol.*, 2007, 170(5), 1435–1444.

Rittirsch, D; Hoesel, LM; Ward, PA. The disconnect between animal models of sepsis and human sepsis. *J. Leukoc. Biol.*, 2007, 81(1), 137–143.

Schabbauer, G. Polymicrobial sepsis models: CLP versus CASP. *Drug Discovery Today: Disease Models*, 2012, 9(1), e17–e21.

Scheer, C; Fuchs, C; Rehberg, S. Biomarkers in severe sepsis and septic shock: just listen to the heart? *Crit. Care Med.*, 2016, 44(4), 849–850.

Schöneborn, S; Vollmer, C; Barthel, F; Herminghaus, A; Schulz, J; Bauer, I; Beck, C; Picker, O. Vasopressin V1A receptors mediate the stabilization of intestinal mucosal oxygenation during hypercapnia in septic rats. *Microvasc. Res.*, 2016, 106, 24–30.

Schultz, MJ; van der Poll, T. Animal and human models for sepsis. *Ann. Med.*, 2002, 34(7-8), 573–581.

Semeraro, N; Ammollo, CT; Semeraro, F; Colucci, M. Coagulopathy of acute sepsis. *Semin. Thromb. Hemost.*, 2015, 41(6), 650–658.

Sharkey, P; Judges, D; Driedger, AA; Cheung, H; Finley, RJ; Sibbald, WJ. The effect of an infusion of zymosan-activated plasma on hemodynamic and pulmonary function in sheep. *Circ. Shock*, 1984, 12(2), 79–93.

Shibayama, Y; Urano, T; Nakata, K. Changes in hepatic lymph vessels in endotoxaemia. *J. Pathol.*, 1992, 168(3), 325–330.

Shrum, B; Anantha, RV; Xu, SX; Donnelly, M; Haeryfar, SMM; McCormick, JK; Mele, T. A robust scoring system to evaluate sepsis severity in an animal model. *BMC Research Notes*, 2014, 7, 233. http://www.biomedcentral.com/1756-0500/7/233.

Siempos, II; Lam, HC; Ding, Y; Choi, ME; Choi, AM; Ryter, SW. Cecal ligation and puncture-induced sepsis as a model to study autophagy in mice. *J. Vis. Exp.*, 2014, 84, e51066–e51072. [article with video link: http://www.jove.com/video/51066/].

Singer, M; Deutschman, CS; Seymour, CW; Shankar-Hari, M; Annane, D; Bauer, M; Bellomo, R; Bernard, GR; Chiche, JD; Coopersmith, CM; Hotchkiss, RS; Levy, MM; Marshall, JC; Martin, GS; Opal SM; Rubenfeld, GD; van der Poll, T; Vincent, JL; Angus, DC. The Third International Consensus Definitions for Sepsis and Septic Shock (Sepsis-3). *JAMA.*, 2016, 315(8), 801–810.

Singleton, KD; Wischmeyer, PE. Distance of cecum ligated influences mortality, tumor necrosis factor-alpha and interleukin-6 expression following cecal ligation and puncture in the rat. *Eur. Surg. Res.*, 2003, 35(6), 486–491.

Smith, AL; Greenfield, MD; Toothaker, RD. Experimental meningitis in the rat: Haemophilus influenzae. *Infection*, 1984, 12(Suppl 1), S11–S22.

Smith, L; Andreasson, S; Saldéen, T; Risberg, B. Combined monitoring of thoracic duct and lung lymph during E. coli sepsis in awake sheep. *Lymphology*, 1988, 21(3), 169–177.

Sordia, T; Tatarishvili, J; Mchedlishvili, G. Hemorheological disorders in the microcirculation during septic shock in rats. *Clin. Hemorheol. Microcirc.*, 2006, 35(1-2), 223–226.

Spronk, PE; Zandstra, DF; Ince, C. Bench-to-bedside review: Sepsis is a disease of the microcirculation. *Crit. Care*, 2004, 8(6), 462–468.

Starr, ME; Saito, H. Sepsis in old age: review of human and animal studies. *Aging Dis.*, 2014, 5(2), 126–136.

Thorgersen, EB; Hellerud, BC; Nielsen, EW; Barratt-Due, A; Fure, H; Lindstad, JK; Pharo, A; Fosse, E; Tonnessen, TI; Johansen, HT; Castellheim, A; Mollnes, TE. CD14 inhibition efficiently attenuates early inflammatory and hemostatic responses in Escherichia coli sepsis in pigs. *FASEB J.*, 2010, 24(3), 712–722.

Toscano, MG; Ganea, D; Gamero, AM. Cecal ligation puncture procedure. *J. Vis. Exp.*, 2011, 51, 2860–2864. [article with video link: http://www.jove.com/video/2860/].

Traber, DL; Schlag, G; Redl, H; Strohmair, W; Traber, LD. Pulmonary microvascular changes during hyperdynamic sepsis in an ovine model. *Circ. Shock*, 1987, 22(2), 185–193.

Trzeciak, S; Cinel, I; Dellinger, PR; Shapiro, NI; Arnold, RC; Parrillo, JE; Hollenberg, SM. Microcirculatory Alterations in Resuscitation and Shock (MARS) Investigators. Resuscitating the microcirculation in sepsis: the central role of nitric oxide, emerging concepts for novel therapies, and challenges for clinical trials. *Acad. Emerg. Med.*, 2008, 15(5), 399–413.

Trzeciak, S; Dellinger, RP; Parrillo, JE; Guglielmi, M; Bajaj, J; Abate, NL; Arnold, RC; Colilla, S; Zanotti, S; Hollenberg, SM. Early microcirculatory perfusion derangements in patients with severe sepsis and septic shock: relationship to hemodynamics, oxygen transport, and survival. *Ann. Emerg. Med.*, 2007, 49(1), 88–98.

Turnbull, IR; Wlzorek, JJ; Osborne, D; Hotchkiss, RS; Coopersmith, CM; Buchman, TG. Effects of age on mortality and antibiotic efficacy in cecal ligation and puncture. *Shock*, 2003, 19(4), 310–313.

Tyagi, A; Sethi, AK; Girotra, G; Mohta, M. The Microcirculation in Sepsis. *Indian J. Anaesth.*, 2009, 53(3), 281–293.

van der Poll, T. Preclinical sepsis models. *Surg. Infect. (Larchmt).*, 2012, 13(5), 287-292.

Vincent, JL; Moreno, R; Takala, J; Willatts, S; De Mendonça, A; Bruining, H; Reinhart, CK; Suter, PM; Thijs, LG. The SOFA (Sepsis-related Organ Failure Assessment) score to describe organ dysfunction/failure. *Intensive Care Med.,* 1996, 22(7), 707–710.

Volman, TJ; Hendriks, T; Goris, RJ. Zymosan-induced generalized inflammation: Experimental studies into mechanisms leading to multiple organ dysfunction syndrome. *Shock,* 2005, 23(4), 291–297.

Walker, H; Mason, Ad; Jr. Raulston, G. Surface infection with *Pseudomonas aeruginosa. Ann. Surg.,* 1964, 160, 297–305.

Wang, P; Chaudry, IH. Mechanism of hepatocellular dysfunction during hyperdynamic sepsis. *Am. J. Physiol.,* 1996, 270(5 Pt 2), R927–R938.

Ward, PA. New approaches to the study of sepsis. *EMBO Mol. Med.,* 2012, 4(12), 1234–1243.

Watters, JM; O'Rourke, K. Effects of age and gender. In: Souba WW, Wilmore DW, editors. *Surgical Research.* Amsterdam: Elsevier Academic Press, 2001, pp. 167–174.

Wester, T; Häggblad, E; Awan, ZA; Barratt-Due, A; Kvernebo, M; Halvorsen, PS; Mollnes, TE; Kvernebo, K. Assessments of skin and tongue microcirculation reveals major changes in porcine sepsis. *Clin. Physiol. Funct. Imaging,* 2011, 31(2), 151–158.

Wichterman, KA; Baue, AE; Chaudry, IH. Sepsis and septic shock: a review of laboratory models and a proposal. *J. Surg. Res.* 1980, 29(2), 189–201.

Williams, JS; Clermont, HG. Thoracic duct lymph flow and acid phosphatase response to steroid in experimental shock. *Ann. Surg.,* 1973, 178(6), 777–780.

Wolfard, A; Kaszaki, J; Szabo, C; Balogh, Z; Nagy, S; Boros, M. Effects of selective nitric oxide synthase inhibition in hyperdynamic endotoxemia in dogs. *Eur. Surg. Res.,* 1999, 31(4), 314–323.

Wynn, JL; Wong, HR. Pathophysiology and treatment of septic shock in neonates. *Clin. Perinatol.,* 2010, 37(2), 439–479.

Wyrzykowski, AD; Feliciano, DV; George, TA; Tremblay, LN; Rozycki, GS; Murphy, TW; Dente, CJ. Emergent right hemicolectomies. *Am. Surg.,* 2005, 71(8), 653–656.

Yang, S; Chung, CS; Ayala, A; Chaudry, IH; Wang, P. Differential alterations in cardiovascular responses during the progression of polymicrobial sepsis in the mouse. *Shock,* 2002, 17(1), 55-60.

Yang, S; Cioffi, WG; Bland, KI; Chaudry, IH; Wang, P. Differential alterations in systemic and regional oxygen delivery and consumption during the early and late stages of sepsis. *J. Trauma,* 1999, 47(4), 706–712.

Yodice, PC; Astiz, ME; Kurian, BM; Lin, RY; Rackow, EC. Neutrophil rheologic changes in septic shock. *Am. J. Respir. Crit. Care Med.,* 1997, 155(1), 38–42.

Young, JD; Cameron, EM. Dynamics of skin blood flow in human sepsis. *Intensive Care Med.,* 1995, 21(8), 669–674.

Zanotti-Cavazzoni, SL; Guglielmi, M; Parrillo, JE; Walker, T; Dellinger, RP; Hollenberg, SM. Fluid resuscitation influences cardiovascular performance and mortality in a murine model of sepsis. *Intensive Care Med.,* 2009, 35(4), 748–754.

Zantl, N; Uebe, A; Neumann, B; Wagner, H; Siewert, JR; Holzmann, B; Heidecke, CD; Pfeffer, K. Essential role of gamma-interferon in survival of colon ascendens stent peritonitis, a novel murine model of abdominal sepsis. *Infect. Immun.,* 1998, 66(5), 2300–2309.

Ziaja, M. Sepsis and septic encephalopathy: characteristics and experimental models. *Folia Neuropathol.,* 2012, 50(3), 231–239.

Zimmermann, T; Laszik, Z; Nagy, S; Kaszaki, J; Joo, F. The role of the complement system in the pathogenesis of multiple organ failure in shock. *Prog. Clin. Biol. Res.*, 1989, 308, 291–297.

Zsikai, B; Bizanc, L; Sztanyi, P; Vida, G; Nagy, E; Jiga, L; Ionac, M; Erces, D; Boros, M; Kaszaki, J. [Clinically relevant sepsis model in minipigs]. *Magy Seb.*, 2012, 65(4), 198–204. [Article in Hungarian].

In: Advances in Experimental Surgery. Volume 2
Editors: Huifang Chen and Paulo N. Martins
ISBN: 978-1-53612-773-7
© 2018 Nova Science Publishers, Inc.

Chapter 3

BARIATRIC EXPERIMENTAL SURGERY MODELS

Osman Bilgin Gulcicek[*], *MD*

University Of Health Sciences
Istanbul Bagcilar Training and Research Hospital,
Department of General Surgery,
Istanbul, Turkey

ABSTRACT

Obesity has recently become a major health problem. To treat obesity, there are non-surgical and surgical methods. However, surgical methods are more effective in managing obesity. Bariatric surgical methods are classified as restrictive, malabsorptive and combined methods. But sleeve gastrectomy and gastric plication are the most popular methods.

These techniques are easily applicable in clinic and have fewer complications. Both methods provide sufficient weight loss and decrease ghrelin and leptin levels. To plan an experimental surgery study for treating obesity, especially in small animals, these two techniques should be preferred for success of the experiments.

Keywords: obesity, sleeve gastrectomy, gastric plication, experimental

INTRODUCTION

Obesity is defined as accumulation of abnormal or excessive fat tissue leading to cardiovascular system diseases, diabetes mellitus, metabolic syndrome, musculoskeletal disorders and psychiatric problems. Obesity is recognized as a major health problem today (Ewing 2011; Blackburn 1987).

---

[*] E-mail: drosmanbilgin@hotmail.com, Phone: +90532 610 69 66, Fax: +90212 440 42 42.

The diagnosis of obesity is done by calculating body mass index (BMI; weight in kilograms divided by length in squared meters, kg/m^2). Patients with a BMI of over 40 kg/m^2 are considered morbidly obese (National Institutes of Health 2010).

To treat obesity, there are non-surgical modalities like diet, changes in habits and medical treatment. But these approaches have limited effects on weight loss (Lo´pez-NavaBrevie`re 2015). Additionally, these strategies are not affecting obesity continuously. However, surgery is considered to be effective in managing obesity (Benaiges 2015).

Bariatric surgery can be classified as restrictive (gastric plication, sleeve gastrectomy, adjustable gastric banding, intragastric balloon), malabsorptive (biliopancreatic diversion, biliopancreatic diversion with duodenal switch) and combined methods (Roux-en-Y gastric bypass, mini gastric bypass).

All these surgical procedures are conducted according to the recommendations of the American Society of Bariatric Surgery (Gastrointestinal surgery for severe obesity 1992).

Adjustable gastric banding was first applied in 1980s by Kuzmak. Gastric band is wrapped around the proximal stomach and there is a small gastric pouch on the upper side. This gastric band is connected to the port, placed under the skin through the catheter (Kuzmak 1991).

Intragastric balloon is a method which is based on inflating the balloon inserted into the stomach endoscopically and thus reducing the stomach volume (Benjamin 1988).

Biliopancreatic diversion was popularized first by Italian surgeon Scopinaro in 1979. This procedure reduces the duration of food interaction with digestive enzymes and absorption surface and abbreviates the transit time of food through the stomach.

It includes partial distal gastrectomy, transection of the small bowel approximately halfway between the ligament of Treitz and ileocecal valve, roux-en-Y gastroenterostomy and an anastomosis of biliopancreatic limb with the alimentary limb 50 cm before the ileocecal valve forming a common channel (Kamal 2012).

Biliopancreatic diversion with duodenal switch was described by Tom R. De Meester. İt is actually an anti-reflux surgery. In this procedure, anastomosis is made between roux leg and first part of duodenum. So biliopancreatic diversion is modified by preserving pyloric sphincter (Alan 2008).

Roux-en-Y gastric bypass was developed from the weight loss that was observed in patients undergoing surgery (partial stomach resection and Billroth-2 anastomosis) for ulcers. Today, it is the most commonly used bariatric method in United States. It was performed as a loop bypass with a larger stomach. In this procedure, stomach is divided horizontally and jejunum is transected from 40–50 cm distal part of Treitz ligament. There is an anastomosis between distal jejunum and new gastric pouch. The other anastomosis is performed between the proximal jejunum and distal jejunum, 75–150 cm away from the first anastomosis. This prevents the bile reflux to the esophagus and new stomach pouch after the surgery (Mason 1967).

Mini gastric bypass was first developed by Robert Rutledge in 1997. It is a simplified form of roux-en-Y gastric bypass. İn this procedure, a long narrow tube of the stomach along the lesser curvature is created. A loop of the small intestine is brought up and hooked to this tube at about 180–200 cm from the Treitz ligament (Rutledge 2001).

There are two important hormones in obesity surgery: Ghrelin and leptin. Ghrelin was discovered by Davis and described by Kojima in 1991.

It is expressed by specialized enterochromaffin cells located in the fundal region of the stomach. There is a proportional correlation between BMI and ghrelin decrease (Davis 1954; Kojima 2001).

Leptin is produced by adipocytes and secreted into blood. It is directly proportional with BMI and amount of body fat. Plasma leptin level is reduced in people who lose weight (Tadokoro 2015; Dagogo 1996). Decreasing plasma leptin and ghrelin levels by the operations of sleeve gastrectomy and gastric plication are shown in an experimental study (Gulcicek 2016). Sleeve gastrectomy and gastric plication have been performed with gradually increasing frequency in recent years. Both procedures can also be applied laparoscopically (Shen 2013).

Sleeve gastrectomy was first described in 1993 by Marceau et al. It was initially applied as a first stage of biliopancreatic diversion, duodenal switch and gastric bypass operations. Until 2003, it has been applied alone. It is a two-stage operation; dissection of the stomach and resection of the stomach. Greater curvature of the stomach is mobilized by the division of gastrocolic and gastrosplenic ligaments.

This dissection should be extended to the left crus of the diaphragm for the complete resection of the fundus. The second stage involves resection of the greater curvature of the stomach from antrum to angle of His throughout latarjet nerve. About 2/3 of the stomach is removed with this surgery (Figure 3.1) (Marceau 1998). Two mechanisms are judged with the weight loss after sleeve gastrectomy: Mechanical restriction by reducing the volume of the stomach and a decline in appetite by subtracting the fundus where ghrelin is produced (Weiner 2007).

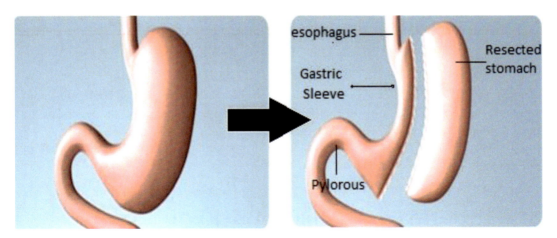

Figure 3.1. Sleeve gastrectomy.

Gastric plication was first described by Taleppour and Amoli in 2007. In this technique, as in sleeve gastrectomy, gastrocolic omentum is divided and the short gastric arteries are dissected.

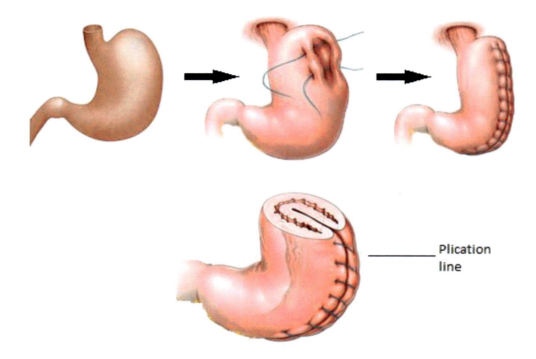

Figure 3.2. Gastric plication.

Then, greater curvature of stomach is plicated over itself by two layered continuous non-absorbable sutures with the help of 32–36 F plug catheters. By this way, the lumen of the stomach is reduced (Figure 3.2) (Talebpourand 2007).

The amount of ghrelin production is reduced in the fundus because of the dissection of short gastric arteries in gastric plication.

ANATOMY OF THE STOMACH IN RATS

General anatomical features of the rat stomach are similar to those of human stomach. It is located in the left side of the abdominal cavity as in humans and adjacent to the left lobe of the liver, esophagus, colon and spleen.

When observed with the naked eye, it consists of two main sections of different colors: Cutan section and glandular section (Figure 3.3).

Cutan section forms the proximal part of the stomach; it is adjacent to the esophagus and its color is lighter. Cutan part is thin-walled and lined with keratinized squamous epithelium. It is responsible for storage and digestion of food. The section which constitutes the large part of the stomach is glandular section.

Glandular section is thick-walled and consists of columnar epithelium. In lamina propria of this section, there are pepsin and HCl secreting cells. This section continues to the duodenum and small intestine as in human (Barlow 2009).

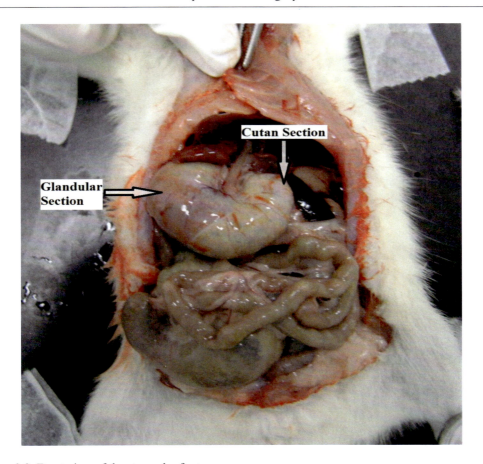

Figure 3.3. Front view of the stomach of rat.

HOW TO CREATE OBESE RATS?

For bariatric experimental surgery, obese rats should be used. Therefore we need to select the rats which are already obese or we need to create obese rats.

Standard diet of experimental animals includes 50% carbohydrates, 25% protein and 5% fat. If we use high-fat diet (35% carbohydrates, 20% protein and 45% fat; d12451, Research Diets, New Brunswick, NJ, USA) for about 28 days, we can get obese rats (Tuncer 2007).

Another method is that when we add 25 grams of butter into 100 grams of standard diet, we'll get diet containing 65% fat. Daily weights of animals are recorded. When the desired weight is reached, we could use these animals for experimental obesity models (XZhou 1998).

BARIATRIC SURGICAL MODELS OF THE RATS

All surgical procedures for obesity mentioned above can be applied to rats.

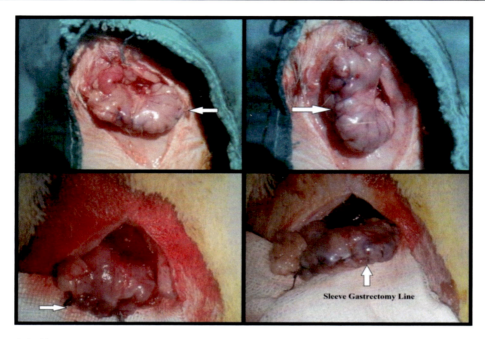

Figure 3.4. Sleeve gastrectomy on rat stomach.

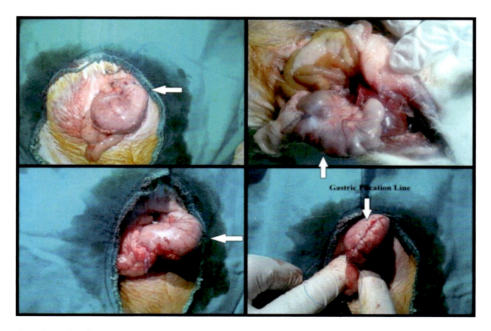

Figure 3.5. Gastric plication on rat stomach.

For sleeve gastrectomy, 3 cm midline incision is done under sterile conditions. Gastrocolic and gastrosplenic ligaments and short gastric arteries are dissected from 0.5cm proximal to the pylorus to diaphragmatic crus. 50–70% of the stomach is excised. Then, the inner layer is closed by continuous 5/0 polypropylene sutures and the outer layer is closed with continuous extramucosal sutures by 5/0 polypropylene (Figure 3.4) (Gulcicek 2016).

For gastric plication, the same steps are done. Stomach is not excised. After the dissection of ligaments, plication of the greater curvature is done with two layered extramucosal continuous sutures by 5/0 polypropylene (Figure 3.5) (Gulcicek 2016).

After the operation, abdomen layers are closed duly and after 5 hours, all rats are fed ad libitum.

CONCLUSION

All surgical procedures for obesity mentioned above for humans can be applied on rats. However, gastric plication and sleeve gastrectomy are the most popular bariatric surgical methods used in recent years.

Technically, it is easier to apply these methods on small experimental animals and complication rates are much less than the other methods. The short operation time and optimal use of anesthetic agents increase the success rate of the experiments.

REFERENCES

Barlow, Z., Cairl, B. (2009) Rat Anatomy.

Benaiges, D., Goday, A., Pedro-Botet, J., Ma´s, A., Chillaro´n, J. J., Flores-Le Roux, J. A. Bariatric surgery: to whom and when? *Minerva Endocrinol,* 2015; 40(2): 119−28.

Benjamin, S. B., Maher, K. A., Cattau, E. L. Jr., Collen, M. J., Fleischer, D. E., Lewis, J. H. (1988) Double-blind controlled trial of the Garren- Edwards gastric bubble: an adjunctive treatment for exogenous obesity. *Gastroenterology,* 95: 581−588.

Blackburn, G. L., Kanders, B. S. Medical evaluation and treatment of the obese patients with cardiovascular disease. *Am. J. Cardiol.,* 1987; 60: 55−8.

Dagogo, J. S., Fanelli, C., Paramore, D., Brothers, J., Landt, M. Plasma leptin and insulin relationships in obese and nonobese humans (abstract). *Diabetes,* 1996; 45: 695−8.

Davis, J. C. The relation between the pancreatic alpha cells and certain cells in the gastric mucosa. *J. Pathol. Bacteriol.,* 1954; 67: 237−40.

Ewing, B. T., Thompson, M. A., Wachtel, M. S., Frezza, E. E. A cost-benefit analysis of bariatric surgery on the South Plains region of Texas. *Obes. Surg.,* 2011; 21: 644−9.

Gastrointestinal surgery for severe obesity: National Institutes of Health Consensus Development Conference Statement. *Am. J. Clin. Nutr.,* 1992; 55 (2 Suppl.):615S−619S.

Gulcicek, O. B., Ozdogan, K., Solmaz, A., Yigitbas, H., Altınay, S., Gunes, A., Celik, D. S., Yavuz, E., Celik, A., Celebi, F. Metabolic and histopathological effects of sleeve gastrectomy and gastric plication: an experimental rodent model. *Food and Nutrition Research,* 2016, 60: 30888.

Kojima, M., Hosoda, H., Date, Y. Ghreline: discovery of natural endogenous ligand for the growth hormone secretgogue receptor. *Trends Endocrinol. Metab.,* 2001; 12: 118−22.

Kuzmak, L. I., Rickert, R. R. Pathologic Changes in the Stomach at the Site of Silicone Gastric Banding. *Obes. Surg.,* 1991;1: 63−68.

Lo´pez-NavaBrevie`re, G., Bautista-Castan͂o, I., Jimenez, A., de Grado, T., Fernandez-Corbelle, J. P. The Primary Obesity Surgery Endolumenal (POSE) procedure: one-year patient weight loss and safety outcomes. *Surg. Obes. Relat. Dis.*, 2015; 11(4): 861–5.

Marceau, P., Hould, F. S., Simard, S., Lebel, S., Bourque, R. A., Potvin, M., Biron, S. Biliopancreatic diversion with duodenal switch. *World J. Surg.*, 1998; 22: 947–54.

Mahawar, K. Bariatric Surgery: The Past, the Present, and the Future. Webmed Central, *Bariatric and Metabolic Surgery*, 2012; 3(7): WMC003610.

Mason, E. E., Ito, C. Gastric bypass in obesity. *Surg. Clin. North. Am.*, 1967; 47: 1345–1351.

National Institutes of Health (2010) NIH consensus statement Gastrointestinal surgery for severe obesity.

Rutledge, R. The mini-gastric bypass: experience with the first 1,274 cases. *Obes. Surg.*, 2001;11: 276–280.

Shen, D., Ye, H., Wang, Y., Ji, Y., Zhan, X., Zhu, J., Li, W. Comparison of short-term outcomes between laparoscopic greater curvature plication and laparoscopic sleeve gastrectomy. *Surg. Endosc.*, 2013; 27(8): 2768–74.

Saber, A. A., Elgamal, M. H., McLeod, M. K. Bariatric Surgery: The Past, Present, and Future. *Obes. Surg.*, 2008; 18(1):121–128.

Tadokoro, S., Ide, S., Tokuyama, R., Umeki, H., Tatehara, S., Kataoka, S., Satomura, K. Leptin promotes wound healing in the skin. *PLoS One*, 2015; 10(3): 1–16.

Talebpourand, M., Amoli, B. S. Laparoscopic total gastric vertical plication in morbid obesity. *J. Laparoendosc. Adv. Surg. Tech. A*, 2007; 17(6): 793–8.

Tuncer, B. B., Barış, E. et al. Evaluation Of Tooth And Surrounding Tissues In Experimental Induced Obese Rats With High Fat İntake A Pilot Study. *GU Diş Hek Fak Derg.*, 2007; 24(3):167–171.

Weiner, R. A., Weiner, S., Pomhoff, I., Jacobi, C., Makarewicz, W., Weigand, G. Laparoscopic sleeve gastrectomy influence of sleevesize and resected gastric volume. *Obes. Surg.*, 2007; 17: 1297–1305.

Zhou, X., De Schepper, J., De Craemer, D., Delhase, M., Gys, G., Smitz, J., and Hooghe-Peters, E. L. (1998) Pituitary growth hormone release and gene expression in cafeteria-diet-induced obese rats. *Journal of Endocrinology*, 1998; 159: 165–72.

In: Advances in Experimental Surgery. Volume 2
Editors: Huifang Chen and Paulo N. Martins
ISBN: 978-1-53612-773-7
© 2018 Nova Science Publishers, Inc.

Chapter 4

ANIMAL MODELS OF HEART FAILURE

Mouer Wang[*], *MD*
Cardiovascular Institute, Stanford University, Stanford, California, US

ABSTRACT

Cardiovascular diseases (CVD) often lead to heart failure (HF). HF prevalenceis continuously rising and represents one of the leading causes ofdeath and an economic burden in the western societies. The study of potential novel therapeutic options and interventions requires reliable animal models to evaluate myocardial progressive structural and functional changes. Indeed, during the past 40 years, basic and translational scientists have used small animal models to understand the pathophysiology of HF and improve prevention and treatment of patients suffering from congestive HF (CHF). Each species and animal model has advantages and disadvantages and the choice of one model over another should take them into account for a good experimental design.

The aim of this chapter is to describe and highlight the features of some commonly used small animal (rats and mouse) surgical models of cardiovascular diseases leading to HF.

Keywords: heart failure, rat, mouse, left anterior descending (LAD) artery ligation, aortic banding, aorto-caval fistula (ACF)

ABBREVIATIONS

ACF: aorto-caval fistula
CVD: cardiovascular diseases
CHF: chronic heart failure
HF: heart failure
LAD: left anterior descending
LV: left ventricle

---

[*]Correspondingauthor: Mouer Wang, M.D. E-mail: mouerw@yahoo.com.

INTRODUCTION

Heart failure is a clinical syndrome characterized by cardiac dysfunction and myocardial structural abnormality (e.g., hypertrophy and dilated cardiomyopathy) resulting in inability of the heart to eject sufficient blood to the metabolizing tissues. Heart failure is a leading cause of morbidity and mortality, posing a major health and economic burden in the western world. Nearly 5 million Americans and 6.5 million Europeans suffer from heart failure, which accounts for 20% of all hospitalizations among patients over the age of 65, and its related complications result in one million admissions with an annual mortality rate of 8–10%. Moreover, heart failure has enormous economic impact because of the high costs of the treatment, frequent hospitalizations, and poor quality of life. Therefore, understanding the basic mechanisms leading to the development of heart failure and its complications, as well as the discovery of innovative adequate treatment for heart failure are crucial in order to improve the outcome of this devastating disease.

Humans present with heart failure of varying severity and of uncertain duration, produced by a wide variety of causes. This variability, and confounding effects of treatment, complicates the study of the pathophysiology and progression of the heart failure.

The ideal model should be able to reproduce each of the aspects of the progression of clinical heart failure. However, none of the models available is able to entirely reproduce heart failure. While some models reproduce neuroendocrine changes, others better reproduce the remodeling that occurs during chronic heart failure. Nevertheless, the progress that has been made so far and the expected future achievements in this field would not have been possible without the continuous development of experimental models of heart failure and hypertrophy in small and large animals, where each one has its unique advantages and limitations. There are three main surgical models of heart failure in rodents: coronary artery ligation to induce myocardial infarction; transverse aortic constriction to create a model of pressure overload; and aortocaval fistula to increate a model of volume overload.

RAT LEFT ANTERIOR DESCENDING (LAD) ARTERY LIGATION

The surgical method, first developed by Pfeffer and coworkers, consists of ligating the left coronary artery (Pfeffer 1979). In this procedure, left thoracotomy is performed on the anesthetized rat, and the heart is rapidly exteriorized by gentle pressure on the right side of the thorax. The left coronary artery is either ligated or heat cauterized between the pulmonary artery outflow tract and the left atrium. The heart is then returned to its normal position and the thorax immediately closed. Several modifications have been introduced to improve performance and to reduce animal mortality, and left coronary artery ligation is the most common method used to induce acute myocardial damage in rat and other animal models. If the left coronary artery is not completely ligated, heart failure may occur as a consequence of chronic myocardial ischemia. Complete occlusion of the left coronary artery results in myocardial infarction of variable sizes with occurrence of overt heart failure after 3–6 weeks in a subset of animals with large infarcts. The impairment of left ventricular function is related to the loss of myocardium. Failure is associated with left ventricular dilatation, reduced systolic function and increased filling pressures. The progression of left ventricular dysfunction and myocardial failure is associated with neurohumoral activation similar to that seen in patients with chronic heart failure (CHF). In particular, it was shown that ACE (angiotensin-converting-enzyme) activity in the left ventricle correlated inversely with left ventricular function and that ACE activity in the kidney was only increased late after the induction of heart failure. Depressed myocardial function is associated with altered calcium transients. The density of L-type calcium channels, as evaluated by antagonist binding was shown to be decreased in moderate to severe stages of congestive heart failure. Furthermore, it was shown that after 4, 8 and 16 weeks following coronary artery ligation, SR (sarcoplasmic reticulum)-Ca^{2+}-ATPase mRNA and protein levels decrease continuously with increasing severity of congestive heart failure. Interestingly, SR-Ca^{2+}-ATPase activity was found to be more depressed than expected from the reduction in protein levels. Although a high initial mortality and induction of mild failure in most cases may be a disadvantage of this model, it seems to be very useful for long-term studies of pharmacological interventions on the neurohumoral activation.

One important modification is temporary occlusion followed by reperfusion, allowing flow recovery through the previously occluded coronary artery bed. Left coronary artery ligation can thus be used to evaluate diverse parameters resulting from either permanent ischemia or ischemia/reperfusion.

Preparation of the Operation

The operating surface is first prepared by disinfecting the area with 70% ethanol.

All surgical instruments are to be sterilized with a hot bead sterilizer before surgery (and in between individual rat surgeries). These instruments include: surgical scissors (2), forceps (1), curved forceps (1), needle holder (2), and a chest retractor.

Adjust the temperature of a homeothermic blanket system (heating pad), to be used to maintain the body temperature of the animal at $37 \pm 1°C$, in order to prevent a dramatic fall in body temperature; the size of an infarct is dependent on the duration of occlusion as well as body temperature. Prior to the induction of anesthesia, animals will be examined to identify any pre-existing conditions that may complicate surgical outcome; physical examination will include visual inspection and measurement of heart rate, respiratory rate, and body temperature and body weight. Prior to anesthesia, each animal will receive a dosage of buprenorphine (0.1–2.5 mg/kg SQ).

Operative Steps

1. Rats are then anesthetized with 80 mg/kg of pentobarbital; the correct level of anesthesia is verified through the limb withdrawal response by applying pressure of the rat nail bed (toe-pinch reflex) and periodically throughout the procedure.
2. An electric shaver is then used to shave the fur form the neck and chest areas.
3. The shaved areas are to be scrubbed and disinfected with beta dinesolution followed by wiping the area with 70% alcohol; this betadine and alcohol scrub and disinfection procedure is to be repeated three times (Figure 4.1).

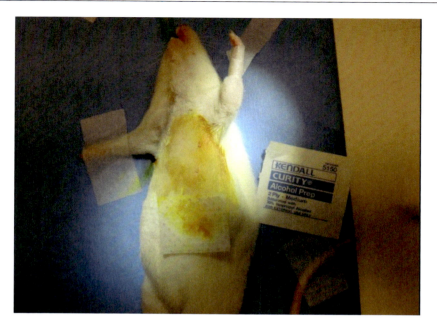

Figure 4.1. Disinfection of surgical field.

4. The anesthetized animal is then placed in a supine position on a homeothermic blanket system (heating pad) in order to maintain body temperature.
5. Intubation is then performed by insertion of the endotracheal tube (polyethylene size 90; PE 90) where the tubing is beveled on the edge for ease of entrance through the larynx.

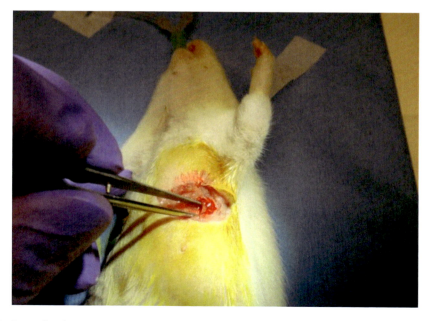

Figure 4.2. Open the thorax.

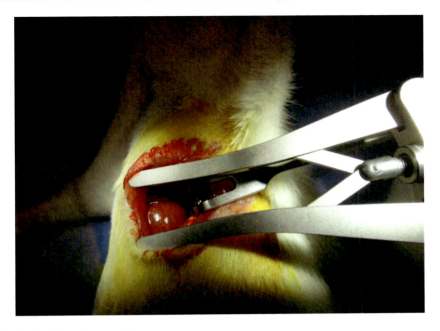

Figure 4.3. Pericardium is opened.

6. Mechanical ventilation is then achieved by connecting the endotracheal tube to Kent Scientific ventilator (TOPO Dual Mode) cycling at 80 breaths per minute and a tidal volume of 1.2 ml per 100 gram body weight.
7. Once steady breathing is established, the chest is opened at the left fourth intercostal space, by using hemostats or round end scissors to open the space, but without cutting the tissue so that the risk of bleeding can be reduced (Figure 4.2).

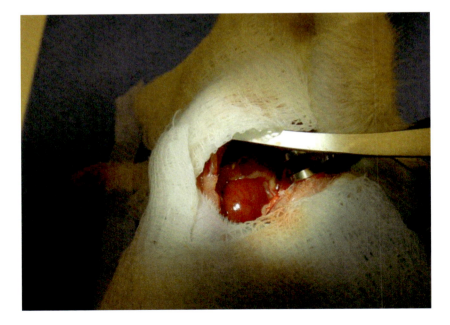

Figure 4.4. LAD is identified.

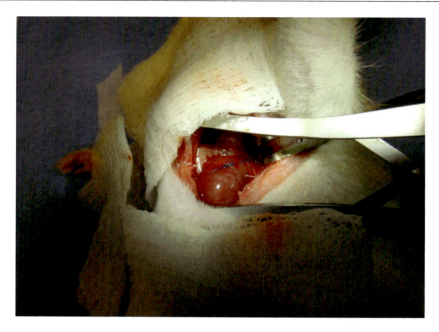

Figure 4.5. LAD is ligated using a 6-0 proline suture.

8. A chest retractor is then positioned within the fourth intercostal space in order to spread the ribs so that the left ventricle (LV) is exposed, taking maximal care not to damage the lung.
9. The pericardium is then opened, but left in place if possible (Figure 4.3).

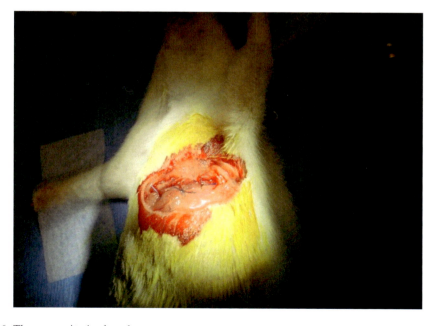

Figure 4.6. Thorax cavity is closed.

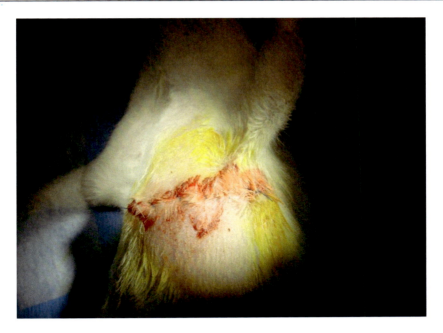

Figure 4.7. Skin is closed using 6-0 proline suture.

10. The proximal left anterior descending (LAD) artery will be identified with the use of a surgical stereo microscope, and the LAD is then ligated using a 6-0 proline suture. Proper ligation of the LAD will be confirmed by observing blanching of myocardial tissue distal to the suture as well as dysfunction of the anterior wall; as observed during the transient LAD ligation (Figure 4.4 and Figure 4.5).
11. The chest retractor is then removed and the ribs are drawn together using a 2-0 proline suture with an interrupted suture pattern.
12. Once the ribs are closed, the outflow of the ventilator is again briefly (1–2 seconds) pinched off to ensure proper breathing (Figure 4.6).

The skin is closed using 6-0 proline suture with a continuous suture pattern (Figure 4.7).

Post-Operative Recovery

Once the surgery is complete, the body temperature (by a rectal thermometer), respiratory rate (by visual inspection), heart rate (by palpitation), and abnormal signs of pain are to be monitored until the animal becomes ambulatory. The rat will be removed from the ventilator and then be placed in an animal cage and allowed to recover from anesthesia.

RAT AORTIC BANDING

Placing a ligature around the ascending aorta induces pressure overload of the left ventricle, eventually resulting in left ventricular hypertrophy and failure. Aortic coarctation results in a very short reactive hyperreninemia of less than 4 days. Thereafter, the circulating renin–angiotensin system is no longer activated, but the ventricular ACE activity begins to rise. After a period of several weeks, ventricular ACE activity may decrease again to normal values which may be related to normalization of wall stress with increasing hypertrophy. Numerous studies have been performed using aortic banding in rats to evaluate different aspects of left ventricular hypertrophy. Furthermore, after several months, a subset of animals goes into failure. In a recent study, chronic experimental aortic constriction imposed by banding of the ascending aorta in weanlings resulted in compensated left ventricular hypertrophy of the adult rats for several weeks. After 20 weeks of aortic banding, two distinct groups could be identified: rats without change in LV systolic pressure development and those with a significant reduction in left ventricular systolic pressure. The latter group exhibited increased left ventricular volumes, reduced ejection fraction and clinical signs of overt heart failure. Left ventricular hypertrophy and failure was associated with increased beta-myosin heavy chain mRNA and atrial natriuretic factor mRNA. Interestingly, a decrease in SR-Ca-ATPase mRNA levels by the polymerase chain reaction occurred in left ventricular myocardium from failing animals after 20 weeks of banding but not in nonfailing hypertrophied hearts. From this data, it was suggested that the decrease in SR-Ca-ATPase mRNA levels may be a marker of the transition from compensatory hypertrophy to failure in these animals. During compensated hypertrophy, while catecholamine levels are normal, there is activation of the local myocardial renin-angiotensin system, which may be important for the development of myocardial failure. With the development of heart failure, plasma catecholamine levels can increase.

This model seems to be well suited for studying the transition from hypertrophy to failure at the level of the myocardium. Nevertheless, one should keep in mind that considerable differences in the function of subcellular systems exist between rat and human myocardium.

Preparation of the Operation

Keep rat (approximately 200 g body weight) under antibiotic umbrella 24 hrbefore surgery by administering amoxicillin orally (dose: 500 mg/L of water). Sterilize all surgical tools (such as scissors, forceps, clip applicator, suture needles, and needle holder) by autoclaving at 121°C for 15 min. Use a heating pad to maintain the animal body temperature around 37°C to avoid a rapid decrease in heart rate. Keep the rat on top of a temperature controlled heating pad in the supine position.

Remove fur from the neckline and left chest region of the rat (preferably using an electric shaver).Disinfect surgical site with povidone-iodine solution and then with 70% ethyl alcohol. Use a sterile drape to expose only the surgical site during the operative procedure. Note: As an additional option for the animal care, 0.25% Bupivicaine ID (2.5 mg/kg) can be incorporated prior to incising at each incision site for local anesthesia/analgesia.

Insert a 16 G I.V. Catheter into the rat's trachea through mouth. Connect the tracheal cannula to a rodent ventilator for maintaining a respiratory rate of 50 breaths/min, tidal volume of 1.70 ml and inspiration time of 0.60 sec (for rat with 200 g body weight).

Operative Steps

1. After skin incision, the upper half of the sternum was divided in the midline using scissors.

2. The thymus was removed and aortic arch was carefully dissected free of the surrounding tissues (Figure 4.8 and Figure 4.9).

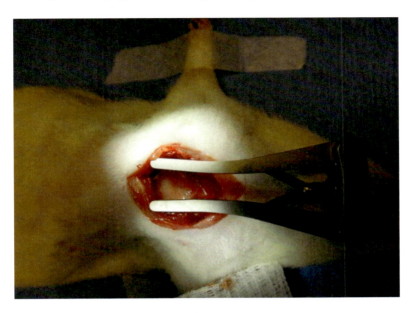

Figure 4.8 Upper half of the sternum was divided.

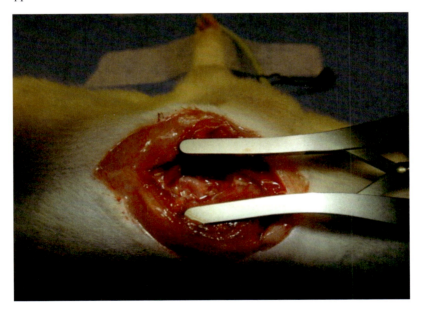

Figure 4.9. Thymus was removed and aortic arch exposed.

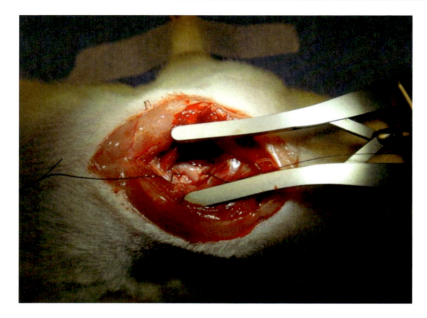

Figure 4.10. Suture is placed between the innominate and left carotid arteries.

3. Following identification of the transverse aorta, a small piece of a 5.0 silk suture is placed between the innominate and left carotid arteries (Figure 4.10).
4. Two loose knots are tied around the transverse aorta and a small piece of a 26½ gauge blunt needle is placed parallel to the transverse aorta. The first knot is quickly tied against the needle, followed by the second and the needle promptly removed in order to yield a constriction (Figure 4.11 and Figure 4.12).

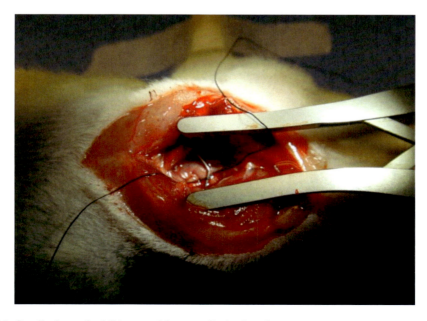

Figure 4.11. Small piece of a 26½ gauge blunt needle is placed.

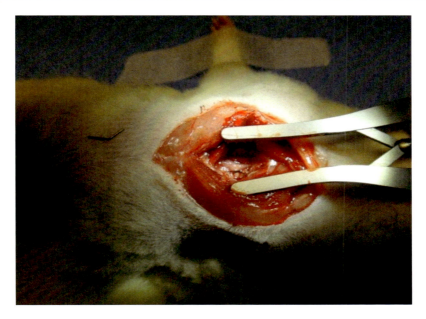

Figure 4.12. Needle removed.

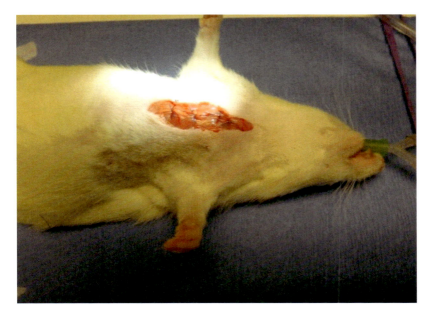

Figure 4.13. Sternotomy closed.

5. The sternotomy and the skin incision were closed with 5-0 sutures (Figure 4.13).

Post-Operative Recovery

Remove tracheal cannula from the rat once spontaneous breathing is re-established.

Allow the animal to recover on the heating pad by gradually lowering the anesthesia and ventilator assisted respiration.

Postoperatively, the animals were kept in separate cages and allowed free access to water and standard laboratory diet. Analgesia with buprenorphine 0.05 mg/kg subcutaneously was provided every 12 hour for 48 hours.

MOUSE CORONARY LIGATION MODEL

One of the most widely used models of heart failure in mice is the left coronary artery ligation procedure, adapted from rat. In some protocols, the artery is occluded permanently, but recently procedures for temporary occlusion have been introduced to reproduce human ischemia/reperfusion injury (Michael 1995). In this method the left anterior descending coronary artery is occluded and then reperfused, allowing flow recovery through the previously occluded coronary artery bed. Reperfusion is monitored visually, and the infarct can be analyzed by histopathological techniques, and can be documented in real time by noninvasive high frequency. The areas at risk and the infarct size are revealed by staining with Evans blue dye and triphenyltetrazolium chloride and are assessed by computerized planimetry. This model has confirmed the benefits of reperfusion, since infarct size was found to be significantly lower than after permanent occlusion of the coronary artery. The method has been further modified to analyze ischemic preconditioning of the heart. In this method, the left coronary artery is repeatedly occluded to subject the heart to several rounds of brief ischemia and reperfusion followed by permanent occlusion. This approach has identified several ischemia-induced genes that confer tolerance to a subsequent ischemic event (West 2008).

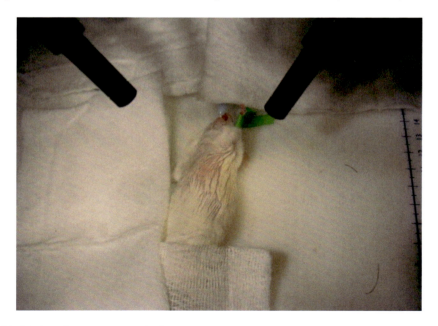

Figure 4.14. Intubated mouse on surgical area.

Preparation of the Operation

Before proceeding to surgery, anesthetize mouse that is 6 weeks of age or older by inhalation of 2–5% isoflurane. Perform a toe pinch to confirm that the animal is sufficiently anesthetized.

The unconscious mouse is placed on its back on a warm pad to maintain a constant temperature of 37°C. The precordial chest on the left side is shaved.

Secure the mouse to an intubation device with an isoflurane-filled chamber. Insert a tube of 0.2 inner diameter into the mouse's trachea through mouth, then place the intubated mouse on an aseptic surgical area (37°C by a temperature controller) and connect the endotracheal tube to a ventilator (rate of 120 per min, pressure of 4–6 mmH$_2$O) (Figure 4.14); disinfect the area with betadine and 75% ethanol.

Apply ophthalmic ointment to the mouse's eyes.

Operative Steps

1. Use sterile scissors to make a 1.5 cm incision along the mid-axillary line. Scissors are used rather than a scalpel to avoid injury to the underlying tissue in mice (Figure 4.15). Then, use blunt-tip vessel scissors to dissect and retract the precordial muscle from the chest wall.
2. Perform a left thoracotomy between the third and fourth ribs to visualize the anterior surface of the heart and left lung.
3. Further retract the thoracic wall using a suitable retractor in order to improve visualization and accessibility. Remove the pericardium by using toothed forceps and blunt-tipped scissors (Figure 4.16).

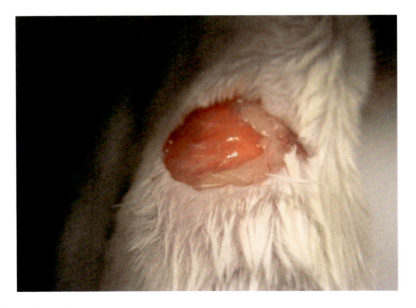

Figure 4.15. Section of skin.

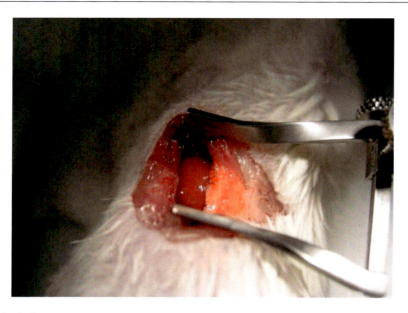

Figure 4.16. Left thoracotomy.

4. Ligate the left coronary artery by placing the needle (attached with 7-0 suture) beneath the artery with a band of myocardium between the ligature and the artery (Figure 4.17). A successful occlusion of coronary artery is verified by hypokinesis/akinesis of the anterior left ventricular wall and by the alterations of ECG recording (*e.g.* ST segment elevation, QRS broadening)
5. Close the chest by placing two stitches (6-0 suture) on the third and fourth ribs.

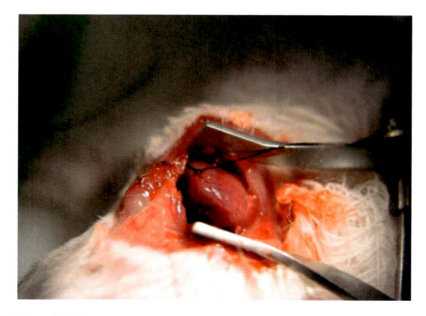

Figure 4.17. Ligate the left coronary artery.

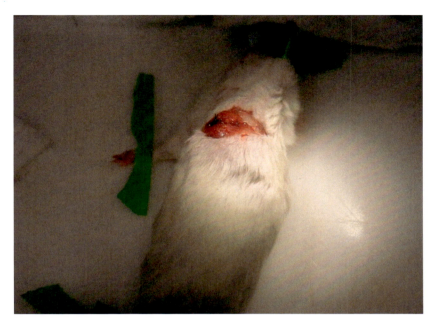

Figure 4.18. Close chest.

Use 5-0 suture to close the skin (Figure 4.18).

Post-Operative Recovery

For post-operative analgesia, administer a single intraperitoneal injection of buprenorphine (0.05 mg/kg). The animals will spontaneously recover within 2–5 min after stopping isoflurane anesthesia. Finally, place the mouse in a warm cage and provide 0.6 mg/ml of buprenorphine in the drinking water to prevent post-operative distress. Closely monitor the mouse for the first 24 hours after surgery.

Echocardiography is performed to evaluate cardiac function 3 days after myocardial infarction.

MOUSE AORTIC BANDING

The technique for transverse aortic constriction has also been adapted for use in mice (Rockman 1991). After anesthetic and thoracotomy of an adult mouse (an 8-week-old mouse is most commonly used), a 27-gauge needle is placed alongside the transverse aorta between the innominate and left carotid arteries. A nylon suture is tied around the vessel and needle, which is then withdrawn, leaving a 0.4-mm-diameter aperture. By this method, a stable, relatively reproducible 35–45 mm Hg gradient can be introduced across the experimental constriction. The intraoperative mortality reported in the original paper was around 10%, which remains the approximate value in current studies. Crucially, Rockman et al. have been able to show that the molecular pathways activated in their postoperative mouse hearts were identical to other animal and cellular models of cardiac hypertrophy (Rockman 1994). The disadvantages of this approach are that, in absolute terms, intraoperative mortality is high, and as aortic banding is more technically demanding in the mouse than the rat, results are operator-dependent, with heart failure developing within weeks of the procedure in the surviving mice. However, the cost savings by using mice, and the huge range of genetic reagents available, may mitigate these disadvantages. It is not clear how applicable this system is to cardiac hypertrophy/failure due to aortic stenosis in humans, but it has allowed several advances in understanding the molecular control mechanisms underlying left ventricular hypertrophy.

Preparation of the Operation

The operating field is disinfected with 75% isopropyl alcohol. Make sure the heating pad is on and at the right temperature. A recommended system is a circulating water pump connected to a therapy pad that is maintained at 37°C ± 1°C. It is important to maintain normal body temperature during surgery as to avoid a rapid decrease in heart rate. Surgical tools are sterilized in a hot bead sterilizer before surgery. For this procedure, you will need the following surgical instruments: blunt scissors, course curved forceps × 2, fine 45° angled forceps × 2, angled spring scissors, chest retractor, and needle holder.

Cotton applicators should be on hand in case of bleeding.

Mice are anesthetized in an induction chamber with 2% isoflurane mixed with 0.5–1.0 L/min 100% O_2. Hair clippers are used to shave the fur from the neckline to mid chest level. The mouse is placed in a supine position atop a heating pad in order to maintain body temperature. A rubber band is placed over the animal's front teeth to extend the neck. Using curved forceps in one hand, the tongue is gently manipulated to the side. With the other hand, endotracheal intubation is performed using PE 90 tubing. The endotracheal tube is then connected to a Harvard volume-cycled rodent ventilator cycling at 125–150 breaths/minute and a tidal volume of 0.1–0.3ml. During the surgical procedure, anesthesia is maintained at 1.5–2% isoflurane with 0.5–1.0 L/min 100% O_2. Correct level of anesthesia is verified by applying pressure on the mouse nail bed (toe-pinch reflex).

The surgical field is disinfected with beta dinesolution followed by 70% alcohol. This procedure is repeated three times.

To prevent contamination of the surgical field during the operation, a sterile drape is placed over the mouse leaving only the operation field exposed.

A set of sterile gloves is used for each individual mouse.

Operative Steps

1. Partial thoracotomy to the second rib is performed under a surgical microscope and the sternum retracted using a chest retractor (Figure 4.19).

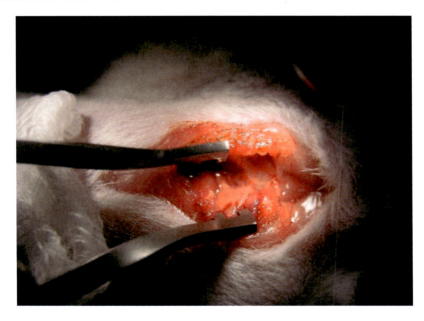

Figure 4.19. Partial thoracotomy.

2. Fine tip 45° angled forceps are used to gently separate the thymus and fat tissue from the aortic arch.
3. Following identification of the transverse aorta, a small piece of a 6.0 silk suture is placed between the innominate and left carotid arteries (Figure 4.20; 4.21).

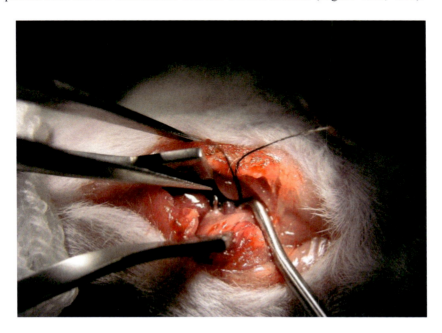

Figure 4.20. Identification of the transverse aorta.

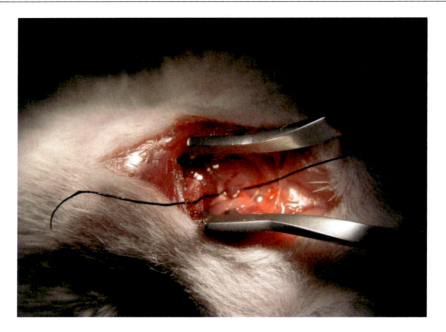

Figure 4.21. Suture is placed between the innominate and left carotid arteries.

4. Two loose knots are tied around the transverse aorta and a small piece of a 27½ gauge blunt needle is placed parallel to the transverse aorta (Figure 4.22). The first knot is quickly tied against the needle, followed by the second (Figure4.23) and the needle promptly removed in order to yield a constriction of 0.4 mm in diameter (Figure 4.24).

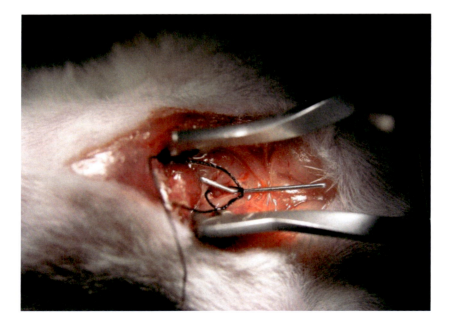

Figure 4.22. Small piece blunt needle is placed parallel to the transverse aorta.

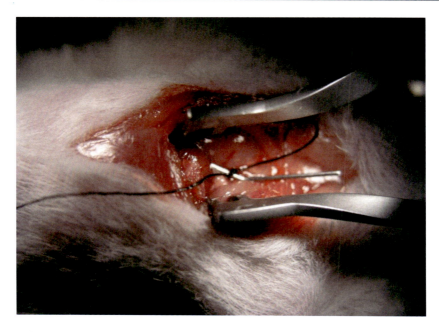

Figure 4.23. The second knot.

5. The chest retractor is removed and the outflow of the ventilator pinched off for 2 seconds to re-inflate the lungs (Figure 4.25).

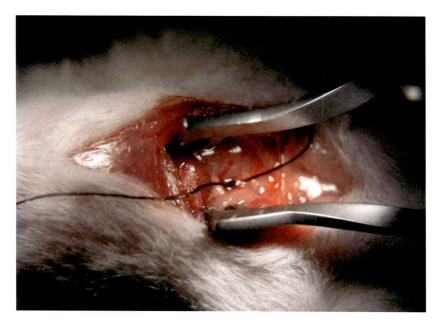

Figure 4.24. Needle removed and yield a constriction of 0.4 mm in diameter.

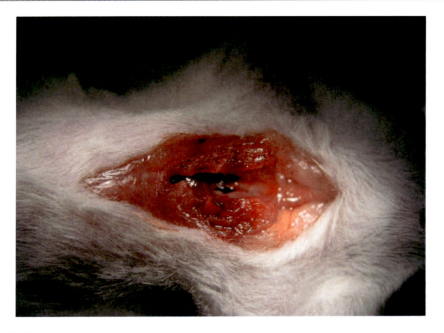

Figure 4.25. Chest retractor is removed.

6. The chest cage is closed using a 6.0 proline suture with an interrupted suture pattern (Figure 4.26).
7. The skin is closed using a 6.0 proline suture with a continuous suture pattern (Figure 4.27).

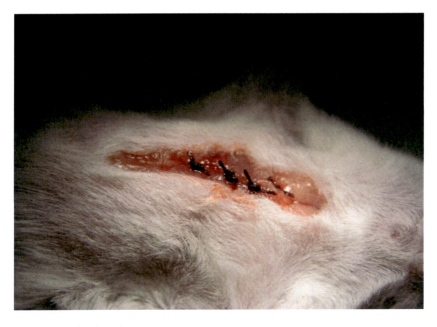

Figure 4.26. Chest cage is closed.

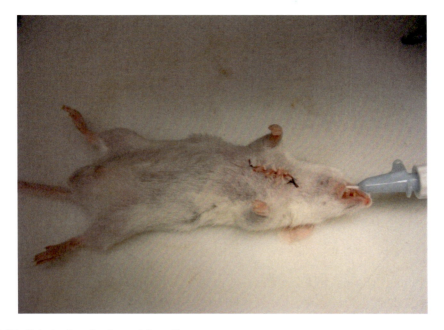

Figure 4.27. Skin is closed using a 6.0 proline suture.

Post-Operative Recovery

For post-operative analgesia, the mouse is injected with buprenorphine (0.1 mg/kg) intraperitoneally. If there are signs of dehydration after surgery, sterile saline is given intraperitoneally.

Anesthesia is gradually lowered to the off position and the endotracheal tube removed when signs of spontaneous breathing occur.

The mouse is moved to the prone position and allowed to recover on a heating pad.

AORTO-CAVAL FISTULA (ACF)

The rat aorto caval fistula (ACF) model is considered to be a model of high-output heart failure, its long-term renal and cardiac manifestations are similar to those seen in patients with low-output heart failure. These include Na^+-retention, cardiac hypertrophy and increased activity of both vasoconstrictor/anti-natriuretic neurohormonal systems and compensatory vasodilating/natriuretic systems. Progression of cardio renal pathophysiology in this model is largely determined by balance between opposing hormonal forces, as reflected in states of heart failure decompensation that are characterized by over activation of vasoconstrictive/Na^+-retaining systems.

Since this model mimics high cardiac output clinical heart failure, it may be suitable to study myocardial alterations, mainly cardiac hypertrophy characterizing these patients.

Thus, ACF serves as a simple, cheap, and reproducible platform to investigate the pathogenesis of heart failure and to examine efficacy of new therapeutic approaches (Liu 1991).

Preparation of the Operation

Male Sprague-Dawley rats weighing 250 to 300 g were anesthetized with pentobarbital sodium (40 mg/kg of body weight).Use a heating pad to maintain the animal body temperature around 37°C to avoid a rapid decrease in heart rate. Take care to avoid dehydration of the animal before and during surgery, check the pedal reflex to confirm successful anesthesia.

Operative Steps

1. Dissecting the vena cava and the aorta from the surrounding tissues, but not from each other (Figure 4.28).
2. Miniature vessels clamp was placed approximately 10 mm distal to the origin of the renal arteries (Figure 4.29).
3. 1.5 mm opening was cut into the lateral wall of the vena cava and the aorta.

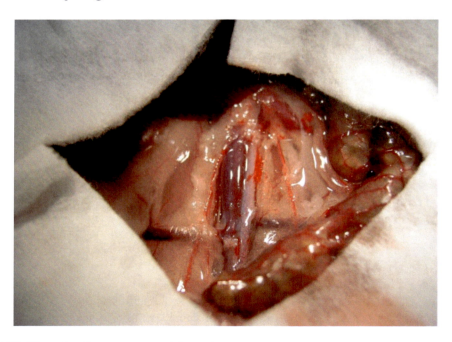

Figure 4.28. Dissecting the vena cava and the aorta.

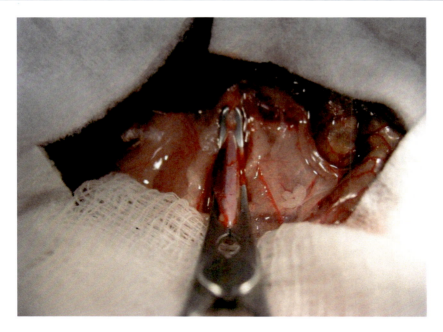

Figure 4.29. Clamp was placed on vena cava and aorta.

4. Vena cava to aorta side-to-side anastomosis was made by continuous 0.6 size proline suture (Figure 4.30).
5. After the vessel clamps were released, arterial blood could be seen vigorously entering the vena cava through the fistula and mixing with the darker venous blood (Figure 4.31).

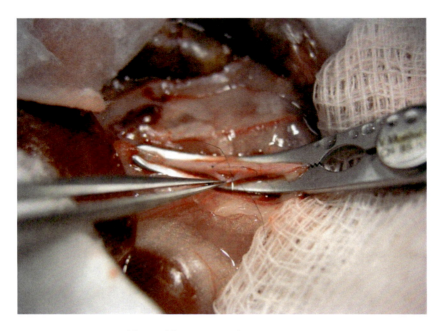

Figure 4.30. Vena cava to aorta side-to-side anastomosis.

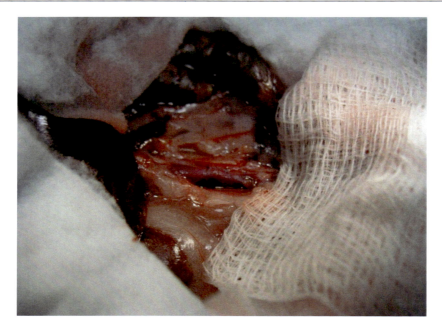

Figure 4.31. Vessel clamps are released.

6. Time of occlusion of both vessels did not exceed 10 minutes.

POST-OPERATIVE RECOVERY

For post-operative analgesia, administer a single intraperitoneal injection of buprenorphine (0.05 mg/kg). Place the rat in a warm cage and closely monitor the rat for the first 24 hours after surgery.

CONCLUSION

The use of animal models has proven to be an extremely valuable tool in understanding the pathophysiology of complex cardiovascular disease mimicking congestive HF. The ideal animal model of cardiovascular disease will mimic the human subject metabolically and pathophysiologically, will be large enough to permit physiological and metabolic studies, and will develop end-stage disease comparable to those in humans. Given the complex multifactorial nature of CVD, no species or animal model will be similar to the human disease and thus the models should be chosen according to the study aim. Animal models may also be relevant to study the effects of new pharmacological interventions on hemodynamics, neurohumoral activation and survival under preclinical conditions. At present, transgenic models of congestive HF are essential for understanding the molecular alterations underlying the development of the disease, as they allow the identification of genes that are causative for HF and to characterize molecular mechanisms responsible for the development and progression of the disease. Animal models which mimic distinct features of human HF will play an important role in unravelling the consequences of gene transfer and molecular techniques to correct disturbed subcellular processes in the failing heart. These experiments are indispensable and these rodent models will continue to held an important role, not only in expanding our knowledge about the mechanisms underlying HF, but also in developing novel therapeutic strategies for this syndrome.

REFERENCES

Michael LH, Entman MI, Hartley CJ, Youker KA, Zhu J, Hall SR, Hawkins HK, Berens K, Ballantyne CM. Myocardial ischemia and reperfusion: a murine model. *American Journal of Physiology* 1995; 269(6):H2147–H2154.

Liu Z, Hilbelink DR, Crockett WB, Gerdes AM. Regional changes in hemodynamics and cardiac myocyte size in rats with aortocaval fistulas. Developing and established hypertrophy.*Circ. Res.* 1991; 69: 52–58.

Pfeffer MA, Pfeffer JM and Fishbein MC. Myocardial infarct size and ventricular function in rats. *Circulation Research* 1979; 44 (4):503–512.

Rockman HA, Ross RS, Harris AN, Knowlton KU, Steinhelper ME, Field LJ, et al. Segregation of atrial-specific and inducible expression of an atrial natriuretic factor transgene inan *in vivo* murine model of cardiac hypertrophy. *Proc. Natl. Acad. Sci. USA* 1991; 88(18):8277–81.

Rockman HA, Wachhorst SP, Mao L, Ross Jr J. ANG II receptor blockade prevents ventricular hypertrophy and ANF gene expression with pressure overload in mice. *Am. J. Physiol.* 1994; 266(6 Pt 2):H2468–75.

West MB, Rokosh G, Obal D, et al. Cardiac myocyte specific expression of inducible nitric oxide synthase protects against ischemia/reperfusion injury by preventing mitochondrial permeability transition, *Circulation* 2008; 118(19):1970–1978.

In: Advances in Experimental Surgery. Volume 2
Editors: Huifang Chen and Paulo N. Martins
ISBN: 978-1-53612-773-7
© 2018 Nova Science Publishers, Inc.

Chapter 5

HEPATOPANCREATOBILIARY SURGERY EXPERIMENTAL MODELS

Paulo N. Martins MD, PhD[*], *Natalie Bath MD and Adel Bozorgzadeh MD*

Department of Surgery, Division of Organ Transplantation,
UMass Memorial Medical Center, University Campus, Worcester, MA

ABSTRACT

Well-characterized animal models of human diseases are fundamental for the analysis of pathophysiologic mechanisms and the development of new treatment strategies. A better understanding of the underlying pathophysiology of hepatopancreatobiliary (HPB) disease may lead to more targeted therapeutic options, potentially leading to improved survival. We will focus this chapter on rodent HPB models. Owing to the low cost of experiments, easily handling, and availability of a variety of genetically modified strains, rodents have become a popular model organism for such experiments.

Despite some limitations, the use of rodent models in HPB surgery provides essential investigative tools to study many important phenomena in HPB research. Due to the availability of large varieties of genetically modified species and monoclonal antibodies, more relevant and more specific questions can be answered utilizing rodent models. Most of these procedures only require basic surgical skills, and they have been performed with high reproducibility, which has been tolerated very well with minimal operative mortality. However, some procedures require microsurgical skills to be performed accurately and reproducibly. Increased knowledge of the rat and mouse liver surgical anatomy and more advanced microsurgical skills permit individualized dissection, and individual ligature of vascular and biliary branches.

Here we will review the HPB anatomy; techniques for hepatectomy, bile duct ligation, and portal systemic shunts; models of cirrhosis; models of acute liver failure; models of hepatocellular carcinoma (HCC) and cholangiocarcinoma (CCC); model of hepatic metastases of colon carcinoma; pancreatitis; and common bile duct (CBD) stricture.

---

[*] Corresponding author: Paulo N. Martins MD., PhD., FAST, FACS., Assistant Professor of Surgery, Department of Surgery, Division of Organ Transplantation, UMass Memorial Medical Center, University Campus, Worcester, MA, Fax: 508-856-1102, Email: paulo.martins@umassmemorial.org.

Keywords: hepatopancreatobiliary surgery, hepatectomy technique, cirrhosis, acute liver failure

ABBREVIATIONS

CBD	common bile duct
CBDL	common bile duct ligation
CCC	cholangiocarcinoma
CCL4	carbon tetrachloride
CDL	closed duodenal loop
CL	caudate lobe
CP	caudate process
DEN	diethylnitrosamine
DMNA	dimethylnitrosamine
FL	falciform ligament
GB	gallbladder
HCC	hepatocelular carcinoma
HCV	hepatitis C virus
HPB	hepatopacreaticobiliary
IRL	inferior right lobe
LLL	left lateral lobe
LML	left middle lobe
ML	middle lobe
PVL	portal vein ligation
PB	phenobarbital
PH	partial hepatectomy
RLL	right lower lobe
RML	right middle lobe
RL	right lobe
SRL	superior right lobe
TAA	thioacetamide

LIVER ANATOMY

Introduction

The rat is the most used experimental model in hepatopancreatobiliary (HPB) surgical research because of many factors, in particular because it is easy to handle and inexpensive (Rodriguez 1999; Martins 2003). In hepatic regeneration, liver metastasis, transplantation immunology and hepatic disease studies, the rat is by far the most frequently used model. On the other hand, the majority of studies that led to advances in techniques of liver resection and transplantation have used the porcine and canine model. Virtually all procedures in liver surgery can be performed in the rat including segmental liver resections, porto-systemic shunts, transplantation of full and partial organs, and vascular embolizations. As a result of the great anatomical variability of liver anatomy such as its extrahepatic biliary tract and vascularization, the knowledge of anatomy is advantageous because it permits individualized dissection, parenchymal section, ligature of specific vascular and biliary branches, and avoids damage of other structures.

The objective of this study was to systematically describe and illustrate the surgical anatomy of the rat liver to facilitate the planning and performance of HPB surgery studies in this animal.

Liver Anatomy

The rat and mouse livers are multi-lobulated as in other mammals (Lorente 1995; Flower 1872; Martins 2007). In rats, the liver mass represents approximately 5% of the total body weight compared to 2.5% in adult humans.

Surfaces

With the rat placed in decubitus position, the rat liver has three surfaces: superior, inferior and posterior. A sharp, well-defined margin divides the inferior from the superior surface. Unique from the human liver, the other margins of the liver are also sharp. Although the rat liver is lobulated, it has rather uniform surfaces since the lobes lie flat against each other as seen in Figure 5.1A. The only exception to this is the posterior caudate lobe, which is separated from the remainder liver by the stomach.

The *superior (parietal) surface*, convex as a whole, comprises a part of the left lateral and medial lobes and fits under the vault of the diaphragm. It is completely covered by peritoneum except along the line of attachment of the falciform ligament. The line of attachment of the falciform ligament divides the liver into two parts, termed the right and left lobes. In comparison to the human liver in which the right lobe is much larger than the left, the rat left and right liver have approximately the same volume.

The *inferior (visceral) surface* is uneven, concave, and it is in close proximity to the stomach, duodenum, right colic flexure, the superior part of the pancreas, the right kidney and suprarenal gland. The rat liver inferior surface does not have the fossae in the shape of the letter "H" as in humans. This surface is almost completely invested by peritoneum. Through the porta (transverse fissure) travels the portal vein, the hepatic artery and nerves, the hepatic duct and lymphatics. Liver impressions (colic, renal, duodenal, and suprarenal) are not as evident as in human livers.

The *posterior surface* it is not covered by peritoneum over some part of its extent, and it is in direct contact with the diaphragm. It extends obliquely between the caudate lobe and the bare area of the liver. The inferior vena cava is completely intrahepatic.

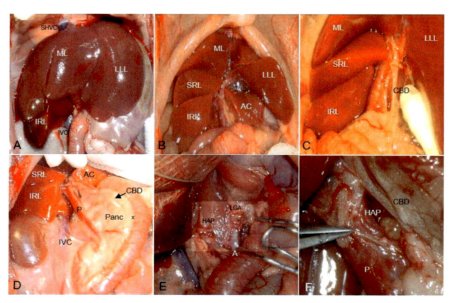

Abbreviations: AC: anterior caudate lobe, CBD common bile duct, Panc pancreas, CT celiac trunk, PHA proper hepatic artery, SA splenic artery, A aorta, LGA left gastric artery, Ly lymph node, S stomach, D duodenum, RK right kidney, SHVC supra-hepatic vena cava, GB gallbladder, FL falciform ligament, P portal vein, IVC inferior vena cava, RLL right lower lobe, ML middle lobe, RML right middle lobe, LML left middle lobe, CL caudate lobe, LLL left lateral lobe, RL right lobe.

Figure 5.1. Rat liver "in-situ". (A) Anterior view, (B) Anterior view after separating the lobes, (C) Porta hepatis, (D) Portal vein and common bile duct descending in the pancreatic tissue along the duodenum (the point of insertion of the CBD in the duodenum is marked with a X), (E) Celiac trunk and its branches: proper hepatic, left gastric and splenic arteries. (F) Magnification of the portal triade: portal vein, CBD, proper hepatic artery and a hilar lymph node.

Ligaments

Similar to the human liver, the rat liver is connected to the under surface of the diaphragm and to the anterior wall of the abdomen by five ligaments: the *falciform*, the *coronary*, two *lateral* which are peritoneal folds, and the *round ligament* – a fibrous cord which represents the obliterated umbilical vein. The liver is also attached to the lesser curvature of the stomach by the hepatogastric ligament and to the duodenum by the hepatoduodenal ligament.

Liver Lobes

The rat's liver lobes, like the human liver, are named after the portal branches that supply them due to the fact that the portal system is the most constant anatomical reference among mammals (Flower 1872; Lorente 1995; Martins 2007) (See Figures 5.1–5.6).

The *middle* or *median lobe* is the largest lobe, accounting for approximately 38% of the liver weight. It is fixed between the diaphragm and abdominal wall by the falciform ligament. It is in continuity with the left lateral lobe and is subdivided by a vertical fissure (main fissure or umbilical fissure) into a large right medial lobe (2/3 of the volume of the medial lobe) and a smaller left medial lobe (1/3 of the volume). The right medial lobe has both left and right hepatic vascular components. (Lorente 1995; Kogure 1999; Martins 2007).

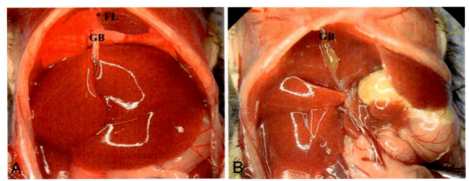

Abbreviations: GB: gallbladder, FL: falciform ligament.

Figure 5.2. A, B. Anterior view of the mouse liver showing the location of the gallbladder and falciform ligament. B) Visceral view of the mouse liver.

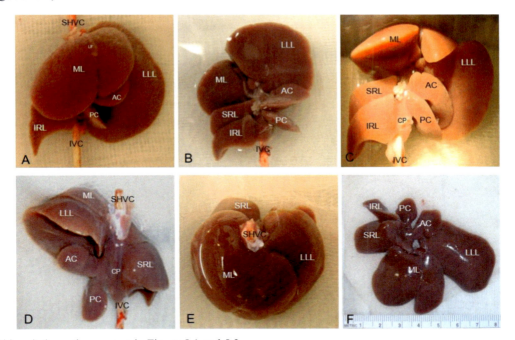

Abbreviations: the same as in Figure 5.1 and 5.2.

Figure 5.3. Rat liver "*ex situ*". (A) Anterior view, (B) Inferior (visceral) view, (C) Anterior after separating the lobes, (D) posterior view, (E) Superior view with the lobes in normal position, (F) Superior view with lobes flattened and separated from each other (note here a millimetric scale on the bottom). When the liver is *ex situ*, the anterior and posterior caudate lobes are on the same plane (see in E), and the anterior lobe lies superiorly. Note in D that the inferior vena cava is completely intrahepatic, a plastic catheter is inside the inferior vena cava.

The *right lobe*, located to the right of the vena cava and posteriorly in the right hypochondrium, is almost completely covered by the medial lobe. It comprises approximately

22% of the liver weight and is divided by a horizontal fissure into two pyramidal-shaped lobules, the superior (SRL, superior right lobe, also called right posterior lobe) and inferior (IRL, inferior right lobe, also called right anterior lobe) lobules.

The *left lateral lobe* is flattened and situated in the epigastric and left hypochondriac regions over the anterior aspect of the stomach. Its medial portion is covered by the left part of the medial lobe. Its upper surface is slightly convex and is molded on the diaphragm. It has no fissures.

The *caudate lobe* is situated behind the left lateral lobe and to the left of the vena porta and inferior cava vein. It comprises 8 to 10% of the liver weight and is divided into two portions: the *paracaval portion (caudate process)* - which accounts for 2 to 3% of the liver mass, encircles the inferior vena cava and bridges the caudate lobes and the right lateral lobe; and the *Spiegel lobe*, which has an *anterior* (superior) and a *posterior* (inferior) portion in form of discs, each representing 4% of the liver mass. The anterior part of the caudate lobe is located anterior to the esophagus and stomach and its pedicle lies superior, while the posterior is located behind these structures and its pedicle lies inferior (Figure 5.3). Both are covered by a very thin layer of peritoneum, the hepatoduodenal and hepatogastric ligaments.

Liver Vasculature

The origin and course of the major vessels are similar to those of humans; no variability in vessel origin was identified in this small number of animals. However, there have been many variations of the liver vasculature described (Flower 1872; Greene 1963; Castaing 1980; Brand 1995; Lorente 1995; Wu 2005; Martins 2007). The most common anatomy of liver vasculature and biliary system is shown on Figure 5.4.

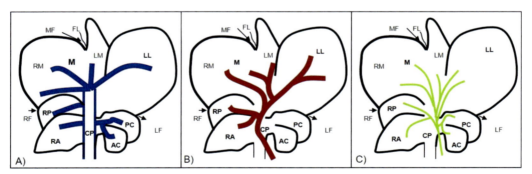

Abbreviations: the same as in Figure 5.2.

Figure 5.4. Most common anatomy of the hepatic veins (A), portal vein (B) and biliary system (C) of the rat.

Hepatic Artery

The liver is supplied by the hepatic artery proper, which originates from the common hepatic artery. The celiac trunk, which is relatively longer in rats than in humans, originates at the anterior or right aspect of the abdominal aorta just below the diaphragm pillars, ascends closely to the aorta for 5 to 7 mm and branches into the common hepatic, left gastric and splenic arteries (Brand 1995) (Figure 5.1E). The common hepatic artery runs within the pancreas and bifurcates at the level of the portal vein into hepatic artery proper and gastroduodenal artery. The hepatic proper artery has a diameter between 0.2 to 0.5 mm and length between 4 to 5 mm. The hepatic artery proper runs at the posterior surface of the portal vein, and at the liver hilum it divides into the right and left branches (Figure 5.1F). The arterial branches run on the anterior surface of the portal vein, pass behind the major hepatic ducts and follow a parallel course with the portal vein branches as they divide into their main lobar ramifications. Sometimes two lobar arteries accompany one single lobar portal vein. The most visible branches are for the superior right lateral, inferior right lateral and medial lobes. In addition to the four branches to the main hepatic lobes, the hepatic artery proper gives off a branch, which can be difficult to visualize, called hepato-esophageal artery. This branch arises on the hepatic pedicle between the caudate and left lobes measuring 10 to 12 mm in length and 0.1 mm in diameter and supplies the lower two-thirds of the esophagus (Leneman 1967). It was not found in the literature description of the intrahepatic arterial branches.

Portal Vein

The extrahepatic portal vein is located posterior and lateral to the hepatic artery and common bile duct (Figure 5.1C–D). It is formed from the superior mesenteric vein, the gastrosplenic vein, and the gastroduodenal vein Innocenti P (1978). The pancreaticoduodenal vein and inferior mesenteric vein drain into the superior mesenteric vein. In this series, the range of diameter and length of the portal vein was 2 to 4 mm and 4 to 7 mm, respectively.

The rat liver has three main portal branches, which determine the following fissures: left portal fissure, right portal fissure and main portal fissure. The left portal fissure separates the right lower lobe (RLL) from the middle lobe (ML), the main fissure separates the right middle lobe (RML) from the left middle lobe (LML), and the left fissure (corresponding to the fossa for the ductus venosus in the human liver), which separates the caudate lobe (CL) from the left lateral lobe (LLL). At the porta hepatis the common portal vein gives branches first to the right lobe (RL), then to the CL, then to ML and last to the LLL (Lorente 1995; Martins 2007). The left, right, and caudate lobes have one primary portal branch, whereas the middle lobe has two portal branches. The right portal vein immediately divides into two branches, one for the superior right lobule and inferior right lobule. The portal branch to the caudate lobe is very short, branching into two main veins, one for anterior and one for the posterior Spiegel lobe. Other very small veins, originating directly from the main portal vein and its left and right branches, supply the paracaval portion (caudate process).

Hepatic Veins

The inferior right lobe and the superior right lobe drain into the inferior vena cava in most cases by one branch each, but each of them can be drained by two veins. In humans, they correspond to the right hepatic and inferior right hepatic vein, the latter representing a variation of the normal anatomy. The middle lobe has two or three large hepatic veins (right, middle and left median veins) (Lorente 1995; Kogure 1999; Martins 2007). The right and left portions of the middle lobe are drained each by one vein. As in humans, the vein draining the left portion of the middle lobe (left medial vein) may enter the vena cava separately or may join the vein draining left lateral lobe (left hepatic vein) to form a common trunk before joining the suprahepatic cava vein (Gershbein 1954; Lorente 1995). The left and caudate lobes are drained in most cases by two large hepatic veins (left and right) that open separately into the vena cava, but in some cases they can be united by a common trunk. The caudate process drains into the intrahepatic vena cava through multiple branches (Figure 5.4).

Biliary Tract

While the mouse has a gallbladder, the rat does not. The extrahepatic biliary ducts of the rat are formed by first order branches of each liver lobe. Second order branches exist for the superior and inferior caudate lobes, right middle lobe and caudate process. The rat biliary tract has many anatomical variations.

Most commonly each lobe is drained by its own bile ducts. The left lateral lobe is most frequently (in 62.5% of cases) drained by two biliary branches. The middle lobe is drained by branches from the right middle lobe (1 to 4 branches) and left medial lobe. In 57.5% of cases each caudate lobe has one branch that join together to form a common branch before draining into the common bile duct (CBD) (Lorente 1995). The superior part of the caudate process drains into branches of the right lateral lobe or the main biliary trunk, while the inferior part of it drains into the branches of the caudate process or to the branch of the right lateral lobe. (Figure 5.4) (Lorente 1995; Martins 2007).

The common bile duct is formed by the junction of the main hepatic ducts. The main hepatic ducts join together on the caudate process (Figure 5.1C). In this series, the CBD ranged from 12 to 16 mm of length and from 0.6 to 1 mm of diameter, but it can be up to 45 mm long (Mann 1920; Hebel 1976; Lorente 1995). The CBD descends to the left of the hepatic artery and the portal vein on the surface of the caudate process and portal vein, then along the right border of the lesser omentum, keeping some distance from them (Figure 5.1D). A long extent of the CBD is completely imbedded in the pancreas, which has a diffuse and lobulated appearance. The CBD opens at the medial side of the descending portion of the duodenum, a little below its middle and about 10 to 22 mm from the pylorus (Figure 5.1C, D and F). The extrahepatic biliary system of the rat has also small intercommunicating branches.

Correlation between Rodent and Human Liver Anatomy and Limitations

The anatomical relationship between the human and rat liver is still undefined (Kogure 1999; Kano 2000). The phylogenetic distance between primates and rodents is more than 80 million years. The functional anatomy of the liver in the rat has been considered different from humans but similar to the pig (Lorente 1995). The classical description of the human liver segmentation by Couinaud divided the human liver into eight segments, and this constitutes the basis of hepatic resections (Figure 5.6B). Three hepatic veins divide the liver into four sectors (right lateral sector, right paramedian sector, left paramedian sector, and left lateral sector) and each sector receives a portal pedicle, which bifurcates and supplies each lobe (I-VIII). Later, Couinaud classified the paracaval portion of the caudate lobe as an independent segment (IX) (Bismuth 1982; Couinaud 1994; Kogure 1999).

The nomenclature of the rat liver lobes is not uniform (Gershbein 1954; Nettelblad 1954; Lorente 1995; Kogure 1999). Most authors consider the rat liver to be divided into four lobes: *left lateral lobe*, *medial lobe* (left medial and right medial), *caudate lobe* (anterior or inferior, and posterior or superior), and *right lobe*. Lorente et al. divided the rat liver into two parts, superior liver and inferior liver, and six sectors: sector 1 or caudate process (CP), sector 2 or caudate lobe (CL), sector 3 or right liver lobe (RLL), sector 4 or right portion of right medial lobe (RML), sector 5 central and left part of the right medial lobe (RML) plus the left medial lobe (LML), and sector 6 made up by the left lateral lobe (LLL) (Figure 5.1–6) (Lorente L 1995). In a recent study from Kongure et al., comparing the rat and human liver, it was shown that the hepatic lobes of the rat are equivalent to the human liver. The rat caudate lobe (Spiegel lobe and paracaval portion) corresponds to segments I and IX, the rat left lobe corresponds to segment II, the rat middle lobe corresponds to segments III, IV, V, and VIII, and the right lobe to segments VI and VII (Kogure 1999). The human caudate lobe, although seems to be only one structure, is functionally divided into three parts (Couinaud 1994). In the rat, the three functional subdivisions of the caudate lobe are individualized structures.

In the rat, the mass of each lobe is relatively constant. Thus, the two anterior lobes, the two right liver lobes, and the two omental lobes (forming the caudate lobe) comprise approximately 70%, 22%, 8% of the liver, respectively (Figure 5.6A). Additionally, each lobe has its own pedicle containing a portal triad. These unique aspects of rat liver anatomy make resections of various extents simple and highly reproducible when performing experiments (Rodriguez 1999). In the rat, the left hemi-liver consists of the LLL, CL and LML while the right hemi-liver represents RL (SRL+IRL) and the RML. In comparison to the human liver in which the right hemi-liver has a greater volume than the left, the left and right hemi-livers in rats have similar volumes (Figure 5.6).

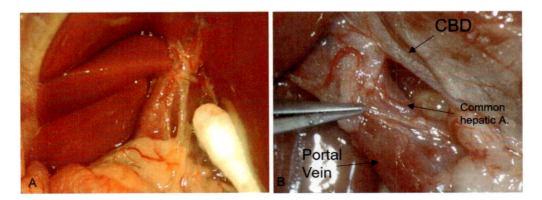

Figure 5.5. A, B Liver hilum.

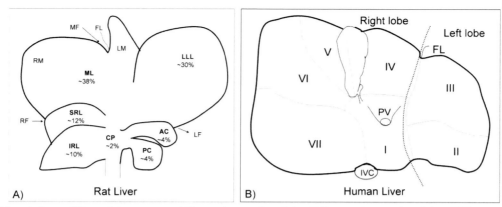

Abbreviations: CP caudate process, AC anterior caudate lobe, PC posterior caudate lobe, SRL superior right lateral lobe, IRL inferior right lateral lobe, ML median lobe, RML right portion of the medial lobe, LML left portion of the medial lobe, LLL left lateral lobe, MF median fissure, LF left fissure, RF right fissure and FL falciform ligament, PV portal vein, IVC inferior vena cava.

Figure 5.6. A) Visceral surface of the rat liver showing lobes and their mean relative weight. The liver mass of which lobe in the rat is quite constant. The caudate lobe is formed by the CP, AC and PC, the right liver lobe is formed by SRL and IRL, and the medial lobe formed by LM and RM. B) Visceral surface of a human liver showing division into segments according to Couinaud's nomenclature. The segment VIII is superior to the segment V and cannot bee see in this figure. According to Kongure K, in the rat, CL, LLL, LML, RML, (IRL+SRL) represent in humans segments I and IX, the segment II, segments III, IV, V, and VIII; and the segments VI and VII, respectively. In the rat, the left hemi-liver consists of the LLL, CL and LML while the right hemi-liver represents RL (SRL+IRL) and the RML.

Differently from humans, dogs, pigs and mice, rats do not have gallbladders. However, other mammals, like the horse and deer, do not have it either. The functional implications of that are not known (Mann 1920). Small intrahepatic bile ducts in rats are thought to correspond to bile ductules in humans and large bile ducts in rats may correspond to human interlobular bile ducts (Alpini 1996). The extrahepatic biliary ducts of the rat are more superficial and the CBD is proportionally longer compared to the human liver. Second order branches exist for the superior and inferior caudate lobes, right middle lobe and caudate process. There are many anatomical variations. For a thorough description of the rat biliary system, see Lorente (Lorente 1995). The extrahepatic biliary system of the rat has also intercommunicating branches that implies existence of a biliary network (Lorente 1995). This also implies that it may be difficult to produce cholestasis selectively in one of the hepatic lobes. The branches of the left middle lobe generally drain into branches of the left lateral lobe, implying the existence of a biliary functional inter-relationship between the left middle lobe and the left lateral lobe. The resection of the left lateral lobe can result in extrahepatic cholestasis of the left middle lobe in some animals. Thus, caution is necessary when trying to translate conclusions from hepatic resection models to humans (Lorente 1995; Lorente 1995; Martins 2007).

Unique from the human CBD, which has a short intra-pancreatic course and lies to the right of the portal vein and in close proximity to it and the hepatic artery, the rat CBD has a long trajectory inside the pancreas and to the left of the hepatic artery and the portal vein, which results in some distance between it and the hepatic artery and portal vein (Figure 5.1D). The CBD can be easily cannulated for experiments to measure bile flow, liver function or for anastomosis using a splint in liver transplantation. Most studies that cannulated the common bile duct used a polyethylene tubing (PE-10, inner diameter of 0.28 mm, outer diameter of 0.61 mm). However, a 24 gauge catheter can also be inserted into the CBD.

The origin and course of the major extrahepatic vessels are similar to humans. However, the branching pattern of the rat portal vein is different from humans. In the rat, the portal vein trifurcates, while in humans it bifurcates (Kogure 1999). Due to the fact that the rat liver is lobulated, there is no interdigitation between portal and venous pedicles; however, each one of the six sectors receives a portal pedicle and has its own venous pedicle (Lorente 1995). However, at microscopic level interdigitations may occur (Gershbein 1954). The inferior vena cava, differently from humans, is completely intrahepatic. The hepato-esophageal artery provides the liver with supra and infra-diaphragmatic systems of collateral circulation, once its ascending branches anastomose with branches of the mediastinal arteries and its descending branches communicate with the cardiac branches of the gastric artery. Thus, in experiments designed to provide arterial supply deprivation to the liver, the hepato-esophageal artery as a collateral route should be considered and previously ligated (Delong 1953).

Pancreas Anatomy

Rats are commonly used as experimental models for partial and total pancreatectomy. It is important to note that the biliary system in rats has numerous anatomical variations. After introducing latex dye into the biliopancreatic duct, portal vein and arteries, pancreas anatomy present in rats was further delineated as seen in a study by ME Kara, et al. (Kara 2005). The pancreas was subsequently divided into three parts following latex injection: biliary, duodenal, and gastrosplenic. The biliopancreatic and pancreatic ducts, biliary, and duodenal portions of the pancreas can be visualized with relative ease by retracting the duodenum caudally. The gastrosplenic portion of the pancreas was seen between the descending duodenum and transverse colon on the right side just caudal to the liver. In order to visualize the pancreas in its entirety, it was necessary to remove the stomach and duodenum. This maneuver also permitted visualization of the pancreaticoduodenal, right gastroepiploic and splenic vessels, and portal vein.

In the study by Kara, et al., the biliopancreatic duct diameter and length of ducts was found to be 1.01 ± 0.03 and 28.86 ± 0.59 mm, respectively. The anterior pancreatic duct originated from the biliopancreatic duct on different sides and was found to drain the entire gastrosplenic portion and part of the duodenal portion of the pancreas. The posterior pancreatic duct opened into the biliopancreatic duct and was found to do this at the level of the papilla in more than 1/3 of specimens, which is an important consideration when ligating the biliopancreatic duct at the level of the duodenal opening. The posterior pancreatic duct also carries the exocrine secretion from the duodenal portion of the pancreas to the biliopancreatic duct. Numerous minor ducts were also noted that drained all three portions of the pancreas directly into the biliopancreatic duct (Kara 2005). A thorough understanding of the anatomy found in the rat pancreas is imperative when using this model to study pancreatic transplantation and regeneration, treatment of pancreatitis, and metabolic or endocrine studies (Figures 5.7–5.11).

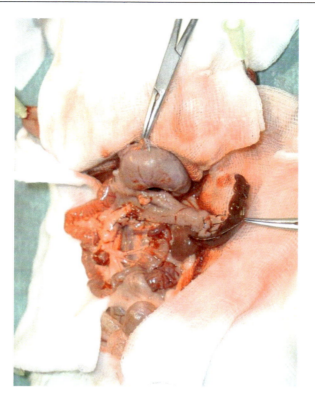

Figure 5.7 Rat pancreas.

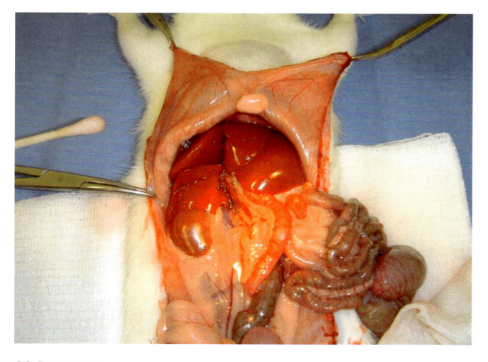

Figure 5.8. Rat pancreas.

Hepatopancreatobiliary Surgery Experimental Models 119

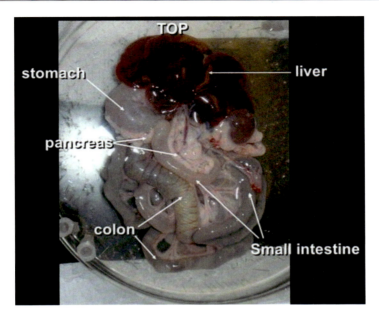

Figure 5.9. Image of rat pancreas illustrating the viscera, immediately post-harvest, in the dissection dish. Note the pins located around the edge of the dish and the black acrylic sheet under the dish. Schloithe AC, Woods CM, Saccone GTP. An isolated rat pancreas preparation for studying pancreatic spinal mechanosensitive and chemosensitive afferent activity. Version 1.0, April 26, 2011 [DOI: 10.3998/panc.2011.13]. The Pancreapedia. www.pancreapedia.org. Free use under Creative Commons Sharealike license.

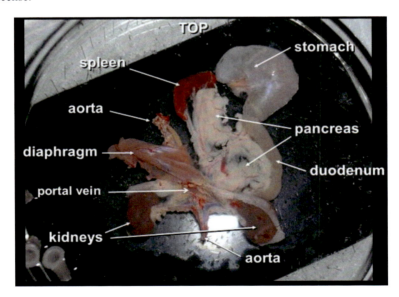

Figure 5.10. Image of a preliminary dissection of rat pancreas. Note that the aorta is oriented roughly north-south with the kidneys on either side. The stomach is positioned upper most, the duodenal segment on the right, the pancreas central and the spleen on the upper left. Schloithe AC, Woods CM, Saccone GTP. An isolated rat pancreas preparation for studying pancreatic spinal mechanosensitive and chemosensitive afferent activity. Version 1.0, April 26, 2011 [DOI: 10.3998/panc.2011.13]. The Pancreapedia. www.pancreapedia.org. Free use under Creative Commons Sharealike license.

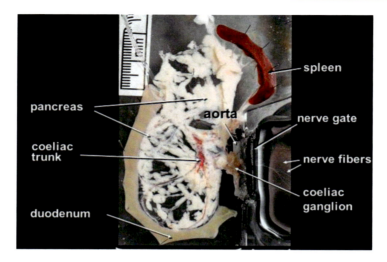

Figure 5.11. Image of the final preparation of rat pancreas (with duodenal segment retained for orientation) pinned in the Krebs-bath. Note that the duodenal segment is normally removed. The spleen is usually retained as it provides a means of maintaining the pancreas in a stretched state without the direct insertion of pins in the pancreas. The nerve trunks with teased bundles and fibers are visible in the nerve-bath. A scale bar is included in the image (1 division = 1 mm). Schloithe AC, Woods CM, Saccone GTP. An isolated rat pancreas preparation for studying pancreatic spinal mechanosensitive and chemosensitive afferent activity. Version 1.0, April 26, 2011 [DOI: 10.3998/panc.2011.13]. The Pancreapedia. www.pancreapedia.org. Free use under Creative Commons Sharealike license.

HEPATECTOMY MODELS

Introduction

Hepatic resections in rodents are performed to study liver regeneration, acute liver failure, tumor dormancy of hepatic metastasis, hepatic function, and response to stress and trauma (Higgins 1931; Bucher 1964; Weinbren 1965; Aleksandrowicz 1981; Rozga 1986; Lin 1990; Panis 1990; de Jong 1995; de Jong 1998; Lu 1999; Fausto 2005). Each lobe has its own pedicle containing a portal triad, and as a result hepatic resections of various extents in rodents are simple and highly reproducible. Hepatectomies both in the rat and mouse require basic surgical skills and have been performed with high success rates (Higgins 1931; Weinbren 1965; Pinto 1987; Lorente 1995; Rodriguez 1999; Fausto 2005; Madrahimov 2006; Martins 2007). In this review, we outline various models, different techniques and limitations of hepatic resections.

Models of Liver Resection

The classic rat model of partial hepatectomy in rats is based on the seminal experiments by Higgins and Anderson from 1931 (Higgins 1931). These investigations demonstrated that resection of the two anterior lobes (median and left lateral lobes) is easy to perform and creates a highly standardized liver reduction of approximately 70%. The classical 70% hepatectomy model in rats is the most popular because it has been extensively studied and can be accomplished in an expedited fashion with a single ligature of the common pedicle (Higgins 1931; Rodriguez 1999). It is also commonly employed in auxiliary liver transplantation models (Wang 2002).

In other models, 90%, 95% and 97% liver tissue resections are employed to study liver regeneration and acute liver failure (Gaub 1984; Emond 1989; Madrahimov 2006). In the 90% hepatectomy the right lobes, median lobe, and the left lateral lobe are resected. In the 95% hepatectomy model, the anterior caudate lobe is also removed, while in the 97% hepatectomy the anterior and posterior caudate lobes are removed, and only the paracaval portion remains. Other extents of resection can also be performed, however with more technical difficulty and higher complication rates (Figure 5.12).

In the mouse the relative volume of the lobes slightly differs from the rat. The right superior lobe represents 16.6 ± 1.4%, the right inferior 14.7 ± 1.4%, the median lobe 26.2 ± 1.9%, and the left lateral lobe represents 34.4 ± 1.9% (Inderbitzin 2004), while in the rat it represents approximately 22%, 10%, 38%, 30%, respectively (Lorente 1995; Madrahimov 2006; Martins 2007). On the other hand, in humans, the average volume ratios of the left lateral segments (II and III), left medial segment (IV), caudate lobe (I and IX), right anterior segments (V and VIII), and right posterior segments (VI and VII) are 17%, 14%, 2%, 37%, and 30%, respectively (Leelaudomlipi 2002).

Commonly performed partial hepatectomies in mice remove 60% (ML+LL), 75% (ML+LL+IRL) and 83% (ML+LL+IRL+CL) of the liver parenchyma (Inderbitzin 2004, Inderbitzin 2006). Twenty-one days after resection of the ML and LL in the mouse, the remaining lobes IRL, SRL, AC, and PC represent 55%, 26%, 9%, and 10%, respectively (Nikfarjam 2004).

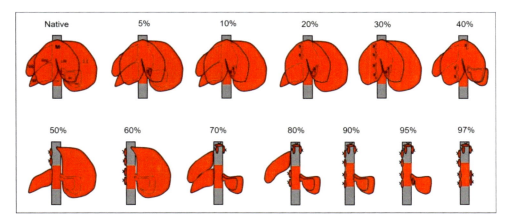

Figure 5.12. Schematic description of partial hepatectomies in the rat (anterior view of the liver) and approximate parenchymal volumes. These values slightly change in the mouse (refer to the text). Hepatectomies ranging from 5 to 95% of total liver weight can be easily performed with high reproducibility using microsurgical techniques, since the parenchymal mass of which lobe is relatively constant. Approximately, the percentages of liver weight per lobe are: SRL 12%, IRL 10%, ML 38% (RML 25% and LML 13%), LLL 30%, AC 4%, PC 4%, CP 2–3%. In the classic 70%-hepatectomy, the left lateral (LL) and the medial (ML) lobes are removed. Isolated resections of the MLL or LLL should preferentially not be performed since cholestatic and vascular complications are more common.

The Liver Regeneration Model

The process of hepatic regeneration in rodents and humans are similar, and the results obtained from rodents are applicable to the human liver (Fausto 2001). The rat 70% hepatectomy is the most valuable and most extensively studied animal model for liver regeneration (Higgins 1931; Rodriguez 1999; Fausto 2005).

The hepatic regeneration process is triggered promptly after injury, and in the rat, the DNA replication begins as early as 16 hours after resection. After a 70%-hepatectomy in the rat, the weight of the liver remnant at 24 and 72 hours is 45% and 70% of the original liver weight, respectively. Between 7 and 14 days, the liver volume is 93%, and by day 20 it completely recovers its original volume by hyperplasia of the remaining lobes (Higgins 1931). Also in humans, the regeneration process occurs quickly. The liver mass doubled at 7 days in the donor liver and 14 days in the recipient after right-lobe transplantation. Donor and recipient livers reached their original weight by 60 days after surgery. However, despite recovery of parenchymal weight the regeneration and remodeling processes continue.

The speed of liver regeneration is proportional to the amount of hepatic tissue resected. (Marcos 2000). Interestingly, it has also been shown that the regenerative capacity of individual remnant lobes is significantly different (Inderbitzin 2006). In addition, too large (> 85%) or too small (< 30%) resections may result in slow cell proliferation (Fausto 2001).

Models for Assessment of Hepatic Metastasis

Models of hepatectomy have been used in studies of liver metastasis after direct hepatic inoculation, or after intraportal or intra-splenic injection of tumor cells. The induction of tumor by carcinogens in the rat with spontaneous liver metastases closely mimics the natural history of colon cancer. However, only a low yield of primary cancer, e.g., colonic cancer (in less than 50% of cases) and liver metastases (approx. 25%) is obtained after 6 months of latency. Direct intraportal injection of colon carcinoma cells is the most frequently used model. Although it bypasses the natural evolution of colon cancer, this simple model produces liver metastases 6 weeks after injection of tumor cells in up to 100% of cases. This model has been used to study tumor biology, tumor induced angiogenesis, surgical and adjuvant therapy for liver metastasis, as well as the influence of hepatic regeneration on reactivation of dormant metastases and tumor growth (Panis 1990).

In this model, 8 weeks after injection of colon carcinoma cells (DHD K12 cells) into the portal vein of BD IX rats, 60% of animals did not show apparent liver metastases. However, after a 70% hepatectomy, 12 weeks after the injection of colon carcinoma cells, 62% of these animals developed macroscopic metastases compared to 20% in sham operated controls. This means that liver micrometastases may have been present at 8 weeks and had not developed until stimulation by liver regeneration after hepatectomy (Panis 1990; Panis 1992). In cases of random spread of hepatic metastases, tumorectomy alone, non-anatomical resections (wedge resection), and segmentectomies may be employed.

Models of Acute Liver Failure

Models of acute liver failure are important to investigate the underlying molecular mechanisms and to test liver-support strategies. These models are divided into: toxic-induced, surgically induced (partial hepatectomy, clamping) or mixed. Surgical models of acute liver failure are divided into: total hepatectomy, partial hepatectomy, and partial or total liver devascularization (Rahman 2000).

Small-for-Size Syndrome

Models of hepatic resection and partial liver transplantation have also been used to study small for size syndrome. One study showed that immediately after classical 70% hepatectomy the hepatic arterial blood flow decreased (from 0.4 ± 0.12 to 0.33 ± 0.03 ml/min/g liver), the portal venous inflow increased (from 0.90 ± 0.30 to 2.20 ± 0.26 ml/min/g liver), the total hepatic blood flow increased (from 1.30 ± 0.39 to 2.53 ± 0.26 ml/min/g liver), and the portal pressure elevated (from 8.80 ± 0.7 to 11.9 ± 1.7 cm H_2O) (Lin 1990).

Portal hyperperfusion in small-for-size livers, in cases of major hepatic resections or transplantation, may seriously impair postoperative liver regeneration. The altered physiologic state results in increased portal blood flow, which induces shear stress and damage to sinusoidal endothelial cells and Kupffer cell activation which contributes to acute liver failure (Glanemann 2005). In these models, a major hepatic resection (e.g., 90%) or a total hepatectomy followed by small-for-size graft (25 to 30% of original volume) liver transplantation are performed (Panis 1997; Glanemann 2005; Yao 2007; Zhong 2007). When transplantation is used as a model, a classical 70% hepatectomy is performed in the donor animal before harvesting the organ.

Following a 70% resection, nearly 100% of rats survive (Emond 1989). Larger resections result in hyperperfusion of the remnant liver and ischemia/reperfusion injury (small-for-size syndrome) with subsequent massive fatty change, congestion, and centrilobular necrosis (Panis 1997). Panis and colleagues showed increased necrosis following progressive increase in the hepatectomy extent (Panis 1997). Following a 75%, > 85%, and > 90% hepatectomy, survival rates were 100%, 18% and 0%, respectively. The increased mortality associated with large resections can be reduced by administration of glucose solution (Gaub 1984; Roger 1996). The survival rate of 90%-hepatectomy could be increased from 5% to 60% by addition of glucose 20% in drinking water (Gaub 1984, Emond 1989). Roger introduced the 95% hepatectomy with survival rate of only 20%, even with addition of glucose (Roger 1996). Madrahinov reported a 1-week survival rate of 100% and 66% following a 90% and 95%, respectively. However, in this study, all animals died of liver failure within 4 days after a 97% hepatectomy (Madrahimov 2006).

Eguchi et al. described a model of resection-ligation (Eguchi 1997). In this model, the left lateral and median lobes (68%) were resected, and the ligated right liver lobes (24%) were left in place; the caudal lobes (8%) were left intact. They reported a 90% mortality rate at 48hr after surgery, proceeded by grade III encephalopathy beginning at 22−24hr, and associated with deterioration of liver function tests, and increased ammonia and lactate levels.

In the mouse, Inderbitzin et al. showed that liver regeneration was excellent in up to 75% partial hepatectomy. On the other hand, 83% resection resulted in animal death after 2–4 days (Inderbitzin 2006). However, in this experiment only one subcutaneous dose (1 ml) of glucose 1% was given postoperatively. One other study showed that all of the 70%-hepatectomized mice were alive at 1 week, but the 90%-hepatectomized mice all died within 24 hours after hepatectomy despite free access to glucose 10% (Makino 2005).

Techniques of Liver Resection

Liver resections in rodents are very well tolerated with minimal operative mortality. So far, four techniques for hepatic resection in rodents have been described:

1. *The classical technique* (Ligature *en-bloc* at the base of the lobe). Although this is the most commonly used technique, it carries the highest risk for injuries because the mass ligature may compromise elements of other pedicles. The risk of vena cava stenosis and liver congestion is particularly high when only one ligature for both the median and left lateral lobes' pedicles is performed, due to compression of the vein after mass ligation. This procedure can be performed through conventional (open), or laparoscopic technique (Higgins 1931; Ralli 1951; Krahenbuhl 1998). However, the laparoscopic approach does not seem to provide any advantage over other techniques. It is time-consuming and requires specialized and costly equipment.
2. *The hemostatic clip technique.* This is a slight modification of the classical technique, where titanium clips are applied to the pedicle instead of using sutures. This procedure is fast, but is associated with similar complications of the mass ligature technique. In addition, concerns with interference on the regeneration process have been raised, although this has not been confirmed in subsequent investigations (Schaeffer 1994; Nikfarjam 2004).
3. *The vessel-oriented parenchyma-preserving technique.* This technique reported by Madrahimov requires no prior ligation at the liver hilum (Madrahimov 2006). Sequential piercing sutures, proximal to clamp, are positioned according to topographic vascular anatomy. Although this technique is faster than the microsurgical technique (described below), it may cause injury of other vascular branches since vessels are not individually visualized. Therefore, it is not recommended for resection of the right or left segments of the median lobe.
4. *The vessel-oriented microsurgical technique.* This technique, first reported by Kubota et al., is similar to the technique for clinical hepatectomies (Kubota 1997). The portal vein and hepatic artery branches are ligated prior to the resection of the lobe, and the hepatic veins are ligated within the lobe during parenchyma resection (in a similar fashion of the parenchyma preserving technique). The advantages of this technique are reduced risk of bleeding from the stump and reduced risk of vena cava constriction. It is also more appropriate for segmental hepatectomies, e.g., resection of the right or left portion of the median lobe, after delineation of the ischemic line following the ligature. The disadvantages include requirement of microsurgical skills and equipment, risk of portal vein injury during dissection, and its more time-consuming nature (Kubota 1997).

Liver Resections Using Microsurgical Techniques

Hepatic resection may be improved by microsurgical techniques because they permit individualized dissection and ligature of small vascular and biliary branches of the median and left lateral liver lobes, while avoiding damage to the remaining lobes and other complications (tear of extra-hepatic biliary tree and biliary fistula, vena cava stenosis). This contributes to reduce complications and make results more homogenous.

To our knowledge, the first description of the use of microsurgery to perform hepatectomy in rodents was from Holmin in 1982. However, he used a microscope (10x magnification) not to perform the parenchymal dissection and resection but to perform a portacaval shunt before a total hepatectomy in a rat model of acute liver failure (Holmin 1982). In fact, Rodriguez in 1999 was the first to report the use of a microscope to perform vascular isolation of individual pedicles for partial hepatectomies in the rat (Rodriguez 1999). In a study from Higgins, utilizing the classical technique without optical magnification, the postoperative mortality rate following a 70% hepatectomy was 25% (n = 220), Rodriguez reported no morbidity and 0% mortality (n = 20) utilizing the microscopic approach (Higgins 1931, Rodriguez 1999). Another study published by Greene et al. obtained 96% survival rate after 70% hepatectomy in the mouse model using magnifying operative loupes (Greene 2003).

Non-Conventional Anatomical Resections

Microsurgical techniques permit anatomical segmentectomies. Isolated resection of the left lateral lobe or median lobe as well as segmental resections of the left or right portion of the median lobe represents a technical challenge. Although the left lateral lobe is easily resectable, care should be taken to avoid ligature of the branches to the median lobe, which will lead to ischemia of the lateral aspect of this lobe. In addition, some biliary ducts of the left median lobe may drain into branches of the left lateral lobe, implying the existence of a biliary functional interrelationship between the left medial lobe and the left lateral lobe. Thus, the isolated resection of either the left lateral lobe or median lobe may sometimes result in cholestasis of the adjacent lobe (Lorente 1995; Lorente 1995).

Isolated resection of the right or left sectors of the median lobe and resection of the superior or inferior aspect of the left lateral lobe requires delicate dissection of the hilar region and intrahepatic ligation of individual vascular and biliary branches. For resection of the right portion of the median lobe (which represents segments IV, V and VIII in humans according to Kongure), the inferior pedicle of the median lobe (which is the first portal branch to the median lobe together with the arterial branch) should be ligated *en-bloc* and divided (Kogure 1999). The superior pedicle of the median lobe lies close to the superior aspect of the superior right lobe. For resection of the left portion of the median lobe (which represents segments III in humans), the second portal branch (superior pedicle) to this lobe should be ligated and divided (Kogure 1999). It lies in close proximity to the hepatic vein draining the left portion of this lobe and can be easily visualized after removal of the overlying peritoneum (Figure 5.13).

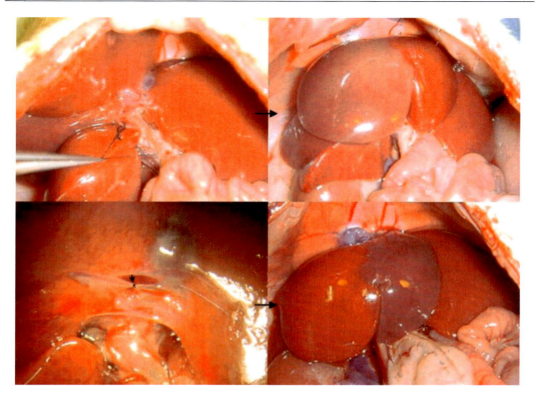

Figure 5.13. Ligature of the inferior pedicle of the median lobe of the rat liver. This pedicle (shown here suture ligated) supplies the right portion of the right median lobe (RML). The superior pedicle of the median lobe is depicted here by the asterisk (*). C and D) Ligation of the superior pedicle of the median lobe (in Figure C, magnification 20X). The superior pedicle of the median lobe supplies the left portion (LML) and is shown here suture ligated (arrow). The location of inferior pedicle of the median lobe is marked here by the asterisk (*). Shortly after these ligations, an ischemic line (dotted line) on the medial lobe ML (B and D) equivalent to the Cantlie's line can be seen on the falciform ligament insertion line, from the suprahepatic vena cava to the main liver fissure (umbilical fissure). The resection of the RML (equivalent in humans to segments IV, V and VIII) and the LML (equivalent to segment III in humans) can only be performed using microsurgical techniques. Dissection and ligation should be very careful to avoid injuries of the vascular and biliary system of the adjacent segment. Scale bar 0.6 cm.

The left lateral lobe also has two vascular pedicles (inferior and superior) and two independent venous drainages, which permits anatomical segmentectomies in this lobe (Lorente 1995; Madrahimov 2006; Martins 2007). The first vascular pedicle, inferior to part of the LLL, lies on the bottom of this lobe while the second is located superior-posterior and close to the left hepatic vein (Figure 5.14). In either one of these segmentectomies (left medial or right medial), after ligating the vascular pedicle, the ischemic line can be visualized on both surfaces of the liver. Then, the parenchyma can be resected 2 mm away from the perfused area. These segmentectomies are more difficult to perform in the mouse because the structures are much smaller and more delicate (the mouse is in average 20 times smaller than a rat).

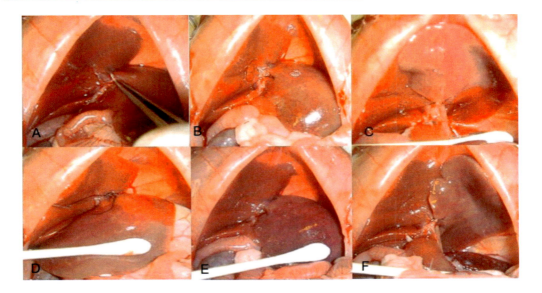

Figure 5.14. A–C) Ligature of the inferior vascular pedicle of the left lateral lobe (arrow) of the rat liver demarcates an ischemic line (dotted line) on the anterior (B) and posterior (C) surface of this lobe. This ischemic area represents ¾ of the LLL and either represents an individual segment, equivalent to the human segment III, or is a subsegment of the LLL. D–F) After ligature of the inferior pedicle (arrow), the superior vascular pedicle was ligated (*) and the whole left lateral lobe turned to be ischemic. The area supplied by the superior pedicle may be the equivalent of the segment II in humans. Magnification 2X.

The individual isolation of the portal vein branch from the arterial branch and bile duct may be necessary in some experiments that investigate individual effects of arterial or portal isolation. This dissection is difficult to perform, since they are fragile and closely adherent and surrounded by connective tissue. One maneuver that helps this dissection is flushing pressured saline solution with a syringe close to the pedicle elements. The author successfully used this technique to perform vascular dissection in a kidney transplantation model (Martins 2006). Hydrodissection can display the correct plane of dissection while reducing risks of injuries.

The main advantage of hepatectomies employing microsurgical techniques is that it is possible to perform several extents of hepatectomy, including segmental resections, while reducing the risks of vascular and cholestatic complications.

Limitations of Rodent Models of Hepatic Resections

The use of rat and mouse models in liver surgery research is limited by their small size and limited knowledge on the liver anatomy (Lorente 1995; Lorente 1995; Martins 2007). As in humans, the rat and mouse liver vasculature and biliary system show a great anatomical variability. In addition, the liver anatomy of rodents and its correlation to the human liver is not completely understood.

Table 5.1. Comparison of rat and human liver

RAT LIVER	HUMAN LIVER
Multi-lobulated liver	Liver lobes have no clear anatomical divisions (liver appears to be single anatomic unit)
Long celiac trunk	Short celiac trunk
Inferior vena cava is intra-hepatic	Inferior vena cava is retroperitoneal
Gallbladder absent	Gallbladder present
CBD lies to the left of portal vein and has a long intra-pancreatic trajectory	CBD lies to the right of the portal vein and has a short pancreatic trajectory
Collateral arterial circulation is common (Hepato-esophageal artery)	Collateral arterial circulation is uncommon
Intercommunications between portal and venous pedicle is common	Vein intercommunications is not common
Divisions of the caudate lobe is distinct	Caudate lobe has no clear-cut anatomical subdivisions
Trifurcation of the portal vein	Bifurcation of the portal vein
"Left-" and "right liver" have similar volume	"Right liver" volume is superior to the "left liver"

The best anatomical model proposed so far is from Kongure and colleagues. In this model, the whole left lateral lobe corresponds to the human segment II and the left median lobe corresponds to segment III. However, his study did not consider that the left lateral lobe has two individual vascular supplies and drainages, which are prerequisites for segmental denomination. Based on topography and proportions, the small superior segment of the left lateral lobe could be considered equivalent to the human segment II and the larger inferior segment to the human segment III. If this is the case, the left median lobe would be equivalent to the segment IV, while the right median lobe would be equivalent only to segments V and VIII. The falciform ligament in humans runs from a point to the left of the vena cava to a point to the left of the gallbladder, and the area between the falciform ligament and the Cantlie's line (imaginary line from the vena cava to the gallbladder) represents the segment IV. Kongure proposed the equivalence of the rat segments assuming that the location of the rat falciform ligament is the same as in humans. If we consider the falciform ligament to define the nomenclature of the rat liver lobes, the left median lobe could be the equivalent to segment III because it lies directly to the left of the falciform ligament. However, in the mouse, which is phylogenetically much closer to the rat, the falciform ligament lies between the vena cava and gallbladder, located in the main liver fissure (Figure 5.2). The main fissure marks the division of the medial lobe into left and right portions. Similarly, to the mouse, the rat falciform ligament runs between the vena cava and the main liver fissure (the rat has no gallbladder) and may have the equivalent position to the Cantlie's line in humans. Taking these facts into consideration, the rat left median lobe could be the equivalent to segment IV, and not to segment III.

One pitfall of segmentectomies of the right or left portion of the median lobe is that they may be associated with liver congestion in the animals in which the vein draining the left portion of the median lobe joins the left hepatic vein (draining the left lateral lobe) to form a common trunk before draining to the vena cava. In addition, some biliary ducts of the left median lobe may drain into branches of the left lateral lobe, implying the existence of a biliary functional interrelationship between the left medial lobe and the left lateral lobe. Thus, the isolated resection of either the left lateral lobe or median lobe may sometimes result in cholestasis of the adjacent lobe (Lorente 1995; Lorente 1995; Martins 2007).

Results obtained in rodent models cannot be fully translated to humans because the kinetics of liver regeneration in different species is not the same. The amount of remnant hepatic tissue compatible with life in rodents seems to be less than in humans. While in humans the maximum amount of liver that can be tolerated is 70−80% of the original volume, rodents can survive even after a 90−95% hepatectomy (Shirabe 1999; Fan 2000; Renz 2000; Leelaudomlipi 2002; Schindl 2005; Madrahimov 2006). Table 5.1 compares rat to human livers.

Models of acute liver failure based only on reduction of liver mass (hepatectomy) are in general not reversible and not associated with the same level of tissue damage and necrosis commonly seen in clinical setting (caused by toxic and viral agents). In order to overcome this problem one can subsequently add liver stress after liver resection with tissue ischemia (clamping) or toxic agents. Another model proposed a combination of major liver resection with hepatocyte transplantation as a possible approach to recover liver function (Roger 1996).

CIRRHOSIS, PORTAL HYPERTENSION MODELS, AND PORTACAVAL SHUNTS

Portal hypertension models are important to the study of the pathophysiology of liver disturbances, liver regeneration, complications and treatment approaches. The models can be categorized as toxic (e.g., carbon tetrachloride (CCl_4), alcohol), nutritional (feeding choline deficient or methionine deficient diet), surgical (partial portal vein ligation, bile duct ligation), immunological (heterologous serum, schistosomiasis), and genetic (Rhino mice) (Tsukamoto 1990; Orloff 2001; Abraldes 2006; Abraldes 2006) (Table 5.2). Other toxic agents that have been used in diverse animal models to produce cirrhosis, include carbon tetrachloride, dimethylnitrosamine, thioacetamine, monocrotaline, and alcohol (Groszmann 1982; Proctor 1984; Tsukamoto 1985; Dashti 1989; Perazzo 1999). Rodents are the most utilized models because of low cost and easy handling. The most common model of cirrhosis is the CCL_4 model. It can be given via injection, inhalation, or orally. Liver cirrhosis is expedited by giving phenobarbital added to the drinking water (cirrhosis obtained in 4 to 6 weeks).

Acute administration of carbon tetrachloride induces acute hepatitis. Continuous administration induces chronic liver injury that leads to cirrhosis. Route of administration varies among laboratories, but the most effective are oral, intraperitoneal or inhalatory routes. Twelve to 15 weeks after CCl_4 administration, the rats develop micronodular cirrhosis (Proctora 1982; Kobayashi 2000; Hernandez-Munoz 2001; Constandinou 2005; Abraldes 2006).

Cirrhosis induced by thioacetamide (TAA) is another widely used model of toxic cirrhosis. The toxin affects both perivenular and periportal areas. It has been used in rats and mice (Li 2002, Okuyama 2005). TAA can be administered in drinking water or by intraperitoneal injection (Li 2002; Luo 2004; Popov 2006). Intraperitoneal injection offers much more consistent results (Popov 2006). This model develops macronodular cirrhosis with portal hypertension in 12 weeks (Abraldes 2006).

Table 5.2. Experimental Models of Hepatic Fibrosis/Cirrhosis. Adapted from Tsukamoto H, et al.

Species		Method	Fibrosis	Cirrhosis
Toxic				
• Carbon tetrachloride (CCl₄)	Rats	Subcutaneous injection, 0.1-0.2ml/100g of body weight twice weekly	>6 weeks	>12 weeks
	Rats	Inhalation twice weekly plus sodium phenobarbital in drinking water	>1-2weeks	>4 weeks
• Dimethylnitrosamine (DMNA)	Rats	Intraperitoneal injection 3 days weekly	>4 weeks	>13 weeks
	Dogs			
• Thioacetamide (TAA)	Rats	Oral administration 2 days weekly TAA in drinking water (300mg/L)	>3-4weeks >2-3 months	>13 weeks >3months
Nutritional	Rats/mice	High-fat/low-choline, low-protein diet	>6weeks	>12-24 weeks
Immunologic				
• Heterologous serum	Rats	Low-protein/low-methionine diet plus ethionine (0.5%)	>4weeks	>12weeks
• Bacterial cell wall	Rats	Swine serum, intraperitoneal injection twice weekly	>5 weeks	>10 weeks
• Marine schistosomiasis	Rats	Streptococcal cell wall, single intraperitoneal injection (20mg/g of body weight)	>6weeks	--
• Endotoxin	Mice	Subcutaneous injection, 50 *cercariae* of *Schistosoma mansoni*	>6weeks	--
	Rabbits	*E. coli* endotoxin injection into the common bile duct (0.2/mg) followed 24 h later by 0.1/mg via marginal ear vein	--	>9 days
Biliary				
	Rats	Common bile duct ligation	>4 weeks	--
	Dogs	Common bile duct ligation	>4 weeks	--
	Monkeys	Common bile duct ligation	>2months	>6 months
Alcoholic				
	Baboons	Ethanol-containing liquid diet, *ad lib*	>6 months	>24 months
	Rats	Continuous intragastric infusion of ethanol and a high-fat diet	>3 months	--
Genetic				
	Rhino mice	Mutant with the anatomical recessive gene	>6 months	--

Dimethilnitrosamine induced cirrhosis (DMNA) DMNA is another hepatotoxin that induces hepatocellular necrosis. After continuous administration (generally intraperitoneal) the rats develop fibrosis with portal hypertension, which may be present as early as 5 weeks despite the fact that animals do not have cirrhosis nor features of hyperdynamic circulation (Veal 2000). Overt cirrhosis with ascites develops in 13 weeks (Jenkins 1985; Tsukamoto 1990).

Diet induced cirrhosis is seen in diets deficient in choline and methionin, or a diet with low protein and choline and enriched with fat, induces liver steatosis associated with marked oxidative stress that induces inflammation and fibrosis (Tsukamoto 1990; Nanji 2004). Cirrhosis develops after 12 to 24 weeks.

Partial Portal Vein Ligation

Partial portal vein ligation model (PVL) has been widely used in the study of the pathophysiology of portal hypertension. This model has been developed in rats, mice, and rabbits (Vorobioff 1983; Colombato 1992; Castaneda 2000; Iwakiri 2002; Fernandez 2004). The portal vein is freed from surrounding tissue after a midline abdominal incision. A ligature (silk 3-0) is placed around a blunt-tipped needle lying along the portal vein. Subsequent removal of the needle yields a calibrated stenosis of the portal vein that has the diameter of the needle. In the conventional rat PVL model a 20G needle is used (0.889 mm diameter) (Vorobioff 1983, Colombato 1992, Castaneda 2000). By using needles of greater caliber, less severe stenosis and thus less severe degrees of portal hypertension are induced (Lozeva 2004, Abraldes 2006). The diameters of the needles and resulting levels of stenosis are as follows: 16G: 1.651 mm, 18G: 1.270 mm, 20G: 0.889 mm. The conventional needles for mice and rabbits are 27G (Iwakiri 2002; Fernandez 2004).

Bile Duct Ligation

Cholestasis is a common pathological condition that can be reproduced in rodents by surgical ligation of the common bile duct. Common bile duct ligation (CBDL) is a model of secondary biliary cirrhosis. Evaluation of the various time-related changes after BDL is paramount for the interpretation of available data as well as for the design of future studies.

A Systematic Chronological Evaluation of Hepatocellular Injury and Proliferation, Hepatic Inflammation or the Development of Liver Fibrosis Following BDL

The intervention consists of the isolation of the common bile duct followed by a double ligature. The first ligature is made below the junction of the hepatic ducts and the other above the pancreatic duct. The portion of the bile duct between the two ligatures can be resected to avoid recannulation. Mortality is high after the fifth week (20%). The use of prophylactic antibiotics (Ampicilin 100 mg/kg s.c. or similar) before surgery and weekly administration of vitamin K (50 mcg subcutaneous) notably improve the survival of CBDL rats. At 2 weeks rats develop mild portal hypertension and at 4 weeks severe portal hypertension, hyperdynamic circulation and portal-systemic shunting of 30−60% (Franco 1979; Beck 1995).

Serum levels of ALT and biliary infarcts increased after BDL, peaking at days 2 and 3 respectively. Following acute or chronic tissue loss, hepatocytes mount a proliferative response. BDL induced a distinct peak of hepatocellular proliferation at day 5, approximately 48 hours after the peak of histologically detectable hepatocellular injury. After the initial peak on day 5, continuous proliferation was observed at a low level. The proportion of continuously proliferating hepatocytes is in the range of 1 to 3% (Ezure 2000; Georgiev 2008).

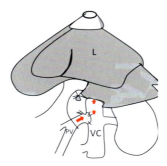

Figure 5.15. End-to-side portacaval shunt. *Abbreviations:* L liver. VC vena cava, PV portal vein. Adapted from Castaing D, et al.

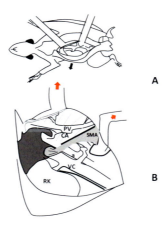

Figure 5.16. A) Ventral view of rat abdomen with retractors in place. The median lobe of the liver, the abdominal viscera and the mesoduodenum are covered with a wet gauze and retracted to the left. Vena cava, portal vein, right kidney and celiac area are exposed. B) Right lateral view of the infra-hepatic area. CA celiac axis, RK right kidney, VC vena cava, PV portal vein, A aorta, SMA superior mesenteric artery. Adapted from Castaing D, et al.

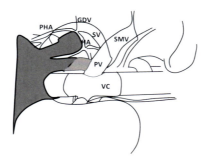

Figure 5.17. Anatomical configuration after the shunt. GDV gastroduodenal vein, HA hepatic artery, LGA left gastric artery, PV portal vein, SV splenic vein, VC vena cava. Adapted from Castaing D, et al.

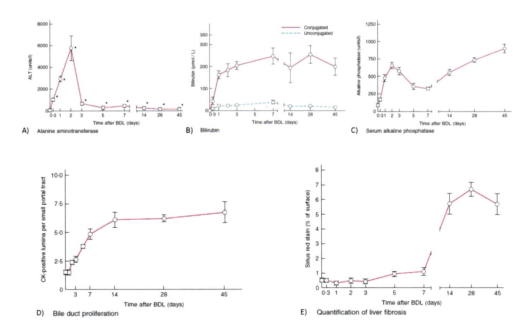

Figure 5.18. Liver injury was determined by A) serum alanine aminotransferase (ALT) levels. Serum levels of A) conjugated and unconjugated bilirubin and B) alkaline phosphatase. Percentage of liver surface stained with Sirius red. Values are mean (s.e.m.) for five to six individual animals per time point. *$P < 0.050$ *versus* sham-operated control (two-tailed Mann–Whitney test). Adapted from Georgiev, et al.

Serum levels of alkaline phosphatase and bilirubin are classical markers of obstructive cholestasis in the clinical setting (Pratt 2005). Raised serum levels of alkaline phosphatase are due to *de novo* synthesis in the liver (Kaplan 1970). Interestingly, serum levels of alkaline phosphatase were not found to increase progressively after BDL. A first peak during the acute phase was followed by decreasing levels from day 3 to day 7, indicating that the acute injury triggers a massive production and release of this enzyme.

BDL results in an increase in serum markers of cholestasis such as bilirubin and alkaline phosphatase. Conjugated and unconjugated bilirubin levels increased steadily and in parallel until day 7 and remained high thereafter (Figure 5.18). Alkaline phosphatase production is induced after BDL in rats and its release from the canalicular membrane of hepatocytes is modulated by bile acids. Serum levels of alkaline phosphatase showed a biphasic course, peaking on day 2 and then increasing steadily from day 7 onwards; cell proliferation reached a steady state in the biliary epithelial cells (BEL) compartment by day 1.

Neutrophils contribute to cholestatic liver injury after BDL for 3 days, whereas Kupffer cells are believed to abrogate acute cholestatic liver injury through the release of interleukin 6 (Gujral 2003; Gujral 2004; Gehring 2006). Little attention has been paid to the role of lymphocytes, which are known to modulate liver fibrosis in other models of liver disease (Wynn 2004; Novobrantseva 2005). The histological analysis indicated that both B and T cells were present in the portal tracts of mice after day 5 of BDL. Interestingly, both cell types accumulated mainly during the phase of collagen deposition and thus may also be involved in the process of fibrogenesis following BDL (Gujral 2003; Georgiev 2008).

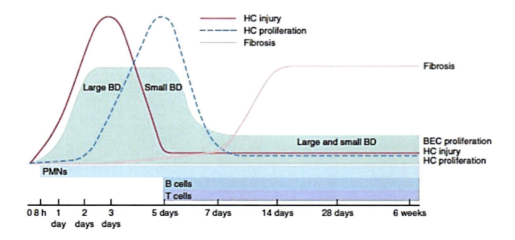

Figure 5.19. Overview of dynamic changes following bile duct ligation in mice. BD, bile duct; BEC, biliary epithelial cell; HC, hepatocyte; PMN, polymorphonuclear leucocyte.

This model develops biliary fibrosis-cirrhosis in 4 to 6 weeks. Histology shows marked cholangiolar proliferation and expansive portal fibrosis (Figure 5.19), but the architectural disturbances typical of cirrhosis are seldom found (Kountouras 1984). See Figures 5.18–5.19.

PORTACAVAL SHUNTS

In 1877, Dr. Eck described experiments using portacaval shunt in dogs (Eck fistula) (Rocko 1985). Lee and Fisher in 1961 perfected the technique of portacaval shunt in the rat so that it became a reproducible model (Lee 1961). Before this technique was established, others have tried to interpose prosthetic tubes between the portal vein and IVC with high mortality rates (Whitaker 1946; Bernstein 1954).

Technique

The peritoneum over the inferior IVC is cut. Then, with a curved forceps the vena cava is mobilized from the inferior aspect of the liver to the right renal vein. Next, the peritoneum covering the portal vein is open, the portal vein is mobilized, and the gastroduodenal vein is doubly ligated and cut. A small vascular spoon clamp is placed on the IVC between the liver and the renal veins, partially obstructing its flow. A 4–5 mm incision is made on the IVC and flushed with heparinized saline. Next, the distal portal vein is ligated with 6-0 silk tie flush to the liver. The proximal portal vein is clamped with a small vascular clip, and the portal vein is cut above the stump of the gastroduodenal vein. The portal vein lumen is flushed with saline and two 7-0 prolene sutures are placed on the corners. The anastomosis is completed on a running fashion. First the posterior wall, followed by the anterior wall. After completion of the anastomosis the caval clamp is released and hemostasis accomplished with gentle compression with cotton swabs. The portal clamping time is of critical importance for the success of the procedure and it should be less than 30 minutes (see Figures 5.15–5.17) (Castaing 1980).

PANCREATITIS MODEL

A better understanding of the underlying pathophysiology of severe acute pancreatitis may lead to more targeted therapeutic options, potentially leading to improved survival. Animal models of acute pancreatitis are therefore an essential investigative tool for these aims to be achieved.

There are several models of acute pancreatitis, and they can be divided as invasive and non-invasive (Su 2006). Non-invasive models of acute pancreatitis are: hormone-induced, alcohol induced, immune-mediated, diet-induced, gene knockout and L-arginine; while invasive models are: and invasive models including closed duodenal loop, antegrade pancreatic duct perfusion, biliopancreatic duct injection, combination of secretory hyperstimulation with minimal intraductal bile acid exposure, vascular-induced, ischemia/reperfusion and duct ligation (Su 2006).

Independent of the model used, the pathophysiology event of experimental acute pancreatitis consists of the activation of pancreatic enzymes within acinar cells, the release of these activated enzymes in the interstitium, the autodigestion of the pancreas, and the release of activated pancreatic enzymes and other factors into the circulation that result in the development of systemic effects. An ideal model of acute pancreatitis should be easily reproducible, be able to adjust the severity of the inflammation and, and the morphology and pathophysiology should resemble that of the human situation.

Animal models of acute pancreatitis, induced by acute ethanol application alone, have been difficult to produce and require prior sensitization with other agents to allow significant pancreatic damage to occur (Letko 1991; Siech 1991; Quon 1992; Foitzik 1994; Luthen 1994; Andrzejewska 1998). Existing alcohol-induced models are relatively simple and cheap to perform. Acute ethanol administration selectively lessened pancreatic blood flow and microcirculation, suggesting that the effect of alcohol might increase ischemia damage during the evolvement of acute pancreatitis with or without underlying chronic disease. Another advantage of this model is that it allows alcohol to directly damage the pancreas by the influence of toxic ethanol metabolites, and perhaps by limitations of pancreatic regeneration. Reproducibility, however, has not been successfully achieved. Furthermore, there is a lack of correlation with the clinical setting.

Closed Duodenal Loop Model

Experimental acute pancreatitis in animals may be produced by creating a closed duodenal loop (CDL). This technique involves surgically closing above and below the duodenal papilla while bile is diverted into the jejunum via an implanted cannula. Evidence of edema, hemorrhage and necrosis of the pancreas developed within 9 to 11 hours. The model was first developed by Pfeffer et al. (Pfeffer 1957). It is relatively simple and is reproducible.

Since the permanent ligation of the duodenum often caused death of the animal within a short period, some investigators have attempted temporary ligation of the duodenum in rats (Ferrie 1978, Orda 1980). This allowed them to examine the progression of acute pancreatitis at an extended time and to investigate potential therapies. In a study by Orda et al., the authors injected a mixture of sodium taurocholate and trypsin into a temporary CDL to induce acute pancreatitis in rats (Orda 1980). They found that the acute pancreatitis induced was mild, associated with a mortality rate of 45%.

Antegrade Pancreatic Duct Perfusion Model

The main pancreatic duct can be made permeable by the perfusion of glycodeoxycholic acid (GDOC) along the main pancreatic duct. Other methods include the administration of intragastric ethanol, the stimulation of pancreatic secretion into an obstructed duct, or causing acute hypercalcemia (Farmer 1983; Wedgwood 1986; Widdison 1992).

The advantages of the pancreatic duct perfusion model are its reliability and reproducibility. The severity of the acute pancreatitis may be varied within well-defined time intervals according to the volumes and perfusion pressures. The etiology and the morphological changes closely resemble the human situation. This model is suitable for studying the early pathophysiology and subsequent progression of the disease. It is the ideal model to assess potential therapeutic agents. The major disadvantage of this model is its complexity (ductal cannulation and perfusion). Other disadvantages include the need to use large animals.

Biliopancreatic Duct Injection Model

Various compounds have been infused into the pancreatic duct to induce acute pancreatitis (EL 1901; Beck 1964; Papp 1966; Sum 1970; Aho 1980). Following a duodenotomy, a retrograde injection of bile salts (with or without activated pancreatic enzymes) into the pancreatic duct at the ampulla leads to severe acute pancreatitis. The severity of the disease can be manipulated by changing either the pressure or the concentration of bile salt used. Acute severe pancreatitis develops within 2 to 24 hours and is characterized by edema, necrosis and hemorrhage. Almost any form of detergent injected into the pancreatic duct under pressure will cause acute pancreatitis in laboratory animals such as dogs and rats (Musa 1976; Aho 1980; Aho 1980; Aho 1983). One of the best standardized compounds to use to develop acute pancreatitis is sodium taurocholate. Infusion of 0.2 ml/kg of 3%, 4.5% or 5% solution induced acute hemorrhagic pancreatitis with 72 hour mortality rates of 24%, 71% and 100%, respectively (Aho 1980; Aho 1980; Aho 1983). This model is appropriate for studies of systemic issues.

The retrograde injection of bile salts into the pancreatic duct of animals is an easy, effective and reproducible model for creating a severe, rapidly evolving and lethal variety of acute hemorrhagic pancreatitis.

It is also technically challenging to control constant pressure recordings and hence produce a standard degree of injury. Another disadvantage of this technique is the injection pressure with which the solution is applied to cause severe acute pancreatitis (Arendt 1993).

Ischemia/Reperfusion Model

In 1995, Hoffman et al. developed a model to study the microcirculation of the pancreas in the rat after complete (interruption of arterial blood supply to the pancreas) and reversible ischemia of the pancreas using intravital fluorescence microscopy (Hoffmann 1995). Complete ischemia of the pancreas was achieved by isolating arteries from surrounding tissue of gastroduodenal artery, left gastric artery, splenic artery and caudal pancreaticoduodenal artery. Complete but reversible ischemia of the pancreas was induced by occluding the four vessels using microvascular clips. The clips were taken out at 30 minutes, 1 hour or 2 hours after ischemia to produce reperfusion.

The duration of ischemia and of reperfusion is responsible for the severity of post-ischemic inflammatory reaction. In addition, there was a rise in the concentration of serum amylase after 1 and 2 hours of ischemia (Hoffmann 1995). Similar results were observed by another group after 2 hours of ischemia and 4 hours of reperfusion (Broe 1982).

Duct Ligation Model

Acute pancreatitis may be induced by ligating the distal bile duct at the level of the duodenum (Baxter 1985). This creates an early development of acute pancreatitis, obstructive jaundice and cholangitis in the rat. The duct ligation model was developed in an attempt to resemble the clinical situation of gallstones, motility disorders of the sphincter, edema and strictures at the papilla, tumors of the papilla, and parasites impacting the terminal biliopancreatic duct. Surgical ligation of the pancreatic duct alone has not been successful in inducing acute pancreatitis.

Most laboratory animals developed chronic lesions in the pancreas characterized by atrophy and apoptosis of acinar and ductal tissue but not significant necrosis or inflammation (Walker 1987). The ligation of the pancreatic duct in rodents has become an established model for chronic pancreatic atrophy and is often used for studying pancreatic regeneration (Lerch 1993; Lerch 1994). Ligation of this common biliopancreatic duct in the rat, however, causes a clinical syndrome resembling the multi-system organ failure observed in man.

Ligation of the pancreatic duct alone, bile and pancreatic duct separately, or the common biliopancreatic duct leads to severe acute pancreatitis with mortality rates approaching 100% within 2 weeks of induction (Senninger 1986; Cavuoti 1988) (See Table 5.3).

Models of chronic pancreatitis in rodents do not closely resemble the same process in humans. Prolonged feeding with ethanol to rodents does not induce chronic pancreatitis and alternative approaches have been suggested (Goto 1995; Van Laethem 1996; Puig-Divi 1999; Vaquero 1999; Gonzalez 2011).

Table 5.3. Summary of non-invasive experimental models of acute pancreatitis

Model	Advantages	Disadvantages	Clinical relevance
Hormone-induced	• Causes acute pancreatitis in animals (e.g., rats, mice, dogs, Syrian hamsters) • Can induce acute pancreatitis by various routes such as IV (preferred), subcutaneous or intraperitoneal • Allows accurate control of infusion rate, thereby enabling control of timing and severity of acute pancreatitis • Useful for studying cell biology, gut endocrine interactions (secretin, CCK levels), pathogenesis of acute pancreatitis-related pulmonary pathology, systemic disease manifestation, and healing and regeneration of damaged tissue after toxic substance has been discontinued • Simple; inexpensive	• Only mild acute pancreatitis develops • Negligible mortality • High variability in course and severity of underlying acute pancreatitis; unsuitable for controlled studies	• Pulmonary injury in rats resembles early stages of ARDS in humans • Structural changes of acinar cells are similar to human acute pancreatitis • Specific changes to intracellular membrane systems of acinar cells resemble acute pancreatitis in humans • Simulates acute pancreatitis induced by anti-cholinesterase insecticide poisoning in humans
Alcohol-induced	• Useful for studying changes to pancreatic blood flow and microcirculation, effect on pancreatic acinar damage by alcohol-related free oxygen radical generation, metabolites and effect on pancreatic regeneration • Used in several animal models (rats, cats, dogs) • Various routes of ethanol administration (IV, oral, direct intragastric instillation) • Simple, inexpensive • Selectively decreases pancreatic blood flow and microcirculation • Gene knockout animals may be used to determine effect of genetic factors on development of acute alcohol-related pancreatic injury	• Animal models of pancreatitis, induced by acute ethanol application alone, have been difficult to produce significant pancreatic damage, thus require prior sensitization with other agents • Lack of reproducibility	• Lack of correlation with clinical situation
Immune-mediated	• Possible application in field of drug or toxin-induced acute pancreatitis	• Difficult to set up in laboratory • Time-consuming • Limited reproducibility • Expensive • High early mortality rate, difficult for studying pathogenesis or treatment options • Development of secondary diabetes due to the involvement of islets of Langerhans	• Uncertain
Diet-induced	• Simplest method to study acute hemorrhagic pancreatitis • Well-established • Inexpensive	• Species-specific; may only be used in mice, whose small size causes technical difficulties	• Produces severe necrotizing pancreatitis similar to that seen in humans

Model	Advantages	Disadvantages	Clinical relevance
	• High reproducibility • No surgical procedure involved • Mortality rate can be controlled at any desired level between 0% and 100% by modifying feeding protocol • Useful for studying pathophysiology for acute pancreatitis and potential experimental treatment by measuring survival, biochemistry, histology, changes in hematocrit, pH and blood gases • Produces hemorrhage and necrosis with lethal course • Inflammatory lesions are homogeneously distributed	• Sex-specific; female mice • Variable onset of acute pancreatitis • Requires careful monitoring to ensure that intake of CDE diet is same in different experimental groups	• Gross and histological appearance of pancreatic and peripancreatic inflammation, and clinical and biochemical course of diet-induced pancreatitis, resemble human disease • Ascites, acidosis, hypoxia, hypovolemia similar to human acute pancreatitis'
Gene knockout	• Useful for studying function or effect of specific gene of interest • Avoids use of pharmacological manipulations that often cause side effects	• Time-consuming • Expensive • Complex • Altering specific gene from time of its conception could mean that other protein expressions may result to compensate for mutation • Mutation may stimulate unforeseen phenotypic changes if gene is expressed in different tissues • Expression of two genes may overlap and the alteration in single gene may mask abnormal phenotype	• Extrapolation of experimental data to humans is difficult
L-arginine (Arg)	• High reproducibility • Ability to achieve selective dose-dependent pancreatic acinar cell necrosis • Suitable for investigating early and late phases of acute pancreatitis • Useful for investigating insulo-acinar axis, extrapancreatic organ damage and its mechanisms	• Long-term administration of Arg produces chronic pancreatitis induction	• In clinical situation, circulatory, pulmonary, renal and hepatic failure (multi-organ failure) significantly affects morbidity and mortality of acute pancreatitis

Adapted from Su KH, et al.

CHOLELITHIASIS

There are several models in animals that are used to study the pathophysiology and treatment of gallstones (Brenneman 1972; MacPherson 1987; Rege 1993; Cona 2016). However, there is no animal model that forms spontaneous gallstones like in humans. Most of them involve dietary manipulation. The most popular is the hamster (*Mesocricetus auralus*) model. The diet in this model consists in fat-free, high sugar, and adequate protein. Ninety percent of these animal develop gallstones in 3 months (Dam 1952). Rats are not commonly used for gallstone research because they do not have a gallbladder. Mouse models are become more popular because the extensive genetic characterization, the availability of knockout, transgenic and inbred strains. The incidence of gallstones in mice treated with lithogenic diet is very variable. While only 14% of C57BL/6J mice fed with diet consisting of 15% dairy fat, 50% sucrose, 20% casein, 1% cholesterol, 0.5% cholic acid, cellulose, vitamins and mineral for 18 weeks developed gallstones, 100% of C57L/J and A/J mice developed gallstones after the same time (Paigen 1995).

HEPATOCELLULAR CARCINOMA (HCC) MODELS

Hepatocellular carcinoma (HCC) is the most common primary malignancy of the liver. Establishing animal models of HCC is essential to study the pathophysiology of carcinogenesis, perform drug screening, and conduct various therapeutic experiments. A wide range of HCC animal models are currently available: chemically induced models, xenograft models, and genetically modified models in mice (Schotman 1998; Heindryckx 2009; Li 2011). No model, however, is ideal for all purposes. This review analyses several mouse models useful for HCC research and points out their advantages and weaknesses. Chemically induced HCC mice models mimic the injury-fibrosis-malignancy cycle by administration of a genotoxic compound alone or, if necessary, followed by a promoting agent.

Chemically Induced

Several chemical agents can promote tumor formation when administered in high doses and long duration. The advantage of chemically induced models is the similarity with the injury-fibrosis-malignancy cycle seen in humans. This makes them the favorite models for HCC research.

Diethylnitrosamine

N-nitrosodiethylamine (DEN) is often used as a carcinogenic reagent. Mouse tumors induced by DEN harbour activating mutations in the *H-ras* proto-oncogene. Administration of a high dose induces HCC after a period of latency. The time needed after a single DEN-injection to develop HCC does not only depend on the administered dose, but also on sex, age and strain of mice. A dose-dependent formation of carcinomas after a single injection (5–90 mg/kg) of DEN in 15-day-old mice is observed after 45–104 weeks. When B6C3F1 mice are exposed to a single dose of 5.0 mg/kg DEN, it takes approximately 64 weeks to develop HCC (Heindryckx 2009).

A two-stage model in which the initiation by a genotoxic compound is followed by a promotion phase is often used for inducing HCC. DEN can be used as an initiator and phenobarbital (PB) as a promoting agent. Several mechanisms might be responsible for the tumour promoting effect of PB. First, PB can increase the expression of cytochrome P-450 a 100-fold, leading to an enhanced effect of DEN. Another two-step carcinogenesis model is known as the Solt-Farber protocol (Farber 1977). In this model, initiation by a hepatocarcinogenic compound is followed by a partial hepatectomy (PH). Partial hepatectomy induces hepatic cell proliferation of the liver, leading to a fast expansion of the initiated cells (See Table 5.4).

Table 5.4. Summary of chemically induced HCC-models

	Time to develop tumors	Percent of mice with HCC	Remarks	References
Single administration	45-104 weeks (dose dependent)	80-100% in male	Poorly reproducible	Chen et al. (1993); Frey et al. (2000); Hacker et al. (1991); Park et al. (2008); Teoh et al. (2008); Zimmers et al. (2008)
Short-term administration	40-60 weeks	100% in male		Shiota et al. (1999)
Long-term administration	20-35 weeks	100% in male. 30% in female	Very aggressive tumors (H-ras mutations)	Finnberg et al. (2004)
+ Pentobarbital	20-40 weeks		B-catenin activation	Goldsworthy and Fransson-Steen (2002); Klaunig et al. (1988); Weghorst and Klaunig (1989)
+ Partial hepatectomy	4-8 weeks (in rats)			Farber et al. (1977); Klinman and Erslev (1963)
Peroxisome proliferators	50-100 weeks (dose dependent)	Depends on strain, dose and PP-agent	PP tumorigenicity in humans not known	Hays et al. (2005); Reddy et al. (1976); Takashima et al. (2008)
Aflatoxine	Early HCC in 52 weeks. High grade HCC 92-110 weeks	Considerable interstrain differences: DBA/2J: 90% C57BL/N: 25-66%	Suitable model for AFB-induced HCC in humans	McGlynn et al. (2003); Ghebranious and Sell (1998)
CCl4	104 weeks	50-94% (dose dependent) in male and female		Confer and Stenger (1966); Farazi et al. (2006); Weisburger (1977)
Choline deficient diet	50-52 weeks	100%	Steatohepatitis	De Lima et al. (2008); Knight et al. (2000); Liquori et al. (2009)
Thioacetamide	50-80 weeks	70-100%		

Adapted from Heindryckx F et al.

Peroxisome Proliferators

Peroxisome proliferators (ethyl clofenapate ciprofibrate, fenofibrate, clofibrate) induce hepatomegaly, peroxisome proliferation in hepatocytes and induction of several hepatic enzymes.

Aflatoxin B₁

The hepatotoxin aflatoxin B_1 (AFB), produced by certain fungi of the *Aspergillus* genus such as *Asparagillus flavum*, is known to be a hepatic carcinogen. When 7-day-old mice are exposed to 6 mg/kg body weight of AFB, in a bolus injection, HCC is developed after 52 weeks (McGlynn 2003). In 90% of the DBA/2J mice (susceptible strain for HCC) HCC occurs after AFB exposure, while only 25% of the C57BL/N mice (relatively resistant strain for HCC) develop HCC after AFB exposure.

Xenograft Models

In xenograft models, the tumors are formed by injecting human cancer cells from a lab culture in immune deficient mice. Athymic (nude) or severe combined immune deficient (SCID) mice are often used as hosts. Tumor xenografts can be established either by direct implantation of biopsy material or by inoculation of human tumor cell lines. First, the ectopic model, in which human tumor cells are injected subcutaneously in the flank of mice. Second, the orthotopic model, where tumor cells are injected intrahepatically into the mice. The advantage of xenograft mouse models is the short time span needed for the development of tumors. However, the resemblance between xenograft tumors and human tumors is rather poor. Thus, most researchers prefer to use models in which tumors arise in a background that resembles the natural history of HCC (Heindryckx 2009).

Transgenic Mouse Models

Genetically modified mouse models are engineered to reproduce pathophysiological and molecular features of human HCC (by simulating hepatitis B or C, over-expressing growth factors, or induction of oncogenes) (Heindryckx 2009). It is a unique model for assessing the effects of oncogenes either alone or in combination with other oncogenes or carcinogenic agents. The transgenic mouse models are the ones that most resemble the human HCC. Transgenic mouse models of HBV or HCV infection have provided reliable experimental proof that viral genes could initiate or promote liver carcinogenesis. Most HBV transgenic mouse models focus on the HBx gene, which encodes HBV X protein (HBx)–a transcriptional transactivator that stimulates expression of a broad range of proto-oncogenes, including c-fos, c-myc and c-jun (Li 2011).

In contrast to wild-type CD1 mice, which do not normally develop spontaneous liver tumors and have a lifespan of approximately 24 months, the majority of HBx transgenic mice died from clear cell HCC at 11 to 15 months of age.

In a similar fashion, Sell et al. constructed HBsAg transgenic C57BL/6 mice (Table 5.4). The 50-4 strain of these mice had a high HBsAg content in hepatocytes, premalignant changes, nodules, adenomas and HCC; exposure to diethylnitrosamine or aflatoxin accelerated the development of HCC, and produced considerably more tumor nodules in the liver.

HBV and HCV Transgenic Mice do not Develop Liver Cirrhosis

To avoid such problems, Yang et al. developed a modified surgical technique, in which a piece of Gelfoam is inserted into the liver incision after delivery of HCC cells. The Gelfoam both facilitates hemostasis and forms a pocket that secures the injected tumor cells (Yang 1992). These techniques have the major disadvantage of possible inadvertent tumor seeding along the needle track or into the bloodstream.

To reproduce the extensive liver disease that is associated with advanced HCC, Tang et al. developed another orthotopic mouse model. HCC cells transfected with vectors carrying the gene for the [beta]-subunit of human choriogonadotropin ([beta]-hCG) were injected into the left liver lobe of SCID mice. In this model, urine levels of [beta]-hCG can be used as a surrogate marker of tumor burden (Tang 2010).

Several HCV transgenic mouse model systems have been established expressing HCV structural proteins (core, E1, E2 and p7) or nonstructural proteins (NS2, NS3, NS4A, NS4B, NS5A and NS5B) individually or in various combinations are available (Li 2011). As early as 3 months of age, HCV core gene transgenic mice developed hepatic steatosis. In mice aged up to 12 months, steatosis slowly progressed without neoplastic changes. At month 16, 25% of the male transgenic mice of the C21 line had developed HCC, but no female mice of the C21 line had developed tumors (Moriya 1998).

Animal models of spontaneous HCC development and metastasis can be used to study the mechanism of HCC progression as well as the best mode of intervention. Futakuchi et al. have established a rat model of *in vivo* HCC lung metastasis based on sequential intraperitoneal injection of diethylnitrosamine and administration of drinking water containing the carcinogen N-nitrosomorpholine for 16 weeks, by which time all animals had developed HCC. By week 23, lung metastasis had occurred in 100% of these animals (Futakuchi 1999).

Most experiments to test the effects of potential drug treatments in animal models of HCC involve the subcutaneous implantation of human hepatoma cells in immunocompromised mice (e.g., SCID mice). Although researchers have expressed doubts and criticisms about the validity of using effects on tumor xenografts to predict clinical activity

Establishing high-quality orthotopic models is, however, technically more challenging than the construction of subcutaneous xenograft models. Conventional techniques of intrahepatic tumor implantation involve direct placement of tumor fragments or injection of free tumor cells.

Cholangiocarcinoma Models

Several carcinogenesis models of cholangiocarcinoma (CCC) have been established in animals (Thamavit 1978; Elmore 1993; Cheifetz 1996; Sirica 1996; Lee 1997; Lai 1999; Al-Bader 2000; Yeh 2004; Sirica 2008; Yang 2011; Ko 2013; Ikenoue 2016). There are several CCC animal models: xenograft and orthotopic models, carcinogen-induced CCC model, and genetically engineered mouse model for CCA. Recent advancements in cell and molecular biology make it possible to mimic the pathogenicity of human cholangiocarcinoma using various animal models.

One model obtained CCC using Syrian hamsters being treated with *Clonorchis sinensis* or *Opisthorchis viverrini* followed by dimethylnitrosamine (DMN) (Thamavit 1978; Flavell 1983; Lee 1997). In another model Syrian hamsters were treated with DMN followed by bile duct ligation also develop CCC (Cheifetz 1996). In these models, CCC develops about 24 weeks after the initial insult, with a yield rate of only 10%. One of the better characterized rat models of CCC has been the furan model described by Sirica et al., which leads to the development of intestinal-type CCC in the caudate lobe of the liver (Elmore 1993; Sirica 1996).

Oral administration of thioacetamide (TAA) in drinking water to male Sprangue-Dawley rats provides a reproducible animal model for development of CCC with a high yield rate. Drinking water with TAA 300 mg/l was administered orally. Multifocal bile ductular proliferation with intestinal metaplasia (presence of goblet cells) and increasing histologic atypia (biliary dysplasia) was observed by the 9th week of TAA administration. Biliary cytokeratin (CK19)-expressing invasive intestinal-type CCC with stromal desmoplasia was evident at the 16th week, and by the 22nd week the yield rate for CCCs had increased to 100%. The progression from normal cholangioles to biliary dysplasia to invasive CCC was accompanied by up-regulation of the proto-oncogenes c-met and c-erbB-2, tyrosine kinase receptors over-expressed in human CCCs. In the first 6 months of follow-up, no systemic metastases or tumor-related deaths were observed in this model. (Yeh 2004).

Yamada and coworkers created a mouse CCC model that transfected the biliary epithelium directly with plasmids containing oncogenes. The common bile duct located below the liver was clamped with a small animal surgical clip to prevent the injected material from rapidly flowing into the duodenum. The bile duct draining the left lateral liver lobe was identified, and a ligature (6-0 silk) was placed loosely around the duct. Another ligature was placed around the base of the gallbladder where it meets the cystic duct. Ectopic oncogene expression in the biliary tract was achieved by the SB transposon transfection system with transduction of murine constitutively active AKT and human YAP. The solution was injected into the gallbladder with enough pressure to allow the solution to distend the biliary system and reach the whole the intrahepatic biliary tree. The ligature around the left lateral liver lobe duct was then tied off so as not to allow the plasmid solution to flow from this bile duct to the common bile duct. Following plasmid injection and the left lateral bile duct ligation, the common bile duct was unclamped. The ligature around the base of the gallbladder was then tied and a cholecystectomy performed. Then, each animal was injected with 1 µg of IL-33 for 3 days (Leake 2015; Yamada 2015).

COLON CARCINOMA METASTASES

Tumor models have a key role in oncology. They are powerful tools guiding clinical research and practice (Demicheli 2001). Most transplantable tumor therapy experiments utilize ectopic (usually subcutaneous) injection of tumor cells. Ectopically transplanted tumors do not necessarily reproduce the biology of orthotopically grown tumors. The response of the primary tumor to therapy is usually what is evaluated in most tumor models. There is a need to place more emphasis on tumor models in which metastases are the primary target to therapy.

The limitations of animal models are that they usually respond better to anti-cancer therapy than in the clinical settings.

Most transplantable tumors are very fast growing (doubling times measured in days) while human tumors (with doubling times measured in months). Experimental tumors tend to be highly responsive to cytotoxic anti-cancer drugs, since this drugs target rapidly dividing cells. Most transplantable tumors are highly immunogenic because it is difficult to obtain truly syngeneic tumors. These tumors therefore become especially vulnerable to various host immune effector mechanisms.

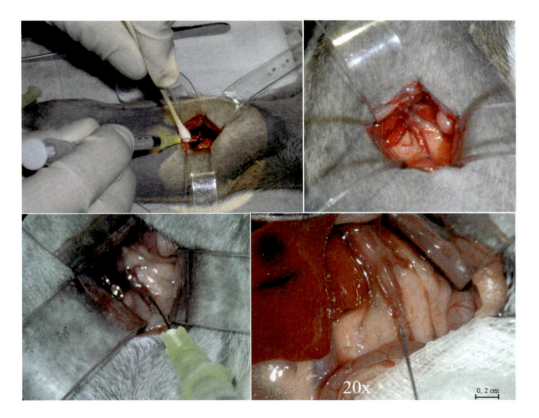

Figure 5.20. Technique of portal injection to inoculate colon cancer cells DKDK12 (CAMR, Salisburg-Withshire, UK) in the rat liver. This reproduces the metastatic process of colon cancer. A 30G needle is used to minimize bleeding.

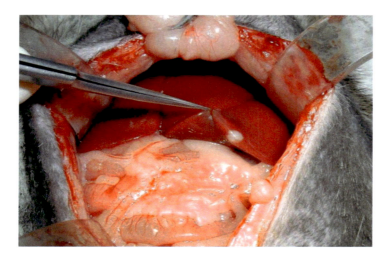

Figure 5.21. Isolated liver tumor of colon cancer cells DKDK12 (CAMR, Salisburg-Withshire, UK) injected in the rat portal vein 2 weeks prior.

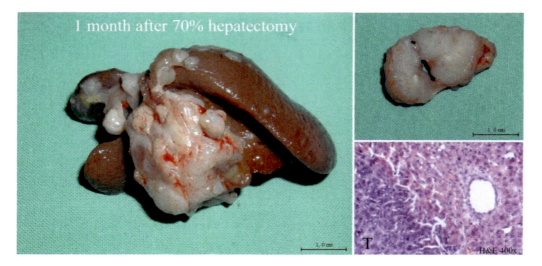

Figure 5.22. Metastatic tumor of colon cancer cells DKDK12 (CAMR, Salisburg-Withshire, UK) injected in the rat portal vein 4 weeks prior.

Over recent years, the interest in the development of experimental models for colorectal liver metastases has increased due to the need for new adjuvant therapies to improve the treatment of both colorectal cancer and liver metastases. The induction of colon cancer by carcinogens in the rat with spontaneous liver metastases closely mimics the natural history of colon cancer but only a low yield of both colonic cancer (less than 50%) and liver metastases (approx. 25%) is obtained after 6 months of latency. Direct intraportal injection of colon carcinoma cells is the most used model. Although it bypasses the natural history of colon cancer, this simple model produces up to 100% of liver metastases 6 weeks after injection of cells. This model has been used to study morphology, neovascularization, surgical and adjuvant therapy (Panis 1991). See Figures 5.20–5.22.

In using animal models for preclinical assessment of anti-metastatic agents, it is necessary that appropriate cell lines, routes of administration and target organs used, be appropriately matched for the information sought (Chambers 1999).

REFERENCES

Abraldes, JG; Iwakiri, Y; Loureiro-Silva, M; Haq, WC; Sessa, Groszmann RJ. Mild increases in portal pressure upregulate vascular endothelial growth factor and endothelial nitric oxide synthase in the intestinal microcirculatory bed: leading to a hyperdynamic state. *Am. J. Physiol. Gastrointest. Liver Physiol.*, 2006, 290(5), G980−987.

Abraldes, JG; Pasarin, M; Garcia-Pagan, JC. Animal models of portal hypertension. *World J. Gastroenterol.*, 2006, 12(41), 6577−6584.

Aho, HJ; Koskensalo, SM; Nevalainen, TJ. Experimental pancreatitis in the rat. Sodium taurocholate-induced acute haemorrhagic pancreatitis. *Scand. J. Gastroenterol.*, 1980, 15(4), 411−416.

Aho, HJ; Nevalainen, YJ. Experimental pancreatitis in the rat. Ultrastructure of sodium taurocholate-induced pancreatic lesions. *Scand. J. Gastroenterol.*, 1980, 15(4), 417−424.

Aho, HJ; Nevalainen, YJ; Aho, AJ. Experimental pancreatitis in the rat. Development of pancreatic necrosis; ischemia and edema after intraductal sodium taurocholate injection. *Eur. Surg. Res.*, 1983, 15(1), 28−36.

Al-Bader, A; Mathew, TC; Abul, H; Al-Sayer, H; Singal, PK; Dashti, HM. Cholangiocarcinoma and liver cirrhosis in relation to changes due to thioacetamide. *Mol. Cell. Biochem.*, 2000, 208(1−2), 1−10.

Aleksandrowicz, R; Gawlik, Z; Wisniewska, IE; Tarlowska, H. Physiological aspects of the partial hepatectomy in rats. *Acta. Physiol. Pol.*, 1981, 32(6), 681−692.

Alpini, G; Roberts, S; Kuntz, SM; Ueno, Y; Gubba, S; Podila, PV; LeSage, G; LaRusso, NF. Morphological, molecular, and functional heterogeneity of cholangiocytes from normal rat liver. *Gastroenterology*, 1996, 110(5), 1636−1643.

Andrzejewska, A; Dlugosz, JW; Jurkowska, G. The effect of antecedent acute ethanol ingestion on the pancreas ultrastructure in taurocholate pancreatitis in rats. *Exp. Mol. Pathol.*, 1998, 65(2), 64−77.

Arendt, T. Bile-induced acute pancreatitis in cats. Roles of bile, bacteria, and pancreatic duct pressure. *Dig. Dis. Sci.*, 1993, 38(1), 39−44.

Baxter, JN; Jenkins, SA; Day, DW; Roberts, NB; Cowell, DC; Mackie, CR; Shields, R. Effects of somatostatin and a long-acting somatostatin analogue on the prevention and treatment of experimentally induced acute pancreatitis in the rat. *Br. J. Surg.*, 1985, 72(5), 382−385.

Beck, IT; Kahn, DS; Solymar, J; McKenna, RD; Zylberszac, B. The role of pancreatic enzymes in the pathogenesis of acute pancreatitis. III. Comparison of the the pathological and biochemical changes in the canine pancreas to intraductal injection with bile and trypsin. *Gastroenterology*, 1964, 46, 531−542.

Beck, PL; Lee, SS. Vitamin K1 improves survival in bile-duct-ligated rats with cirrhosis. *J. Hepatol.*, 1995, 23(2), 235.

Bernstein, DECS. Simple technique for portacaval shunt in the rat. *J. Appl. Physiol.*, 1954, 14, 469.

Bismuth, H. Surgical anatomy and anatomical surgery of the liver. 1982; *World J. Surg.*, 6(1), 3–9.

Brand, MI; Kononov, A; Vladisavljevic, A; Milsom, JW. Surgical anatomy of the celiac artery and portal vein of the rat. *Lab. Anim. Sci.*, 1995, 45(1), 76–80.

Brenneman, DE; Connor, WE; Forker, EL; DenBesten, L. The formation of abnormal bile and cholesterol gallstones from dietary cholesterol in the prairie dog. *J. Clin. Invest.*, 1972, 51(6), 1495–1503.

Broe, PJ; Zuidema, GD; Cameron, JL. The role of ischemia in acute pancreatitis: studies with an isolated perfused canine pancreas. *Surgery*, 1982, 91(4), 377–382.

Bucher, NL; Swaffield, MN. The rate of incorporation of labelled thymidine into the deoxyribonucleic acid of regenerating rat liver in relation to the amount of liver excised. *Cancer. Res.*, 1964, 24, 1611–1625.

Castaing, DHD; Bismuth, D (1980). *Anatomy of the liver and portal system of the rat*. Paris, Masson Co.

Castaneda, B; Debernardi-Venon, W; Bandi, JC; Andreu, V; Perez-del-Pulgar, S; Moitinho, E; Pizcueta, P; Bosch, J. The role of portal pressure in the severity of bleeding in portal hypertensive rats. *Hepatology*, 2000, 31(3), 581–586.

Cavuoti, OP; Moody, FG; Martinez, G. Role of pancreatic duct occlusion with prolamine (Ethibloc) in necrotizing pancreatitis. *Surgery*, 1988, 103(3), 361–366.

Chambers, AF. The metastatic process: basic research and clinical implications. *Oncol. Res.*, 1999, 11(4), 161–168.

Cheifetz, RE; Davis, NL; Owen, DA. An animal model of benign bile-duct stricture, sclerosing cholangitis and cholangiocarcinoma and the role of epidermal growth factor receptor in ductal proliferation. *Can. J. Surg.*, 1996, 39(3), 193–197.

Colombato, LA; Albillos, A; Groszmann, RJ. Temporal relationship of peripheral vasodilatation, plasma volume expansion and the hyperdynamic circulatory state in portal-hypertensive rats. *Hepatology*, 15(2), 323–328.

Cona, MM; Liu, Y; Yin, T; Feng, Y; Chen, F; Mulier, S; Li, Y; Zhang, J; Oyen, R; Ni, Y. Rat model of cholelithiasis with human gallstones implanted in cholestasis-induced virtual gallbladder. *World J. Methodol.*, 2016, 6(2), 154–162.

Constandinou, C; Henderson, N; Iredale, JP. Modeling liver fibrosis in rodents. *Methods Mol. Med.*, 2005, 117, 237–250.

Couinaud, C. The paracaval segments of the liver. *Journal of Hepato-Biliary-Pancreatic Surgery*, 1994, 1(2), 145–151.

Dam, H; Christensen, F. Alimentary production of gallstones in hamsters. *Acta. Pathol. Microbiol. Scand.*, 1952, 30(2), 236–242.

Dashti, H; Jeppsson, B; Hagerstrand, I; Hultberg, B; Srinivas, U; Abdulla, M; Bengmark, S. Thioacetamide- and carbon tetrachloride-induced liver cirrhosis. *Eur. Surg. Res.*, 1989, 21(2), 83–91.

de Jong, KP; Brouwers, MA; Huls, GA; Dam, A; Bun, JC; Wubbena, AS; Nieuwenhuis, P; Slooff, MJ. Liver cell proliferation after partial hepatectomy in rats with liver metastases. *Anal. Quant. Cytol. Histol.*, 1998, 20(1), 59–68.

de Jong, KP; Lont, HE; Bijma, AM; Brouwers, MA; de Vries, EG; van Veen, ML; Marquet, RL; Slooff, MJ; Terpstra, OT. The effect of partial hepatectomy on tumor growth in rats: *in vivo* and *in vitro* studies. *Hepatology*, 1995, 22(4 Pt 1), 1263–1272.

Delong, RP. Revascularization of the rat liver following interruption of its arterial supply. *Surg. Forum*, 1953, 4, 388–392.

Demicheli, R. Tumour dormancy: findings and hypotheses from clinical research on breast cancer. *Semin. Cancer Biol.*, 2001, 11(4), 297–306.

Eguchi, S; Lilja, H; Hewitt, WR; Middleton, Y; Demetriou, AA; Rozga, J. Loss and recovery of liver regeneration in rats with fulminant hepatic failure. *J. Surg. Res.*, 1997, 72(2), 112–122.

EL, O. The etiology of acute hemorrhagic pancreatitis. *Johns Hopkins Hosp. Bull.*, 1901, 12, 182–190.

Elmore, LW; Sirica, AE. Intestinal-type" of adenocarcinoma preferentially induced in right/caudate liver lobes of rats treated with furan. *Cancer Res.*, 1993, 53(2), 254–259.

Emond, J; Capron-Laudereau, M; Meriggi, F; Bernuau, J; Reynes, M; Houssin, D. Extent of hepatectomy in the rat. Evaluation of basal conditions and effect of therapy. *Eur. Surg. Res.*, 1989, 21(5), 251–259.

Ezure, T; Sakamoto, T; Tsuji, H; Lunz, 3rd JG; Murase, N; Fung, JJ; Demetris, AJ. The development and compensation of biliary cirrhosis in interleukin-6-deficient mice. *Am. J. Pathol.*, 2000, 156(5), 1627–1639.

Fan, ST; Lo, CM; Liu, CL; Yong, BH; Chan, JK; Ng, IO. Safety of donors in live donor liver transplantation using right lobe grafts. *Arch. Surg.*, 2000, 135(3), 336–340.

Farber, E; Solt, D; Cameron, R; Laishes, B; Ogawa, K; Medline, A. Newer insights into the pathogenesis of liver cancer. *Am. J. Pathol.*, 1977, 89(2), 477–482.

Farmer, RCMS; Reber, HA. Acute pancreatitis: the role of duct permeability. *Surg. Forum*, 1983, 34, 224–227.

Fausto, N. Liver regeneration: from laboratory to clinic. *Liver Transpl.*, 2001, **7**(10), 835–844.

Fausto, N; Riehle, KJ. Mechanisms of liver regeneration and their clinical implications. *J. Hepatobiliary Pancreat. Surg.*, 2005, 12(3), 181–189.

Fernandez, M; Vizzutti, F; Garcia-Pagan, JC; Rodes, J; Bosch, J. Anti-VEGF receptor-2 monoclonal antibody prevents portal-systemic collateral vessel formation in portal hypertensive mice. *Gastroenterology*, 2004, 126(3), 886–894.

Ferrie, MM; O'Hare, R; Joffe, SN. Acute and chronic pancreatitis in the rat caused by a closed duodenal loop. *Digestion*, 1978, 18(3–4), 280–285.

Flavell, DJ; Lucas, SB. Promotion of N-nitrosodimethylamine-initiated bile duct carcinogenesis in the hamster by the human liver fluke, Opisthorchis viverrini. *Carcinogenesis*, 1983, 4(7), 927–930.

Flower, MW. Sur la disposition et la nomenclature des lobes du foi chez les mammifères. [On the disposition and nomenclature of the lobes of faith in mammals] *J. de Zool.*, 1872, 1, 420–425.

Foitzik, T; Lewandrowski, KB; Fernandez-del Castillo, C; Rattner, DW; Klar, E; Warshaw, AL. Exocrine hyperstimulation but not pancreatic duct obstruction increases the susceptibility to alcohol-related pancreatic injury. *Arch. Surg.*, 1994, 129(10), 1081–1085.

Franco, D; Gigou, M; Szekely, AM; Bismuth, H. Portal hypertension after bile duct obstruction: effect of bile diversion on portal pressure in the rat. *Arch. Surg.*, 1979, 114(9), 1064–1067.

Futakuchi, M; Hirose, M; Ogiso, T; Kato, K; Sano, M; Ogawa, K; Shirai, T. Establishment of an *in vivo* highly metastatic rat hepatocellular carcinoma model. *Jpn. J. Cancer Res.*, 1999, 90(11), 1196–1202.

Gaub, J; Iversen, J. Rat liver regeneration after 90% partial hepatectomy. *Hepatology*, 1984, 4(5), 902−904.

Gehring, S; Dickson, EM; San Martin, ME; van Rooijen, N; Papa, EF; Harty, MW; Tracy, Jr. TF; Gregory, SH. Kupffer cells abrogate cholestatic liver injury in mice. *Gastroenterology*, 2006, 130(3), 810−822.

Georgiev, P; Jochum, W; Heinrich, S; Jang, JH; Nocito, A; Dahm, F; Clavien, PA. Characterization of time-related changes after experimental bile duct ligation. *Br. J. Surg.*, 2008, 95(5), 646−656.

Gershbein, LL; Elias, H. Observations on the anatomy of the rat liver. *Anat. Rec.*, 1954, 120(1), 85−98.

Glanemann, M; Eipel, C; Nussler, AK; Vollmar, B; Neuhaus, P. Hyperperfusion syndrome in small-for-size livers. *Eur. Surg. Res.*, 2005, 37(6), 335−341.

Gonzalez, AM; Garcia, T; Samper, E; Rickmann, M; Vaquero, EC; Molero, X. Assessment of the protective effects of oral tocotrienols in arginine chronic-like pancreatitis. *Am. J. Physiol. Gastrointest. Liver Physiol.*, 2011, 301(5), G846−855.

Goto, M; Nakano, I; Kimura, T; Miyahara, T; Kinjo, M; Nawata, H. New chronic pancreatitis model with diabetes induced by cerulein plus stress in rats. *Dig. Dis. Sci.*, 1995, 40(11), 2356−2363.

Greene, AK; Puder, M. Partial hepatectomy in the mouse: technique and perioperative management. *J. Invest. Surg.*, 2003, 16(2), 99−102.

Greene, E. C. (1963). *Anatomy of the rat*. New York, Hafner Publishing Company.

Groszmann, RJ; Kravetz, D; Bosch, J; Glickman, M; Bruix, J; Bredfeldt, J; Conn, HO; Rodes, J; Storer, EH. Nitroglycerin improves the hemodynamic response to vasopressin in portal hypertension. *Hepatology*, 1982, 2(6), 757−762.

Gujral, JS; Farhood, A; Bajt, ML; Jaeschke, H. Neutrophils aggravate acute liver injury during obstructive cholestasis in bile duct-ligated mice. *Hepatology*, 2003, 38(2), 355−363.

Gujral, JS; Liu Farhood, A; Hinson, JA; Jaeschke, H. Functional importance of ICAM-1 in the mechanism of neutrophil-induced liver injury in bile duct-ligated mice. *Am. J. Physiol. Gastrointest. Liver Physiol.*, 2004, 286(3), G499−507.

Hebel, RSM. (1976). *Anatomy of the Laboratory Rat*. Baltimore, Williams and Wilkins Co.

Heindryckx, F; Colle, I; Van Vlierberghe, H. Experimental mouse models for hepatocellular carcinoma research. *Int. J. Exp. Pathol.*, 2009, 90(4), 367−386.

Hernandez-Munoz, R; Diaz-Munoz, M; Suarez-Cuenca, JA; Trejo-Solis, C; Lopez, V; Sanchez-Sevilla, L; Yanez, L; De Sanchez, VC. Adenosine reverses a preestablished CCl4-induced micronodular cirrhosis through enhancing collagenolytic activity and stimulating hepatocyte cell proliferation in rats. *Hepatology*, 2001, 34 (4 Pt 1), 677−687.

Higgins, GMAR. Restoration of the liver of the white rat following partial surgical removal. *Arch. Path. Lab. Med.*, 1931, 12, 186−202.

Hoffmann, TF; Leiderer, R; Waldner, H; Arbogast, S; Messmer, K. Ischemia reperfusion of the pancreas: a new *in vivo* model for acute pancreatitis in rats. *Res. Exp. Med. (Berl)* 1995, 195(3), 125−144.

Holmin, T; Alinder, G; Herlin, P. A microsurgical method for total hepatectomy in the rat. *Eur. Surg. Res.*, 1982, 14(6), 420−427.

Ikenoue, T; Terakado, Y; Nakagawa, H; Hikiba, Y; Fujii, T; Matsubara, D; Noguchi, R; Zhu, C; Yamamoto, K; Kudo, Y; Asaoka, Y; Yamaguchi, K; Ijichi, H; Tateishi, K; Fukushima, N; Maeda, S; Koike, K; Furukawa, Y. A novel mouse model of intrahepatic cholangiocarcinoma induced by liver-specific Kras activation and Pten deletion. *Sci. Rep.*, 2016, 6, 23899.

Inderbitzin, D; Gass, M; Beldi, G; Ayouni, E; Nordin, A; Sidler, D; Gloor, B; Candinas, D; Stoupis, C. Magnetic resonance imaging provides accurate and precise volume determination of the regenerating mouse liver. *J. Gastrointest. Surg.*, 2004, 8(7), 806−811.

Inderbitzin, D; Studer, P; Sidler, D; Beldi, G; Djonov, V; Keogh, A; Candinas, D. Regenerative capacity of individual liver lobes in the microsurgical mouse model. *Microsurgery*, 2006, 26(6), 465−469.

Innocenti, PCR; Falcone, A; Gargano, E; Piattelli, E. Anatomia chirurgica del sistema portale nel rato. *Boll. Soc. It. Biol. Sper.*, 1978, 54, 2421−2425.

Iwakiri, Y; Cadelina, G; Sessa, WC; Groszmann, RJ. Mice with targeted deletion of eNOS develop hyperdynamic circulation associated with portal hypertension. *Am. J. Physiol. Gastrointest. Liver Physiol.*, 2002, 283(5), G1074−1081.

Jenkins, SA; Grandison, A; Baxter, JN; Day, DW; Taylor, I; Shields, R. A dimethylnitrosamine-induced model of cirrhosis and portal hypertension in the rat. *J. Hepatol.*, 1985, 1(5), 489−499.

Grisham, JW. A morphologic study of deoxyribonucleic acid synthesis and cell proliferation in regenerating rat liver: autoradiography with thymidine-H3. *Cancer Res.*, 1996, 22, 842−849.

Kanno, N; LeSage, G; Glaser, S; Alvaro, D; Alpini, G. Functional heterogeneity of the intrahepatic biliary epithelium. *Hepatology*, 2000, 31(3), 555−561.

Kaplan, MM; Righetti, A. Induction of rat liver alkaline phosphatase: the mechanism of the serum elevation in bile duct obstruction. *J. Clin. Invest.*, 1970, 49(3), 508−516.

Kara, ME. The anatomical study on the rat pancreas and its ducts with emphasis on the surgical approach. *Ann. Anat.*, 2005, 187(2), 105−112.

Ko, KS; Peng, J; Yang, H. Animal models of cholangiocarcinoma. *Curr. Opin. Gastroenterol.*, 2013, 29(3), 312−318.

Kobayashi, N; Ito, M; Nakamura, J; Cai, J; Gao, C; Hammel, JM; Fox, IJ. Hepatocyte transplantation in rats with decompensated cirrhosis. *Hepatology*, 2000, 31(4), 851−857.

Kogure, K; Ishizaki, M; Nemoto, M; Kuwano, H; Makuuchi, M. A comparative study of the anatomy of rat and human livers. *J. Hepatobiliary Pancreat. Surg.*, 1999, 6(2), 171−175.

Kountouras, J; Billing, BH; Scheuer, PJ. Prolonged bile duct obstruction: a new experimental model for cirrhosis in the rat. *Br. J. Exp. Pathol.*, 1984, 65(3), 305−311.

Krahenbuhl, L; Feodorovici, M; Renzulli, P; Schafer, M; Abou-Shady, M; Baer, HU. Laparoscopic partial hepatectomy in the rat: a new resectional technique. *Dig. Surg.*, 1998, 15(2), 140−144.

Kubota, T; Takabe, K; Yang, M; Sekido, H; Endo, I; Ichikawa, Y; Togo, S; Shimada, H. Minimum sizes for remnant and transplanted livers in rats. *Journal of Hepato-Biliary-Pancreatic Surgery*, 1997, 4(4), 398−404.

Lai, GH; Sirica, AE. Establishment of a novel rat cholangiocarcinoma cell culture model. *Carcinogenesis*, 1999, 20(12), 2335−2340.

Leake, I. Biliary tract. A new mouse model that closely resembles human cholangiocarcinoma. *Nat. Rev. Gastroenterol. Hepatol.*, 2015, 12(3), 122.

Lee, JH; Rim, HJ; Sell, S. Heterogeneity of the "oval-cell" response in the hamster liver during cholangiocarcinogenesis following Clonorchis sinensis infection and dimethylnitrosamine treatment. *J. Hepatol.*, 1997, 26(6), 1313−1323.

Lee, SH; Fisher, B. Portacaval shunt in the rat. *Surgery*, 1961, 50, 668–672.

Leelaudomlipi, S; Sugawara, Y; Kaneko, J; Matsui, Y; Ohkubo, T; Makuuchi, M. Volumetric analysis of liver segments in 155 living donors. *Liver Transpl.*, 2002, 8(7), 612–614.

Leneman, F; Burton, S. The hepato-esophageal artery of the rat. Brief report. *Acta. Anat. (Basel)*, 1967, 68(3), 334–343.

Lerch, MM; Adler, G. Experimental pancreatitis. *Current Opinion in Gastroenterology*, 1993, 9(5), 752–759.

Lerch, MM; Adler, G. Experimental animal models of acute pancreatitis. *Int. J. Pancreatol.*, 1994, 15(3), 159–170.

Letko, G; Nosofsky, T; Lessel, W; Siech, M. Transition of rat *pancreatic* juice edema into acute pancreatitis by single ethanol administration. *Pathol. Res. Pract.*, 1991, 187(2–3), 247–250.

Li, X; Benjamin, IS; Alexander, B. Reproducible production of thioacetamide-induced macronodular cirrhosis in the rat with no mortality. *J. Hepatol.*, 2002, 36(4), 488–493.

Li, Y; Tang, ZY; Hou, JX. Hepatocellular carcinoma: insight from animal models. *Nat. Rev. Gastroenterol. Hepatol.*, 2011, 9(1), 32–43.

Lin, PW. Hemodynamic changes after hepatectomy in rats studied with radioactive microspheres. *J. Formos. Med. Assoc.*, 1990, 89(3), 177–181.

Lorente, LAM; Duran, HJ; Cejalvo, D; Lloris, JM; Arias, J. Extrahepatic biliary anatomy in wistar rats. *Surg. Res. Comm.*, 1995, 17, 31–38.

Lorente, LAM; Rodriguez, J; Duran, MC; Duran, HJ; Alonso, S; Arias, J. Surgical Anatomy of the liver in Wistar rats. *Surg. Res. Comm.*, 1995, 17, 113–121.

Lozeva, V; Montgomery, JA; Tuomisto, L; Rocheleau, B; Pannunzio, M; Huet, PM; Butterworth, RF. Increased brain serotonin turnover correlates with the degree of shunting and hyperammonemia in rats following variable portal vein stenosis. *J. Hepatol.*, 2004, 40(5), 742–748.

Lu, MD; Chen, JW; Xie, XY; Liang, LJ; Huang, JF. Portal vein embolization by fine needle ethanol injection, experimental and clinical studies. *World J. Gastroenterol.*, 1999, 5(6), 506–510.

Luo, B; Liu, L; Tang, L; Zhang, J; Ling, Y; Fallon, MB. ET-1 and TNF-alpha in HPS, analysis in prehepatic portal hypertension and biliary and nonbiliary cirrhosis in rats. *Am. J. Physiol. Gastrointest. Liver Physiol.*, 2004, 286(2), G294–303.

Luthen, RE; Niederau, C; Grendell, JH. Glutathione and ATP levels, subcellular distribution of enzymes; and permeability of duct system in rabbit pancreas following intravenous administration of alcohol and cerulein. *Dig. Dis. Sci.*, 1994, 39(4), 871–879.

MacPherson, BR; Pemsingh, RS; Scott, GW. Experimental cholelithiasis in the ground squirrel. *Lab. Invest.*, 1987, 56(2), 138–145.

Madrahimov, N; Dirsch, O; Broelsch, C; Dahmen, U. Marginal hepatectomy in the rat: from anatomy to surgery. *Ann. Surg.*, 2006, 244(1), 89–98.

Makino, H; Togo, S; Kubota, T; Morioka, D; Morita, T; Kobayashi, T; Tanaka, K; Shimizu, T; Matsuo, K; Nagashima, Y; Shimada, H. A good model of hepatic failure after excessive hepatectomy in mice. *J. Surg. Res.*, 2005, 127(2), 171–176.

Mann, FCBS; Forster, JP. The extrahepatic biliary tract in common domestic and laboratory animals. *Anat. Rec.*, 1920, 18, 47–66.

Marcos, A; Fisher, RA; Ham, JM; Shiffman, ML; Sanyal, AJ; Luketic, VA; Sterling, RK; Fulcher, AS; Posner, MP. Liver regeneration and function in donor and recipient after right lobe adult to adult living donor liver transplantation. *Transplantation*, 2000, 69(7), 1375−1379.

Martins, PN. Kidney transplantation in the rat: a modified technique using hydrodissection. *Microsurgery*, 2006, 26(7), 543−546.

Martins, PN; Neuhaus, P. Surgical anatomy of the liver, hepatic vasculature and bile ducts in the rat. *Liver Int.*, 2007, 27(3), 384−392.

Martins, PNA; Filatenkov, A. Microsurgical techniques for experimental kidney transplantation and general guidelines to establish studies about transplantation immunology. *Acta Cirurgica Brasileira*, 2003, 18, 355−380.

McGlynn, KA; Hunter, K; LeVoyer, T; Roush, J; Wise, P; Michielli, RA; Shen, FM; Evans, AA; London, WT; Buetow, KH. Susceptibility to Aflatoxin B$_1$-related Primary Hepatocellular Carcinoma in Mice and Humans. *Cancer Research*, 2003, 63(15), 4594−4601.

Moriya, K; Fujie, H; Shintani, Y; Yotsuyanagi, H; Tsutsumi, T; Ishibashi, K; Matsuura, Y; Kimura, S; Miyamura, T; Koike, K. The core protein of hepatitis C virus induces hepatocellular carcinoma in transgenic mice. *Nat. Med.*, 1998, 4(9), 1065−1067.

Musa, BE; Nelson, AW; Gillette, EL; Ferguson, HL; Lumb, WV. A model to study acute pancreatitis in the dog. *J. Surg. Res.*, 1976, 21(1), 51−56.

Nanji, AA. Animal models of nonalcoholic fatty liver disease and steatohepatitis. *Clin. Liver Dis.*, 2004, 8(3), 559−574, ix.

Nettelblad, SC. (1954). *Die Lobierung und innere Topographie der Säugerleber; nebst Beiträgen zur Kenntnis der Leberentwicklung beim Goldhamster* [The Lobung and inner topography of the mammalian liver; in addition to contributions to the knowledge of the liver development in the golden hamster] *(Cricetus auratus)*, Karger.

Nikfarjam, M; Malcontenti-Wilson, C; Fanartzis, M; Daruwalla, J; Christophi, C. A model of partial hepatectomy in mice. *J. Invest. Surg.*, 2004, 17(5), 291−294.

Novobrantseva, TI; Majeau, GR; Amatucci, A; Kogan, S; Brenner, I; Casola, S; Shlomchik, MJ; Koteliansky, V; Hochman, PS; Ibraghimov, A. Attenuated liver fibrosis in the absence of B cells. *J. Clin. Invest.*, 2005, 115(11), 3072−3082.

Okuyama, H; Nakamura, H; Shimahara, Y; Uyama, N; Kwon, YW; Kawada, N; Yamaoka, Y Yodoi, J. Overexpression of thioredoxin prevents thioacetamide-induced hepatic fibrosis in mice. *J. Hepatol.*, 2005, 42(1), 117−123.

Orda, R; Hadas, N; Orda, S; Wiznitzer, T. Experimental acute pancreatitis. Inducement by taurocholate sodium-trypsin injection into a temporarily closed duodenal loop in the rat. *Arch. Surg.*, 1980, 115(3), 327−329.

Orloff, WD; in Souba, WW. Portal hypertension and portacaval shunt. *Surgical Research.*. Academic Press. San Diego, 2001.

Paigen, B. Genetics of responsiveness to high-fat and high-cholesterol diets in the mouse. *Am. J. Clin. Nutr.*, 1995, 62(2), 458s−462s.

Panis, Y; McMullan, DM; Emond, JC. Progressive necrosis after hepatectomy and the pathophysiology of liver failure after massive resection. *Surgery*, 1997, 121(2), 142−149.

Panis, Y; Nordlinger, B. Experimental models for hepatic metastases from colorectal tumors. *Ann. Chir.*, 1991, 45(3), 222−228.

Panis, Y; Nordlinger, B; Delelo, R; Herve, JP; Infante, J; Kuhnle, M; Ballet, F. Experimental colorectal liver metastases. Influence of sex, immunological status and liver regeneration. *J. Hepatol.*, 1990, 11(1), 53−57.

Panis, Y; Ribeiro, J; Chretien, Y; Nordlinger, B. Dormant liver metastases: an experimental study. *Br. J. Surg.*, 1992, 79(3), 221-223.

Papp, M; Makara, GB; Hajtman, B; Csaki, L. A quantitative study of pancreatic blood flow in experimental pancreatitis. *Gastroenterology* 1966, 51(4), 524-528.

Perazzo, J; Eizayaga, F; Romay, S; Bengochea, L; Pavese, A; Lemberg, A. An experimental model of liver damage and portal hypertension induced by a single dose of monocrotaline. *Hepatogastroenterology*, 1999, 46(25), 432-435.

Pfeffer, RB; Stasior, O; Hinton, JW. The clinical picture of the sequential development of acute hemorrhagic pancreatitis in the dog. *Surg. Forum*, 1957, 8, 248-251.

Pinto, M; Herzberg, H; Barnea, A; Shenberg, E. Effects of partial hepatectomy on the immune responses in mice. *Clin. Immunol. Immunopathol.*, 1987, 42(1), 123-132.

Popov, Y; Patsenker, E; Bauer, M; Niedobitek, E; Schulze-Krebs, A; Schuppan, D. Halofuginone induces matrix metalloproteinases in rat hepatic stellate cells via activation of p38 and NFkappaB. *J. Biol. Chem.*, 2006, 281(22), 15090-15098.

Pratt, DS. *Harrison's Principles of Internal Medicine.* F. A. Kasper DL, Longo DL, Braunwald E, Hauser SL, Jameson JL. New York, McGraw-Hill, 1813-1816. 2005

Proctor, E; Chatamra, K. High yield micronodular cirrhosis in the rat. *Gastroenterology*, 1982, 83(6), 1183-1190.

Proctor, E; Chatamra, K. Standardized micronodular cirrhosis in the rat. *Eur. Surg. Res.*, 1984, 16(3), 182-186.

Puig-Divi, V; Molero, X; Vaquero, E; Salas, A; Guarner, F; Malagelada, J. Ethanol feeding aggravates morphological and biochemical parameters in experimental chronic pancreatitis. *Digestion*, 1999, 60(2), 166-174.

Quon, MG; Kugelmas, M; Wisner, JR; Chandrasoma, P; Valenzuela, JE. Chronic alcohol consumption intensifies caerulein-induced acute pancreatitis in the rat. *Int. J. Pancreatol.*, 1992, 12(1), 31-39.

Rahman, TM; and Hodgson, HJ. Animal models of acute hepatic failure. *Int. J. Exp. Pathol.*, 2000, 81(2), 145-157.

Ralli, EPDM. Simplified technique of partial hepatectomy in the rat with fat liver. *Proc. Soc. Exp. Biol.*, 1951, 77, 188-190.

Rege, RV; Dawes, LG; Ostrow, JD. Animal models of pigment gallstones. *Adv. Vet. Sci. Comp. Med.*, 1993, 37, 257-287.

Renz, JF; Busuttil, RW. Adult-to-adult living-donor liver transplantation: a critical analysis. *Semin. Liver Dis.*, 2000, 20(4), 411-424.

Rocko, JM; Swan, KG. The Eck-Pavlov connection. *Am. Surg.*, 1985, 51(11), 641-644.

Rodriguez, G; Lorente, L; Duran, HJ; Aller, MA; Arias, J. A 70% hepatectomy in the rat using a microsurgical technique. *Int. Surg.*, 1999, 84(2), 135-138.

Roger, V; Balladur, P; Honiger, J; Delelo, R; Baudrimont, M; Robert, A; Calmus, Y; Capeau, J; Nordlinger, B. A good model of acute hepatic failure: 95% hepatectomy. Treatment by transplantation of hepatocytes. *Chirurgie*, 1996, 121(6), 470-473.

Rozga, J; Jeppsson, JB; Bengmark, S. Portal branch ligation in the rat. Reevaluation of a model. *Am. J. Pathol.*, 1986, 125(2), 300-308.

Schaeffer, DO; Hosgood, G; Oakes, MG; St Amant, LG; Koon, CE. An alternative technique for partial hepatectomy in mice. *Lab. Anim. Sci.*, 1994, 44(2), 189-190.

Schindl, MJ; Redhead, DN; Fearon, KC; Garden, OJ; Wigmore, SJ. The value of residual liver volume as a predictor of hepatic dysfunction and infection after major liver resection. *Gut*, 2005, 54(2), 289−296.

Schotman, SN; Schraa, EO; Marquet, RL; Zondervan, PE; Ijzermans, JN. Hepatocellular carcinoma and liver transplantation: an animal model. *Transpl. Int.*, 1998, 11 Suppl 1, S201−205.

Senninger, N; Moody, FG; Coelho, JC; Van Buren, DH. The role of biliary obstruction in the pathogenesis of acute pancreatitis in the opossum. *Surgery*, 1986, 99(6), 688-693.

Shirabe, K; Shimada, M; Gion, T; Hasegawa, H; Takenaka, K; Utsunomiya, T; Sugimachi, K. Postoperative liver failure after major hepatic resection for hepatocellular carcinoma in the modern era with special reference to remnant liver volume. 1999; *J. Am. Coll. Surg.*, 188(3), 304−309.

Siech, M; Heinrich, P; Letko, G. Development of acute pancreatitis in rats after single ethanol administration and induction of a pancreatic juice edema. *Int. J. Pancreatol.*, 1991, 8(2), 169−175.

Sirica, AE. Biliary proliferation and adaptation in furan-induced rat liver injury and carcinogenesis. *Toxicol. Pathol.*, 1996, 24(1), 90−99.

Sirica, AE; Zhang, Z; Lai, GH; Asano, T; Shen, XN; Ward, DJ; Mahatme, A; Dewitt, JL. A novel "patient-like" model of cholangiocarcinoma progression based on bile duct inoculation of tumorigenic rat cholangiocyte cell lines. *Hepatology*, 2008, 47(4), 1178−1190.

Su, KH; Cuthbertson, C; Christophi, C. Review of experimental animal models of acute pancreatitis. *HPB (Oxford)*, 2006, 8(4), 264−286.

Sum, PT; Bencosme, SA; Beck, IT. Pathogenesis of bile-induced acute pancreatitis in the dog. Experiments with detergents. *Am. J. Dig. Dis.*, 1970, 15(7), 637−646.

Tang, TC; Man, S; Lee, CR; Xu, P; Kerbel, RS. Impact of metronomic UFT/cyclophosphamide chemotherapy and antiangiogenic drug assessed in a new preclinical model of locally advanced orthotopic hepatocellular carcinoma. *Neoplasia*, 2010, 12(3), 264−274.

Thamavit, W; Bhamarapravati, N; Sahaphong, S; Vajrasthira, S; Angsubhakorn, S. Effects of dimethylnitrosamine on induction of cholangiocarcinoma in Opisthorchis viverrini-infected Syrian golden hamsters. *Cancer Res.*, 1978, 38(12), 4634−4639.

Tsukamoto, H; French, SW; Benson, N; Delgado, G; Rao, GA; Larkin, EC; Largman, C. Severe and progressive steatosis and focal necrosis in rat liver induced by continuous intragastric infusion of ethanol and low fat diet. *Hepatology*, 1985, 5(2), 224−232.

Tsukamoto, H; Matsuoka, M; French, SW. Experimental models of hepatic fibrosis: a review. *Semin. Liver Dis.*, 1990, 10(1), 56−65.

Van Laethem, JL; Robberecht, P; Resibois, A; Deviere, J. Transforming growth factor beta promotes development of fibrosis after repeated courses of acute pancreatitis in mice. *Gastroenterology*, 1996, 110(2), 576−582.

Vaquero, E; Molero, X; Tian, X; Salas, A; Malagelada, JR. Myofibroblast proliferation, fibrosis, and defective pancreatic repair induced by cyclosporin in rats. *Gut*, 1999, 45(2), 269−277.

Veal, N; Oberti, F; Moal, F; Vuillemin, E; Fort, J; Kaassis, M; Pilette, C; Cales, P. Spleno-renal shunt blood flow is an accurate index of collateral circulation in different models of portal hypertension and after pharmacological changes in rats. *J. Hepatol.*, 2000, 32(3), 434−440.

Vorobioff, J; Bredfeldt, JE; Groszmann, RJ. Hyperdynamic circulation in portal-hypertensive rat model: a primary factor for maintenance of chronic portal hypertension. *Am. J. Physiol.*, 1983, 244(1), G52−57.

Walker, NI. Ultrastructure of the rat pancreas after experimental duct ligation. I. The role of apoptosis and intraepithelial macrophages in acinar cell deletion. *Am. J. Pathol.*, 1987, 126(3), 439−451.

Wang, J; Tahara, K; Hakamata, Y; Mutoh, H; Murakami, T; Takahashi, M; Kusama, M; Kobayashi, E. Auxiliary partial liver grafting in rats: effect of host hepatectomy on graft regeneration, and review of literature on surgical technique. *Microsurgery*, 2002, 22(8), 371−377.

Wedgwood, KR; Farmer, RC; Reber, HA. A model of hemorrhagic pancreatitis in cats−role of 16,16-dimethyl prostaglandin E2. *Gastroenterology*, 1986, 90(1), 32−39.

Weinbren, K; Taghizadeh, A. The mitotic response after subtotal hepatectomy in the rat. *Br. J. Exp. Pathol.*, 1965, 46(4), 413−417.

Whitaker, WL. Portal vein ligation and the Eck fistula in the rat. *Proc. Soc. Exp. Biol. Med.*, 1946, 61, 420−423.

Widdison, AL; Alvarez, C; Reber, HA. The low-pressure duct perfusion model of acute pancreatitis. *Eur. Surg. Res.*, 1992, 24 Suppl 1, 55−61.

Wu, SH; Xu, YX; Yin, T; Song, XH; Wang, JJ; Li, R. Fabrication and data harvesting of casting sample of rat liver blood vessels. *Hepatobiliary Pancreat. Dis. Int.*, 2005, 4(4), 582−584.

Wynn, TA. Fibrotic disease and the T(H)1/T(H)2 paradigm. *Nat. Rev. Immunol.*, 2005, 4(8), 583−594.

Yamada, D; Rizvi, S; Razumilava, N; Bronk, SF; Davila, JI; Champion, MD; Borad, MJ; Bezerra, JA; Chen, X; Gores, GJ. IL-33 facilitates oncogene-induced cholangiocarcinoma in mice by an interleukin-6-sensitive mechanism. *Hepatology*, 2005, 61(5), 1627−1642.

Yang, H; Li, TW; Peng, J; Tang, X; Ko, KS; Xia, M; Aller, MA. A mouse model of cholestasis-associated cholangiocarcinoma and transcription factors involved in progression. *Gastroenterology*, 2011, 141(1), 378−388, 388.e371−374.

Yang, R; Rescorla, FJ; Reilly, CR; Faught, PR; Sanghvi, NT; Lumeng, L; Franklin, TD; Jr. Grosfeld, JL. A reproducible rat liver cancer model for experimental therapy: introducing a technique of intrahepatic tumor implantation. *J. Surg. Res.*, 1992, 52(3), 193−198.

Yao, A; Li, X; Pu, L; Zhong, J; Liu, X; Yu, Y; Zhang, F; Kong, L; Sun, B; Wang, X. Impaired hepatic regeneration by ischemic preconditioning in a rat model of small-for-size liver transplantation. *Transpl. Immunol.*, 2007, 18(1), 37−43.

Yeh, CN; Maitra, A; Lee, KF; Jan, YY; Chen, MF. Thioacetamide-induced intestinal-type cholangiocarcinoma in rat: an animal model recapitulating the multi-stage progression of human cholangiocarcinoma. *Carcinogenesis*, 2004, 25(4), 631−636.

Zhong, Z; Theruvath, TP; Currin, RT; Waldmeier, PC; Lemasters, JJ. NIM811, a mitochondrial permeability transition inhibitor, prevents mitochondrial depolarization in small-for-size rat liver grafts. *Am. J. Transplant.*, 2007, **7**(5), 1103−1111.

Section II. Other Experimental Models

In: Advances in Experimental Surgery. Volume 2
Editors: Huifang Chen and Paulo N. Martins
ISBN: 978-1-53612-773-7
© 2018 Nova Science Publishers, Inc.

Chapter 6

ANIMAL MODELS OF ACUTE GRAFT-VERSUS-HOST AND HOST-VERSUS-GRAFT RESPONSES AND DISEASE

*Abraham Matar[1] and Raimon Duran-Struuck[2],**

[1]Department of Surgery, Emory University School of Medicine, Atlanta, GA, US
[2]Department of Pathobiology, University of Pennsylvania School of Veterinary Medicine. Philadelphia, PA, US

ABSTRACT

This chapter aims to provide insight into the strengths and weaknesses of animal models for the study of host-versus-graft (HVG) and graft-versus-host (GVH) responses and disease. As with any complex biological process in which animal models are used, careful assessment of their strengths and weaknesses is paramount. There is no one Universal or "best" animal model. Large animal models such as the dog, pig, or non-human primate, approximate the clinical scenario with much higher fidelity than rodents. However, rodents can be genetically manipulated with ease for the understanding of mechanistic processes that are difficult to investigate in large animals. This chapter will address both large and small animal models used to examine GVH and HVG responses/disease. We will also discuss how these approaches have reached impacted the bedside after being tested at the bench side and cage side.

Keywords: host-versus-graft (HVG), graft-versus-host (GVH) responses, mouse, dog, pig, nonhuman primate, bone marrow transplantation, liver, spleen, small bowel transplantation

---

* Corresponding author: Raimon Duran-Struuck D.V.M. Ph.D. University of Pennsylvania School of Veterinary Medicine, 3800 Spruce Street, Old Veterinary Quadrangle, Suite 177E, (215) 573-3625, E. Mail: rdura@upenn.edu.

ABBREVIATIONS

ALS	anti-lymphocyte serum
BMT	bone marrow transplantation
CyA	cyclosporine A
DLA	Dog leukocyte antigen
GVHR	Graft-versus-host responses
GVHD	Graft-versus-host disease
HSCT/HCT	hematopoietic stem cell transpolantation/hematopoietic cell transplantation
H2	histocompatibility system
HVG	Host-versus-graft
KI	knockin
KO	knockout
miHA	minor histocompatibility antigens
MTX	methotrexate
MMF	mycophenolate mofetil
MHC	Major histocompatibility complex
PBCs	Peripheral blood cells
SBT	Small bowel transplantation
SOT	Solid organ transplantation
TBI	total body irradiation

INTRODUCTION

"It should be noted that marrow grafting could not have reached clinical application without animal research, first in inbred rodents and then in outbred species." E. Donnall Thomas, was the Nobel Prizes winner in 1990.

Animal research, as mentioned by Dr. E. Donnall Thomas in 1990 during his Nobel Prize award, has been crucial for the understanding of bone marrow transplantation (BMT) as a clinical therapy (Ladiges 1990). His studies extensively used both mice and dogs as animal models. Other important models used in BMT research are rats, cats, pigs and non-human primates. The mouse is an excellent animal model because of the similarities in physiological and pathological traits that it shares with other animals and humans. The field of BMT research has taken full advantage of these qualities, and mice have become one of the most commonly used BMT animal models.

Transplantation (organ and hematopoietic) began in the early 20th century. Several studies published between 1949–1953 (Owen 1945; Billingham 1953) documented that organs removed and immediately transplanted back into the same individual (autotransplants) were not rejected. However, organs from genetically different animals but from the same species (allografts) would eventually fail several days after transplantation. After the identification of the antigens that comprise the major histocompatibility complexes (MHC) in the 1960's, transplantation between genetically different individuals became feasible (Copelan 2006). In the veterinary medical field, it was observed that freemartin cattle (a cow with masculinized behavior and non-functioning ovaries that is genetically a female, but is sterilized *in utero* by the hormones from a male twin) did not exhibit similar rejection patterns as observed in allogeneic transplantation (1945). This led to studies that hypothesized the presence of "tolerance" *in utero* which was lost soon after birth. Years later (1956–1959), the immune system was identified as the responsible mechanism for differentiating between "self" and "non-self."

GVHD AFTER BONE MARROW TRANSPLANTATION

Mice and other rodents were first used as animal models for BMT research when scientists and physicians began investigating irradiation-induced bone marrow injury after the World War II. It was observed that after lethal total body irradiation (TBI), restoring bone marrow would rescue the animal's immune system (Thomas 1975a; Thomas 1975b; Jacobson 1951). With the development of inbred strains of mice, many discoveries in the field of immunology, immunogenetics, and radiation oncology have taken place. Important early transplant studies by Van Bekkum and de Vries were summarized by E. Donnall Thomas and Rainer Storb (Thomas 1975a; Thomas 1975b). They discovered that: (1) the delivery of bone marrow intravenously was efficient in rescuing the immunoablated recipient animal; (2) donor bone marrow would cause a "secondary disease" or "runt disease" in mice from which the recipient animals would die unless they were genetically identical [This disease was later identified as GVHD]; (3) genetic factors dictated the severity of GVHD; and (4) the use of immunosuppressive agents (such as methotrexate) was able to ameliorate the GVHD reaction in allogeneic transplants, implicating the immune system as the culprit in GVHD (Thomas 1975a; Thomas 1975b).

Hematopoietic stem cell transplantation (HSCT) is most commonly used for the treatment of hematologic and lymphoid neoplasias and less commonly for non-neoplastic diseases. Mice are the premier animal model for researching novel therapies for the cure of many of these neoplastic and non-neoplastic diseases. Furthermore, mice are used extensively for the study of BMT-related complications such as GVHD. Acute GVHD and leukemic relapse remain the two major obstacles to successful outcomes after allogeneic bone marrow transplantation. We will concentrate on common mouse models that are used to understand the major factors governing graft versus host responses (GVHR) and its side effect, GVHD. These effects are closely intertwined with GVL effects.

Although HSCT is a lifesaving treatment for many patients, the side effects limit its success and wider application. Graft versus host disease (GVHD) is the most common complication and can affect up to 75% of patients. First described in 1962, GVHD was later classically characterized by Billingham as a syndrome in which a graft from an immunocompetent donor recognizes non-self antigens and attacks the immunocompromised cells of the allogeneic recipient (Shlomchik 2007). GVHD can present both acutely and chronically. Acute GVHD (aGVHD) is most often categorized as disease onset within 100 days of transplant, and is a rapidly progressive illness with a strong inflammatory component. In addition to the significant morbidity and mortality of aGVHD, it has also been found to be a powerful predictor of chronic GVHD risk (Copelan 2006), which displays more autoimmune and fibrotic features (Martin 2004). Chronic GVHD was categorized when the disease developed 100 days post-BMT. Clearly this method of categorization of GVHD has had to be modified with the much-improved post-transplant pharmacological approaches where acute GVHD has been observed beyond 100 days. Acute and chronic GVHD is being divided nowadays based on their immunological profiles. While acute GVHD is a CD8 T cell driven, chronic GVHD has been dominated by the generation of allo-antibody and resembles more an antibody-mediated auto-immune condition.

ACUTE GVHD

The induction of acute GVHD is a stepwise process divided into an afferent and an efferent phase (Ferrara 2009). Multiple well-written reviews have been published (Copelan 2006; Shlomchik 2007; Duran-Struuck 2008a). The afferent phase is characterized by donor T cell activation which can be broken down into three steps. First, an inflammatory environment is propagated as a direct result of the pre-transplant conditioning protocol (Ferrara 2009). Next, MHC-peptide complexes are presented on the surface of host antigen presenting cells (APCs) and recognized by mature T cells through the T cell receptor (TCR). Once engaged with the TCR, host APCs produce co-stimulatory signals which activate the T cells. Activated T cells then produce further cytokines, such as IL-2, which act in an autocrine manner to induce clonal expansion. In the efferent phase, these activated T cells produce inflammatory cytokines, recruit additional effector cells, induce the expression of HLA proteins and focus the attack on target organs. This is a self-perpetuating disease state that is difficult to control. 15% of annual HSCT patients die from aGVHD, and this mortality rate can reach 50% for chronic GVHD (Copelan 2006; Ferrara 2009). For these reasons, it is imperative that we develop a better understanding of the mechanism of induction and the factors underlying the severity of disease.

Crucial insights into the pathophysiology of GVHD have been provided by both small and large animal models of GVHD. These insights have in turn, led to improved clinical outcomes of patients suffering from GVHD.

There are multiple approaches to mitigate GVHD. These combine the use of pharmacological and biologicals (Table 6.1). In general, all of these are aimed at targeting T cells but often impact more than one immunological cell subset rendering the animal (or patient) significantly immunossupressed.

MURINE MODELS OF BONE MARROW TRANSPLANTATION AND ACUTE GVHD

Murine animal models have been crucial for the elucidation of immunobiology questions related to bone marrow transplantation. When compared to other species, mice have several advantages that have facilitated these advances. Mouse models are attractive because of their small mass, large litter size, short pregnancy period, the availability of diverse stocks and strains as well as the use of transgenic, knockout (KO) and knock-in (KI) mice have made them the most valuable and versatile experimental animal model for biomedical research. Additionally, mice are relatively inexpensive. Large populations of mice can be maintained in facilities designed specifically for rodents. Several inbred strains are available and have been well characterized; inbred strains have allowed for large experiments where all individuals are genetically identical (as compared to outbred stocks). Knockout and transgenic technology has enabled the study of specific immunological mechanisms by providing a tool that keeps most genetic factors constant. Of all animals, the murine immune system is the best defined. In fact, the major histocompatibility factor (H2) system, was discovered in mice in the 1940's (Snell 1980). Besides man, mice have the highest number of available biological reagents. Some of these reagents include, but are not limited to, monoclonal antibodies, cytokines and growth factors.

Table 6.1. GVHD treatment/sparing strategies

Biologicals		CELLULAR TARGETS	EFFECT
a)Cells	Regulatory T cells (Tregs)	T cells, B cells and innate cells	Direct cell:cell contact immunosuppression/kill and cytokine mediated
	Mesechymal stromal cells	T cells and innate cells	Cytokine mediated and through indirect increases of Tregs
	Chimeric antigen Receptors on T cells (CARs)	Tumor targets	Direct cytotoxicity and kill of tumors
b)Antibodies	Anti-thymocyte globulin (ATG)	T-cell	Apoptosis
	Anti-CD52	T cell & B cell	Apoptosis
	Anti-CD20 (Rituximab)	B-cell	Apoptosis
	Anti-CD2, CD3, CD5 monoclonal antibodies	T-cell	Apoptosis
	Infliximab (monoclonal antibody)	TNF-a	Anti-TNF
Non-pharmacological	Reduced intensity conditioning	Decreased pre-transplant organ damage	Decreased TNF-α, IL-1 and LPS translocation
	Extra-corporeal photopheresis	T-cell apoptosis	8-MOP T cell sensitization
Pharmacological	Glucocorticoids (1st line)	Lymphocytes, monocytes	Anti-inflammatory and apoptosis
	Mycophenolate mofetil (MMF)	T-cell	Inhibition of monophosphate dehydrogenase
	Rapamycin (Sirolimus)	T-cell	Inhibits (G1→S) phase transition
	Cyclosporine	T-cell	Calcineurin inhibitor through cyclophilin
	Tacrolimus	T-cell	Calcineurin inhibitor through FK506 binding protein
	Etanercept (Enbrel)	TNF-α	Soluble TNF-α receptor

Mouse models of GVHD can be separated into animals in which GVHD is directed to either MHC class I or class II, both, or isolated to multiple minor antigens (miHAs). Although multiple miHA mismatches are present across major MHC mismatches, their impact is usually limited relative to that induced by full MHC disparities (Reddy 2008). The GVHD that develops in response to a full (class I and II) MHC disparity is dependent on CD4 T cells and CD8 T cells. These systems result in an inflammatory "cytokine storm," capable of inducing GVHD in target tissues without the requirement for cognate T cell interaction with MHC on tissue (Teshima 2002). In contrast to CD4-dependent GVHD, CD8 T cells induce GVHD primarily by using their cytolytic machinery, which requires the TCR to engage MHC on target tissue (Duran-Struuck 2008a). The induction of GVHD to multiple miHAs results in a process that involves either CD8 T cells, CD4 T cells, or both, depending on the strain combination (Table 6.2).

Table 6.2. H2 haplotypes of common used mouse strains

Strain	H-2 complex			
	MHC-I		MHC-II	
	K	D	A	E
Common strains				
AKR/J	k	k	k	k
C3H/HeJ	k	k	k	k
BALB/c	d	d	d	d
C57BL/6	b	b	b	b
CBA/J	k	k	k	k
DBA/2	d	d	d	d
Congenic strains				
BALB.B	b	b	b	b
BALB.K	k	k	k	k
C3H.SW	b	b	b	b
B6.C-H2 [BM1]	bm1	b	b	b
B6.C-H2 [BM12]	b	b	bm12	b
Recombinant strains				
A	d	k	k	k
B10a	k	d	k	k

These mouse models have helped dissect and shape the complex immunopathology of GVHD. It is critical to understand that no single mouse model can be considered the most appropriate for clinical BMT, because clinical BMT recipients that are MHC matched with the donor also have multiple miHA disparaties. In the laboratory, both MHC and miHA disparate systems can induce aspects of GVHD which are clinically relevant. These permit the isolation of immunological pathways for understanding the mechanisms of GVHD.

Radiation, as a form of myeloablation, is most commonly utilized in mice. Inbred mouse strains (including congenics) demonstrate variable sensitivity to radiation (Duran-Struuck 2008b). The higher the TBI dose, the more intense the inflammatory arm (cytokine storm) of GVHD will be. BMT models utilizing low TBI doses and high donor T cell doses result in GVHD dominated by later onset T cell-dependent pathology (Reddy 2008). Other forms of chemotherapy conditioning with cyclophosphamide, fludarabine, and busulfan can also be delivered in mouse systems, however, these are more commonly used in large animal studies.

Like many animal models, mice have limitations and major differences. First, mouse BMTs are usually supplemented with T cells from the spleen in order to induce GVHD. This is because

BM itself, even across MHC barriers, does not cause GVHD. In larger species, such as humans and pigs, BM-derived T cells are sufficient for inducing GVHD (Duran-Struuck 2015; Duran-Struuck 2016; Duran-Struuck 2017). Currently, most of the BMTs in humans are performed with peripheral blood cells (PBCs) only. PBC transplants in mice are rarely used because of size limitations and blood volume limitations. Second, mouse pre and peri-transplant preparatory regimens do not follow the protocols used in humans, who are gradually rendered immunosuppressed over a number of days. Mice are generally given a myeloablative irradiation dose 2–24 hours prior to the intravenous delivery of the bone marrow graft.

BMT and its applications in mice have been used in a plethora of research fields. Here we will concentrate on the use of these animal models for BMT biomedical research and immunobiology. More specifically, we discuss the use of BMT for the study of GVHD and for its anti-leukemia (GVL) effects, since leukemia relapse and GVHD, as mentioned before, remain the two major obstacles for successful BMT.

Many of the pivotal concepts in BMT have been elucidated by studying the donor: recipient combinations in mice. As described by Shlomchik (Shlomchik 2007), these can be divided into: (a) MHC identical, minor histocompatibility antigen (b) MHC disparate in different background strains (c) MHC disparate in identical background strains (d) the use of strains where single MHC-I or MHC-II alleles differ by a small number of peptides (e) Parent to F1 models.

These combinations have been very important in addressing the involvement of specific cell subsets causing GVHD. T cells have been identified to be important factors for the development of GVHD (Ferrara 1999). As an example, different transplant combinations have induced immune responses mediated by $CD4^+$ T cells, $CD8^+$ T cells, or a combination of both. It should be noted that besides effector T cells, other cell lines such as B cells (Rowe 2006), natural Killer cells (NKCs) (Sentman 1989), and T regulatory cells (Tregs) (Nguyen 2006) have been identified to have an impact in the development or protection of the GVH response. Therefore, the use of mouse models has aided in polarizing the immune system in an effort to dissect the involvement of each one of the multiple factors involved in GVHD. Such "clean" studies, most likely, would have not been able in larger, outbred species because of the genetic variability between animals.

In summary, mouse models, including KI and KO systems, and the use of phenotyping markers (monoclonal antibodies), availability of agonist/antagonists of chemokines, cytokines, co-stimulatory molecules, have proven to be crucial for the elucidation of BMT engraftment and GVHD pathophysiological processes. Clinical applications of many of the concepts discovered in mice have proven to be necessary in pre-clinical large animal models. In our case, we used the pig.

LARGE ANIMAL MODELS OF GVHD

1. Canine Models

Progress in experimental bone marrow transplantation in canines has provided for the translation of dog experimental findings to the clinic. The therapeutic application of marrow grafting in dog has been applied to a variety of human diseases. Dog models of total body irradiation, engraftment and graft-versus-host disease have been (and continue to be) used to address existing clinical problems of hematopoietic cell transplantation and GVHD. Domestic dogs with spontaneously occurring lymphomas and other cancers are used for cellular therapies (as an example, at the University of Pennsylvania (Panjwani 2016) novel chimeric antigen receptor (CARs) T cell approaches are being studied in domestic dogs). Clinical parameters necessary for implementing safe autotransplant approaches in conjunction with high dose radiation and/or chemotherapy have been studied in dogs. Chemicals, radiation, antisera and monoclonal antibodies have been (and continue to be) developed in laboratory bred dogs as a model for human transplantation. Interestingly, the demand for enhanced clinical medical care in domestic dogs has pushed this model beyond experimental use. As a GVHD model, the refinement of approaches that suppress the immune system either nonspecifically using radio/chemo ablation, or directed to specific immune cells continues to be an area of research in which the dog continues to play a big part.

Much of the early work in large animals studying GVHD was at first performed in canines. The Seattle group led the way with early experiments demonstrating the importance of HLA matching in preventing GVHD after BMT. Crucial to these efforts was the development of a reproducible model of lethal acute GVHD in which dogs receiving between 8.5 – 9.2 Gy TBI and dog leukocyte antigens (DLA)-nonidentical unrelated marrow grafts without any immunosuppression died shortly after transplant due to effects of GVHD (Atkinson 1982). Using this model as a foundation, a major contribution to the understanding of GVHD by the Seattle group was studying the effects of different immune suppression regimens on GVHD. Many of these early immunosuppressants tested in the canine model are the same ones used today in clinical BMT, including cyclosporine A (CyA), mycophenolate mofetil (MMF), and methotrexate (MTX) (Table 6.1).

In the early 1980s, E. Donald Thomas and colleagues reported GVHD-free survival in 12/13 animals receiving treatment with methotrexate following supralethal levels of TBI and hematopoietic grafts from DLA matched littermates. This was compared to animals who did not receive methotrexate, in which 16/28 animals developed and died of GVHD. Thomas went on to examine the effect of combination Cyclosporin A and methotrexate (MTX) as a prophylaxis against GVHD (Deeg 1984). They showed that combination MTX and CyA was superior to MTX alone in prophylaxing against GVHD in recipients conditioned with 9 Gy of TBI and receiving DLA-haploidentical transplants (Deeg 1984). This initial work sparked controlled clinical trials assessing the efficacy of combination MTX and CyA for GVHD prophylaxis. Yu et al. demonstrated the synergistic effect of mycophenolate mofetil (MMF) and cyclosporine for the prevention of GVHD in this model (Yu 1998). Dogs receiving either MMF or CyA alone after transplant had increased survival compared to control dogs not receiving any immunosuppression, but all dogs eventually died secondary to GVHD. Groups of animals receiving combination MMF and CyA had greater than 50% survival. Kuhr et al. tested RDP58, a novel anti-inflammatory peptide derived from the HLA class I heavy chain, in prophylaxing against GVHD in this model (Kuhr 2006). Unfortunately, in five dogs that engrafted after transplant, all five developed acute GVHD and were euthanized at 20 days after HCT, not significantly prolonging survival compared to control animals. Similarly, FTY720, also known as Fingolimod, which is the first oral disease modifying drug for the treatment of multiple sclerosis, did not significantly increase survival after the development of GVHD in this model (Lee 2003). Denileukin diftitox, also known as Ontak, an anti-IL2 receptor immunotoxin was unable to mitigate GVHD or increase survival (Mielcarek 2006). The addition of glucocorticoids to tacrolimus or tacrolimus/MTX combination did not show a synergistic effect with respect to the prevention of GVHD or increasing survival compared to tacrolimus or tacrolimus/MTX combination alone (Yu 1997).

More recently, Zorn et al. showed the reduced incidence of GVHD in a canine model of DLA-homozygous donor and DLA-heterozygous recipient transplant using CD6-depleted bone marrow (Zorn 2009). In a control group of 7 canines treated with 10 Gy TBI and receiving unmanipulated bone marrow, all animals died of GVHD within 1 month of transplantation. Animals treated with the same preparatory regimen but receiving CD6-depleted bone marrow using a mouse-anti-human antibody which cross reacts with the canine CD6 antigen, had a significantly reduced incidence of GVHD without jeopardizing the engraftment.

2. Primate Models

Non-human primates (NHP) have been used in transplantation for several decades. Leukaphoresis can be performed in NHPs (Pathiraja 2013) as an alternative to BMT. Not until relatively recently have been MHC-characterized colonies made available for experimental purposes (to mimic allogeneic BMT has been performed like in mice or humans). Two NHP models, one in *cynomolgus macaques (cynos)* and one in *rhesus macaques (rhesus)* have genotyped and characterized their MHC to better design transplant studies. A population of cynos has been naturally isolated on the small island of Mauritius. The Mauritian Islands have been naturally separated from the main land Asia for hundreds of thousands of years. Over five hundred years ago Asian cynos were brought by settlers to the islands from Asia as few founder animals. This geographic isolation has allowed for some natural inbreeding to occur, narrowing their genetic MHC diversity to 6 different haplotypes (PHS 1996; O'Connor 2007). This makes the Mauritius cyno a particularly attractive model for immunological studies. No studies focusing in GVHD have yet been reported using these animals, but have been recently made available commercially and will be an invaluable tool for studies of GVHD biology. There is a recent study which extensively describes the leukocyte populations within the lymphohematopoietic organs (bone marrow, peripheral blood, thymus, lymph nodes and spleen) from these animals providing a platform upon which to build from (Duran-Struuck 2017; Zitsman 2016). No other study exists to date that describes in such careful detail all these cell subsets in GVHD target organs. It is a matter of time that these are further utilized for studies of GVHD.

Under a closely managed breeding program at Yerkes National Primate Research Center and the direction of Kean and colleagues, the NHP GVHD model has been established. This new model is currently being used as a valuable tool to pre-clinically screen novel checkpoint blockade immunotherapies (Kaliyaperumal 2014; Miller 2010). As an example, studies from Miller et al. reported that 100% of animals conditioned with 8 – Gy TBI on day 0 developed rapid-onset of severe GVHD involving the skin, GI system, and liver (Miller 2010). Two of three animals receiving leukapheresis-derived grafts succumbed within 7 days, and 1 animal who received a BM-derived graft succumbed at day 22. Clinical disease correlated closely with $CD8^-$ predominant lymphocyte expansion and activation. In these animals, expanding $CD4^+$ and $CD8^+$ lymphocytes expressed a memory phenotype as indicated by $CD95^+$ cells. Interestingly, the majority of expanding $CD4^+$ cells expressed a central memory phenotype ($CD28^+/CD95^+$) compared to expanding $CD8^+$ cells which predominantly expressed an effector memory phenotype (CD28⁻/CD95⁺). Regardless, both expanding CD4⁺ and CD8⁺ lymphocytes significantly upregulated expression of Ki67, an intra-nuclear marker of proliferation, and downregulated expression of BCl-2, an antiapoptotic protein. Furthermore, untreated animals developing GVHD accumulated high levels of IL-1RA, IL-18, IFNy, and CCL4. Alternatively, five animals treated with 8 Gy TBI in addition to costimulation blockade (CTLA4Ig and anti-CD40L monoclonal antibody) and sirolimus were initially protected from the severe GVHD observed in the untreated recipients and showed 100% survival at day 30, compared with 0% 30 day survival among the untreated animals. T cell activation in treated animals was significantly reduced, and treated animals retained a cohort of naïve CD4 and CD8 T cells (CD95⁻) despite alloantigen exposure that was essentially absent in untreated animals. Despite early protection from GVHD, all treated animals did eventually succumb to GVHD. This was hypothesized to be due to a subset of CD8⁺ T cells (CD28⁻/CD95⁺) exhibiting breakthrough immune activation despite treatment with costimulation blockade and sirolimus. This subset of CD8⁺ T cells exhibited an activated phenotype as evidenced by Ki67 upregulation and BCl-2 downregulation.

3. Swine Models

Studies and descriptions of GVHD in swine have mostly been performed by Sachs and colleagues. The pig is arguably one of the best models for the study GVHD, in particular skin GVHD (Duran-Struuck 2016). To date, the most extensive swine studies of HSCT and GVHD come from the Massachusetts General Hospital (MGH). Over a period of 40 years, David Sachs has developed a herd of partially inbred, MHC-defined miniature swine that have allowed for the study of different clinical HSCT scenarios including minor antigen mismatch, haploidentical match, and full MHC mismatch (Cina 2006). The development of acute GVHD in swine involves the same organ systems as in humans, including skin, liver, gastrointestinal system, and bone marrow (Duran-Struuck 2015). Skin GVHD is the earliest and most common manifestation in swine. Lesions usually involve the neck, back and abdomen of animals, often becoming confluent and ulcerative in nature. Histologically, a differentiating feature of swine GVHD is a denser infiltrate of neutrophils into the skin. This is seen in addition to the classic lymphocytic infiltrate seen in human. An extensive review of swine as a model for GVHD has recently been published (Duran-Struuck 2015).

Early studies from MGH showed that in a haploidentical model (parent to F1), 100% of recipients (n = 18) irradiated with 900 cGY of TBI successfully engrafted after allogeneic BMT. All but one recipient developed varying intensities of skin GVHD, which directly correlated with the degree of T cell depletion in the infused marrow. Similarly to humans, attempts at preventing GVHD by depleting the graft of T cells led to graft failure (Pennington 1988; Popitz-Bergez 1988; Sakamoto 1988).

Table 6.3. Major histocompatibility complexes in mice, pigs and men

Species	MHC-I	MHC-II
Mouse	H2-K, D, L	H2- A, E, O
Human	HLA- A, B, C	HLA- DR, DQ, DP

In mice, the administration of IL-2 post BMT between HLA-mismatched recipient/donor pairs reduces the incidence of GHVD. The effect of high dose IL-2 therapy on GHVD in swine was studied in a series of single haplotype mismatch and full haplotype mismatch transplants (Kozlowski 2000). In fully mismatched bone marrow transplants, high dose IL-2 therapy had no effect on the development of GVHD, and all swine eventually succumb to severe GVHD. However, in the context of single haplotype (class II) mismatched BMT, high dose IL-2 significantly reduced the incidence and severity of GVHD, which translated into increased survival.

Over time, the MGH group has developed a model of haploidentical hematopoietic cell transplantation using a novel reduced intensity conditioning regimen consisting of low dose total body irradiation, T cell depletion using a CD3 immunotoxin, and a short course of cyclosporine. This regimen results in stable multilineage chimerism without significant GVHD, and can induce immunological tolerance to solid organ grafts including kidney, lung, and vascularized composite allografts (Cina 2006; Hettiaratchy 2004).

GVHD AFTER SOLD ORGAN TRANSPLANTATION

The first description of GVHD after solid organ transplantation (SOT) in the literature was by Starzl et al. in 1984, who described GVHD in a patient after undergoing a combined pancreas and splenic transplant (Starzl 1984). Since then, there have been a number of case series retrospectively analyzing GVHD after SOT, specifically liver and small bowel allografts. However, due to the relatively rare incidence of GVHD after SOT, prospective studies of GVHD in humans are impractical. To date, no dedicated large animal model of acute GVHD after SOT exists, most likely related to its rare clinical incidence. Several rat models of GVHD after liver transplantation exist, and we will review those here.

1. Liver

1.1. Experimental

Xue et al. established a reproducible model of acute GVHD after liver transplantation and donor splenocyte infusion in Lewis rats. In this model, the level of chimerism after liver transplantation was shown to correlate with the development of acute GVHD (Xue 2009). Another subsequent study by the same group assessed the effect of tacrolimus vs. rapamycin on GVHD in this model (Xu 2010). They found that rapamycin significantly increased survival compared to tacrolimus, and this survival was associated with higher percentages of CD4+CD25+FoxP3+ T regulatory cells in the circulation and tissues. Finally, the infusion of either donor or recipient derived mesenchymal stem cells (MSCs) prior to the development of aGVHD symptoms (days 0–6) led to the abrogation of typical aGVHD symptoms seen in this model and led to significantly increased survival (Xia 2012). Interestingly, MSCs infused between days 8–14, after the typical symptoms of aGVHD started, had no effect on GVHD or survival. The group hypothesized that the mechanism of MSC protection against aGVHD was via the induction of Tregs, as MSC-infused rats had higher amounts of Tregs in the blood and intestines.

Another recent model of aGVHD after liver transplantation in rats involved preconditioning recipients with sublethal irradiation plus treatment with anti-CD8a mAB to deplete radioresistant NK cells (Yu 2016). Subsequent transplantation of liver allografts alone without a cellular graft consistently resulted in lethal aGVHD. Interestingly, in an attempt to abrogate aGVHD in this model, donor livers were perfused *ex vivo* with a media containing a TCRab mAB, and then transplanted using the same preparatory regimen. *Ex vivo* T cell depletion of liver grafts prevented aGVHD without any accompanying effect on graft function. This strategy may be a viable clinical option in high risk donor and recipient pairs undergoing liver transplantation.

1.2. Clinical

It has been almost 30 years since a case of acute GVHD after orthotopic liver transplant (OLT) was first described in the literature by Burdick et al. (Burdick 1988). Since that sentinel report in 1988, there have been numerous case reports describing GVHD after OLT, as well as several large series reporting on incidence and outcomes (Taylor 2004a; Taylor 2004b; Smith 2003). The three prerequisites that Billingham set forth in his initial description of GVHD after *bone marrow transplant* hold true for the development of GVHD after solid organ transplant. It is estimated that a donor liver graft retains between 1×10^9 and 1×10^{10} passenger leukocytes within its parenchyma and portal tracts even after aggressive flushing with cold preservative solution. This is equivalent or greater to the number of donor lymphocytes transplanted during an HSCT. In the first few weeks following OLT, these donor leukocytes can often be detected in the recipient blood.

As expected, compared to cell transplantation, GVHD after OLT has a much lower incidence, estimated at 1–1.5% (Akbulut 2012). Despite its low incidence, GVHD after OLT carries a dismal prognosis, with a mortality of 85–90% (Smith 2003). GVHD after OLT manifests anywhere between 1–8 weeks following transplantation and produces a similar clinical picture of GVHD after HSCT with symptoms including rash, fevers, diarrhea, and pancytopenia. Marked neutropenia and thrombocytopenia can often precipitate life-threatening infection or hemorrhage. One notable difference is the absence of hepatic and biliary dysfunction as GVHD is restricted to host derived tissues.

Several retrospective analyses have identified risk factors for the development of GVHD after OLT. The most important risk factor appears to be the sharing of HLA antigens between recipient and donor, specifically the use of an HLA homozygous donor. This results in complete one way HLA antigen match in the GVH direction, predisposing to GVHD. Kamei et al. analyzed 8 cases of fatal GVHD after OLT in Japan, and found that all eight cases had one-way HLA matching in the GVH direction in the three loci, HLA-A, HLA-B, and HLA-DR (Kamei 2006). The authors concluded that the risk of fatal GVHD after OLT was likely associated with the number of loci (with the one-way HLA matching) and those with mismatching at all 3 loci (HLA-A, -B, -DR) were at highest risk. In another retrospective series of 12 patients who developed GVHD after OLT by Smith et al. identified several risk factors including close matching at HLA antigens, recipient age >65, and age difference >40 years between donor and recipient (Smith 2003).

Due to the rare incidence of GVHD after OLT and its generally vague presenting symptoms of fever, rash, and diarrhea, the diagnosis of GVHD is not always made immediately. Often times, drug reactions and infectious processes, such as cytomegalovirus (CMV) are investigated first as these are much more common. The strongest supportive evidence for a diagnosis of GVHD, short of a biopsy, is a large number of circulating donor derived T cells in the peripheral blood, referred to as chimerism. These donor cells may be identified by flow cytometry, serologic typing, or PCR-based analysis. In the case of sex differences between donor and recipient, fluorescence in situ hybridization (FISH) analysis can distinguish donor and recipient lymphocytes (Kanehira 2009). It is important to remember that the majority of liver transplant recipients will have detectable donor-derived lymphocytes in the peripheral blood for the first two weeks, but usually taper off by that time (Schlitt 1993). Therefore, the presence of large numbers of donor-derived lymphocytes several weeks after transplant in the setting of fever, rash, diarrhea, etc. should prompt immediate investigation.

Due to the rare incidence of GVHD after OLT and variable patient scenarios, a standardized and proven treatment modality is lacking. Instead, the literature contains various case reports reporting on different treatment strategies, often in a small cohort of patients. Nevertheless, the majority of these reports revolve around several different therapeutic approaches including the use of corticosteroids, increasing/reducing the dose of immunosuppression, and the use of antibody preparations such as antithymocyte globulin (ATG) or OKT3 to eliminate donor lymphocytes. Each has had variable success, and as such, not one agreed regimen yet exists.

The use of corticosteroids for the treatment of GVHD is based on the HSCT experience, in which steroids are the mainstay of treatment and have largely been successful. Although the exact mechanism by which corticosteroids dampen the GVH reaction is not completely understood, it is thought to be a combination of their lymphocytic and anti-inflammatory properties. The use of corticosteroids appears to be the first line approach by many clinicians based on a review of the literature. In the most comprehensive literature review to date, Akbulut et al. reviewed 87 cases of GVHD after OLT (Akbulut 2012). They reported the use of corticosteroids in 61 of 87. Of those 61 patients, 43 died. In the majority of patients who had a suboptimal response to corticosteroids, a variety of other agents were added to attempt to control GVHD. Of these agents, ATG and basiliximab were the most commonly used adjuncts. Regardless, mortality rates did not significantly differ based on the treatment regimen used and remained high.

Another approach is to reduce the level of immunosuppression, thereby allowing the host immune system to reconstitute and mount an immune response to eliminate the donor lymphocytes mediating the GVHD response. The theoretical downside to this approach is the risk of liver rejection in the absence of host immunosuppression. A prospective series of three patients by Chinnakolta et al. suggested that later onset of GVHD (>8 weeks) and lower levels of donor chimerism (<20%) may be predictive factors of favorable GVHD response to withdrawal of immunosuppression (Chinnakotla 2007). In that report, two patients with late onset GVHD (10 weeks, 18 weeks) and low levels of peripheral blood donor chimerism (7%, 11%) underwent withdrawal of immunosuppression and experienced reduction of donor chimerism levels and rapid resolution of symptoms. Both patients did experience mild cases of acute cellular rejection in response to immunosuppression withdrawal, but these were successfully treated with a short course of steroids. A third patient who developed symptoms of GVHD at 2 weeks and had 26.5% donor chimerism in the peripheral blood did not immediately respond to withdrawal of immunosuppression and had worsening of clinical symptoms, eventually dying of uncontrolled sepsis on day 63.

2. Intestine

2.1. Experimental

The first published report of intestinal transplantation came in 1959 by Richard Lillehei, who reported an experimental model for isolated intestinal transplantation in canines (Lillehei 1959). With the introduction of cyclosporine and later tacrolimus, intestinal transplantation has now become a viable clinical option for patients with short bowel syndrome (SBS) who are total parenteral nutrition dependent. Early studies by Lillehei demonstrated that some dogs who died early after intestinal transplantation had relatively normal graft histology, but did have enlarged mesenteric lymph nodes, suggesting that GVHD could develop after intestinal transplantation (Lillehei 1963). Later, a heterotopic small bowel transplant model was developed in rats by Monchik at el, in which GVHD reproducibly led to recipient death within 12–20 days (Monchik 1971). That model was used as a foundation for further studies which showed that immunocompetent T cells in the intestinal grafts were necessary for the induction of GVHD (Kirkman 1984). Donor T cells adoptively transferred from recipient spleens of intestinal transplants were able to induce a graft vs. host reaction in animals syngeneic to the recipient (Pomposelli 1985). Deltz et al. also showed that the extent of GVHD correlated closely with the amount of lymphoid tissue contained within the donor intestinal graft (Deltz 1981). Interestingly Shaffer et al. attempted to abrogate the development of GVHD in this model and were able to demonstrate the effectiveness of pretreatment of donor rats with antilymphocyte serum (ALS) prior to small bowl transplantation (SBT) (Shaffer 1988). ALS prior to SBT prevented GVHD in recipient rats without adversely affecting graft function in both heterotopic and orthotopic allograft models.

There are few large animal models of SBT, likely due to the cost and technical difficulty of the operation. Hale et al. developed a model of heterotopic small bowel allotransplantation in non-human primates (rhesus macaque and baboons) that led to long-term graft survival using an immunosuppressive regimen of Cyclosporine 40 mg/kg/day, Solu-Medrol 2 mg/kg/day, and Azathioprine 5 mg/kg/day (Hale 1991). Graft survival using this immunosuppressive regimen was 75.3 days, and three long-term survivors were euthanized for presumed sepsis with viable grafts. Importantly, there was no incidence of GVHD.

Miura et al. compared the efficacy of heterotopic vs. orthotopic small bowel transplantation in MHC inbred miniature swine and found that orthotopic SBT was superior (Miura 2016). All heterotopic grafts underwent ischemic changes soon after transplantation, presumably due to a compartment-syndrome type process in the limited abdominal space. However, when the native small bowel was removed and orthotopic small bowel allografts were transplanted into swine, all grafts were viable on autopsy and showed no signs of ischemia. Furthermore, compared to recipients of orthotopic small bowel allografts, those swine receiving heterotopic allografts had higher elevation of serum inflammatory cytokines and had a significantly faster progression to lethal metabolic acidosis. In both heterotopic and orthotopic SBT, there was no incidence of GVHD.

2.2. Clinical

Clinically, GVHD following small bowel transplant (SBT) is more common than after other solid organ transplants due to the significant amount of lymphoid tissue contained within the small bowel, particularly the ileum. Several case series reporting on GVHD after SBT have described the incidence between 5–10% (Andres 2010; Mazariegos 2004; Wu 2011). However, because SBT is a much more recent endeavor compared to liver transplantation, there is less published literature regarding GVHD after SBT. Therefore, we will focus on three large retrospective analyses describing the incidence of GVHD after intestinal transplantation (ITx).

In 2004, Mazariegos et al. reviewed 250 adult and pediatric patients receiving ITx between 1990 and 2003 at a single transplant center (Mazariegos 2004). There was a mix of isolated small bowel transplants (44.8%), combined liver and small bowel transplants (36.8%), multivisceral transplants (12.8%), and modified multivisceral transplants without liver (5.6%). Immunosuppression regimens were also quite variable and evolved overtime from a baseline tacrolimus and steroid therapy to include cyclophosphamide, daclizumab, or antibody preconditioning with either thymoglobulin or Campath.

Of the 250 patients included in the study, GVHD was clinically suspected in 23 (9.2%) (6 adults, 17 children) patients based on clinical presentation including skin rash, diarrhea, lymphadenopathy, liver dysfunction, or oral mucosal ulceration. The median onset of GVHD was 1.2 months, which is consistent with acute GVHD. Risk factors for the development of GVHD included multivisceral transplantation and crossmatch negative patients. Multivisceral transplant recipients were twice as likely to develop GVHD as those receiving isolated small bowel transplants, most likely related to the increased lymphoid tissues in multivisceral grafts. Crossmatch negative patients were also more likely to develop GVHD as would be hypothesized, as recipient neutralizing antibodies would have a deleterious effect on donor graft T cells.

Of the 14 histopathological confirmed cases of GVHD, seven patients had increased donor-cell chimerism supportive of the GVHD diagnosis. Donor cell chimerism in those 7 patients was a median of 7.9%, and ranged from 0–35.9%. The majority of confirmed cases of GVHD were mild (Grade I-II) and confined to the skin, although several included the GI tract. There was only 1 case of chronic GVHD. Fortunately, of the 23 cases of suspected GVHD, there were only 2 deaths and neither directly attributed to GVHD. GVHD was resolved in the other 21 patients. 4 patients resolved spontaneously without intervention while the others resolved after either steroid boluses or a methylprednisolone taper.

In 2010, Andres et al. reviewed 46 pediatric patients who underwent SBT between 1999 and 2009 (Andres 2010). Of the 46 patients, 5 (10.8%) developed GVHD as determined by clinical diagnosis. Similarly to the previous study, those patients receiving multivisceral transplants were more likely to develop GVHD as two of the five patients received combined liver-intestinal transplants and three patients underwent multivisceral transplants. There was no GVHD observed after isolated SBT. The median time to GVHD was 47 days (16–333 days). All five GVHD patients had skin manifestation, two had concomitant GI symptoms and three interestingly had respiratory symptoms. Histopathological diagnosis of GVHD was made in four of the five patients, and donor chimerism levels were supportive of the diagnosis in two patients. In contrast to the study by Mazariegos et al, the majority of GVHD observed in this study was severe (Grade III-IV). All five patients were initially treated with high dose steroids (HDS), and four of the five patients had a partial response to therapy defined as a decrease in stage of GVHD. Of the five patients who developed GVHD in this study, three died due to complications of GVHD within four months of diagnosis, a stark contrast to previous studies.

In 2011, Wu et al. reviewed 241 adult and pediatric patients who underwent intestinal transplantation during a 13 year time span between 1994 and 2007 (Wu 2011). The incidence of GVHD was 9.1% (22/241) as determined by clinical diagnosis and confirmed by histopathological evidence. Of the 10 patients with available flow cytometric analysis, four had confirmed macrochimerism (>1%) and the remaining six had detectable microchimerism (<1%). The median onset was twice that of the previous study by Mazariegos et al. (2.5 months vs. 1.2 months). Risk factors associated with the development of GVHD included age, diagnosis, type of graft, and the presence of splenectomy. Children less than 5 years of age were more likely to develop GVHD than were adults (13.2% vs. 4.7%). Interestingly, patients requiring transplant for intestinal atresia were more likely to develop GVHD than those with other diagnoses including gastroschisis, necrotizing enterocolitis, or Hirschsprung's disease (22.2% vs. 2.6%). Consistent with previous studies, recipients of multivisceral transplants were at higher risk of GVHD than those recipients of isolated SBT (12.4% vs. 4.6%). Finally, the addition of recipient splenectomy was also associated with a higher rate of GVHD (13.6 vs. 6.8%). Crossmatch status was not associated with GVHD in this study. Of the 22 cases of GVHD, all involved the skin and all but three were considered mild (grade I-II). Despite the majority of GVHD cases being grade I-II, 17/22 patients died in follow-up, with infection being the most common cause of mortality. The authors concluded that treatment with corticosteroids and increased immunosuppression was inadequate to control GVHD in this series.

Although younger age appears to be associated with a higher chance of developing GVHD and a higher GVHD-associated mortality, it is unclear in these studies whether age is an independent risk factor or whether this association is affected by other variables. In Wu et al. children < 5 were more likely to receive a multivisceral transplant which may have been a factor. Alternatively, one hypothesis to the association between younger age and GVHD could be the underdeveloped immune system of children and their inability to mount an immune response. Similarly, the inability to mount an immune response could be the mechanism by which recipients of recipient splenectomy seem to be more prone to GVHD as in the study by Wu et al.

The most glaring difference between the results of Mazariegos et al. and Wu et al. were the responses to treatment after development of GVHD as well as the GVHD-associated mortality. The vast majority of patients reviewed by Mazariegos et al. that were suspected of having GVHD (n=23), either resolved spontaneously or responded promptly to corticosteroids and adjustment of tacrolimus doses. On the other hand, patients treated with corticosteroids and increased immunosuppression in the series by Wu et al. did not respond to conventional therapy and 77% of patients died of GVHD-related complications according to the authors.

SPLEEN

Small and large animal models of spleen transplantation are uncommon due to the fact that clinical splenic transplantation is rare. The spleen is not a vital organ for survival, and thus justifying long term immunosuppression for splenic transplantation is difficult. However, there have been several studies in large animals assessing the use of splenic transplantation to induce mixed hematopoietic chimerism and immunological tolerance. The rationale is that the spleen is a relatively rich source of hematopoietic progenitor cells. Dor et al. showed that spleen allografts can be accepted across full MHC mismatch barriers in miniature swine (Dor 2005). The acceptance of splenic allografts and continued viability was associated with multilineage chimerism in thymus, bone marrow and blood. Importantly, this multilineage chimerism was associated with donor-specific hyporesponsiveness and did not cause GVHD. Interestingly, two swine that were tolerant of splenic grafts were then transplanted with donor-MHC matched kidney allografts without immunosuppression which were both accepted. The authors concluded that splenic transplantation in miniature swine could result in hematopoietic cell engraftment in the absence of GVHD.

HOST-VERSUS-GRAFT (HVG) RESPONSES

Very few studies have investigated the causality of host-versus-graft responses after BMT. In general, graft loss has always been considered an unwelcomed outcome of BMT, especially when the anti-leukemia graft-versus-host responses sought were not harnessed. Host-versus-graft responses are known as rejection (in solid organ transplantation) or marrow failure/loss (in BMT patients). Little is known about the immunological processes involved in loss of donor bone marrow. The use of reduced intensity conditioning (RIC) regimens in BMT has facilitated the transplantation of patients who previously would have not been considered suitable candidates due to the toxicity of the myeloablative preparatory regimens (Li 2012). Although the risk of complications due to conditioning is decreased with non-myeloablative conditioning, the risk of graft loss is increased. Graft loss can be caused by several factors; i) rejection, ii) the inability of the stem cells (SCs) to engraft due to the lack of "space" (Salomon 1990) or iii) poor donor graft quality (Zeng 1997). These causes may lead to different immunological responses. Rejection of the donor graft implies an active immunological process whereby donor cells sensitize the host (through cellular and/or humoral mechanisms). Conversely, if the loss of donor cells is not immunological, but due to a deficiency in stem cell "fitness" or stem cell quality, there may not be immunological consequences (e.g., sensitization). Some factors related to graft loss include donor/recipient MHC mis/match, the degree of host myeloablation, the level of immunosuppression post-HCT, the degree of host immune competence related to immediate preparatory regimens, the level of T cell depletion of the donor graft and pre-sensitization to donor antigens as is seen in aplastic anemia patients. Clinical studies assessing immune responses of patients following graft loss and after re-exposure of donor antigen have not been extensively investigated. A recent study investigated the immunological responses after graft loss in the MGH MHC defined miniature swine (Duran-Struuck 2012). In this study, recipients underwent reduced intensity conditioning and received cytokine mobilized peripheral blood mononuclear cells (PBMCs) which were haplo-mismatched at both MHC I and II. The RIC regimen consisted of CD3-immunotoxin, 100cGy of TBI and 45 days of cyclosporine A. Cellular and humoral anti-donor responses were studied before and after re-exposure to donor antigen and anti-donor (HVG) immune responses among transplanted and naïve animals exposed to donor antigen were compared. The data this study presented highlighted two important findings. First, peri-transplant conditioning could modify how the immune system responded to a graft and that not all graft rejection was the same. Second, absence of *in vitro* evidence of sensitization by the means utilized (MLRs and antibody binding) did not correlate with absence of a sensitized response leading to the loss of the donor graft. Animals that lost their HCT graft following conditioning regained normal cellular proliferative and cytotoxic allo-responses to donors. These responses were similar in quality to a naïve animal and without any detectable anti-donor antibody responses. Interestingly and to the authors' surprise, whereas animals that lost chimerism might have been expected to have immune responses to donor antigen comparable to naïve animals, this was incorrect. Only after a second donor antigen exposure (without immunosuppression and in the form of a donor leukocyte infusion) in animals which lost chimerism, eventually induced a sensitized cellular immune response that differed from naïve animals. The studies suggested that the initial exposure to donor cells induced an immune response that may have contributed to graft loss but were not detectable with the immunological tools commonly used.

Immunologically, HCT recipients which presumably rejected their grafts, had a much higher host $CD8^+/CD4^+$ Tc ratio when measured by CFSE assays. Sensitized animals at a cellular level had very low $CD4^+$ T cell proliferation. It was postulated that lack of antibody production in animals that rejected their graft was that $CD8^+$ T cell responses may have overwhelmed the ability of $CD4^+$ T cells to provide sufficient B cell help (also known as immune deviation). Similar to the findings reported in the swine studies, immunological responses with a dominant $CD8^+$ T cell population have been observed in patients that rejected their grafts (Kraus 2003).

In conclusion, and of clinical importance, a remarkable finding was the observation that allo-antibodies were never induced after graft loss or after leukocyte infusions. This does have important clinical implications since allo-antibodies are generally tested in the clinic to assess for sensitization (Gandini 2000). Hence, the data supporting allo-antibodies following graft loss may not be a reliable indicator for lack of sensitization and re-transplantation decisions based on their presence may be misleading. More studies are needed to provide further insight into the immunological responses after graft loss which may serve as a guide for modifications of preparatory regimens when subsequent re-transplantation of immune-sensitized hosts is considered.

CONCLUSION

We hope that this chapter provides insight of the strengths and weaknesses of animal models to study HVG and GVH responses and disease. There is no one best animal model. They all have their advantages and disadvantages. Clearly, large animal models (dog, pig, NHP) approximate the clinical scenario with more fidelity than rodents do for the reasons discussed. The most important factor for the researcher will remain to identify the pre-clinical model that can best answer the experimental question. Often, more than one model may be necessary prior to translation to the bedside and begin clinical trials.

REFERENCES

Akbulut S, Yilmaz M, Yilmaz S. Graft-versus-host disease after liver transplantation: a comprehensive literature review. *World Journal of Gastroenterology* 2012; 18(37):5240–5248.

Andres AM, Santamaria ML, Ramos E, Sarriá J, Molina M, Hernandez F, Encinas JL, Larrauri J, Prieto G, Tovar JA. Graft-vs-host disease after small bowel transplantation in children. *J. Pediatr. Surg.* 2010; 45(2):330–336; discussion 336.

Atkinson K, Shulman HM, Deeg HJ, Weiden PL, Graham TC, Thomas ED, Storb R. Acute and chronic graft-versus-host disease in dogs given hemopoietic grafts from DLA-nonidentical littermates. Two distinct syndromes. *The American Journal of Pathology* 1982; 108(2):196–205.

Billingham RE, Brent L, Medawar PB. Actively acquired tolerance to foreign cells. *Nature* 1953; 172:603–606.

Burdick JF, Vogelsang GB, Smith WJ, Farmer ER, Bias WB, Kaufmann SH, Horn J, Colombani PM, Pitt HA, Perler BA, Merritt WT, Williams GM, Boitnott JK, Herlong HF. Severe graft-versus-host disease in a liver-transplant recipient. *The New England Journal of Medicine* 1988; 318(11):689–691.

Chinnakotla S, Smith DM, Domiati-Saad R, Agura ED, Watkins DL, Netto G, Uemura T, Sanchez EQ, Levy MF, Klintmalm GB. Acute graft-versus-host disease after liver transplantation: role of withdrawal of immunosuppression in therapeutic management. *Liver transplantation: official publication of the American Association for the Study of Liver Diseases and the International Liver Transplantation Society.* 2007; 13(1):157–161.

Cina RA, Wikiel KJ, Lee PW, Cameron AM, Hettiarachy S, Rowland H, Goodrich J, Colby C, Spitzer TR, Neville DM Jr, Huang CA. Stable multilineage chimerism without graft versus host disease following nonmyeloablative haploidentical hematopoietic cell transplantation. *Transplantation* 2006; 81(12):1677–1685.

Copelan EA. Hematopoietic stem-cell transplantation. *N Engl J Med.* 2006; 354(17):1813–1826.

Deeg HJ, Storb R, Appelbaum FR, Kennedy MS, Graham TC, Thomas ED. Combined immunosuppression with cyclosporine and methotrexate in dogs given bone marrow grafts from DLA-haploidentical littermates. *Transplantation* 1984; 37(1):62–65.

Deltz E, Muller-Hermelink HK, Ulrichs K, Thiede A, Muller-Ruchholtz W. Development of graft-versus-host reaction in various target organs after small intestine transplantation. *Transplantation Proceedings* 1981; 13(1 Pt 2):1215–1216.

Dor FJ, Tseng YL, Kuwaki K, Gollackner B, Ramirez ML, Prabharasuth DD, Cina RA, Knosalla C, Nuhn MG, Houser SL, Huang CA, Ko DS, Cooper DK. Immunological unresponsiveness in chimeric miniature swine following MHC-mismatched spleen transplantation. *Transplantation* 2005; 80(12):1791–1804.

Duran-Struuck R, Hartigan A, Clouthier SG, Dyson MC, Lowler K, Gatza E, Tawara I, Toubai T, Weisiger E, Hugunin K, Reddy P, Wilkinson JE. Differential susceptibility of C57BL/6NCr and B6.Cg-Ptprca mice to commensal bacteria after whole body irradiation in translational bone marrow transplant studies. *J. Transl. Med.* 2008b; 6:10.

Duran-Struuck R, Huang CA, Orf K, Bronson RT, Sachs DH, Spitzer TR. Miniature Swine as a Clinically Relevant Model of Graft-Versus-Host Disease. *Comp. Med.* 2015; 65(5):429–443.

Duran-Struuck R, Matar A, Crepeau R, Gusha A, Schenk M, Hanekamp I, Pathiraja V, Spitzer TR, Sachs DH, Huang CA. Lack of antidonor alloantibody does not indicate lack of immune sensitization: studies of graft loss in a haploidentical hematopoietic cell transplantation Swine model. *Biol. Blood Marrow Transplant* 2012; 18(11):1629–1637.

Duran-Struuck R, Matar AJ, Crepeau RL, Teague AG, Horner BM, Pathiraja V, Spitzer TR, Fishman JA, Bronson RT, Sachs DH, Huang CA. Donor Lymphocyte Infusion-Mediated Graft-versus-Host Responses in a Preclinical Swine Model of Haploidentical

Hematopoietic Cell Transplantation. *Biol. Blood Marrow Transplant.* 2016; 22(11):1953–1960.

Duran-Struuck R, Reddy P. Biological advances in acute graft-versus-host disease after allogeneic hematopoietic stem cell transplantation. *Transplantation* 2008a; 85(3):303–308.

Duran-Struuck R, Sondermeijer HP, Buhler L, Alonso-Guallart P, Zitsman J, Kato Y, Wu A, McMurchy AN, Woodland D, Griesemer A, Martinez M, Boskovic S, Kawai T, Cosimi AB, Wuu CS, Slate A, Mapara MY, Baker S, Tokarz R, D'Agati V, Hammer S, Pereira M, Lipkin WI, Wekerle T, Levings MK, Sykes M. Effect of Ex Vivo-Expanded Recipient Regulatory T Cells on Hematopoietic Chimerism and Kidney Allograft Tolerance Across MHC Barriers in Cynomolgus Macaques. *Transplantation* 2017; 101(2):274–283.

Ferrara JL, Levine JE, Reddy P, Holler E. Graft-versus-host disease. *Lancet* 2009; 373(9674):1550–1561.

Ferrara JL, Levy R, Chao NJ. Pathophysiologic mechanisms of acute graft-vs.-host disease. Biol *Blood Marrow Transplant.* 1999; 5(6):347–356.

Gandini G, Franchini M, de Gironcoli M, Vassanelli A, Benedetti F, Turrini A, Benini F, Aprili G. Detection of an anti-RhD antibody 2 years after sensitization in a patient who had undergone an allogeneic BMT. *Bone Marrow Transplant.* 2000; 25(4):457–459.

Hale DA, Waldorf KA, Kleinschmidt J, Pearl RH, Seyfer AE. Small intestinal transplantation in nonhuman primates. *Journal of Pediatric Surgery.* 1991; 26(8):914–920.

Hettiaratchy S, Melendy E, Randolph MA, Coburn RC, Neville DM Jr, Sachs DH, Huang CA, Lee WP. Tolerance to composite tissue allografts across a major histocompatibility barrier in miniature swine. *Transplantation* 2004; 77(4):514–521.

Jacobson LO, Simmons EL, Marks EK, Eldredge JH. Recovery from radiation injury. *Science.* 1951; 113 (2940):510–511.

Kaliyaperumal S, Watkins B, Sharma P, Furlan S, Ramakrishnan S, Giver C, Garcia A, Courtney C, Knight H, Strobert E, Elder E, Crenshaw T, Blazar BR, Waller EK, Westmoreland S, Kean LS. CD8-predominant T-cell CNS infiltration accompanies GVHD in primates and is improved with immunoprophylaxis. *Blood* 2014; 123(12):1967–1969.

Kamei H, Oike F, Fujimoto Y, Yamamoto H, Tanaka K, Kiuchi T. Fatal graft-versus-host disease after living donor liver transplantation: differential impact of donor-dominant one-way HLA matching. *Liver transplantation: official publication of the American Association for the Study of Liver Diseases and the International Liver Transplantation Society.* 2006; 12(1):140–145.

Kanehira K, Riegert-Johnson DL, Chen D, Gibson LE, Grinnell SD, Velgaleti GV. FISH diagnosis of acute graft-versus-host disease following living-related liver transplant. *The Journal of Molecular Diagnostics: JMD* 2009; 11(4):355–358.

Kirkman RL, Lear PA, Madara JL, Tilney NL. Small intestine transplantation in the rat--immunology and function. *Surgery* 1984; 96(2):280–287.

Kozlowski T, Sablinski T, Basker M, Kitamura H, Spitzer TR, Fishman J, Sykes M, Cooper DK, Sachs DH. Decreased graft-versus-host disease after haplotype mismatched bone marrow allografts in miniature swine following interleukin-2 treatment. *Bone Marrow Transplantation* 2000; 25(1):47–52.

Kraus AB, Shaffer J, Toh HC, Preffer F, Dombkowski D, Saidman S, Colby C, George R, McAfee S, Sackstein R, Dey B, Spitzer TR, Sykes M. Early host CD8 T-cell recovery and sensitized anti-donor interleukin-2-producing and cytotoxic T-cell responses associated with marrow graft rejection following nonmyeloablative allogeneic bone marrow transplantation. *Exp. Hematol.* 2003; 31(7):609–621.

Kuhr CS, Lupu M, Little MT, Zellmer E, Sale GE, Storb R. RDP58 does not prevent graft-versus-host disease after dog leukocyte antigen-nonidentical canine hematopoietic cell transplantation. *Transplantation* 2006; 81(10):1460–1462.

Ladiges WC, Storb R, Thomas ED. Canine models of bone marrow transplantation. *Lab. Anim. Sci.* 1990; 40:11–15.

Lee RS, Kuhr CS, Sale GE, Zellmer E, Hogan WJ, Storb R, Little MT. FTY720 does not abrogate acute graft-versus-host disease in the dog leukocyte antigen-nonidentical unrelated canine model. *Transplantation* 2003; 76(8):1155–1158.

Li HW, Sykes M. Emerging concepts in haematopoietic cell transplantation. *Nat. Rev. Immunol.* 2012; 12(6):403–416.

Lillehei RC, Goldberg S, Goott B, Longerbeam JK. The present status of intestinal transplantation. *American Journal of Surgery* 1963; 105:58–72.

Lillehei RC, Goott B, Miller FA. The physiological response of the small bowel of the dog to ischemia including prolonged *in vitro* preservation of the bowel with successful replacement and survival. *Annals of Surgery* 1959; 150:543–560.

Martin PJ, Carpenter PA, Sanders JE, Flowers ME. Diagnosis and clinical management of chronic graft-versus-host disease. *Int. J. Hematol.* 2004; 79(3):221–228.

Mazariegos GV, Abu-Elmagd K, Jaffe R, Bond G, Sindhi R, Martin L, Macedo C, Peters J, Girnita A, Reyes J. Graft versus host disease in intestinal transplantation. *Am. J. Transplant.* 2004; 4(9):1459–1465.

Mielcarek M, Georges GE, Storb R. Denileukin diftitox as prophylaxis against graft-versus-host disease in the canine hematopoietic cell transplantation model. *Biol. Blood Marrow Transplant.* 2006; 12(9):899–904.

Miller WP, Srinivasan S, Panoskaltsis-Mortari A, Singh K, Sen S, Hamby K, Deane T, Stempora L, Beus J, Turner A, Wheeler C, Anderson DC, Sharma P, Garcia A, Strobert E, Elder E, Crocker I, Crenshaw T, Penedo MC, Ward T, Song M, Horan J, Larsen CP, Blazar BR, Kean LS. GVHD after haploidentical transplantation: a novel, MHC-defined rhesus macaque model identifies CD28- CD8+ T cells as a reservoir of breakthrough T-cell proliferation during costimulation blockade and sirolimus-based immunosuppression. *Blood* 2010; 116(24):5403–5418.

Miura K, Sahara H, Waki S, Kawai A, Sekijima M, Kobayashi T, Zhang Z, Wakai T, Shimizu A, Yamada K. Development of the Intestinal Transplantation Model With Major Histocompatibility Complex Inbred CLAWN Miniature Swine. *Transplant. Proc.* 2016; 48(4):1315–1319.

Monchik GJ, Russell PS. Transplantation of small bowel in the rat: technical and immunological considerations. *Surgery* 1971; 70(5):693–702.

Nguyen VH, Zeiser R, Negrin RS. Role of naturally arising regulatory T cells in hematopoietic cell transplantation. *Biol. Blood Marrow Transplant*. 2006; 12(10):995–1009.

O'Connor SL, Blasky AJ, Pendley CJ, Becker EA, Wiseman RW, Karl JA, Hughes AL, O'Connor DH. Comprehensive characterization of MHC class II haplotypes in Mauritian cynomolgus macaques. *Immunogenetics* 2007; 59(6):449–462.

Owen RD. Immunogenetic consequences of vascular anastomoses between bovine twins. *Science* 1945; 102:400–401.

Panjwani MK, Smith JB, Schutsky K, Gnanandarajah J, O'Connor CM, Powell DJ Jr, Mason NJ. Feasibility and Safety of RNA-transfected CD20-specific Chimeric Antigen Receptor T Cells in Dogs with Spontaneous B Cell Lymphoma. *Mol. Ther.* 2016; 24(9):1602–1614.

Pathiraja V, Matar AJ, Gusha A, Huang CA, Duran-Struuck R. Leukapheresis protocol for nonhuman primates weighing less than 10 kg. *J Am Assoc Lab Anim Sci.* 2013 Jan; 52(1):70-7.

Pennington LR, Sakamoto K, Popitz-Bergez F, Pescovitz MD, McDonough MA, MacVittie TJ, Gress RE, Sachs DH. Bone marrow transplantation in miniature swine. I. Development of the model. *Transplantation* 1988; 45:21–26.

PHS. Public Health Service. Draft Public Health Service Guideline on Infectious Disease Issues in Xenotransplantation, *Fed. Regist.* 1996; 61(185): 49920–49932.

Pomposelli F, Maki T, Kiyoizumi T, Gaber L, Balogh K, Monaco AP. Induction of graft-versus-host disease by small intestinal allotransplantation in rats. *Transplantation* 1985; 40(4):343–347.

Popitz-Bergez FA, Sakamoto K, Pennington LR, Pescovitz MD, McDonough MA, MacVittie TJ, Gress RE, Sachs DH. Bone marrow transplantation in miniature swine. II. Effect of selective genetic differences on marrow engraftment and recipient survival. *Transplantation* 1988; 45:27–31.

Reddy P, Negrin R, Hill GR. Mouse models of bone marrow transplantation. *Biol. Blood Marrow Transplant* 2008; 14(1 Suppl 1):129–135.

Rowe V, Banovic T, Macdonald KP, Kuns R, Don AL, Morris ES, Burman AC, Bofinger HM, Clouston AD, Hill GR. Host B cells produce IL-10 following TBI and attenuate acute GVHD after allogeneic bone marrow transplantation. *Blood* 2006; 108(7):2485–2492.

Sakamoto K, Sachs DH, Shimada S, Popitz-Bergez FA, Pennington LR, Pescovitz MD, McDonough MA, MacVittie TJ, Katz SI, Gress RE. Bone marrow transplantation in miniature swine. III Graft-versus-host disease and the effect of T cell depletion of marrow. *Transplantation* 1988; 45:869–875.

Salomon O, Lapidot T, Terenzi A, Lubin I, Rabi I, Reisner Y. Induction of donor-type chimerism in murine recipients of bone marrow allografts by different radiation regimens currently used in treatment of leukemia patients. *Blood* 1990; 76(9):1872–1878.

Schlitt HJ, Kanehiro H, Raddatz G, Steinhoff G, Richter N, Nashan B, Ringe B, Wonigeit K, Pichlmayr R. Persistence of donor lymphocytes in liver allograft recipients. *Transplantation* 1993; 56(4):1001–1007.

Sentman CL, Kumar V, Koo G, Bennett M. Effector cell expression of NK1.1, a murine natural killer cell-specific molecule, and ability of mice to reject bone marrow allografts. *J. Immunol.* 1989; 142:1847–1853.

Shaffer D, Maki T, DeMichele SJ, Karlstad MD, Bistrian BR, Balogh K, Monaco AP. Studies in small bowel transplantation. Prevention of graft-versus-host disease with preservation of allograft function by donor pretreatment with antilymphocyte serum. *Transplantation* 1988; 45(2):262–269.

Shlomchik WD. Graft-versus-host disease. *Nat. Rev. Immunol.* 2007; 7(5):340–352.

Smith DM, Agura E, Netto G, Collins R, Levy M, Goldstein R, Christensen L, Baker J, Altrabulsi B, Osowski L, McCormack J, Fichtel L, Dawson DB, Domiati-Saad R, Stone M, Klintmalm G. Liver transplant-associated graft-versus-host disease. *Transplantation* 2003; 75(1):118–126.

Snell GD. The major histocompatibility complex: its evolution and involvement in cellular immunity. *Harvey Lect.* 1980; 74:49–80.

Starzl TE, Iwatsuki S, Shaw BW, Jr., Greene DA, Van Thiel DH, Nalesnik MA, Nusbacher J, Diliz-Perez H, Hakala TR. Pancreaticoduodenal transplantation in humans. *Surg Gynecol Obstet.* 1984; 159(3):265–272.

Taylor AL, Gibbs P, Bradley JA. Acute graft versus host disease following liver transplantation: the enemy within. *American journal of transplantation: official journal of the American Society of Transplantation and the American Society of Transplant Surgeons.* 2004a; 4(4):466–474.

Taylor AL, Gibbs P, Sudhindran S, Key T, Goodman RS, Morgan CH, Watson CJ, Delriviere L, Alexander GJ, Jamieson NV, Bradley JA, Taylor CJ. Monitoring systemic donor lymphocyte macrochimerism to aid the diagnosis of graft-versus-host disease after liver transplantation. *Transplantation* 2004b; 77(3):441–446.

Teshima T, Ordemann R, Reddy P, Gagin S, Liu C, Cooke KR, Ferrara JL. Acute graft-versus-host disease does not require alloantigen expression on host epithelium. *Nat. Med.* 2002; 8(6):575–581.

Thomas ED, Storb R, Clift RA, Fefer A, Johnson FL, Neiman PE, Lerner KG, Glucksberg H, Buckner CD. Bone marrow transplantation. *N. Engl. J. Med.* 1975a; 292:832–843.

Thomas ED, Storb R, Clift RA, Fefer A, Johnson L, Neiman PE, Lerner KG, Glucksberg H, Buckner CD. Bone-marrow transplantation (second of two parts). *N. Engl. J. Med.* 1975b; 292(17):895–902.

Wu G, Selvaggi G, Nishida S, Moon J, Island E, Ruiz P, Tzakis AG. Graft-versus-host disease after intestinal and multivisceral transplantation. *Transplantation* 2011; 91(2):219–224.

Xia X, Chen W, Ma T, Xu G, Liu H, Liang C, Bai X, Zhang Y, He Y, Liang T. Mesenchymal stem cells administered after liver transplantation prevent acute graft-versus-host disease in rats. *Liver Transpl.* 2012; 18(6):696–706.

Xu G, Wang L, Chen W, Xue F, Bai X, Liang L, Shen X, Zhang M, Xia D, Liang T. Rapamycin and tacrolimus differentially modulate acute graft-versus-host disease in rats after liver transplantation. *Liver Transpl.* 2010; 16(3):357–363.

Xue F, Chen W, Wang XG, Liang L, Bai XL, Wang LY, Wang HP, Liang TB. Establishment of an acute graft-versus-host disease model following liver transplantation in donor-dominant one-way major histocompatibility complex matching rats. *Transplant. Proc.* 2009; 41(5):1914–1920.

Yu C, Seidel K, Fitzsimmons WE, Sale G, Storb R. Glucocorticoids fail to enhance the effect of FK506 and methotrexate in prevention of graft-versus-host disease after DLA-nonidentical, unrelated marrow transplantation. *Bone Marrow Transplantation* 1997; 20(2):137–141.

Yu C, Seidel K, Nash RA, Deeg HJ, Sandmaier BM, Barsoukov A, Santos E, Storb R. Synergism between mycophenolate mofetil and cyclosporine in preventing graft-versus-host disease among lethally irradiated dogs given DLA-nonidentical unrelated marrow grafts. *Blood* 1998; 91(7):2581–2587.

Yu E, Ueta H, Kimura H, Kitazawa Y, Sawanobori Y, Matsuno K. Graft-Versus-Host Disease Following Liver Transplantation: Development of a High-Incidence Rat Model and a Selective Prevention Method. *Am. J. Transplant.* 2017; 17(4):979–991.

Zeng D, Dejbakhsh-Jones S, Strober S. Granulocyte colony-stimulating factor reduces the capacity of blood mononuclear cells to induce graft-versus-host disease: impact on blood progenitor cell transplantation. *Blood* 1997; 90(1):453–463.

Zitsman JS, Alonso-Guallart P, Ovanez C, Kato Y, Rosen JF, Weiner JI, Duran-Struuck R. Distinctive Leukocyte Subpopulations According to Organ Type in Cynomolgus Macaques. *Comp. Med.* 2016; 66(4):308–323.

Zorn J, Herber M, Schwamberger S, Panzer W, Adler H, Kolb HJ. Tolerance in DLA-haploidentical canine littermates following CD6-depleted marrow transplantation and donor lymphocyte transfusion. *Exp. Hematol.* 2009; 37(8):998–1006.

In: Advances in Experimental Surgery. Volume 2
Editors: Huifang Chen and Paulo N. Martins

ISBN: 978-1-53612-773-7
© 2018 Nova Science Publishers, Inc.

Chapter 7

MICROFLUIDIC DEVICES AND MICRO-DISSECTED TISSUE TO PREDICT THERAPEUTIC RESPONSE IN PATIENTS WITH PROSTATE CANCER

*Robin Guay-Lord[*], Muhammad Abdul Lateef[*], PhD,
Kayla Simeone[*], Benjamin Péant, PhD,
Jennifer Kendall-Dupont, Anne-Marie Mes-Masson, PhD,
Thomas Gervais, PhD and Fred Saad[†], MD*

CRCHUM, Departments of Molecular Biology, Surgery and Medicine,
Faculty of Medicine, University of Montreal, Montreal, Quebec, Canada

ABSTRACT

Given the genetic and epigenetic diversity of prostate tumors and their variable response to chemotherapy, therapeutic strategies against prostate cancer have experienced a framework shift from broad cytotoxic drugs to a more personalized level of medicine. This personalized approach not only results in superior medical care by improving effectiveness while diminishing toxicities, but it also directly impacts health economics and patient quality of life. In this scope, we present a novel model that allows empirical testing of therapeutic agents on *ex vivo* patient-derived tissues, cultured in a non-perfused microfluidic device. The proposed model relies on the micro-dissection of tumor biopsies and samples obtained through surgical resection of the prostate (radical prostatectomy or transurethral resection of the prostate) to produce micro-dissected tissue (MDT) samples, which are trapped in a microfluidic device and exposed to various combinations of drugs. Confocal microscopy and flow cytometry analysis are used to determine the viability of the drug-treated MDTs. These analytical methods are a promising way to determine therapeutic response or resistance and to help identify the optimal treatment plan for an individual patient in less than two weeks after tissue procurement. The presented model is simple to operate, cost effective, offers high-throughput potential through multiplexing,

---

[*] Each author contributed equally to this project.
[†] Corresponding Author Email: fred.saad@umontreal.ca.

and is clinically relevant to predict *in vivo* therapeutic response, thus making it a new tool with the potential to significantly improve the current treatment of prostate cancer.

Keywords: microfluidics, micro-dissected tissue, prostate cancer, therapeutic response, lab-on-a-chip, organotypic tissue

ABBREVIATIONS

LOC	Lab-on-a-Chip
MEMS	Microelectromechanical System
PDMS	Poly (dimethylsiloxane)
CSRA	Chemosensitivity and Resistance Assay
2D	two-dimensional
3D	three-dimensional
ECM	Extracellular Matrix
PDX	Patient-Derived Xenograft
MDT	Micro-Dissected Tissue
PMMA	Poly (methylmethacrylate)
CNC	Computer Numerical Control
TURP	Transurethral Resection of the Prostate
BPH	Benign Prostate Hyperplasia
SOP	Standard Operating Procedure
HBSS	Hanks' Balanced Salt Solution
HBSS $_{complete}$	HBSS, 10% FBS, 55 mg/L gentamicin and 0.6 mg/L amphotericin
HBSS $_{antibio}$	HBSS, 55 mg/L gentamicin and 0.6 mg/L amphotericin
PBS	Phosphate-Buffered Saline
FBS	Fetal Bovine Serum
RPMI	Roswell Park Memorial Institute
CTO	Cell Tracker Orange CMTMR
SG	Sytox Green

INTRODUCTION

Despite the impressive stride forward in early diagnostics, prostate cancer remains the second leading cause of death by cancer in western countries. Given the genetic and epigenetic diversity of prostate tumors and their variable response to different agents, therapeutic treatment plan efficacy has become a challenge. Recently, therapeutic strategies against prostate cancer have experienced a framework shift from broad cytotoxic drugs to a more personalized level of medicine. This personalized approach not only results in superior medical care by enhancing effectiveness while minimizing drug-induced toxicities, but it also directly impacts health economics and potentially improve patient quality of life. To attain this goal, much effort has focused on predictive biomarkers that provide a statistical probability of response, however this approach has proven to be unpredictable and not always straightforward (Ginsburg 2001).

In this context, direct testing of therapeutic agents on the biopsied tumor mass, or on cell cultures derived from tumor tissues, has been proposed as a viable complementary method to predict patient response. So far, preclinical models used to address therapeutic efficacy and specificity have largely relied on monolayer (2D) cultures, either of cell lines or tumor explants. These often provide an imperfect measure of what is observed in xenografts or patients, largely because they do not take into account the tumor heterogeneity and the complexity of the tumor microenvironment (Justice 2009). Considering the limited amount of tissue available from biopsies and the long assay time to execute multiplexed drug resistance tests, the direct testing of treatment on biopsied tumor mass has not been feasible until recently.

In this chapter, we present a new model that relies on the application of microfluidic technologies coupled to micro-dissected tissue (MDT)-based sampling to assess the chemosensitivity profile of tumor tissues in a patient-specific manner. We first review the history and the advantages of microfluidics for drug screening applications in oncology. We then describe the design and fabrication of the microfluidic platform along with the methodology to produce the MDT samples and trap them into the microfluidic device for further culturing and maintenance. Finally, the MDTs can be treated with various therapeutic agents on-chip to allow confocal microscopy and flow cytometry analysis of MDT response to treatment.

EVOLUTIONARY HISTORY OF MICROFLUIDIC TECHNOLOGY

First introduced in 1990 in the seminal work of Manz et al., the concept of lab-on-a-chip (LOC) today has deeply influenced modern analytical chemistry and biology (Manz 1990). The idea behind LOC technologies is to miniaturize and integrate all the necessary steps for a particular assay in a low-cost and portable format, with fast analysis time and digital-like capabilities for efficient processing of biological samples. These LOC systems offer multiple benefits over their macroscale counterparts, including improved throughput and automation, which will be further detailed in this chapter. The history of LOCs is closely related to microfluidics where the science and technologies involve controlling small volumes of fluid at the sub-millimeter scale (Whitesides 2006). Some of the earliest applications integrating the concept of microfluidics and LOCs were used for analytical chemistry techniques: gas-phase chromatography (de Mello 2002; Terry 1979), high-pressure liquid chromatography (de Mello 2002; Manz 1990) and capillary electrophoresis (Kim 1996; Mathies 1992; Woolley 1994). Since then, a great number of biological applications ranging from genomics to cellular assays have been miniaturized and integrated into LOC devices. For instance, in fundamental research, LOC devices, which reproduce organ functionality, have been developed to study human physiology in an organ-specific context (Huh 2011). Often named "organs-on-chips," various new *in vitro* models have been reported to study organ-specific functions of brain (Park 2009), liver (Kane 2006; Lee 2007), kidney (Jang 2010), gut (Kimura 2008), breast (Song 2009), and bone (You 2008). In a clinical context, LOCs have been used to provide a high-throughput platform to manipulate and probe tissue samples for drug screening (Astolfi 2016; Pak 2015).

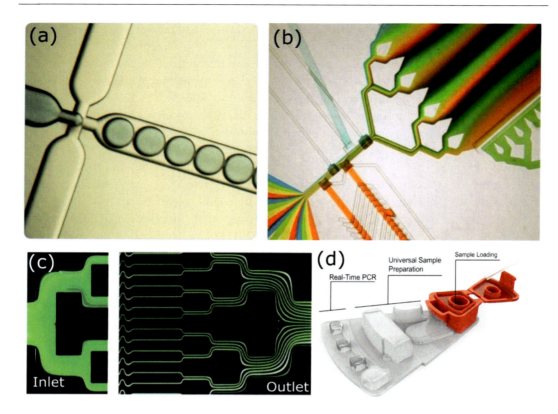

Figure 7.1. Common applications of microfluidics: (a) Droplets-based microfluidics are a promising tool for many chemical and biological assays that require controlled and rapid mixing and accurate temperature control. Image courtesy of Dolomite Microfluidics. (b) Microfluidic devices can be used to generate gradients of reagents with precise spatial and temporal control. Image courtesy of Albert Folch, University of Washington. (c) Inertial microfluidics is frequently used to separate particles or cells in a continuous flow for high-throughput sorting applications. Image reproduced with permission from (Di Carlo, 2009) (d) Lab-on-a-CD devices use the centrifugal force of a rotating compact-disk as pumping force to move the fluid in the device and execute an assay. Image courtesy of GenePoc.

What are the benefits of downsizing these procedures to a micrometer-scale and combining them in a microfluidic device? The most obvious advantage is a reduction in sample size and reagent consumption, which is not trivial when reagents are expensive (e.g., antibodies, chemotherapeutics and small molecules) or when samples are scarce (e.g., tissue biopsies). Furthermore, the high surface-to-volume ratio of the microfluidic channels facilitates heat transfer, enabling quick temperature changes and accurate temperature control. At the small scale of microfluidic devices, diffusive mixing occurs much faster than in a macroscale environment, which yields faster chemical reactions and reduced overall time per analysis. Alternatively, the long and narrow microfluidic channels boast a low Reynolds number (Re <1), resulting in laminar flow that enables precise spatiotemporal control of the fluids in the channels. One could take advantage of the precious characteristic to manipulate, trap and probe cells aggregates or whole-sections of tissues without direct physical contact on the sample reducing potential environmental contamination. Particularly for biological applications, another advantage of microfluidics is the ability to tailor and customize the cellular microenvironment in the device by using micro-fabrication techniques to pattern molecules in the device or by exploiting the laminar nature of the flow to create physiologically relevant gradients (Young 2010). Furthermore, the dimensions of the microfluidic channel can be adjusted to enable precise manipulation of biological samples of varying size ranging from individual cells to sub-milliliter tissues. Few of the most common applications of microfluidics are illustrated in Figure 7.1. Moreover, the small scale of these LOC platforms enables the design of portable, low-cost devices that could be used in a variety of point-of-care applications ranging from bedside care to global healthcare.

The development of soft lithography (Whitesides 2001) techniques using polymers enables the fabrication of microfluidic devices suitable for cell culture by forming the device in an optically transparent, oxygen permeable, cheap and flexible elastomer: poly (dimethylsiloxane) (PDMS). These PDMS devices have already been used as biological platforms to study cells and can be used to provide an *in vitro* framework more representative of the *in vivo* behaviour of cells. The versatile and high-throughput nature of soft lithography microfluidics has been vastly exploited to develop new biological techniques towards expanding our comprehension of human physiology. Particularly in personalized cancer models, microfluidics is emerging as a promising tool to develop new clinically relevant therapeutic models that could improve chemotherapy outcome by minimizing drug-induced toxicities. In the next section, we will review the most commonly used models for drug sensitivity screening in oncology and describe how microfluidics can provide new preclinical models for improved patient-specific prediction of therapeutic outcome of a drug.

General Description of Common Cancer Models

Biological assays that help evaluate the effect of a drug on a patient-derived tissue are generally referred to as chemosensitivity and resistance assays (CSRAs). CSRAs have been developed and used in clinical trials for a few decades as a way to characterize the chemosensitivity of a particular patient in order to prescribe the optimal treatment for that patient (Bellamy 1992). Generally, these assays require patient-derived tumor samples to be preserved, *ex vivo,* and exposed to different therapeutic agents. These assays investigate different clinical end-points (cell-death, tumor growth, ATP production) to determine the patient's chemosensitivity profile.

In Vitro 2D Monolayer Cell Culture Model

Common *in vitro* CSRAs utilize tumor cell monocultures derived from cancer cell lines or patient-specific tumor cells (Figure 7.2A) for anti-cancer drug screening and development (Abaan 2013; Boyd 1997). However, increasing evidence suggest that two dimensional (2D) monoculture models can develop irreversible genetic changes and loss of heterogeneity of the cell populations over time (Bounaix Morand du Puch 2016; Huh 2011; Sung 2013). Furthermore, these 2D models lack key features of *in vivo* tissues such as 3D complex architecture, presence of extracellular matrix as well as immune and stromal components, which have been shown to play a crucial role in cancer progression and drug resistance (Junttila 2013; Morgan 2016).

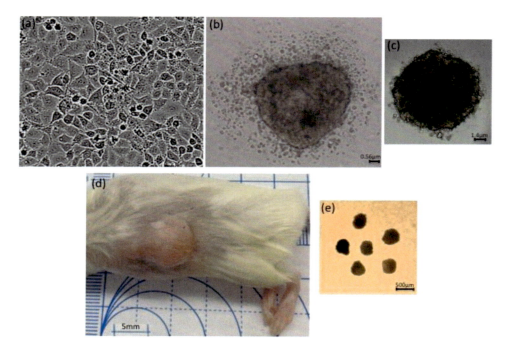

Figure 7.2. Common cancer models used to evaluate chemosensitivity and resistance to therapeutic agents. A) *In vitro* 2D monolayer cell culture B) *In vitro* matrix-assisted 3D culture C) *In vitro* 3D hanging droplet spheroid culture D) *In vivo* patient-derived xenograft model E) *Ex vivo* 3D Microdissected Tissues model. Acknowlegment to Dr Mes-Massons' post-doctorate students, Zied Boudhra and Patra Bishnubrata for the 2D and 3D *in vitro* models.

In Vitro 3D Cell Culture Models

Matrix-Assisted 3D Culture

Natural hydrogels, such as collagen and Matrigel, can be used to produce extracellular matrices (ECMs) acting as scaffolds that provide the cells with 3D growth architecture (Figure 7.2B) close to *in vivo* conditions. The presence of ECM during cellular growth has been reported to have great influence on key cell characteristics such as morphology, differentiation, polarity and gene expression, in comparison to conventional 2D cultures (Kenny 2007; Sung 2013; Yamada 2007). Likewise, co-culturing of cancer cells in ECM conditions with other non-cancerous cellular components present in the cell's microenvironment has been shown to affect the proliferation rate, drug sensitivity and protein secretion of cancer cells (Pak 2015; Sadlonova 2005; Xu 2013). These studies highlight the strong influence of cell-cell and cell-matrix interactions on the cell's response to drugs.

Spheroids

Generally, a spheroid originates from a self-aggregating cell that forms a sphere-like shape (Figure 7.2C). With size varying from a few micrometers up to a few millimeters, spheroids mimic the spatial heterogeneity of tumors, consisting of three primordial layers; proliferating cells on the peripheral layer, quiescent cells in the central layer and necrotic cells in the aggregate center. Furthermore, the 3D nature of the spheroids allows the study of drug response and the effect of hypoxia through its ability to transport natural gradients of oxygen nutrients and metabolic waste.

For those reasons, spheroids have been generally adopted as a new therapeutic model and a number of microfluidic devices have been designed to allow the formation of spheroids as well as to study the chemosensitivity of these spheroids on-chip (Hirschhaeuser 2010; Shield 2009; Weiswald 2015). For instance, Torisawa et al. have reported a microfluidic device that allows on-chip generation of multicellular spheroids and long-term analysis of cellular viability following treatment of the spheroids in the chip (Torisawa 2007). While spheroids provide a 3D structure that better reflects *in vivo* tumor architecture than 2D monocultures, these models still fail to include components of tumor microenvironment that highly influence tumor cell behaviour.

Organoid Culture

Organoid culture models have emerged in effort to include both the *in vivo* microenvironment and the complex architecture of tumors. Organoids are derived from the stem cells that are grown in ECM, which allow the cells to differentiate and migrate to recreate the specific architecture and function of an organ (Morgan 2016). Fully-grown organoids are composed of multiple cell types and exhibit intra- and inter-cellular communication networks as well as cell signalling pathways that reflect the physiological *in vivo* behaviour of organs. Furthermore, the organoids can be cultured for a long period of time while maintaining histological, immunohistological and genetic properties of the tissue, making them ideal for drug sensitivity assays, clearly observed by Santo et al. through the generation gut-specific crypt-villus structures originating from a single intestinal stem cell (Sato 2009).

In Vivo Patient-Derived Xenograft Model

Patient-Derived Xenograft

At the other end of the experimental continuum, *in vivo* CSRAs are most commonly carried out on patient-derived xenografts (PDXs). To generate a PDX, a small portion of a patient's tumor tissue is engrafted subcutaneously in an immune-compromised mouse, where it grows *in vivo* (Figure 7.2D) in conditions that maintain the local human tumor microenvironment. Such models have the advantage of retaining key characteristics of the original tumor tissue such as tumor heterogeneity, complex 3D architecture, and genetic makeup. Furthermore, genetic analysis revealed that the PDX tumors share the same genetic mutations in the stromal cells and immune cells, with some minor exception. These exceptions may be attributed to the fact that PDX tumors are generated in immune-compromised mice and that tumor stromal cells can be infiltrated by host stromal cells (De Wever 2003; Marangoni 2007; Reyal 2012). Recently published reports suggest that the genetic expression profile of the donor and the PDX tumor were similar but those of the cell lines generated from the same donor tumor showed a very different profile (Bertotti 2011; Fichtner 2008; Julien 2012; Zhang 2013). While PDXs are an interesting model for drug screening and studying treatment effects on cancer progression, these models still present limitations that need to be addressed. For instance, it normally takes 3–4 months to generate a PDX tumor model that corresponds to a donor tumor, making it inappropriate to determine the chemosensitivity of a patient before the first treatment is initiated. Additionally, as these mice lack a functional immune system, their use in immune drug screening is impractical. Moreover, these models require a lot of resources and are extremely costly to maintain (Ellis 2010). In effort to bridge the gap between 2D/3D monocultures and PDXs, a wide selection of *in vitro* microfluidics-based assays of varying complexity has been developed to improve our understanding of therapeutic response.

Ex vivo 3D Models

Organotypic Tissue Slices

Although the biological models presented thus far help to understand how the 3D architecture and cell-matrix contacts influence the therapeutic outcome of a drug, matching the *in vitro* complexity of *in vivo* tumors is still an unmet challenge. Instead of artificially recreating the complex microenvironment of a tissue, one step towards this goal is to produce organotypic cultures that preserves both *in vitro* tissue viability and the original structure of the tissue in an *ex vivo* environment. These models generally require the tumor tissue to be extracted by surgery and sectioned in smaller pieces to allow diffusion of oxygen and nutrients to the center of the tissue. As it preserves some of the tissue's original *in vivo* architecture and maintains cell-matrix interactions from the primary tissue, organotypic cultures offer the potential of predicting *in vivo* behaviour of the tissue. It is an outstanding tool used to characterize the therapeutic outcome of a drug for a specific patient tissue. Black first described this tool in 1951 where epithelial carcinomas (breast, colon, kidney, ovary, etc.) are extracted by surgery and sliced free hand to a size of approximately 0.5 cm by 0.5 cm and a thickness of 1 mm (Black 1951). The therapeutic response is evaluated by monitoring dehydrogenase activity of the tissues fragments exposed to various chemotherapy treatments or enzyme inhibitors.

A few years later, Thomlinson and Gray used histological analyses to study the mass transport limitation in human lung tumors and showed that large tumors exhibit a hypoxic core in their center (Thomlinson 1955). Based on the diffusive properties of metabolites and the general intake of nutrients by the tissue, they determined a critical diameter that a tumor core should not exceed: if one dimension of the cultured tissue is inferior to this critical diameter, the diffusion of metabolites through the tissue is enough to prevent depletion of nutrients. In this scope, different research groups began to slice tissue biopsies in thin slices (300–400 µm) before cultivating them to prevent diffusion-limited hypoxia (Figure 7.3). For instance, van Midwoud et al. reported that it is possible to study the metabolism of a precision-cut rat liver slice culture on-chip for a minimum period of 24 hours under continuous perfusion (van Midwoud 2010). Later, Chang et al. introduced a microfluidic device compatible with a 96-well plate allowing long-term culture of mouse brain slices and parallel chemosensitivity testing on the individual slices (Chang 2014).

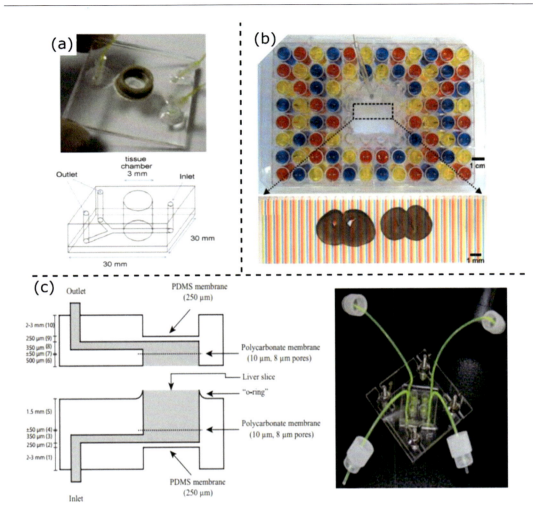

Figure 7.3. Organotypic models published previously in the literature. (a) Microfluidic chip that was used by Hattersley et al. to culture liver tissue biopsies. The device comprises a large tissue chamber where the tissue is perfused and can remain viable for over 70h. Image reproduced with permission from (Hattersley, 2008). (b) Microfluidic device reported by Chang et al. that allows organotypic culture of liver slices and parallel chemosensitivity screening on single liver slices. The multi-layered device is compatible with a 96-wells plate and enables the treatment of the sliced tissue with multiple compounds for high-throughput screening assays. Image reproduced with permission from (Chang, 2014). (c) Microfluidic platform developed by van Midwoud et al. to culture rat liver slices under continuous perfusion to study the metabolism and toxicology of the liver slices. Image reproduced with permission from (van Midwoud, 2010).

The main shortcoming of organotypic slice culture relies on the manipulation of large tissue slices without damaging the structure of the tissue, making such a model inappropriate for high-throughput drug screening on a large number of tissue slices. Moreover, long-term culture of large tissue slices usually requires continuous perfusion of the system to prevent hypoxia and nutrient starvation. Such perfusion and associated fluidic connections are cumbersome thus reducing the number of tissue slices that can be multiplexed in a single device, once again affecting the high-throughput screening capabilities of the model.

Micro-Dissected Tissue Culture

In effort to address these shortcomings, our group developed a new model for high-throughput *in vitro* study of therapeutic drug response on *ex vivo* patient-derived tissues (Figure 7.4). Briefly, tumor samples are micro-dissected and loaded in a microfluidic device where they are trapped and cultured. The micro-dissected tissue (MDT) samples are exposed to various therapeutic agents in the device and therapeutic response is quantified to determine the optimal treatment for that particular patient. The novelty of the presented model relies on the micro-dissection of the patient's tumor biopsy to enable precise spatiotemporal control of MDTs in a microfluidic device. The device consists of parallel fluidic channels to help trap and cultivate multiple MDTs thus assessing chemosensitivity of the tissue in a simple, high-throughput and multiplexed manner. Moreover, the micro-dissection of the tumor sample in sub-milliliter samples eliminates the need for continuous perfusion. The small diameter of the MDTs allows simple diffusion of oxygen through the PDMS matrix, enough to prevent hypoxia in the center. This novel biological model for drug screening combines the physiological relevance of the sliced tissue culture with the simple manipulations of small spheroid-sized tissue sample. The following sections of this chapter will allow in-depth understanding of this new MDT-based organotypic model, highlighting its clinically relevant chemosensitivity screening potential.

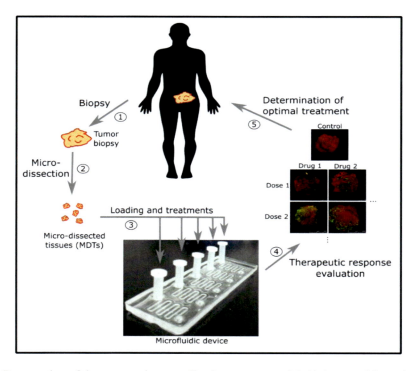

Figure 7.4. Presentation of the proposed personalized treatment model. 1) A tumor biopsy is extracted through biopsy or surgery. 2) Micro-dissection of the tumor biopsy to produce micro-dissected tissues (MDTs). 3) Loading and trapping of the MDTs in the microfluidic device, followed by treatment with different therapeutic agents directly in the device. 4) Evaluation of the therapeutic response with confocal microscopy and fluorescence activated cell sorting. 5) Results are interpreted and used to select the most effective treatment for that patient.

Microfluidic Platform

Design and Fabrication of the Microfluidic Platform

Microfluidic devices dedicated to cell culture have certain requirements that distinguish them from micro-scale devices used commonly for analytical chemistry or physics. In the case of a microfluidic device that traps and preserves *ex vivo* tissues, design considerations of particular importance are: (1) the choice of material for the device, (2) choice of trapping mechanism, and (3) geometry and dimensions of the channels. We will review each of these considerations and present the important design characteristics of the microfluidic device. We will then describe the fabrication process to produce the microfluidic chip.

Description of Polymer Used for Microfluidic Design

The development of soft lithography by Whitesides and his group in the late 1990s opened new avenues for microfluidic-based cellular applications (Whitesides 2001). Soft lithography comprises a set fabrication technique similar to photolithography, but uses silicon rubber instead due to low-cost and easy fabrication than conventional silicon-based materials. PDMS has several unique properties that make it an ideal choice of material for cell culture applications. First and foremost, unlike silicon or glass, PDMS has a high gas permeability that ensures sufficient oxygen supply to the cells in the device, eliminating the need for separate oxygen chambers. This property is particularly important when cultivating cells that have high metabolic demands like cancer cells. Another advantage of PDMS is its optical transparency and low autofluorescence, both in the visible and infrared regions. This property has been vastly exploited to couple microfluidic devices with imaging modalities that allow assessing the viability of the tissue directly on-chip. Moreover, PDMS is fairly cheap and easy to mold, making it ideal for rapid prototyping and mass production of microfluidic devices. Finally, to form enclosed micro-channels, PDMS can be bonded to different materials (e.g., PDMS, glass, polystyrene) using simple methods such as oxygen plasma treatment.

Sample Trapping Mechanism

As mentioned previously, there are numerous advantages provided by microfluidic devices, particularly when working with biological samples. These devices have the ability to enclose a biological sample in a chamber allowing for easy perfusion and use of smaller volumes of reagents than conventional macro-scale techniques (i.e., 96-wells plate). Microfluidic devices are transparent such that samples can be imaged directly on-chip, eliminating the need to manipulate the sample once it is loaded in the device. For all those reasons, research groups have used microfluidic chips to trap and enclose various types of tissue samples of different sizes ranging from single-cells to tissue slices. For specific sub-microliter particle trapping, such as spheroids, cell aggregates and MDTs, numerous trapping mechanisms have been reported. These mechanisms include acoustic (Liu 2007), mechanical (Khoury 2010), resistive (Ruppen 2014) and sedimentation trapping (Ruppen 2015). The latter mechanism seems to be more adapted for clinical applications, as it doesn't require complex instruments and continuous perfusion to operate the trap. Furthermore, when tissues sediment in well-like traps, they are protected from the high sheer stress induced in the main fluidic channel.

Two conditions must be met for sedimentation trapping to occur. First, the tissue sample being trapped needs to be denser than the surrounding medium for it to sediment to the bottom of the trap. Second, the sedimentation time has to be shorter than the travelling time over the trap. Cells are slightly denser than the medium in which they are cultured because the organelles and proteins they contain are denser than water. This is exploited in petri-dish cultures where cells need to sediment to the bottom of the dish and adhere to its surface to form a 2D cell layer. In steady-state regime, bigger spheres of equal density sediment faster, which explains why a tissue sample of 500 microns in diameter sediments roughly 10 000 times faster than single cells of about 5 µm in diameter, allowing the former to be trapped in less than a second in such small wells.

Configuration of the Microfluidic Platform

An example of channel configuration is shown in Figure 5A, where a whole microfluidic platform is seen from the top. The platform is made up of two fluidic levels: the top level shown in black contours where the samples circulate and the bottom level shown in red where the samples sediment. Five independent channels fit on a 2.5 cm by 7.5 cm surface (equivalent to the surface of a standard glass slide), making it possible to trap up to 25 individual tissue samples and to submit them to five different treatment conditions. The channel length was optimized so that the samples could be controlled using a 20 µL micropipette. Some distance was left between the traps so that each sample would have access to a maximum amount of nutrients from the medium in non-perfused conditions. Each channel is laid out in a serpentine fashion and can be viewed entirely in the field of view of a low magnification stereoscope.

As shown in Figure 5B, the inlet of each channel has a micro-reservoir which facilitates the loading of the samples into the system. The bottom of this micro-reservoir is lower than the rest of the inlet, at the same level as the channels to which it directly connects.

In the current design presented within this manuscript, the channel cross-section is 600 µm by 600 µm. The gravitational square-bottom traps are 600 µm in width by 500 µm in height. The total length of the channel is about 78 mm. Each independent system contains a volume of 29 µL. These dimensions have been tested to accommodate cylindrical tissue samples with dimensions of approximately 350 to 400 µm in diameter by 300 µm in height, and could easily be scaled to better accommodate samples of slightly different sizes.

Diffusion is the main transport mechanism *in vivo* between capillaries and the surrounding tissue. Similarly, within the microfluidic platform, the tissue samples access the nutrients from the medium and discard their cellular waste by diffusion between the channel and the traps. When fresh medium is added to the channels, our simulations show that only the channel (top fluidic layer) fills with fresh medium whereas the medium within the traps mostly recirculates (Astolfi 2016). Gradually, nutrients from the channel diffuse into the traps and metabolic waste diffuse into the main channel. Since diffusion times depend on the size of the molecules, small molecules such as oxygen diffuse rapidly into the traps whereas larger molecules such as glucose take more time to reach the tissue. Following Einstein's approximation, $t \approx x^2/2D$, a molecule such as glucose with a diffusion constant (D) in water of 600 µm²/s would take approximately 3.5 minutes to diffuse a 500 µm distance (x) to the bottom of the traps. When the nutrients reach the tissue, it is expected that diffusion also occur within the tissue, as would be the case *in vivo*.

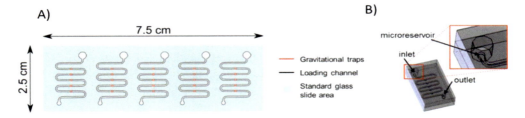

Figure 7.5. Channel Configuration of the microfluidic device. A) Microfluidic platform viewed from the top. The top channels are shown in black contours and the traps are shown in red. B) 3D view of a single assembled system.

Microfluidic Platform Fabrication

The platform fabrication process includes the following steps: mold fabrication, PDMS casting and cooking, assembly of the platform, bubble dislodging, sterilization, surface treatment, and pre-loading of channels with saline solution. Two molds are needed to fabricate the platforms. The first Poly (methyl methacrylate) (PMMA) mold, with features that form both fluidic levels (channels and traps) in the bottom layer of the platform, was fabricated by computer numerical control (CNC) milling using a flat endmill of 1 mm in diameter (Figure 7.5A). The second PMMA mold, with features that form the inlet and outlet holes in the top layer, was also fabricated by CNC milling using a flat endmill of 3.57 mm in diameter (Figure 7.5A). Liquid PDMS is prepared by combining a base polymer to a curing agent at a ratio of 10:1. This carefully mixed liquid PDMS can then be poured in the mold, degassed and cured in the oven for 1 hour. Once the top and bottom layers of the device are unmolded and cleaned, they can be assembled by oxygen plasma treatment. A nylon hollow cylinder is inserted into each inlet hole, acting as a fluid reservoir. A schematic and an actual real life image of the assembled platform are shown in Figure 7.6.

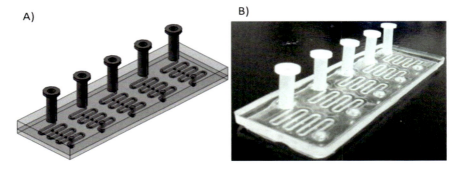

Figure 7.6. Schematic and real life image of the assembled platform.

Experimental Procedure for Preparation, Loading and Treatment of Micro-Dissected Tissue

Micro-dissected tissue (MDT), being the main focus of this chapter, is a new concept that has recently entered the scientific era. The micro-dissection of scarce tumor tissue samples, cut into sub-millimeter size, allows easy handling and tissue maintenance once trapped in microfluidic devices. Given the architecture of the devices, it is possible to simultaneously test multiple therapeutic agents, giving information on specific patient sensitivity or resistance to particular treatments. Furthermore, this high-throughput biological model exhibits a personalized medicine approach technique that will further help clinicians make therapeutic decisions.

The tissue processing of patient samples is organized in multiple steps, which include tissue harvest and acquisition, the production and culturing of the MDTs allowing tissue viability to be maintained. Once the viability of MDTs is attained in cultured conditions, it is possible to proceed to chemotherapy treatment of the samples permitting the ability to determine the chemosensitivity of an individual patient in a time frame suitable for clinical decision-making.

Criteria for Tumor Tissue Resection

There is one major criterion that is common for all MDT processing projects: the targeted tissue must be palpable or must have visible tumor areas present during the surgical procedure. The cancerous regions must be clearly identified by either a pathologist or a clinician performing the surgery.

Other criteria have been established depending on the solid tumor being processed and on the type of study performed. For example, prostate cancer patients may be enrolled in the study when the cancer targeted can be obtained by a biopsy specimen (of the primary tumor or a metastatic lesion) or by a transurethral resection of the prostate (TURP).

Tissue Micro-Sectioning of Prostate Cancer Biopsy Samples

Tissue Acquisition of Patient Samples

From past experiences and after the optimization of multiple conditions to attain maximum cell viability, a standard operating procedure (SOP) has been written to ensure proper procurement of tissue samples from clinicians. This procedure takes into account the collection, detection of malignancy and transportation of cancerous specimens. The sampling procedure has been fabricated to facilitate safe and efficient handling of the tumor sample with high integrity and quality, which is crucial for the preparation of the MDTs.

The SOP for tissue acquisition of prostate cancer specimen:

Tissue procurement of the prostate is usually done by ultrasound guided trans-rectal biopsies or can be done at the time of radical prostatectomy in patients undergoing surgery.

1) By using true-cut biopsy needles one can obtain specimens of 2 mm in diameter × 20 mm in length.
2) 5–6 biopsies of the suspected prostate region with palpable or visible tumor should be obtained.
3) Biopsy specimens should be kept in Hanks' Balanced Salt Solution (HBSS, #311-516-CL, Wisent Inc., Saint-Bruno-de-Montarville, Canada) supplemented with 10% fetal bovine serum (FBS, BD Biosicences) and 55 mg/L gentamicin (Wisent) and 0.6 mg/L amphotericin (Wisent) (HBSS$_{complete}$) and further transported on ice in aseptic conditions.

HBSS is a balanced salt solution that helps maintain tissue pH and osmotic balance. This solution thus provides water and essential inorganic ions such as calcium and magnesium to support vital cellular activity. Additionally, HBSS contains glucose, a main nutrient allowing viability of tissue biopsy to be sustained for a longer period of time. Recent studies have compared HBSS to regular phosphate-buffered saline (PBS) in terms of tissue viability and have shown that HBSS better supports whole tissue maintenance compared to PBS thus making it tissue specific (Astolfi 2016).

For solid tumors that require the identification of cancerous regions by a pathologist, here is the SOP for tissue processing and sectioning by the pathologist:

1) A sterile scalpel is used to cut the tumor where there is suspicion of tumor cells.
2) Freeze a fresh, unfixed tissue sample, up to 2.0 cm in diameter, at optimal cutting temperature (OCT) in a suitable tissue mold onto the specialized metal grids that fit onto the cryostat. NOTE: Approximate freezing times at -24 °C using a cold chuck ranges between 20–60 seconds depending on tissue depth.
3) Cut sections 5–15 μm-thick in the cryostat at -20°C. If necessary, adjust the temperature of the cutting chamber ± 5°C, according to the tissue under study. A hairbrush is useful to help guide the emerging section over the knife blade.
4) Within the first minute of cutting the tissue section, transfer it directly onto a microscope slide at room temperature. By letting the slide touch the tissue, the tissue section will melt onto the slide. This must be accomplished within the first minute of cutting the section to avoid freeze-drying of the tissue. The slide is then coated with Poly-L-lysine to improve adherence of the section to the slide.
5) To evaluate tissue preservation and orientation, stain the first couple of slides with toluidine blue (1–2% w/v in H_2O), hematoxylin, and eosin, or any aqueous stain.
6) The pathologist examines the slides and determines the approximate probability of tumor cell in the sample.
7) Using a clean and sterile blade, the mirror section of the tumor sample is cut and placed in HBSS$_{complete}$.
8) The sample is picked up by a technician and transported on ice to the processing laboratory
9) The tumor tissue is either processed right away or stored at 4 °C for no more than 24 hours in HBSS$_{complete}$.

Microfluidic Chip Preparation

The microfluidic devices must be prepared one day prior to micro-dissection of the patient sample. It is important that the microfluidic chips go through several decontamination and sterilization procedures. Firstly, the devices are treated with 100% ethanol to decontaminate the chips followed by 70% ethanol incubation at room temperature for 15 minutes in to allow sterilization. Next, they are treated overnight in a humidified cell culture incubator (37°C, 5% CO_2, 95% ambient air) with a 10 mg/mL triblock copolymer, Pluronic F-108 (Sigma-Aldrich, St-Louis, USA) to reduce cell adhesion on the PDMS surfaces. The following day, the devices are re-sterilized through 70% ethanol incubation for 15 minutes at room temperature. Lastly, they are thoroughly rinsed using sterile HBSS supplemented with 55 mg/L gentamicin and 0.6 mg/L amphotericin ($HBSS_{antibio}$) and placed at 4°C until the MDTs are produced and ready to be loaded in the devices.

Generation of Micro-Dissected Tumor Tissue

Detail of Micro-Dissection Protocol

Prostate cancer biopsy samples are approximately 2 cm in length and 1 mm in diameter. These fragments are cut into 1 to 2 mm long fragments and immediately embedded in low melting-point agarose supplemented with 10% FBS, which is kept in a liquid form at 40°C. The agarose solidifies on ice to obtain a supporting structure around the tissue. The excess agarose is then removed and the fragments are repositioned vertically and glued to the stage for slicing into 300 µm thick slices using a traditional vibratome. These slices were further punched, using a 400 µm biopsy punch, into disk-like tumor micro-sections, MDTs. On average, a single prostate cancer biopsy can produce 80 MDTs, thus with 5–6 biopsies, we can easily obtain between 400 to 480 MDTs from one single patient sample. The MDTs obtained from each biopsy are pooled together in a petri plate, submerged in $HBSS_{antibio}$, to ensure randomized selection of the MDTs allowing drug testing of heterogeneous tissues. The MDTs obtained are then carefully loaded in the customized microfluidic chips under a stereomicroscope and cultured in specific culture medium, Roswell Park Memorial Institute (RPMI 1640) (#350-045-CL, Wisent Inc.) medium used for prostate cancer sample culturing. For the loading procedure, the hollow nylon cylinders that form the inlet reservoirs are removed and the microfluidic device is placed under a stereomicroscope. For each individual channel, 5 MDTs are collected using a P20 micropipette and introduced in the inlet, where they sediment to the bottom of the channel. By aspirating fluid from the outlet of the device, flow is induced in the microfluidic channels allowing the MDTs to travel in the channel to attain the wells. Once the MDTs are above the wells the flow is stopped for approximately 1 to 2 seconds allowing them to sediment to the bottom of the traps. The same procedure is repeated to fully load the 5 channels of the device, resulting in a total number of 25 MDTs per device (for visual comprehension, the whole process is illustrated in Figure 7.7). Furthermore, This $RPMI_{complete}$ medium used does not contain phenol but is supplemented with L-glutamine, 10% FBS, 55 mg/L gentamicin and 0.6 mg/L amphotericin and allows whole cell overall survival of MDTs in our microfluidic devices to be between 60 to 95% (Astoli, 2016).

Microfluidic Devices and Micro-Dissected Tissue to Predict Therapeutic Response ... 199

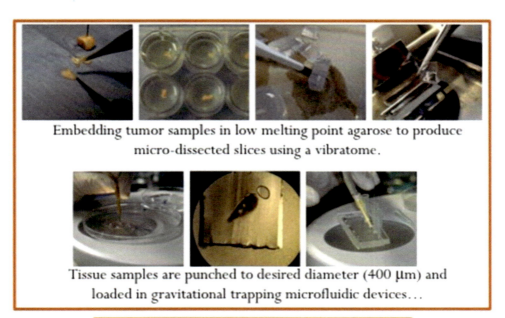

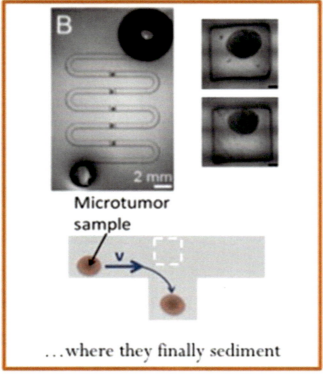

Figure 7.7. Overview of the procedure to produce micro-dissected tissue (MDT), to load them into a microfluidic system and to analyze their viability using two complementary methods.

Tissue Sectioning Reproducibility

The distribution of size of the MDTs produced was determined by confocal microscopy analysis. Using maximum projection imaging, the diameter of each MDT was calculated as the average of two perpendicular diameter measurements. Upon analysis, the diameter of the MDTs remained relatively stable with time and slight variability was detected. This variability was further explained by differences in mechanical properties of the tumor tissues, especially their elasticity, by wear and tear of the biopsy punch and slight differences in sectioning procedure between users. It was clearly noted that tissue with higher elasticity could easily be stretched out during sectioning due to compression force applied by the biopsy punch and can later be brought back into its original configuration.

Irrespective of the tumor type, the diameters of 247 produced MDTs seem to follow a normal distribution with an average (μ) of 380 µm and a standard deviation (σ) of 43 µm (Figure 7.8) (Astolfi 2016). The ratio σ/μ being less than 12% indicates that the sectioning procedure is highly reproducible.

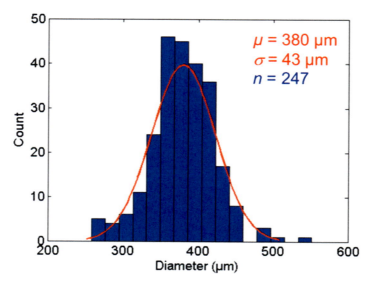

Figure 7.8. Histogram (blue bars) with normal fit (red curve) representing the diameter of microsections of xenograft models of various cell lines.

Culturing of Micro-Dissected Tissues and Chemotherapy Treatments

To ensure cell viability and tumor survival of the MDTs at harvest day, HBSS$_{antibio}$ was replaced by fresh RPMI$_{complete}$ medium. The MDTs are continuously incubated at 37°C, 5% CO_2 for the remaining period. The medium is changed 24 hours subsequent to harvest day to ensure proper circulation of nutrients and avoid glucose deprivation, followed by 24 to 48 hours of recovery period to acclimatize the MDTs within the systems before further treatment with different therapeutic agents.

The concentration of the chemotherapy agents used to treat the MDTs was determined by the IC$_{50}$ obtained by monolayer cell line cultures that are generally used to generate xenografts. Recent studies have demonstrated that at a concentration of 10 times the IC$_{50}$ of chemotherapy agent results in a significant increase in mortality fraction in spheroids compared to lower concentrations and control (Das 2013). The treatment plan for the MDTs may differ depending on the objective of the project and on the solid tumor being processed. Specifically, for prostate cancer samples processed at the CRCHUM, the MDTs were treated with Docetaxel, and/or Bicalutamide, common prostate cancer treatment drugs. The IC_{50} of Docetaxel being 1 nM, was calculated in our lab through a metabolic assay, WST-1-based, using various prostate cell lines, all-resulting in similar values. Additionally, through clonogenic assays our lab has determined the IC_{50} of Bicalutamide for 22RV1 cell line to be 10 μM.

Particularly in our lab, these treatments were given alone, sequentially or in combination at a concentration of 10 nM for Docetaxel and 100 μM for Bicalutamide. Generally, a cycle of chemotherapy includes a 24-hour incubation period with the chemotherapy agent followed by removal of treatment and a 48-hour recovery period. In order to allow comparison with clinical treatment plan and patient survival, two cycles of chemotherapy are completed on the MDTs. Explicitly, after the recovery period from MDT processing, the chemotherapy agents were diluted in $RPMI_{complete}$ medium in order to attain the desired concentrations. The $RPMI_{complete}$ medium previously in the microfluidic devices was replaced with the medium containing the chemotherapy agent. The chemotherapy treatment was removed and replaced with fresh medium after 24 hours of treatment and thus repeated after 24 to 48 hours of recovery period. Many chemotherapy agents take several days before effects are apparent hence why final day analysis are done 48 hours after the second treatment has been completed.

The MDTs are analyzed at different time points in order to determine initial and final viability of the MDTs. In addition, controls are consistently used throughout the procedure to act as a comparable group of untreated samples ensuring reliability of the results. Initial MDT viability measures are determined by confocal imaging and flow cytometry on harvest day (day 0) and then on first cycle treatment day (day 2). Finally, samples are analyzed, by the same two methods, 48 hours after the second cycle (day 8), comparing untreated samples to treated samples being able to estimate the patients' response to treatment.

The complete process takes approximately 8–10 days and the samples are collected and analyzed in less than two weeks. This method utilized as a 3D cancer model can help determine the chemosensitivity of an individual patient in a time frame suitable for clinical decision-making. Furthermore, this method can help decide which treatment plan will be most effective for an individual thus excluding the use of ineffective therapies for that patient.

METHODS FOR ANALYSIS OF TREATMENT RESPONSE

Two methods were developed to follow cancer cell survival and MDT response to treatment over several days: confocal microscopy of live and dead cells (time point assay) and flow cytometry (endpoint assay) to discriminate the MDT cells according to their viability stage (alive, early apoptotic or dead).

An Automated Analysis of Confocal Microscopy Images to Determine Cancer Cell Response to Treatment

Since PDMS is completely transparent, it allows for direct imaging of the MDTs under the microscope. By confocal microscopy, MDTs trapped in the microfluidic platforms were imaged at different time points to follow the evolution of cell viability during the 8-day culture period. The combination of CellTracker™ Orange CMTMR (CTO, Thermo Fisher Scientific), which stains viable cells, and Sytox Green (SG, Thermo Fisher Scientific) which stains nucleic acids of dead cells, gives a measure of the viability of cells (Figure 7.9A). To minimize detection of auto-fluorescence, non-labelled MDTs incubated under the same conditions as the stained MDTs were imaged first to calibrate the upper threshold settings of the microscope (laser power and photomultiplier gains). Labeled MDTs were then imaged directly through the microfluidic platforms using an inverted confocal microscope equipped with a 10X or 20X dry objective (Figure 7.9A).

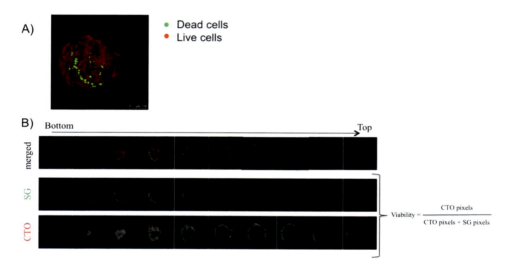

Figure 7.9. *Overview of the confocal microscopy imaging of live and dead cells.* A) 3D projection of a confocal image of an MDT stained with CTO and SG. B) Individual z-stack images used for viability analysis of the same MDT. Top row is the merged color stacks. Middle and lower rows are the Sytox Green (SG = dead cells) and CellTracker Orange (CTO = live cells) channels respectively.

From confocal microscopy images, overall cell viability was evaluated by calculating the ratio of the area of the CTO-positive signal over the summed areas of the CTO- and SG-positive signals. An algorithm applied a median filter to all images to reduce noise and then determined the red and green signal contours in order to apply a threshold algorithm only to those pixels near the contours (Figure 7.9B), for each fluorescent marker. This threshold method separates the pixels in two groups, background and foreground, so that their intra-class variance is minimal. Once both thresholds were applied, the numbers of CTO-positive and SG-positive pixels were calculated. The sample viability was evaluated by the ratio of CTO pixels divided by the sum of CTO and SG pixels [$V_{iability}=CTO/(CTO+SG)$].

Characterization of Treatment Response of Each Cell Type Using Flow Cytometry Assays

Flow cytometry was employed as an endpoint assay to analyze the cell population (epithelial, immune or stromal cells) and their viability before and after the MDTs had been exposed to different chemotherapy agents. MDTs were analyzed at different time points to reflect the evolution of cell death over the 8-day incubation period. All fifteen MDTs from the three channels were pooled in the same tube for analysis. A single cell suspension of MDTs was obtained through enzymatic digestion using a combination of crude and type 1A collagenase and mechanical action of gentle repeated pipetting. The resulting suspension is analyzed by flow cytometry. All medium fractions collected from the three channels during the medium changes and stored at 4°C were also pooled together with the digested MDT suspension. This step was added to take into account all the live and dead cells that had been washed out of the systems during medium changes in the microfluidic platform. Single cells from the homogenous cell suspension were then stained with the apoptotic fluorescent dyes Annexin V for apoptosis and DRAQ7™ for dead cells, unstained cells were considered as viable cells for flow cytometry analyses. The cell survival was gated in forward and side scatter graphs, as shown in Figure 7.10. A survival state was associated for each cell according to its dye staining (live, early apoptotic or dead).

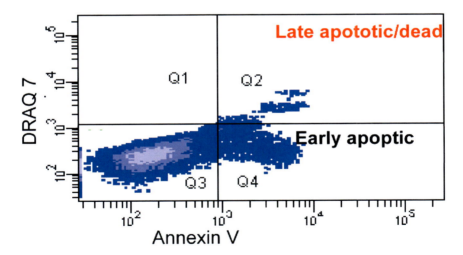

Figure 7.10. Typical representation of flow cytometry analysis. Each cell (represented by a blue dot) obtained from the MDT was associated to one of three viability categories according to its fluorescence intensity in both DRAQ7 and Annexin V detection channels: early apoptotic cells (Annexin V-stained only), late apoptotic / dead cells (DRAQ7-stained), and live cells (non stained).

Preliminary Analysis of Treatment Response

Patient A was a TURP sample that had developed a castration-resistant prostate cancer (CRPC). The MDTs prepared from this patient sample were cultured for 8 days in the microfluidic platforms and received two complete treatment cycles (for details, see section Culturing of Micro-Dissected Tissues and Chemotherapy Treatments). Confocal 3D projection imaging of treated MDTs allowed for quantitative evaluation and effect of two common prostate cancer treatment drugs. The viability of prostate cancer MDTs is shown below with the live cells in red (CTO) and dead cells in green (SG). The percent viability of the control samples at 95.8% ± 3.1% was compared with the 2 treatment conditions, Drug A at 90.5% ± 2.4% and Drug B at 83.1% ± 2.8% (Figure 7.11), indicating a decrease in viability in the Drug B treated samples with respect to the control. In parallel, flow cytometry technique was used to confirm MDT viability and drug sensitivity. The percent viability of the control MDT samples at 62.4% ± 10.1% was compared with the 2 treatment conditions, Drug A at 63.1% ± 4.8% and Drug B at 35.2% ± 2.3% (Figure 7.12). The preliminary results from both techniques show an increase in Drug B sensibility compared to Drug A. However, the viability results of flow cytometry were quite inferior to those obtained by confocal microscopy. Differences between these two techniques were explained by the identification of early apoptotic cells in the flow cytometry analysis (Figure 7.12), which might still appear CTO-positive in the dual-stain confocal microscopy analysis.

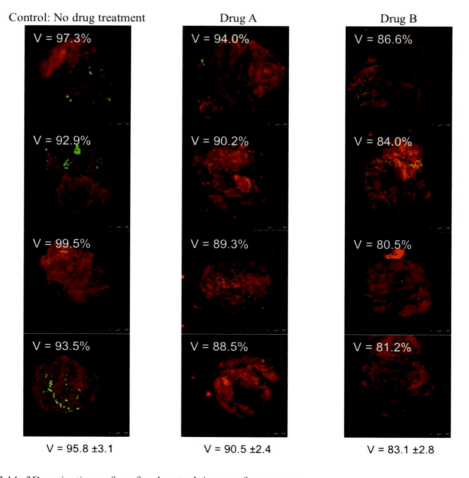

Figure 7.11. 3D projections of confocal z-stack images for prostate

patient A taken 8 days after surgery. Treatment applied for a 24 hr period 2 days and 6 days after surgery. 1) control, 2) Drug A, and 3) Drug B.

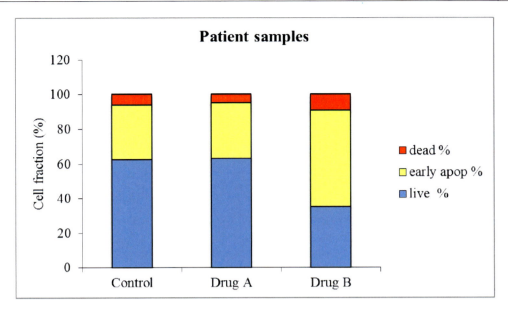

Figure 7.12. Flow cytometry survival analysis of MDTs from patient A. MDTs were treated with Drug A or Drug B. Each treatment was applied for a 24 hr period 2 days and 6 days after surgery.

Advantages and Disadvantages of Each Viability Analysis Technique

To compare the potential of confocal microscopy and flow cytometry to evaluate the cancer cell sensitivity to different treatments, it is necessary to analyze advantages and disadvantages of each technique.

Confocal Microscopy

Confocal microscopy gives information about the spatial distribution and the morphology of MDTs. Since samples are imaged on-chip, this technique is fast and makes it possible to easily follow the treatment effect at different time points and the survival evolution of a single MDT in response to one treatment or to a sequence of treatments. On the other hand, mortality is generally underestimated due to the washing out of dead cells during medium changes and staining protocols as well as the staining of early apoptotic cells by "live" dyes. The limited imaging depth of the confocal microscopy (around 100 μm) creates a "black" unanalyzed region in the center of the MDT. This being a strong limitation to estimate the effect of drugs on the survival of cancer cells in the middle of the MDTs.

Flow Cytometry

Flow cytometry is a better quantitative technique to evaluate the overall survival of cells and to allow the discrimination of early apoptotic cells. These early apoptotic cells are the starting point of cell death processes that are accounted as dead cells for the purpose of evaluating cell survivability fraction. However, this technique is uniquely an endpoint analysis as it necessitates the digestion of MDTs, thus preventing the ability to monitor sample viability over time. This technique also needs a high quantity of cells (at least 15 MDTs) and gives an average reading of the whole microfluidic platforms which reduces the ability to perform statistical analyses.

Overall, these two techniques are complementary to each other and were adapted to measure the overall survival of MDTs within the microfluidic platforms.

CONCLUSION

Strategies toward the management of cancer have changed significantly over the last decade and focused on a personalized medical approach. The major challenge of this approach is to identify treatments that will significantly increase patient survival. One solution proposed is the direct testing of patient tumor material that should allow empirical evaluation of therapeutic responses to a wide concentration and variety of agents. This idea led to the development of a novel high-throughput and low-cost tool for monitoring drug sensitivity of patient tissue. This tool associates a novel technique of micro-dissection, to produce sub-microliter cancer tissue samples, and microfluidic technologies, to generate a biocompatible, gas-permeable and optically transparent platform suitable for cell biology and imaging application. The new *ex vivo* micro-dissected cancer tissue model, which retains the original 3D tumor architecture, should closely mimic the type of responses expected in patients. This rapid and direct approach would influence clinical decision-making and allow the tailoring of therapeutic strategies for individual patients within an acceptable time frame. This would reduce not only the economic burden on the health care system but also the inconvenience and risk of exposing patients to drugs with little chance of response as well as the optimization of therapies in patients more likely to respond.

REFERENCES

Abaan OD, Polley EC, Davis SR, Zhu YJ, Bilke S, Walker RL, Pineda M, Gindin Y, Jiang Y, Reinhold WC, Holbeck SL, Simon RM, Doroshow JH, Pommier Y, Meltzer PS. The exomes of the NCI-60 panel: a genomic resource for cancer biology and systems pharmacology. *Cancer Res.* 2013; 73(14):4372–82.

Astolfi M, Péant B, Lateef MA, Rousset N, Kendall-Dupont J, Carmona E, Monet F, Saad F, Provencher D, Mes-Masson A-M, Gervais T. Micro-dissected tumor tissues on chip: an ex vivo method for drug testing and personalized therapy. *Lab. Chip.* 2016; 16:312–325.

Bellamy WT. Prediction of response to drug therapy of cancer. A review of in vitro assays. *Drugs* 1992; 44(5):690–708.

Bertotti A, Migliardi G, Galimi F, Sassi F, Torti D, Isella C, Corà D, Di Nicolantonio F, Buscarino M, Petti C, Ribero D, Russolillo N, Muratore A, Massucco P, Pisacane A, Molinaro L, Valtorta E, Sartore-Bianchi A, Risio M, Capussotti L, Gambacorta M, Siena S, Medico E, Sapino A, Marsoni S, Comoglio PM, Bardelli A, Trusolino L. A molecularly annotated platform of patient-derived xenografts identifies HER2 as an effective therapeutic target in cetuximab-resistant colorectal cancer. *Cancer Discov.* 2011; 1(6):508–23.

Black MM, Kleiner IS, Speer FD. Effects of enzyme inhibitors on in vitro dehydrogenase activity of cancer tissue slices. *Proc. Soc. Exp. Biol. Med.* 1951; 77(4):611–5.

Black MM, Speer FD. Effects of cancer chemotherapeutic agents on dehydrogenase activity of human cancer tissue in vitro. *Am. J. Clin. Pathol.* 1953; 23(3):218–27.

Bounaix Morand du Puch C, Nouaille M, Giraud S, Labrunie A, Luce S, Preux P-M, Labrousse F, Gainant A, Tubiana-Mathieu N, Le Brun-Ly V, Valleix D, Guillaudeau A, Mesturoux L, Coulibaly B, Lautrette C, Mathonnet M. Chemotherapy outcome predictive effectiveness by the Oncogramme: pilot trial on stage-IV colorectal cancer. *J. Transl. Med.* 2016; 14(1):10.

Boyd MR. The NCI In Vitro Anticancer Drug Discovery Screen. In *Anticancer Drug Development Guide* (pp. 23–42). Totowa, NJ: Humana Press; 1997.

Chang TC, Mikheev AM, Huynh W, Monnat RJ, Rostomily RC, Folch A, Folch A. Parallel microfluidic chemosensitivity testing on individual slice cultures. *Lab. Chip.* 2014; 14(23):4540–51.

de Mello A. On-chip chromatography: the last twenty years. *Lab. Chip.* 2002; 2(3):48N–54N.

De Wever O, Mareel M. Role of tissue stroma in cancer cell invasion. *J. Pathol.* 2003; 200(4):429–47.

Ellis LM, Fidler IJ. Finding the tumor copycat: Therapy fails, patients don't. *Nat. Med.* 2010; 16(9):974–975.

Fichtner I, Rolff J, Soong R, Hoffmann J, Hammer S, Sommer A, Becker M, Merk J. Establishment of patient-derived non-small cell lung cancer xenografts as models for the identification of predictive biomarkers. *Clin. Cancer Res.* 2008; 14(20):6456–68.

Ginsburg GS, McCarthy JJ. Personalized medicine: revolutionizing drug discovery and patient care. *Trends Biotechnol.* 2001; 19(12):491–496.

Hirschhaeuser F, Menne H, Dittfeld C, West J, Mueller-Klieser W, Kunz-Schughart LA. Multicellular tumor spheroids: An underestimated tool is catching up again. *J. Biotechnol.* 2010; 148(1):3–15.

Huh D, Hamilton GA, Ingber DE. From 3D cell culture to organs-on-chips. *Trends Cell Biol.* 2011; 21(12):745–754.

Jang K-J, Suh K-Y. A multi-layer microfluidic device for efficient culture and analysis of renal tubular cells. *Lab. Chip.* 2010; 10(1):36–42.

Johnson JI, Decker S, Zaharevitz D, Rubinstein L V, Venditti JM, Schepartz S, Kalyandrug S, Christian M, Arbuck S, Hollingshead M, Sausville EA. Relationships between drug activity in NCI preclinical in vitro and in vivo models and early clinical trials. *Br. J. Cancer* 2001; 84(10):1424–31.

Julien S, Merino-Trigo A, Lacroix L, Pocard M, Goéré D, Mariani P, Landron S, Bigot L, Nemati F, Dartigues P, Weiswald L-B, Lantuas D, Morgand L, Pham E, Gonin P, Dangles-Marie V, Job B, Dessen P, Bruno A, Pierré A, De Thé H, Soliman H, Nunes M, Lardier G, Calvet L, Demers B, Prévost G, Vrignaud P, Roman-Roman S, Duchamp O, Berthet C. Characterization of a Large Panel of Patient-Derived Tumor Xenografts Representing the Clinical Heterogeneity of Human Colorectal Cancer. *Clin. Cancer Res.* 2012; 18(19):5314–28.

Junttila MR, de Sauvage FJ. Influence of tumour micro-environment heterogeneity on therapeutic response. *Nature* 2013; 501(7467):346–354.

Justice BA, Badr NA, Felder RA. 3D cell culture opens new dimensions in cell-based assays. *Drug Discov. Today* 2009; 14(1–2):102–7.

Kane BJ, Zinner MJ, Yarmush ML, Toner M. Liver-specific functional studies in a microfluidic array of primary mammalian hepatocytes. *Anal. Chem.* 2006; 78(13):4291–8.

Kenny PA, Lee GY, Myers CA, Neve RM, Semeiks JR, Spellman PT, Lorenz K, Lee EH, Barcellos-Hoff MH, Petersen OW, Gray JW, Bissell MJ. The morphologies of breast cancer cell lines in three-dimensional assays correlate with their profiles of gene expression. *Mol. Oncol.* 2007; 1(1):84–96.

Keysar SB, Astling DP, Anderson RT, Vogler BW, Bowles DW, Morton JJ, Paylor JJ, Glogowska MJ, Le PN, Eagles-Soukup JR, Kako SL, Takimoto SM, Sehrt DB, Umpierrez A, Pittman MA, Macfadden SM, Helber RM, Peterson S, Hausman DF, Said S, Leem TH, Goddard JA, Arcaroli JJ, Messersmith WA, Robinson WA, Hirsch FR, Varella-Garcia M, Raben D, Wang XJ, Song JI, Tan AC, Jimeno A. A patient tumor transplant model of squamous cell cancer identifies PI3K inhibitors as candidate therapeutics in defined molecular bins. *Mol. Oncol.* 2013; 7(4):776–90.

Khoury M, Bransky A, Korin N, Konak LC, Enikolopov G, Tzchori I, Levenberg S. A microfluidic traps system supporting prolonged culture of human embryonic stem cells aggregates. *Biomed. Microdevices* 2010; 12(6):1001–1008.

Kim E, Xia Y, Whitesides GM. Micromolding in Capillaries: Applications in Materials Science. *J. Am. Chem. Soc.* 1996; 118(24):5722–5731.

Kimura H, Yamamoto T, Sakai H, Sakai Y, Fujii T. An integrated microfluidic system for long-term perfusion culture and on-line monitoring of intestinal tissue models. *Lab. Chip.* 2008; 8(5):741–6.

Lee PJ, Hung PJ, Lee LP. An artificial liver sinusoid with a microfluidic endothelial-like barrier for primary hepatocyte culture. *Biotechnol. Bioeng.* 2007; 97(5):1340–6.

Liu J, Kuznetsova LA, Edwards GO, Xu J, Ma M, Purcell WM, Jackson SK, Coakley WT. Functional three-dimensional HepG2 aggregate cultures generated from an ultrasound trap: Comparison with HepG2 spheroids. *J. Cell. Biochem.* 2007; 102(5):1180–1189.

Manz A, Graber N, Widmer HM. Miniaturized total chemical analysis systems: A novel concept for chemical sensing. *Sensors Actuators B Chem.* 1990; 1(1–6):244–248.

Manz A, Miyahara Y, Miura J, Watanabe Y, Miyagi H, Sato K. Design of an open-tubular column liquid chromatograph using silicon chip technology. *Sensors Actuators B Chem.* 1990; 1(1–6):249–255.

Marangoni E, Vincent-Salomon A, Auger N, Degeorges A, Assayag F, de Cremoux P, de Plater L, Guyader C, De Pinieux G, Judde J-G, Rebucci M, Tran-Perennou C, Sastre-Garau X, Sigal-Zafrani B, Delattre O, Diéras V, Poupon M-F. A new model of patient tumor-derived breast cancer xenografts for preclinical assays. *Clin. Cancer Res.* 2007; 13(13):3989–98.

Mathies RA, Huang XC. Capillary array electrophoresis: an approach to high-speed, high-throughput DNA sequencing. *Nature* 1992; 359(6391):167–169.

Morgan MM, Johnson BP, Livingston MK, Schuler LA, Alarid ET, Sung KE, Beebe DJ. Personalized in vitro cancer models to predict therapeutic response: Challenges and a framework for improvement. *Pharmacol. Ther.* 2016;165:79-92.

Pak C, Callander NS, Young EWK, Titz B, Kim K, Saha S, Chng K, Asimakopoulos F, Beebe DJ, Miyamoto S. MicroC ^{3}: an ex vivo microfluidic cis-coculture assay to test chemosensitivity and resistance of patient multiple myeloma cells. *Integr. Biol.* 2015; 7(6):643–654.

Pampaloni F, Reynaud EG, Stelzer EHK. The third dimension bridges the gap between cell culture and live tissue. *Nat. Rev. Mol. Cell Biol.* 2007; 8(10):839–845.

Park J, Koito H, Li J, Han A. Microfluidic compartmentalized co-culture platform for CNS axon myelination research. *Biomed. Microdevices* 2009; 11(6):1145–53.

Reyal F, Guyader C, Decraene C, Lucchesi C, Auger N, Assayag F, De Plater L, Gentien D, Poupon M-F, Cottu P, De Cremoux P, Gestraud P, Vincent-Salomon A, Fontaine J-J, Roman-Roman S, Delattre O, Decaudin D, Marangoni E. Molecular profiling of patient-derived breast cancer xenografts. *Breast Cancer Res.* 2012; 14(1):R11.

Ruppen J, Cortes-Dericks L, Marconi E, Karoubi G, Schmid RA, Peng R, Marti TM, Guenat OT. A microfluidic platform for chemoresistive testing of multicellular pleural cancer spheroids. *Lab Chip* 2014; 14(6):1198–1205.

Ruppen J, Wildhaber FD, Strub C, Hall SRR, Schmid RA, Geiser T, Guenat OT. Towards personalized medicine: chemosensitivity assays of patient lung cancer cell spheroids in a perfused microfluidic platform. *Lab. Chip.* 2015; 15(14):3076–3085.

Sadlonova A, Novak Z, Johnson MR, Bowe DB, Gault SR, Page GP, Thottassery J V, Welch DR, Frost AR. Breast fibroblasts modulate epithelial cell proliferation in three-dimensional in vitro co-culture. *Breast Cancer Res.* 2005; 7(7):R46.

Sato T, Vries RG, Snippert HJ, van de Wetering M, Barker N, Stange DE, van Es JH, Abo A, Kujala P, Peters PJ, Clevers H. Single Lgr5 stem cells build crypt–villus structures in vitro without a mesenchymal niche. *Nature* 2009; 459(7244):262–265.

Shield K, Ackland ML, Ahmed N, Rice GE. Multicellular spheroids in ovarian cancer metastases: Biology and pathology. *Gynecol. Oncol.* 2009; 113(1):143–148.

Song JW, Cavnar SP, Walker AC, Luker KE, Gupta M, Tung Y-C, Luker GD, Takayama S. Microfluidic Endothelium for Studying the Intravascular Adhesion of Metastatic Breast Cancer Cells. *PLoS One* 2009; 4(6):e5756.

Sung KE, Su X, Berthier E, Pehlke C, Friedl A, Beebe DJ. Understanding the Impact of 2D and 3D Fibroblast Cultures on In Vitro Breast Cancer Models. *PLoS One* 2013; 8(10):e76373.

Terry SC, Jerman JH, Angell JB. A gas chromatographic air analyzer fabricated on a silicon wafer. *IEEE Trans. Electron Devices* 1979; 26(12):1880–1886.

Thomlinson RH, Gray LH. The histological structure of some human lung cancers and the possible implications for radiotherapy. *Br. J. Cancer* 1955; 9(4):539–49.

Torisawa Y, Takagi A, Nashimoto Y, Yasukawa T, Shiku H, Matsue T. A multicellular spheroid array to realize spheroid formation, culture, and viability assay on a chip. *Biomaterials* 2007; 28(3):559–66.

van Midwoud PM, Groothuis GMM, Merema MT, Verpoorte E. Microfluidic biochip for the perifusion of precision-cut rat liver slices for metabolism and toxicology studies. *Biotechnol. Bioeng.* 2010; 105(1):184–194.

Venditti JM, Wesley RA, Plowman J. Current NCI Preclinical Antitumor Screening in Vivo: Results of Tumor Panel Screening, 1976–1982, and Future Directions. *Adv. Pharmacol.* 1984; 20:1–20.

Weiswald L-B, Bellet D, Dangles-Marie V. Spherical Cancer Models in Tumor Biology. *Neoplasia* 2015; 17(1):1–15.

Whitesides GM. The origins and the future of microfluidics. *Nature* 2006; 442(7101):368–373.

Whitesides GM, Ostuni E, Takayama S, Jiang X, Ingber DE. Soft Lithography in Biology and Biochemistry. *Annu. Rev. Biomed. Eng.* 2001; 3(1):335–373.

Woolley AT, Mathies RA. Ultra-high-speed DNA fragment separations using microfabricated capillary array electrophoresis chips. *Proc. Natl. Acad. Sci. U. S. A.* 1994; 91(24):11348–52.

Xu Z, Gao Y, Hao Y, Li E, Wang Y, Zhang J, Wang W, Gao Z, Wang Q. Application of a microfluidic chip-based 3D co-culture to test drug sensitivity for individualized treatment of lung cancer. *Biomaterials* 2013; 34(16):4109–4117.

Yamada KM, Cukierman E. Modeling Tissue Morphogenesis and Cancer in 3D. *Cell* 2007; 130(4):601–610.

You L, Temiyasathit S, Lee P, Kim CH, Tummala P, Yao W, Kingery W, Malone AM, Kwon RY, Jacobs CR. Osteocytes as mechanosensors in the inhibition of bone resorption due to mechanical loading. *Bone* 2008; 42(1):172–9.

Young EWK, Beebe DJ. Fundamentals of microfluidic cell culture in controlled microenvironments. *Chem. Soc. Rev.* 2010; 39(3):1036–48.

Zhang X, Claerhout S, Prat A, Dobrolecki LE, Petrovic I, Lai Q, Landis MD, Wiechmann L, Schiff R, Giuliano M, Wong H, Fuqua SW, Contreras A, Gutierrez C, Huang J, Mao S, Pavlick AC, Froehlich AM, Wu MF, Tsimelzon A, Hilsenbeck SG, Chen ES, Zuloaga P, Shaw CA, Rimawi MF, Perou CM, Mills GB, Chang JC, Lewis MT. A renewable tissue resource of phenotypically stable, biologically and ethnically diverse, patient-derived human breast cancer xenograft models. *Cancer Res.* 2013; 73(15):4885–97.

In: Advances in Experimental Surgery. Volume 2
Editors: Huifang Chen and Paulo N. Martins
ISBN: 978-1-53612-773-7
© 2018 Nova Science Publishers, Inc.

Chapter 8

OF MICE AND RATS: ANIMAL MODELS FOR USE IN LAPAROSCOPY AND LAPAROTOMY WITH HUMAN OVARIAN CANCER CELL LINE INTRAPERITONEAL XENOGRAFTS

Philippe Sauthier[1,2,3,*], *MD, Anne-Marie Mes-Masson*[1,2,4], *PhD, Louise Champoux*[1,2], *Michèle Bally*[1], *PhD and Diane M. Provencher*[1,2,3], *MD*

[1]Centre de recherche du Centre hospitalier de l'Université de Montréal (CRCHUM), Montreal, Canada
[2]Institut du Cancer de Montréal, Montreal, Canada
[3]Department of Obstetrics and Gynecology, Division of Gynecologic Oncology, Université de Montréal, Montreal, Canada
[4]Department of Medicine, Université de Montréal, Montreal, Canada

ABSTRACT

Experimental models of human diseases are crucial not only for understanding the biological and genetic factors that influence the phenotypic characteristics of the disease but also for developing rational intervention strategies. These models often require trial and error adaptation for which limited guidance exists; for example in epithelial ovarian cancer (EOC), a human disease characterized by intraperitoneal dissemination. In this chapter, we provide a detailed stepwise methodology that facilitates laparoscopic or laparotomy approaches in rodent models with EOC xenograft and report outcomes of our experiments.

We compared two immunocompromised rodent intraperitoneal xenograft models for their suitability for laparoscopic or laparotomy techniques. Intraperitoneal xenografts were obtained by injecting nude rats (HSD: RH−*rnu*) with one of the three human EOC cell lines

---

[*] Corresponding author: Philippe Sauthier, MD. Department of Obstetrics and Gynecology, Gynecologic Oncology Unit 1560 Sherbrooke E., H2L 4M1, Montreal, Quebec, Canada, E-mail: philippe.sauthier@umontreal.ca, Tel.: (514) 890−8000 ext 27244, Fax: (514) 412−7604.

(TOV-112D, TOV-21G, SKOV-3) and nude mice (SWISS-CD-1) with TOV-112D. Laparoscopy or laparotomy was performed using a customized operating table. Rats and mice developed intraperitoneal macroscopic tumors within 2 to 3 months after injection. In some animals, these were associated with hemorrhagic ascites. Anesthesia, when measured by the number of injections, was more difficult in mouse than in rat laparoscopies and, in both animals, an incisional hernia was sometimes observed. The rat tolerated and survived surgical laparoscopy or laparotomy. In contrast, the mouse was more fragile perioperatively, the number of surgical acts was more limited and survival rate was lower. While the nude mouse was most cost-effective, requiring less operative time and smaller volumes of anesthetic. Our results suggest that the nude rat is better suited to oncological experimentation that involves laparotomy or laparoscopy. Further studies are needed to confirm whether the biological characteristics of the disease are similar in rat and mouse models.

Keywords: ovarian cancer, xenograft, rodent models, laparoscopy, laparotomy

ABBREVIATIONS

CIPA   Comité Institutionel de la Protection des Animaux
EOC   Epithelial ovarian cancer
MMP2   Matrix metalloproteinases
VEGF   Vascular endothelial growth factor

INTRODUCTION

Laparoscopic surgery has been applied in oncology for several years. It has remained controversial in animal models as in clinical practice (Dargent 2000; Hopkins 2000; Canis 2001), although in the last two decades it has gained acceptance in defined clinical settings (Barakat 2013). A number of studies have demonstrated the feasibility of this technique, particularly in human epithelial ovarian cancer (EOC) (Deffieux 2006; Nezhat 2013). Laparoscopy can offer highly satisfactory surgical staging of cancer, including human EOC (Pomel 1995; Pratt 2000). The main concerns with laparoscopy have been the implantation of tumors in trocar puncture sites (Childers 1994), peritoneal carcinomatosis (Fondrinier 2002; Ramirez 2003), modification of tumor growth parameters, and the influence of the laparoscopic environment (CO_2) (LeMoine 1998; Shen 2008). A low rate (1%) of parietal implantation was found in early work (Childers 1994) but further studies found variable rates ranging from 1% up to 18% (Ramirez 2003; Curet 2004; Vergote 2005). Of note, over 100 cases of parietal metastases have been reported in the literature after laparoscopic cholecystectomy (Martinez 1995). In gynecological oncology, such metastases have been documented with invasive ovarian cancer (Hopkins 2000), borderline ovarian tumors (Morice 2004), cancer of the cervix (Agostini 2003), cancer of the endometrium (Sanjuan 2005) and even after laparoscopic surgery for benign disease (benign implants) (Carlson 2002). Nevertheless, some would argue that the presence of parietal metastases after laparoscopy or after paracentesis for ovarian cancer in human seems to have no significant impact on survival (Kruitwagen 1996; Vergote 2005).

In an ovarian cancer animal model, the surgical wound resulting from laparoscopy was suggested to induce little surgical stress on enhancing tumor growth compared with laparotomy, possibly because it minimally influences the secretion of VEGF (Vascular Endothelial Growth Factor) and MMP2 (Matrix Metalloproteinases) (Lee 2013). Moreover, in a rat ovarian cancer model, peritoneal closure is reported to reduce port site metastases (Agostini 2002).

Numerous hypotheses have been put forward for explaining wound or port site implants which implicate immune responses, pneumoperitoneum (Lecuru 2002), carbon dioxide (CO2), tumoral laceration, smoke, water vapor and contaminated instruments (Brundell 2002; Ramirez 2003; Curet 2004). However tumor implantation was not affected by CO_2, helium, or nitrous oxide gas in an animal model. Thus, CO_2 insufflation does not appear to increase tumor spread compared with other gasses (Agostini 2002; Hopkins 2002). Further characterization of this phenomenon can only be carried out with an animal model (Canis 1998; Agostini 2001; Lecuru 2001; Bourdel 2008). Use of experimental models for laparoscopy has been reviewed (Canis 2000). The models that are traditionally used are large, (Volz 1996) thereby reproducing conditions of human surgery, including instruments. However these models are expensive and immune-competent and therefore they may reject human tumoral transplants (Reymond 2000). Several immune-incompetent animal models have been developed, such as the nude mouse, the nude rat and the nude rabbit (Hajduch 1992). From an oncological viewpoint, the nude mouse is well characterized, whereas the rat is far less so and the rabbit not at all. Laparoscopy in the rat has been studied for colic resection (Allendorf 1997), rectal tumor resection (Braumann 2008), retroperitoneal dissection (Sandoval 1996) and cecum ligature (Berguer 1997). The metabolic effect of this type of surgery has been described in detail in the rat (Bouvy 1996). In summary, the rat has become an interesting surgical model, primarily owing to its lower cost than that of large animals.

A few animal models develop ovarian tumors spontaneously (Vanderhyden 2003). Intraperitoneal or sub-cutaneous xenograft models have been described for a mouse adenocarcinoma in the previously immune-incompetent rat (Rose 1996), an ovarian adenocarcinoma in a rat of the same species (Sugiyama 1990) and for ovarian tumors of human origin (Sawada 1982; Lecuru 2001; Rubin 2003). The influence of laparoscopy on the tumoral intra-abdominal behavior in the rat was studied after the implantation of mammary cancer (Mathew 1996) and adenocarcinoma of the colon (Jacobi 1997). Likewise, an intraperitoneal xenograft model in the mouse that mimics the dynamic progression of human ovarian cancer might provide a valuable surrogate for studying the biological properties of ovarian cancer as well as for testing new therapeutic strategies in preclinical trials (Lin 2007). In human EOC, a large number of cell lines have been sourced from patient samples, although only a small number is derived solely from chemotherapy- and radiation therapy-naïve women. Our laboratory has previously described such cell lines, which were obtained from solid tumors and readily formed tumors in mice (Provencher 2000). We report details of our procedure for conducting laparoscopy or laparotomy in xenograft rodent models with EOC as well as our findings.

METHODS

Animals

Following approval by the local Institutional Review Board and the Comité Institutionel de la Protection des Animaux (CIPA) animal care guidelines, rodents such as female (Swiss-

CD-1) nude mice (Charles Rivers Laboratories) and female (Hsd:RH-*rnu*) nude rats (Harlan Sprague Dawley Laboratories) were maintained on site at the Hôpital Notre-Dame animal facilities. These rats have a non-functional cystic thymus and accept allografts and xenografts.

Mice were housed in groups of five and rats in groups of four. All animals were acclimatized to a sterile environment controlled for temperature and light cycle. They had access to adequate food and water ad libitum. Tumor cell injections were performed when attained weight was 30 grams in mice and 60 grams in rats. At the time of their surgery, mice weighed approximately 50 grams whereas rats weighed about 200 grams. An ear punch allowed identification and surveillance of each animal.

All animals were clinically evaluated twice weekly and observed for 12 weeks or until there were obvious clinical signs of a tumor. Euthanasia was practiced on animals at 12 weeks or when tumors were larger than 1 cm on clinical examination. During autopsy, the tumors, as well as the trocar and laparotomy scar tissues were excised for pathological analysis (Figure 8.1a, 8.1b).

Human EOC Cell Lines Preparation and Injection

We grew and prepared TOV-21G and TOV-112D EOC cell lines obtained from chemotherapy- and radiotherapy-naïve patients, as previously reported (Provencher 2000). Briefly, TOV-112D was derived from an aggressive FIGO Stage IIIc grade 3 endometrioid adenocarcinoma. TOV-21G was established from a less aggressive FIGO IIIc clear cell carcinoma. The SKOV-3 EOC cell line was derived from ascitic cells of a patient with an ovarian adenocarcinoma previously treated with Thiotepa and obtained from American Type Culture Collection. Before their injection in rodents, tumor cells were diluted in phosphate-buffered saline with a pH of 7.4 containing Mg^+ but without Ca^{++} in a volume of 1 ml for the rats and 0.5 ml for the mice. A total of 14 mice were injected at passage (p66) with 10^6 cells from the TOV-21G cell line as described earlier (Provencher 2000). Rats were injected with one of the three tumoral cell lines. Either 10^6 or 10^7 cells were injected in order to determine optimum seeding of tumors in the rat model. Six (6) rats were injected with TOV-112D cells at passage (p74), 6 were injected with TOV-21G at passage (p56), and 2 were injected with SKOV-3. Intraperitoneal tumor growth was assessed by clinical observation of rodent abdominal distension, which guided the appropriate time for surgery.

EQUIPMENT

Operating Table

We custom built a laparoscopic table for small animals. It is adapted to the size of the animal, its height can be modified, and unlike commercially available laparoscopic tables, it allows for a variable Trendelenburg position (Figure 8.2a, 8.2b and 8.2c). Furthermore, this laparoscopic table is equipped with an optical system that can be fixed to reduce the interference caused by hand shaking movements and it enables one sole operator to work in a sterile environment.

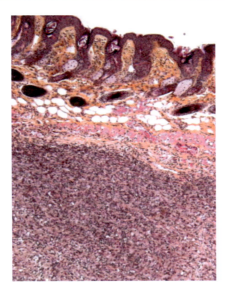

Figure 8.1a. Undifferentiated carcinoma in the scar tissue (low-magnification).

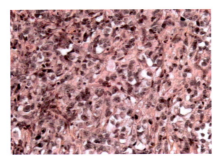

Figure 8.1b. Undifferentiated carcinoma in the scar tissue (high-magnification).

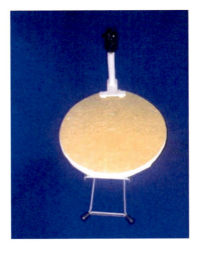

Figure 8.2a. Operating table in horizontal position.

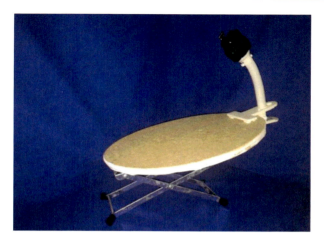

Figure 8.2b. Operating table in Trendelenburg position.

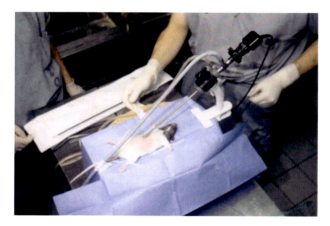

Figure 8.2c. Operating table in action.

Laparoscopy

Surgical laparoscopy was carried out with a conventional system. This consisted of a monitor (Trinitron™, Sony™), a cold light source (Xenon 611™, Karl Storz™), a CO$_2$ insufflator (Cabot Medical™), a camera (Autoexposure™, Karl Storz™), and an optical system with a diameter of 5 mm angled at 30 (Karl Storz™). Alternatively we also tested optical systems of 2 mm and 5 mm in diameter (Origin System). In addition, the instruments for laparoscopic surgery comprised a pair of scissors, prehensile and biopsy forceps, 1.7 mm in diameter (Origin System). We also used #15 scalpel blades, 3-0 absorbable sutures (Vicryl, Ethicon) and non-absorbable sutures (Surgilon™, Davis + Geck™), cutaneous sutures (Steristrips Skin Closures™, 3M™), 22G catheters (Jelco™, Critikon™), compresses, and 1 ml syringes with 26G needles.

Procedure

Anaesthesia

All surgeries were done in a sterile environment. Slow anesthesia was performed on the animals over 15 to 30 minutes. For rats, Pentobarbital 50 mg/kg was given intraperitoneally for induction, and additional doses of 25 mg/kg were injected as necessary. For mice, a combination of Ketamine 100 mg/kg, Xylazine 10 mg/kg and Acepromazine 0.1 mg/kg was administered by intraperitoneal injection, repeating the injection with half the dose as maintenance. Control of the anesthesia was carried out by pinching a hind paw, then observing the animal reactions and monitoring respiratory movements. As soon as the anesthesia was deemed sufficient, the animal was laid out on its back with its forelegs splayed out at right angles and attached with cutaneous sutures (Steristrips™). This procedure was intended to verify for perioperatory respiratory failure.

Laparoscopy

The initial pneumoperitoneum was induced by means of a 22G catheter in the abdominal right lower quadrant of the animal with a CO_2 air flow controlled at 3 to 5 mm Hg. A bursa, 4 mm in diameter and 1 cm below the xiphoid appendix, was created, supported with a 3-0 absorbable suture. The abdominal wall was then incised with a #15 scalpel blade at the centre of the bursa and the optical system was rapidly introduced. The bursa was tightened with a simple knot to ensure that there was no leak. The insufflation system was then fixed to the optical system allowing the surgical instruments to be introduced under direct vision, without trocar, laterally in the left and right iliac fossae. They were made impermeable by an identical bursa to that of the optical system. After the surgery, the instruments were withdrawn while still under direct vision and the bursae were closed. An analgesic (Buprenorphine 0.1 mg/kg) was injected subcutaneously immediately postoperatively and 24 hours later for pain control.

Laparotomy

Laparotomies were carried out with the same operative table under the same anesthesia protocol. In each case, a xyphopubic median incision was made with a cold knife #15 blade. The wound was closed with a continuous plane sunk suture with a 3-0 non-absorbable suture.

Surgery

Surgery, whether by laparotomy or laparoscopy, entailed the observation of the intra-abdominal tumor spread status and the tumor was manipulated and resected when possible. The extent of the tumoral invasion was evaluated according to the peritoneal cancer indexes described by Chauffert (PCIC) (Chauffert 1992) and Eggermont (PICE) (Eggermont 1988) (Table 8.2).

RESULTS

Intraperitoneal xenografts were successfully initiated by injecting one of the three human EOC cell lines (TOV-112D, TOV-21G, SKOV-3) to 14 nude rats (Hsd:RH-*rnu*) and the TOV-21G cell line to 14 nude mice (SWISS-CD-1).

All animals survived the initial tumoral injection but one rat, injected with 10^7 TOV-21G cells, had to be sacrificed early due to rapid and excessive tumor spread. Over the observation period, a total of 6 rats and 2 mice developed an intraperitoneal macroscopic tumor with 6 rats and 5 mice also having a hemorrhagic ascite. At the time of surgery, only 4 rats and 1 mouse had developed a tumor. All tumors were macroscopic with an index of 2 to 3 on the PCIC and PCIE. These tumors appeared in the rat on average 63.5 days after the injection of TOV-112D, 97.3 days after the injection of TOV-21G, and 75 days after the injection of SKOV-3- for an overall mean induction time of 82.3 days (range of 52 to 150 days). In the mouse, the time to development of tumors was on average 83.5 days (range of 58 to 109 days) after the injection of TOV- 21G.

Laparotomies were carried out on 6 rats and 7 mice and laparoscopies on 7 rats and 7 mice. In rats, laparotomy had a mean duration of 15.8 minutes and required a mean anesthetic volume of 0.38 ml/animal and a mean of 2.0 injection/animal whereas laparoscopy had a mean duration of 16.9 minutes and required a mean anesthetic volume of 0.44 ml/animal and a mean of 2.1 injections/ animal. In mice, the comparative mean anesthetic volumes and mean injections required were 0.13 ml and 1.7 injection/animal and 0.21 ml and 2.3 injection/animal, respectively for laparotomy and laparoscopy. Laparotomy took 9.1 minutes on average and laparoscopy 13.4 minutes in mice. The per-operative characteristics are summarized in Table 8.1.

The post-operative observation of animals with tumors at the time of surgery showed progression in 5 out of 7 cases and one case of total spontaneous remission. The existence of tumors in the scar tissue was only confirmed histologically in two cases, in mice operated by laparoscopy. None of these two mice showed signs of visible macroscopic tumors but all had ascites. The analysis of the extracted tumors confirmed the existence of extremely undifferentiated carcinomas. The characteristics and the analysis of the tumors in the scar tissue are shown in (Figure 8.1a and 8.1b) and tumors evaluation after laparoscopy or laparotomy are summarized in Table 8.2.

Complications occurred resulting in the death of one mouse, after laparoscopy, immediately post-operatively with no obvious cause at autopsy. One rat was found dead 72 hours after laparotomy and 2 mice died on the 4th and 6th day after the operation, one for no identifiable reason and the other from complete evisceration. Several post-cicatrical hernias were observed over time. One rat developed a hernia in the 12 hours following the operation. It was treated surgically the following day, but reoccurred several days later. Neither infections nor bleeding were observed. One mouse developed articular swelling of an unknown origin that regressed spontaneously. Another mouse showed signs of cutaneous discoloring with bluish stripes developing over its back. Post-operative evolution is summarized in Table 8.2.

Table 8.1. Types of tumoral lines, number (#) of animals with presence of tumor or ascites and surgical parameters

Lines	Rat model TOV-112D LAP	TOV-112D LSC	TOV-21G LAP	TOV-21G LSC	SKOV-3 LAP	SKOV-3 LSC	Mouse model TOV-21G LAP	TOV-21G LSC
Number of animals	2	2	2*	2	1	1	7	7
Number of cells/injection	10^7	10^7	10^7	10^7	10^7	10^7	10^6	10^6
Number of animals with tumor at time of surgery	2	0	0	0	0	1	1	0
Number of animals with ascites at time of surgery	0	0	0	2	0	0	0	4
Number of animals with cicatrical tumor	0	0	0	0	0	0	0	2
Total number of animals with tumors (at time of surgery or at autopsy)	2	0	1*	1	0	1	2	0
Total number of animals with ascites (at time of surgery or at autopsy)	0	1	0	2	1	0	0	5
Mean number of injections of anesthetic during surgery	2.0	2.1	2.0	2.1	2.0	2.1	1.7	2.3
Mean duration of surgery by type and by cell line (min)	15.8	16.9	15.8	16.9	15.8	16.9	9.1	13.4
Mean volume of anesthetic injected by surgery type and cell line (ml/animal)	0.38	0.44	0.38	0.44	0.38	0.44	0.13	0.21
Number of deaths <48 h of surgery by surgery type and cell line	0	0	0	0	0	0	0	1
Number of deaths > 48 h after surgery by surgery type and cell line	1	0	0	0	0	0	2	0
Number of animals with hernia by surgery type and cell line	1	1	1	0	1	0	0	2

LAP = laparotomy; LSC = laparoscopy.
* One rate was sacrificed.

Table 8.2. Evolution of the models and characteristics of the tumors

Animal #	Lines	No	PCIC[1]	PCIE[2]	Time [days]	Evolution	Death	Time of post–operative death
Rat #3	TOV–112D	10^7	2	2	75	Unknown	Spontaneous	48 h
Rat #5	TOV–112D	10^7	2	2	52	Remission	Autopsy	12th week
Rat #9	TOV–21G	10^7	3	3	67	Progression	Autopsy	No operation
Rat #12	TOV–21G	10^7	2	2	150	Progression	Autopsy	12th week
Rat #7	TOV–21G	10^6	1	1	75	Progression	Autopsy	12th week
Rat #14	SKOV–3	10^7	3	3	75	Progression	Autopsy	2nd week
Mouse #2	TOV–21G	10^6	1	1	58	Progression	Autopsy	4th week
Mouse #3	TOV–21G	10^6	2	2	109	Progression	Autopsy	8th week

[1] Peritoneal Cancer Index of Chauffert (PCIC):

[2] Peritoneal Cancer Index of Eggermont (PCIE):

0 = No tumour 1 = Tumoral nodule < 1 mm.

2 = Tumoral nodule > 1 mm   3 = Diffuse carcinomatosis with ascite.

0 = No tumour.

1 = Nodule of between 1 and 3 mm   2 = Moderate tumour   3 = Abundant tumour replacing the cavity.

DISCUSSION

We described our methods for successful EOC xenograft models amenable to either laparotomy or laparoscopy in rodents. We encountered no problems for injecting animals with tumoral lines extracted from untreated solid ovarian human tumors and animals withstood cell line injection well. The observation of cutaneous discoloring with bluish stripes in one of the mice remains unexplained, however this phenomenon was also observed in an earlier study (Provencher 2000). General anesthesia by subcutaneous injection is preferred by others to avoid any kind of interference with tumor development (Lecuru 2001). Anesthesia posed no particular problem in the rat, neither in laparoscopy nor in laparotomy. The total quantity of anesthetic and number of injections per rat were comparable. In the mouse, the anesthesia was particularly difficult when performing laparoscopy, as evidenced by a high number of re-injections and mean anesthetic volume that was almost twice as high compared with that needed for laparotomy. Nonetheless, mice required smaller anesthetic volumes than rats overall.

As the dimensions of the abdominal cavity in the mouse are small, the number of acts and manipulations remains very limited despite using instruments of 1.7 mm in diameter. We tested an optical system 2 mm in diameter, which frequently had to be repositioned due to its restricted visual field. Nonetheless, this optical system can be useful in diagnostic laparoscopy. The use of a 5 mm optical system and thus vision that extends over the entire pelvic cavity is possible in the rat.

Coagulation attempts with monopolar instruments were carried out and were feasible as long as an isolated 2 mm trocar was used (Veress needle).

Postoperative complications are more serious in mice than in rats. Our results in the rat were similar to those reported by Canis (Canis 1998). The frequently observed incisional hernias are probably explained by the fact that the animals are able to access their abdominal sutures. They can chew and tear off their sutures or their clips. For this reason, it would be preferable to close the wounds without suture material (sutures or clips), possibly using biological glue.

The tumors developed after the injection of 10^7 cells and it appears that this concentration is a minimal concentration required to induce tumors in this animal model. In his study, Rubin (1993) injected 4×10^7 to 2.5×10^9 cells per animal of the SKOV-3 and SKOV-7 lines and Lecuru (2001) injected 27×10^6 IGR-OV1 and 36×10^6 NIH: OVCAR-3 cells per animal. As the volume injected is already 1 ml (maximum injectable intraperitoneal volume tolerated by the rat), we felt that the viscousness would be too high if the number of cells were to exceed 10^7. It would seem preferable to inject 10^7 cells and to repeat the injection 48 hours later. This warrants further consideration.

All the tumors in the rats were sizeable as confirmed by the intraperitoneal cancer indexes, PCIC and PCIE (Table 8.2). They appeared after a relatively long time after injection (mean of 82.3 days in the rats and 83.5 days in the mice). This is significantly longer than in the IGR-OV1 model (7–21 days) and even in the NIH: OVCAR-3 model (14–21 days) (Lecuru 2001). This parameter is important to consider when planning studies of this kind. The rat, contrary to the mouse, tolerates the growth of intraperitoneal tumors well. This enabled us to stagger the surgery, sometimes by a few days, which may be of practical use. In contrast, for mice, abdominal distension quickly progressed to serious deterioration of the animal condition translating into a need for emergency surgery. In rodents the distribution of intraperitoneal tumors was similar to that observed in women with EOC. It should be noted that surgery consisted of a close examination of the cavity and that maximal cytoreduction could only be carried out in a few cases. The examination of the abdominal cavity was more precise with laparoscopy.

Tumoral implants were sometimes found in the laparoscopy incision scars in the mice (Figure 8.1a and 8.1b). These mice showed no signs of visible tumors but had ascites. No rats developed tumors in any incision sites in our pilot study. The number of animals studied is too small to draw conclusions but the presence of tumoral ascite has already been evoked as a factor that favors parietal tumoral implants (Kruitwagen 1996).

The nude rat therefore seems more robust as a model of human ovarian cancer and could enable an in-depth study of the influence of laparoscopy on the *in vivo* and *ex vivo* behavior of tumoral lines. Using rats involves a greater infrastructure in terms of animal husbandry and a higher daily cost. These factors need to be taken into consideration as the animals are generally housed in small sterile units. Furthermore, the acquisition cost of nude rats is higher than that of nude mice.

The operating table we custom built enabled us to carry out all required laparoscopic acts we wanted in a sterile environment. Its size is well adapted to the height of the animals and the adjustable Trendelenburg position was extremely useful allowing leverage for manipulation of the instruments (Figure 8.1a, 8.1b and 8.1c). The camera being fixed, enables stability while providing gentle rotation to visualize the specific operating field. In this respect, our custom table may offer an advantage over the existing commercial operating table (Kaps Co., Frankfurt, Germany™) (Berguer 1997).

CONCLUSION

The use of laparoscopy in oncology today raises certain concerns and requires more detailed investigations. Our experience suggests that the nude rat is a good animal model of human epithelial ovarian cancer. Animals tolerate laparoscopy and laparotomy well and have a high survival rate. Although it is better characterized from an oncological point of view, the nude mouse has proved to be less reliable in terms of tumor growth in our study. Most importantly, it is more fragile perioperatively and its overall survival is not as good as that of the rat. Furthermore, the restricted size of this animal greatly limits the surgical acts as surgical instruments are not very well adapted for this type of animal despite recent development of operating tables for laparoscopy on small animals. The nude rat, therefore, currently appears to be the ideal model for studying the concept of laparoscopy in oncology. Nevertheless, more in-depth studies are needed to fully characterize the biology of xenograft EOC tumorigenesis in the rat.

ACKNOWLEDGMENTS

We are grateful for the support of Jocelyne Gauvin research fund for this project.

REFERENCES

Agostini A, Robin F, Aggerbeck M, Jais JP, Blanc B, Lecuru F. Influence of peritoneal factors on port- site metastases in a xenograft ovarian cancer model. *BJOG* 2001; 108(8):809-812.

Agostini A, Robin F, Jais JP, Aggerbeck M, Vildé F, Blanc B, Lécuru F. Impact of different gases and pneumoperitoneum pressures on tumor growth during laparoscopy in a rat model. *Surg. Endosc.* 2002; 16(3):529-532.

Agostini A, Robin F, Jais JP, Aggerbeck M, Vildé F, Blanc B, Lécuru F. Peritoneal closure reduces port site metastases: results of an experiment in a rat ovarian cancer model. *Surg. Endosc.* 2002; 16(2): 289-291.

Agostini A, Carcopino X, Franchi F, Cravello L, Lecuru F, Blanc B. Port site metastasis after laparoscopy for uterine cervical carcinoma. *Surg. Endosc.* 2003; 17(10):1663-1665.

Allendorf JD, Bessler M, Whelan RL. A murine model of laparoscopic-assisted intervention. *Surg. Endosc.* 1997; 11(6):622-624.

Barakat RR, Berchuck A, Markman M, Randall ME. *Principles and Practice of Gynecologic Oncology.* 6th edition. Philadelphia: Williams and Wilkins. 2013.

Berguer R, Alarcon A, Feng S, Gutt C. Laparoscopic cecal ligation and puncture in the rat. Surgical technique and preliminary results. *Surg. Endosc.* 1997; 11(12):1206-1208.

Bourdel N, Matsuzaki S, Bazin JE, Darcha C, Pouly JL, Mage G, Canis M. Postoperative peritoneal dissemination of ovarian cancer cells is not promoted by carbon-dioxide pneumoperitoneum at low intraperitoneal pressure in a syngenic mouse laparoscopic model with controlled respiratory support: a pilot study. *J. Minim. Invasive. Gynecol.* 2008; 15(3):321-326.

Bouvy ND, Marquet RL, Hamming JF, Jeekel J, Bonjer HJ. Laparoscopic surgery in the rat. Beneficial effect on body weight and tumor take. *Surg. Endosc.* 1996; 10(5):490-494.

Braumann C, Balague C, Guenther N, Menenakos C, Jacobi CA. Application of a solid tumor model to evaluate tumor recurrence after an open or laparoscopic rectal resection in rats. *Surg. Laparosc. Endosc. Percutan. Tech.* 2008; 18(4):348-352.

Brundell SM, Tucker K, Texler M, Brown B, Chatterton B, Hewett PJ. Variables in the spread of tumor cells to trocars and port sites during operative laparoscopy. *Surg. Endosc.* 2002; 16(10):1413-1419.

Canis M, Botchorishvili R, Wattiez A, Mage G, Pouly JL, Bruhat MA. Tumor growth and dissemination after laparotomy and CO2 pneumoperitoneum: a rat ovarian cancer model. *Obstet. Gynecol.* 1998; 92(1):104-108.

Canis M, Botchorishvili R, Wattiez A, Pouly JL, Mage G, Manhes H, et al. Cancer and laparoscopy, experimental studies: a review. *Eur. J. Obstet. Gynecol. Reprod. Biol.* 2000; 91(1):1-9.

Canis M, Rabischong B, Botchorishvili R, Tamburro S, Wattiez A, Mage G, Pouly JL, Bruhat MA. Risk of spread of ovarian cancer after laparoscopic surgery. *Curr. Opin. Obstet. Gynecol.* 2001; 13(1): 9-14.

Carlson NL, Krivak TC, Winter WE, 3rd, Macri CI. Port site metastasis of ovarian carcinoma remote from laparoscopic surgery for benign disease. *Gynecol Oncol* 2002;85(3):529-531.

Chauffert B, Dimanche–Boitrel MT, Genne P, Petit JM, Onier N, Jeannin JF. [Experimental chemotherapy of peritoneal carcinomatosis of colonic origin in rats]. *Gastroenterol. Clin. Biol.* 1992; 16(3):215–219.

Childers JM, Aqua KA, Surwit EA, Hallum AV, Hatch KD. Abdominal–wall tumor implantation after laparoscopy for malignant conditions. *Obstet. Gynecol.* 1994; 84(5):765–769.

Curet MJ. Port site metastases. *Am. J. Surg.* 2004; 187(6):705–712.

Dargent D. [Laparoscopic surgery in gynecologic oncology]. *J. Gynecol. Obstet. Biol. Reprod.* (Paris) 2000; 29(3):282–284.

Deffieux X, Castaigne D, Pomel C. Role of laparoscopy to evaluate candidates for complete cytoreduction in advanced stages of epithelial ovarian cancer. *Int. J. Gynecol. Cancer.* 2006; 16 Suppl 1:35–40.

Eggermont AM, Steller EP, Marquet RL, Jeekel J, Sugarbaker PH. Local regional promotion of tumor growth after abdominal surgery is dominant over immunotherapy with interleukin–2 and lymphokine activated killer cells. *Cancer Detect. Prev.* 1988; 12(1–6):421–429.

Fagotti A, Ferrandina G, Fanfani F, Garganese G, Vizzielli G, Carone V, Salerno MG, Scambia G. Prospective validation of a laparoscopic predictive model for optimal cytoreduction in advanced ovarian carcinoma. *Am. J. Obstet. Gynecol.* 2008; 199(6):642.e1–6.

Fondrinier E, Descamps P, Arnaud JP, Pezet D. [Carbon dioxide pneumoperitoneum and peritoneal carcinosis: review]. *J. Gynecol. Obstet. Biol. Reprod.* (Paris) 2002; 31(1):11–27.

Hajduch M, Kod'ousek R. "Nude rabbit" with aplasia of B–lymphoid structures. *Acta. Univ. Palacki. Olomuc. Fac. Med.* 1992; 134:51–54.

Hopkins MP, von Gruenigen V, Gaich S. Laparoscopic port site implantation with ovarian cancer. *Am. J. Obstet. Gynecol.* 2000; 182(3):735–736.

Hopkins MP. The myths of laparoscopic surgery. *Am. J. Obstet. Gynecol.* 2000; 183(1):1–5.

Hopkins MP, von Gruenigen V, Haller NA, Holda S. The effect of various insufflation gases on tumor implantation in an animal model. *Am. J. Obstet. Gynecol.* 2002; 187(4):994–996.

Jacobi CA, Ordemann J, Bohm B, Zieren HU, Liebenthal C, Volk HD. The influence of laparotomy and laparoscopy on tumor growth in a rat model. *Surg. Endosc.* 1997; 11(6):618–621

Kadar N. Laparoscopic management of gynecological malignancies. *Curr. Opin. Obstet. Gynecol.* 1997; 9(4):247–255.

Kruitwagen RF, Swinkels BM, Keyser KG, Doesburg WH, Schijf CP. Incidence and effect on survival of abdominal wall metastases at trocar or puncture sites following laparoscopy or paracentesis in women with ovarian cancer. *Gynecol. Oncol.* 1996; 60(2):233–237.

Le Moine MC, Navarro F, Burgel JS, Pellegrin A, Khiari AR, Pourquier D, et al. Experimental assessment of the risk of tumor recurrence after laparoscopic surgery. *Surgery* 1998; 123(4):427–431.

Lecuru F, Agostini A, Camatte S, Robin F, Aggerbeck M, Jaiss JP, et al. Impact of pneumoperitoneum on visceral metastasis rate and survival. Results in two ovarian cancer models in rats. *BJOG* 2001; 108(7):733–737.

Lecuru F, Guilbaud N, Agostini A, Augereau C, Vilde F, Taurelle R. Description of two new human ovarian carcinoma models in nude rats suitable for laparoscopic experimentation. *Surg. Endosc.* 2001; 15(11):1346–1352.

Lécuru F, Agostini A, Camatte S, Robin F, Aggerbeck M, Jaïs JP, Vilde F, Taurelle R. Impact of pneumoperitoneum on tumor growth. *Surg. Endosc.* 2002; 16(8):1170−1174.

Lee JW, Park YA, Cho YJ, Kang KH, Choi JJ, Lee YY, Kim TJ, Choi CH, Kim BG, Bae DS. The effect of surgical wound on ovarian carcinoma growth in an animal model. *Anticancer Res.* 2013; (8):3177−3184.

Lin XJ, Chen XC, Wang L, Wei YQ, Kan B, Wen YJ, He X, Zhao X. Dynamic progression of an intraperitoneal xenograft model of human ovarian cancer and its potential for preclinical trials. *J. Exp. Clin. Cancer Res.* 2007; 26(4):467−474.

Martinez J, Targarona EM, Balague C, Pera M, Trias M. Port site metastasis. An unresolved problem in laparoscopic surgery. *A review. Int. Surg.* 1995; 80(4):315−321.

Mathew G, Watson DI, Rofe AM, Baigrie CF, Ellis T, Jamieson GG. Wound metastases following laparoscopic and open surgery for abdominal cancer in a rat model. *Br. J. Surg.* 1996; 83(8):1087−1090.

Morice P, Camatte S, Larregain-Fournier D, Thoury A, Duvillard P, Castaigne D. Port−site implantation after laparoscopic treatment of borderline ovarian tumors. *Obstet. Gynecol.* 2004; 104(5 Pt 2):1167−1170.

Nezhat FR, Pejovic T, Finger TN, Khalil SS. Role of minimally invasive surgery in ovarian cancer. *J. Minim. Invasive Gynecol.* 2013 Nov−Dec; 20(6):754−765.

Pomel C, Provencher D, Dauplat J, Gauthier P, Le Bouedec G, Drouin P, Audet−Lapointe P, Dubuc− Lissoir J.*Gynecol Oncol.* 1995 Sep; 58(3):301−306.

Pratt BL, Greene FL. Role of laparoscopy in the staging of malignant disease. *Surg. Clin. North Am.* 2000; 80(4):1111−1126.

Provencher DM, Lounis H, Champoux L, Tetrault M, Manderson EN, Wang JC, et al. Characterization of four novel epithelial ovarian cancer cell lines. *In Vitro Cell Dev. Biol. Anim.* 2000; 36(6):357−361.

Ramirez PT, Wolf JK, Levenback C. Laparoscopic port−site metastases: etiology and prevention. *Gynecol. Oncol.* 2003; 91(1):179−189.

Reymond MA, Tannapfel A, Schneider C, Scheidbach H, Kover S, Jung A. Description of an intraperitoneal tumour xenograft survival model in the pig. *Eur. J. Surg. Oncol.* 2000; 26(4):393−397.

Rose GS, Tocco LM, Granger GA, DiSaia PJ, Hamilton TC, Santin AD, et al. Development and characterization of a clinically useful animal model of epithelial ovarian cancer in the Fischer 344 rat. *Am. J. Obstet. Gynecol.* 1996; 175(3 Pt 1):593−599.

Rubin SC, Kairemo KJ, Brownell AL, Daghighian F, Federici MG, Pentlow KS, et al. High−resolution positron emission tomography of human ovarian cancer in nude rats using 124I−labeled monoclonal antibodies. *Gynecol. Oncol.* 1993; 48(1):61−67.

Sandoval BA, Sulaiman TT, Robinson AV, Stellato TA. Laparoscopic surgery in a small animal model. A simplified technique of retroperitoneal dissection in the rat. *Surg. Endosc.* 1996; 10(9):925−927.

Sanjuan A, Hernandez S, Pahisa J, Ayuso JR, Torne A, Martinez Roman S. Port-site metastasis after laparoscopic surgery for endometrial carcinoma: two case reports. *Gynecol. Oncol.* 2005; 96(2): 539−542.

Sawada M, Matsui Y, Hayakawa K, Nishiura H, Okudaira Y, Taki I. Human gynecologic cancers heterotransplanted into athymic nude rats. *Gynecol. Oncol.* 1982; 13(2):220−228.

Shen MY, Huang IP, Chen WS, Chang JT, Lin JK. Influence of pneumoperitoneum on tumor growth and pattern of intra-abdominal tumor spreading: in vivo study of a murine model. *Hepatogastroenterology* 2008; 55(84):947-951.

Sugiyama T, Nishida T, Yokota D, Ushijima K, Imaishi K, Hirakawa N, et al. An experimental model for advanced ovarian cancer. *Kurume Med. J.* 1990; 37(1):15-21.

Vanderhyden BC, Shaw TJ, Ethier JF. Animal models of ovarian cancer. *Reprod. Biol. Endocrinol.* 2003; 1:67-82.

Vergote I, Marquette S, Amant F, Berteloot P, Neven P. Port-site metastases after open laparoscopy: a study in 173 patients with advanced ovarian carcinoma. *Int. J. Gynecol. Cancer.* 2005; 15(5):776-779.

Volz J, Koster S, Weiss M, Schmidt R, Urbaschek R, Melchert F. Pathophysiologic features of a pneumoperitoneum at laparoscopy: a swine model. *Am. J. Obstet. Gynecol.* 1996; 174(1 Pt 1):132-140.

Section III. Advance Techniques in Experimental Surgery

In: Advances in Experimental Surgery. Volume 2
Editors: Huifang Chen and Paulo N. Martins
ISBN: 978-1-53612-773-7
© 2018 Nova Science Publishers, Inc.

Chapter 9

ORGAN BIOENGINEERING THROUGH DECELLULARIZATION AND RECELLULARIZATION APPROACHES

Maria Jaramillo, PhD and Basak E. Uygun, PhD*

Center for Engineering in Medicine, Massachusetts General Hospital.
Department of Surgery, Harvard Medical School,
Massachusetts General Hospital, Boston, Massachusetts, US

ABSTRACT

Organ transplantation has been used for over a century for the treatment of end organ failure. Despite vast advances in the field, the main challenge remains the availability of good quality donor organs. Scientists around the world are working on the development of alternative options for donor organs available for transplantation, including development of decellularization-based artificial organs, which is the focus of this chapter.

Organ and tissue decellularization has a number of advantages, including preservation of the extracellular matrix architecture and composition, which provide signals necessary for cell function and survival. The preserved vascular architecture in the scaffolds allows for connecting the bioengineered organ to the blood torrent upon transplantation. In addition, ECM scaffolds have been found to elicit low to negligible immune response which is a major advantage, eliminating the need for long-lasting use of potentially harmful immunosuppression therapy in transplant patients.

While very promising to increase the pool of donor organs, the decellularization/recellularization approach for bioengineered organs has a number of challenges. These include methods for decellularization with minimal damage to the extracellular matrix composition and architecture, choice of cells type and source for replacing the functions of organ in question and achieving long-term viability of the engineered organ *in vivo*. Here, we discuss each of these challenges and present current progress in the field for different organs including liver, heart, kidney and lungs.

---

[*] Corresponding author: Basak E. Uygun, PhD. Center for Engineering in Medicine, Massachusetts General Hospital, Department of Surgery, Harvard Medical School, 51 Blossom St., Boston, MA, Tel: 617-726-3474, E-mail: BUYGUN@mgh.harvard.edu.

Keywords: decellularization, recellularization, organ engineering

ABBREVIATIONS

ECM	Extracellular Matrix
SDS	Sodium dodecyl sulfate
hiPSC	human induced pluripotent stem cells
EPC	endothelial progenitor cells
HUVEC	Human umbilical vein endothelial cells
MSC	Mesenchymal Stem cells

INTRODUCTION

According to the United Network for Organ Sharing (UNOS), there are currently over 120,000 people in need of organ transplants in the United States, from which over 75,000 are on an active waiting list. However, it is estimated that only 30,000 to 35,000 transplants will be performed by the end of this year. This highlights the need for strategies to increase the pool of available organs. Several approaches have been developed to this end, including the formation of organizations devoted to education regarding organ donation to increase donor participation and research in areas including organ preservation, organ rehabilitation and organ engineering.

Organ engineering refers to the development of biological substitutes to replace or aid damaged and diseased tissues, thus maintaining physiological homeostasis in the patient. This involves the use of biomaterials, cells and other microenvironmental signals to mimic the niche of native organs such that their functions are recapitulated and maintained. Several strategies have been adopted for these purposes, including encapsulation of donor cells in biomaterials that provide immunogenic barriers while promoting cell survival and allowing proper cell function. Another approach that is quickly gaining interest is the concept of 3D printing, however, one of the most promising approaches and our main focus for this chapter is the development of artificial organs by decellularization and recellularization of native tissues and whole organs.

Organ decellularization consists of the complete removal of cells and cellular components from native tissues. This offers a number of advantages, including perhaps the closest recapitulation of physical and chemicals microenvironmental signals of tissues as well as low biomaterial immunogenicity. In addition, this offers a potentially abundant source of scaffolds, as, in contrast to organ transplantation, organs used for decellularization do not require such strict parameters such as minimal ischemia time, and preservation of the ECM can be achieved more easily than preservation of cell functions. Organs are then decellularized and repopulated with healthy cells, which can be derived from different sources such as allogeneic primary cells, expanded autologous cells, cells differentiated from different sources of stem cells (embryonic, induced pluripotent, adult) amongst others.

In the next sections, we will talk about different strategies used for tissue decellularization, including methods used to evaluate successful removal of cellular components. We will discuss several approaches for recellularization and will review some of the most notable advances in the field. Because each organ has a different function, organ engineering approaches have to be tailored to satisfy the physical and chemical requirements, therefore we will discuss research work in different organs. Finally, we will review other aspects of decellularization and recellularization organ engineering like introduction of non-parenchymal cells such as endothelial cells for proper vascularization and function of these replacement organs and their immunogenicity.

DECELLULARIZATION

Organ decellularization is typically achieved by subjecting tissues/organs to treatments that disrupt cell integrity, while preserving structure and composition of the extracellular matrix. Most commonly, these treatments are chemical agents, although several physical treatments have been successfully used alone or in combination with chemical treatment to ensure appropriate removal of cellular components from tissues and organs. Ultimately, all methods have a number of advantages and disadvantages, which have to be taken into consideration along with the tissue-specific requirements to come up with the best possible specific strategies for decellularization.

CHEMICAL METHODS

Detergents

Perhaps the most commonly used method for organ and tissue decellularization is the use of detergents that emulsify oils, disrupting the lipid bilayer of the cellular membrane, hence promoting cell lysis. Addition of fluid flow through whole organ perfusion or tissue agitation ensures efficient removal of remaining cellular components. Detergents can be classified into ionic, non-ionic or Zwitterionic detergents.

Ionic detergents have a charged hydrophilic group. They disrupt lipids and proteins, hence strongly disturbing the cellular structures, making them more effective at removing cellular components. Because of the fact that they can interact and denature proteins, they are considered the most destructive and they have a greater effect on the chemical composition of ECM. Additionally, they are harder to "rinse" than other types of detergents, which presents an obstacle to subsequent recellularization of the tissues due to its cytotoxic effects. The most commonly used ionic detergent is sodium dodecyl sulfate (SDS). It is routinely used for decellularization of tissues such as heart valves (Korossis 2002), tubular structures such as trachea (Hung 2016) and blood vessels (Schaner 2004), and whole organs including heart (Oberwallner 2014), liver (Uygun 2010) and kidneys (Wang 2015).

Non-ionic detergents are neutral and hydrophilic. They are highly capable of breaking lipid-lipid interactions, but due to their limited ability to interact with proteins, are unable to break protein-protein interactions and have reduced ability to break lipid-protein interactions. Because of this, they have weaker decellularization potential, but are better at maintaining the chemical composition of the ECM. The most commonly used non-ionic detergent is Triton

X-100, which is typically used in addition to SDS. In a few cases, it has been reported to promote appropriate decellularization alone in tissues such as ligaments (ACL) (Vavken 2009; Xu 2014) and annulus fibrosus (Xu 2014), suggesting to be more appropriate for decellularization of tissues with relatively low cellularity.

Finally, Zwitterionic detergents are considered to be "in between" ionic and non-ionic detergents. They have a net neutral charge, but are able to disturb protein interactions, without altering their native charge, hence are less damaging to the ECM composition than non-ionic detergents. 3-[(3-cholamidopropyl)dimethylammonio]-1-propanesulfonate (CHAPS) is the most widely used Zwitterionic detergent in decellularization approaches, and has been reported to efficiently decellularize tissues such as lung (Tsuchiya 2016). When compared to decellularization with SDS, it has been proven to preserve composition of components such as collagen and elastin, which have a strong effect in mechanical integrity, suggesting that CHAPS may be a better choice for highly cellular tissues whose function is highly dependent on its mechanical properties.

Osmotic Decellularization

Osmotic decellularization, consisting of alternation of hypertonic and hypotonic solution for cell disruption and removal, has been used alone and in combination with other methods such as detergent-based decellularization. Typically, TRIS-based buffers and Phosphate Buffered Saline (PBS) solutions are used. Hypotonic solutions force movement of water into the cell, causing cells to burst, which is followed by use of hypertonic solutions that promote non-histone protein dissociation from DNA. This method is gentler than the use of detergents, and it is considered to lead to better preservation of ECM, so it is typically used for tissue with low cellularity such as heart valves (Meyer 2006), cartilage (Schneider 2016) and cornea (Yam 2016).

Enzymes

Enzymatic decellularization consists of removing cellular components with the aid of enzymes that break down cellular components; some of such enzymes are trypsin, nucleases and dispase. Nucleases are enzymes that break down nucleic acids (DNA and RNA), but usually do not act on other cellular components, therefore are typically used in conjunction with other treatments that aid penetration of nucleases into the cells. There are other enzymes such as trypsin that promote breakdown of serine-containing proteins, which are very efficient at breaking down cells; however, because they are non-specific, they also interact with ECM proteins. Lipases are a good candidate for decellularization as they specifically disrupt the lipid bilayer of the cell membranes without disrupting ECM proteins, however, rather limited success at complete cellular removal has been achieved by the use of lipases alone (Crapo 2011).

PHYSICAL METHODS

Sonication

Sonication has been used mostly in combination with other methods for decellularization of tissues such as larynx (Hung 2013), trachea (Hung 2016), cardiovascular tissues (Azhim 2011), cartilage (Azhim 2013) and small intestine (Oliveira 2013). It has been shown to be advantageous in cases when perfusion decellularization is not possible due to the limited diffusion of chemical agents. In such cases, sonication has shown to enhance the degree of removal of cellular components through passive diffusion of decellularizing agents. It has been observed that sonication greatly speeds up the decellularization process, decreasing exposure time to chemical agents which typically show higher disruption of chemical composition.

Freeze/Thaw

This method is rarely used alone, but typically used as a critical step of decellularization in combination with other methods discussed here. Freezing promotes ice crystal formation of water, which, unlike most other materials, increases volume in its frozen form. This increase in water volume damages cell membrane, leading to break down of the cells. Typically, ice crystal formation can be reduced by cooling at low rates; hence, decellularization by thawing is better achieved by rapid freezing of tissue.

Irreversible Electroporation

Irreversible electroporation (IRE) is a novel technique that is currently being explored. It consists of applying non-thermal pulsed electric fields to disrupt the cellular membrane while maintaining the integrity of the ECM. This method has been explored as an *in vivo* decellularized method (Golberg 2016), where the scaffolds are decellularized in live animals, however, it has also been used in *ex vivo* perfusion models (Sano 2010).

Evaluation and Success Parameters

Biochemical evaluation of decellularization is typically performed by quantifying cellular components such as DNA and actin to estimate the amount of cellular material removed. In addition, preservation of ECM composition is evaluated by estimating concentration of ECM proteins such as laminin, elastin, collagen and fibronectin, or other components such as glycosaminoglycans (GAG). Quantification of these is typically done by standard assays such as ELISA, PicoGreen and immunostaining, however, due to the destructive nature of these methods, recent studies have highlighted the need to develop new methods that do not require damage to the decellularized tissue, thus promoting maintenance of its integrity for subsequent use. Some of the suggested technique include analysis of perfusate (Jörn 2015), but also more sophisticated methods such as computer tomography, which has been used for monitoring DNA content in real time (Geerts 2016).

Another parameter that is typically evaluated in most applications is the maintenance of the microstructural integrity of the scaffolds. For most tissues, the maintenance of a capillary network is essential, and this can be investigated by corrosion casting and a number of microscopy techniques including angiography and scanning electron microscopy. Furthermore, perfusion of dyes that can be removed by additional perfusion can be used to visualize capillary integrity after decellularization. In addition to capillary network integrity, other parameters such as topography have been evaluated through technique such as atomic force microscopy; the significance of it being that material characteristics such as roughness can alter cell behavior.

Additionally, for tissues that serve a mechanical function or tissues that need to be able to withstand mechanical loads, bulk physical parameters need to be evaluated. This is the case for tissues such as bone, tendon, cartilage, cardiac valves, lungs, muscle, blood vessels and many others. Depending on the tissue requirements, stress, strain, tensile strength, elasticity and compliance need to be evaluated.

Overall, there is no standardized set of parameters to define success in decellularization except for DNA content which is defined as 1) less than 50 ng of dsDNA per mg of dry weight; 2) DNA fragments less than 200 bp in length; and 3) no visible nuclear material in histologic analysis with DAPI or H&E, according to Faulk et al. (Faulk 2015). When performing such evaluation, it is important to keep in mind that every tissue serves a different function and hence, preservation of certain characteristics may be more important. For instance, in the case of liver engineering, the conservation of biochemical composition may be of higher importance, as hepatocyte function and viability is highly dependent on the chemical microenvironment. Alternatively, tissues such as cartilage are relatively acellular and the biggest functional requirement is the ability to withstand mechanical loads, hence, higher importance is given to the maintenance of physical characteristics. This highlights the need for a comprehensive compilation of data to define tissue-specific parameters and tolerance levels that will allow optimizing decellularization procedures based on specific requirements.

RECELLULARIZATION

After successful decellularization of organs and tissues, the next step is to repopulate the decellularized scaffolds with cells that will carry out vital functions of the organ. The main challenge in this step is the identification of a reliable and abundant cell source that will replace the functions of the native organ. There are a number of constraints in this step which include development of strategies for cell delivery, retention and maintenance. However, perhaps the biggest challenge is the establishment of an abundant cell source, which we will discuss in the following sections.

In Vitro Expansion and Maintenance of Primary Cells

Most cells in the body have a limited ability to expand and maintain a functional phenotype in an *in vitro* setting. This phenomenon is not well understood but its investigation could lead to the development of strategies to generate an abundance of functional cells to be used in cell/tissue engineering applications. Unfortunately, despite the great promise of this field for regenerative medicine applications, very limited advances have been made in this area.

A recent study describes genetic modification of primary human hepatocytes to express Human Papilloma Virus (HPV) genes, which mediate expression of receptors-associated hepatocyte proliferation *in vivo*. Exposure of the genetically modified hepatocytes to proliferation-inducing cytokines promotes their expansion amounting to up to a trillion cells per single hepatocyte. Removal of proliferation signals leads to polarization and induction of function in the hepatocytes (Levy 2015). Genetic engineering strategies has also been exploited for the expansion and maintenance of beta-cells using Cre/loxP-based reversible immortalization (Kobayashi 2006), however, these approaches rely on use of viral vectors, which could cause activation of oncogenes, hence, tumorigenicity. Other studies have concentrated on manipulation of the *in vivo* microenvironment rather than the cells, including the development of scaffolds with appropriate physical and chemical cues that have been found to promote limited expansion and functionality of cells such as alveolar cells and hepatocytes (Shamis 2011).

A number of tissues rely on progenitor cells with proliferation potential for repair of damaged tissue and cell turnover. Isolation of these cells, with subsequent expansion and induction of terminally differentiated phenotype, constitutes another strategy for organ engineering relying on primary human cells. The difficulty of this approach is isolation and identification of these cells from live patients; however, some advances have been made with the use of progenitor cells derived from stem cells, which will be further discussion in a later section.

To conclude this section, it is important to note that use of primary cells would require immunological matching of cells to patient, and potentially immunosuppression to avoid rejection of the transplanted graft. Recent studies have also explored the possibility of silencing genes involved in immune rejection (Figueiredo 2013), which in conjunction with successful strategies for expansion and maintenance of primary cells, would make the possibility of the creation of universal cell banking for off-shelve regenerative medicine applications a reality.

Cell Recovery from Discarded Organs

A new strategy that has emerged as an alternative approach is to recover cells from marginal organs deemed unacceptable for transplantation. While very little work has been done in this field, a few recent studies have shown that a number of cells including beta cells (Matsumoto 2007) and hepatocytes (Izamis 2013; Izamis 2015; Uygun 2016) can be recovered from organs exposed to warm ischemia for up to one hour by perfusion with preservation solutions that restore ionic concentrations of the cells and ATP generation. The resulting cells have been isolated at yields and levels of functionality comparable to those of primary cells.

Stem Cell Differentiation

Perhaps one of the most explored options is differentiation of functional cells from a number of different stem cell sources. Depending on their origin, cells can be pluripotent, multipotent, or have the ability to become a very limited number of cells. Stem cells are most commonly categorized into pluripotent, mesenchymal or tissue-specific stem cells.

Pluripotent stem cells include embryonic stem cells derived from the inner mass of the embryonic blastocyst and induced pluripotent stem cells, which are somatic cells that have been genetically engineered to express a number of genes characteristic of embryonic stem cells, giving these cells their pluripotency characteristics. Both cell types have two main features: their ability to self-renew indefinitely (making them a potentially unlimited cell source) and to differentiate into cells derived from the three germ layers of embryonic development (mesoderm, ectoderm and endoderm). Differentiation programs are based on developmental studies that identify specific signals that determine their fate, which are then recapitulated in an *in vitro* setting. Most commonly, these signals are chemical cues such as cytokines and small molecules, but can also be in the form of physical cues, such as substrates with varying mechanical properties. Despite their enormous potential, success of pluripotent stem cell differentiation has been limited partly due to the fact that they rely on developmental studies using non-human models; hence translation of these observations into development of human systems is imprecise. Challenges in this field remain, including low functionality and maturity of the resulting cells. In terms of complex cell types, such as hepatocytes, that carry a large number of diverse functions, a challenge has been the recapitulation of all the functions. This last requirement can be bypassed by the alternative strategy of creating auxiliary grafts that instead of replacing the entire organ will aid it by providing the function that is aberrated in the patient. This strategy could be used in deficiency diseases, such as Alpha-1 antitrypsin (AAT) deficiency. Hepatocytes in AAT-deficient patients often carry out other vital functions such as albumin production, lipid metabolism, carbohydrate metabolism and drug metabolism. In such cases, creation of a graft with differentiated cells that produce AAT and be transplanted in the patients, auxiliary to their native liver to aid rather than replace the marginal organ.

Mesenchymal stem cells are naturally occurring adult cells that are not terminally differentiated hence maintain the ability to differentiate into a limited number of tissues within the mesodermal lineage (bone, cartilage, muscle, adipose tissue and blood; although some studies report limited differentiation into ectoderm and endoderm lineages). Their sources include cells derived from adipose tissue, bone marrow, tooth bud and umbilical cord which are readily accessible and can be patient-specific.

Finally, some tissues have fast cell turnover and rely on resident stem cells to continually replace aged or damaged cells. Some of these include oval cells in the liver, epithelial lining of the stomach and intestine and skin. These cells typically can differentiate into just one or two cell types, and can be isolated using cell-specific markers.

ADVANCES

In the following sections, we will discuss and summarize some of the most prominent advances in the field of decellularized tissue-based organ engineering of a number of specific systems.

Liver

First reports of whole liver decellularization date back to 2009 (Baptista 2009). Being a highly cellular organ, and because the lipid content can be higher than in most other tissues, liver decellularization is most often achieved by the use of detergent, which preserves a significant amount of the chemical composition and the architectural integrity of the liver including its vascular network. Because of the highly vascular content, decellularization is typically done by perfusion through one of the main vessels (typically portal vein).

Report of recellularization first appeared in 2010 (Uygun 2010) when rat livers were recellularized using freshly isolated primary rat hepatocytes, which performed hepatic functions (albumin and urea secretion, and drug metabolism protein expression) comparable to those found when hepatocytes were maintained under static collagen sandwich culture conditions, which to date, remains the gold-standard for culture of human hepatocytes. In addition, the recellularized grafts were transplanted into rats that underwent unilateral nephrectomy to prepare a viable site for auxiliary liver graft transplantation. The renal vein and artery were used as ports to create blood source. Efflux was established within 5 min of unclamping and the recellularized graft was kept for 8 h before evaluating damage to the hepatocytes due to the arterial blood flow and the resulting shear stress, which was found to be minimal. A later study showed that the recipient survival could be extended to 24 h by the addition of a heparin layer on recellularized liver grafts (Bruinsma 2015). However, thrombogenicity of the grafts still remains a problem.

Subsequent studies have been conducted in larger animal models including rabbits, sheep, and porcine livers (Kajbafzadeh 2012; Nari 2013; Wang 2015). One study using porcine livers (Barakat 2012) evaluated recellularization using human fetal hepatocytes and stellate cells, and the recellularized grafts were kept under perfusion culture for up to two weeks, during which they showed metabolic activity including oxygen and glucose consumption, lactate and urea production, and albumin secretion.

Several cells have been investigated as potential sources for recellularization. A number of studies have investigated the use of MSC (He 2013; Jiang 2014) and have reported differentiation of these cells within the scaffolds (with addition of soluble chemical cues) to be superior to differentiation of the same cells under 2D culture conditions. However, neither report compared hepatic functions of differentiated cells to those found in primary hepatocytes, making it hard to determine whether maturation is achieved to physiologically-relevant levels. Other studies have used MSC for recellularization in conjunction with primary hepatocytes, and have shown that this co-culture configuration improves engraftment and function of the primary hepatocytes (Kadota 2014).

Finally, there are two alternative approaches to both decellularization and recellularization that are worth discussing. First, there have been a few reports of efficient liver decellularization using IRE (Golberg 2016; Sano 2010). This method has been used for decellularization of livers under *ex vivo* perfusion, which can be subsequently recellularized, however, due to the regenerative potential of liver, has also been explored as a method for *in vivo* decellularization and recellularization, as it has been demonstrated that after IRE treatment, liver regeneration occurs in the absence of scar formation. Other methods for *in vivo* decellularization and recellularization have been developed, including detergent-based decellularization of a single lobe *in vivo* through surgical by-pass circulation with a perfusion chamber system (Pan 2016). In this study, decellularized lobe was subsequently recellularized *in vivo* with primary hepatocytes from donor rats. Alternatively, the idea of transplanting decellularized livers to allow for "spontaneous" *in vivo* recellularization has also been explored, but the resulting grafts were inferior when compared to *in vitro* recellularized grafts (Sabetkish 2015).

Lung

Lung decellularization was first reported in 2010 in studies in mice and rat lungs (Ott 2010; Price 2010) and using a combination of methods, including hypertonic/hypotonic solutions, detergents and enzymes. Because of the function of the lung, preservation of its mechanical integrity is of utmost importance, hence, decellularization protocols have been developed avoiding or minimizing use of ionic detergents, which have been shown to lead to greater loss of elastin and collagen that confer lungs their mechanical properties, including tensile strength and elastic behavior (Petersen 2012). A number of strategies have been developed to maximize cell removal while promoting maximal retention of ECM components, and in turn mechanical properties. These include: use of zwitterionic detergents such as sulfobetaine-10 (Nagao 2013), or non-ionic detergent such as Triton X-100 or CHAPS. Alternative ionic detergents such as ethoxylated sodium lauryl ether sulfate (SLES), have been developed solely for decellularization purposes. SLES is weaker than traditionally used SDS, and because of its ethoxylation, the lauryl alcohol content is reduced, hence exhibiting lower protein denaturation (Kawasaki 2015). Alternative approaches have focused on modification of delivery of decellularization reagents. For instance, it has been suggested that perfusion route has an effect on efficiency of decellularization, with intratracheal route being suggested as the preferred method (Maghsoudlou 2013; Tsuchiya 2016; Wang 2016). In addition, some studies focus on optimization of physical parameters such as flow rate and pressure, which can be increased to speed up the decellularization process, hence, minimize exposure (da Palma 2015; Khalpey 2015). Despite, or partly due to the large number of studies evaluating decellularization methods in lungs, there is little consensus about which method leads to best decellularization. Because these studies are often performed in different animal systems, there is very little real time monitoring of the progression of decellularization, and so much variability in terms of concentrations, physical parameters, and timing used, reports often come to contradicting conclusions, highlighting the need for a comprehensive evaluation of these methods in a systematic way that would allow for standardization of lung decellularization protocols.

Recellularization of lungs has been attempted using adult and fetal alveolar cells (Price 2010; Song 2011), airway epithelial cells (Gilpin 2014), lung cancer cells (Mishra 2012), MSC (Bonvillain 2013), human iPSC-derived alveolar epithelial cells (Ghaedi 2013), hESC (Nakayama 2013), basal epithelial stem cells isolated and expanded from human lungs (Gilpin 2016) and fibroblasts (Sun 2014). In general, these studies have demonstrated that decellularized scaffolds are capable of supporting cell engraftment and in some cases, differentiation. It has also been suggested that when recellularizing lungs with progenitor cells (either fetal or stem cell-derived), the addition of mechanical forces such as stress and strain are important as these provide differentiation signals to the cells (Bonvillain 2013). Interestingly, decellularized rhesus monkey lungs have been used as a model to demonstrate decellularized matrix specificity to cell type by performing differentiation studies of hESC showing that differentiation of these cells in lung scaffolds showed better epithelial airway differentiation than if the cells were seeded on scaffolds derived from other tissues (Nakayama 2013).

Finally, there have been a few reported studies of evaluation of function of the decellularization-based engineered lungs in an *in vivo* setting. This was first attempted in 2010 (Ott 2010) when rat lungs were recellularized with lung endothelial and epithelial cells and transplanted into recipient rats after 5 days of *ex vivo* culture. The rats first underwent pneumonectomy (left lung) and the grafts were transplanted by anastomosis of the graft to pulmonary artery, pulmonary vein and left main bronchus of the recipient. No bleeding, edema or leakage was observed within one hour of transplant, and blood gas levels showed improvement when compared to the levels after pneumonectomy. The grafts were maintained for up to 6 hours, however, complications were observed at this time-point, including edema, which was probably because of pulmonary secretions.

Heart

Heart valves were amongst the first tissues explored for decellularization/recellularization tissue engineering approaches. Despite this, whole heart decellularization was not explored until 2008 (Ott 2008) in a seminal study that produced decellularized hearts from rats via coronary perfusion of SDS. Since then, a number of protocols have been developed exploring different chemical agents (Triton X-100, EDTA, deoxycholic acid, Sodium Azide, Soponin, Glycerol), perfusion routes (pulmonary, aortic or coronary) and physical parameters, however, there is little consensus regarding the best method for whole-heart decellularization.

Decellularization success parameters are typically retention of chemical components, especially, elastin and GAG. Biomechanical characterization often involves stress-relaxation which analyzes elastic moduli and viscosity, and tensile-failure tests which also can be used to estimate elastic modality and viscosity in addition to load limit (Bronshtein 2013).

Recellularization of heart tissue has been explored using a number of cell types, including myoblast cell lines (Akhyari 2011), adult and fetal cardiomyocytes from different sources (Wainwright 2010), as well as supporting cell types present in the heart. Cardiomyocytes recellularization has been attempted using primary rat cardiomyocytes. They have been shown to gain myocardial organization and express cardiac markers, and exhibit synchronized beating (Eitan 2009). A different study using neonatal cardiomyocytes from mouse to recellularize porcine hearts showed maintenance of cell viability and measurable electrical activity within five days of recellularization (Weymann 2014). Similarly, recellularization of human hearts with human cardiomyocytes has shown that the cells align in a muscle-like fiber manner, exhibit calcium dynamics and action potential propagation (Sanchez 2015). Pluripotent stem cells and MSC (Sarig 2012) have been seeded onto decellularized hearts both to test the cytocompatibility of the scaffolds with these cells, but also for their ability to differentiate within the scaffolds. In the absence of differentiation signals, it was shown that hiPSC were able to engrafts and survive for up to seven days, however, it was also observed that by the end of the culture, there was a significant loss of pluripotency markers (Carvalho 2012). In addition, hiPSC-derived cardiomyocytes have been used to recellularize human heart ventricular scaffolds resulting in increased expression of ion channels and increase in electrophysiological responses (Garreta 2016).

Recellularization with fibroblasts was shown to regain some of the lost components during decellularization process such as GAGs, which enabled to gain strength (Eitan 2009). Finally, it has been suggested that recellularization success is dependent on the source of the scaffolding tissue. A recent study compared recellularization success in hearts prepared from adult and fetal rats and found that fetal scaffolds provide better engraftment and proliferation of neonatal cardiomyocytes and adult cardiac progenitor cell (Silva 2016).

Very few translational studies involving transplantation of decellularized matrix-based engineered hearts have been performed. The first reported of such studies involved transplantation of porcine scaffolds using ascending aorta and the superior vena cava as an inlet and outlet of the blood stream, respectively, with closure of vena cava, pulmonary veins and pulmonary artery circulation. The results of this study showed that the scaffold integrity was adequate to endure surgical procedure, and artery perfusion was achieved. Additional procedures were performed with scaffold pre-recellularized with MSC, however, blood flow in this model was not achieved. Alternatively, MSC were injected into the scaffold immediately prior to transplantation, which allowed for establishment of blood flow and some degree of engraftment of the cells was confirmed after 3 days (Kitahara 2016).

Finally, several groups have attempted to engineer bioreactors for cardiac heart engineering in order to ensure small variability in decellularization/recellularization process, but also to efficiently deliver a variety of signals that will promote cell engraftment, viability, proper function and/or differentiation, and in some cases, even provide real time monitoring of the grafts. One example is a modular bioreactor developed to maintain recellularized hearts under controlled perfusion and medium conditioning (oxygenation, temperature and pH control), which also provides myocardial stretching, electrophysiological stimulation and/or monitoring (Hülsmann 2013).

Kidney

Kidney decellularization was first achieved in rat models (Ross 2009) and shortly after tested in large animal models (Nakayama 2010; Vishwakarma 2014). Decellularization of kidneys is typically achieved by detergent-based methods, with SDS being deemed the most successful (Wang 2015), hence the most commonly used. Transplantation studies with SDS-decellularized porcine kidneys have been performed which showed maintenance of vascular structure as suggested by lack of blood extravasation (Orlando 2012), intact microarchitecture of the glomerular structures, and when seeded with primary human cells, promoted their survival and viability (Sullivan 2012). Furthermore, SDS decellularization has been successfully attempted in human kidneys (Orlando 2013), which exhibit preserved vasculature, microstructure and maintenance of growth factors within the matrix (Peloso 2015).

Decellularized kidney recellularization has been performed using murine stem cells (Bonandrini 2014; Guan 2015), iPSC-derived tubular epithelial cells (Caralt 2015), renal epithelial cells (Uzarski 2015) and adipose-derived MSC (Rafighdoust 2015). Addition of chemical signals, such as chondroitin sulfate has been used to improve seeding and differentiation of stem cells into renal epithelial cells (Rafighdoust 2015). In terms of stem cells, it has been found that seeding and culture in decellularized scaffolds promotes a decrease in pluripotency and increase in mesoendodermal markers (Bonandrini 2014). Finally, it has been suggested that recellularization with different cell types can be achieved by perfusion seeding of epithelial cells through the ureter, and non-parenchymal cells through arterial route (Willenberg 2015).

Pancreas

Pancreas is perhaps one of the most complex organs in terms of decellularization, which is probably reflected by the very small number of published studies in the field. It has been suggested that success has been hampered by the complex architecture of pancreas and very delicate vascular structure, which is easily disrupted by common decellularization methods (Willenberg 2015).

Decellularization of rat pancreas was first reported in 2013 (Goh 2013). In this study, decellularization was achieved by perfusion with SDS at low concentration, and the decellularized scaffolds were subsequently seeded with acinar and beta cell lines, which showed an increase in functionality. A very recent study successfully achieved human pancreas recellularization with triton X-100 and recellularized with primary human beta cells and endothelial cells, showing viability and insulin secretion after 4 days in perfusion culture (Peloso 2016).

VASCULARIZATION/ENDOTHELIALIZATION

Every tissue in the body relies in some degree of vascularization for its survival and proper functioning. Vascular structures are in charge of ensuring delivery of nutrients and oxygen to each cell to guarantee its survival, but in many cases, cell signals are also delivered from the cells into the blood-stream through the same capillary structures, for systemic delivery and homeostasis. Liver and pancreas are two organs that are highly vascularized, both due to the high metabolic requirements of the cells and the delivery of cell-products, which include albumin and insulin respectively. This highlights the need for decellularization protocols that maintain the integrity of capillary network.

Blood vessels, regardless of size, are lined by a specialized epithelium that performs a number of functions, from providing a selective barrier between blood and tissues to production of signals that aid functioning of parenchymal cells. Importantly, endothelial cells prevent blood coagulation and fibrinolysis by a number of mechanisms, including the production of prostacyclin and nitric oxide that prevent platelet aggregation, activation of anticoagulation pathways and thrombin inhibition through heparin-rich domains in their cell surface. Transplantation studies have shown that in the absence of endothelium, decellularized scaffolds fail due to blood clot formation. For this and more reasons, in addition to maintenance of capillary structure, it is important to develop approaches for appropriate endothelial coverage of the vasculature of decellularized tissues.

Challenges

Success of decellularization-based artificial organs is highly dependent on the achievement of adequate re-endothelialization of the vascular networks, which remains one of the greatest obstacles in this field. A number of factors contribute to the difficulty of achieving adequate endothelial coverage, including challenges in delivering endothelial cells exclusively to capillary networks, poor engraftment, insufficient spreading of endothelial cells, poor formation of tight junctions and other functional morphological characteristics of endothelial cells and identification of highly available cell sources.

At the initial stages of development of this field, it was hypothesized that decellularized matrix possessed a sort of "postal code" that would allow specific cells to attach to the appropriate locations within the scaffolds (Bonvillain 2012). However, a number of studies found that when a mixed population of cells was seeded onto decellularized organ scaffolds, cell engraftment was heterogeneous. Some studies have nevertheless found that maintenance of phenotype and differentiation into specific cell types is improved when cells are seeded onto their appropriate site (Petersen 2010). Approaches for cell delivery into specific sites vary greatly depending on the organs, with some organs having several routes for cell delivery that can be used to orchestrate the spatial organization of cells. Improved engraftment of endothelial cells can be promoted by a number of approaches including use of capture antibodies that will recruit endothelial cells through surface markers, preparation of coatings that improve endothelial cell attachment, functionalization of matrix with angiogenic factors and signals that promote endothelial cell proliferation and spreading. In addition, it is also important to provide signals that will induce organization of cells into functional structures that will provide barrier functions, including tight junctions, adherent junctions and adhesive structures that regulate specific permeability of cells. Finally, like with other aspects of organ engineering, a significant challenge is the identification of an abundant cell source. In terms of reendothelialization, some of the candidate cell sources include: primary cells from cadaveric tissues, stem cell-derived endothelial cells and progenitor endothelial cells from patient circulation.

Advances

As previously mentioned, one strategy for spatial control of cell organization consists of using specific routes for cell delivery. This can more easily be used in organs with separate luminal networks such as lung that contains circulatory and airway networks. Specifically, re-endothelialization is achieved by perfusion seeding on endothelial cells through pulmonary vein and/or artery (Ren 2015) while alveolar epithelial cells are to be seeded via the trachea (Ott 2010). In cases where multiple routes are not an option, spatial organization was attempted through injection of parenchymal cells into the parenchymal space, in combination with perfusion seeding of endothelial cells through the vasculature (Zhou 2016). Sequential seeding can also be exploited so that parenchymal cells are first introduced through vascular perfusion filling the parenchymal space, followed by perfusion of endothelial cells (Kadota 2014). Finally, it has been suggested that simply adjusting the posture of the decellularized organ during cell-seeding increased cell homogeneity and cell retention (Stabler 2016).

In terms of improved endothelial cell capture, spreading and survival, some strategies have been developed based on previous studies for endothelialization of engineered vascular grafts, valves and devices such as cardiovascular stents. These include CD133 or CD31 antibody conjugation to the decellularized scaffolds to increase capture of endothelial cells through surface marker capture (Jackson 2014; Ko 2015; Vossler 2015). This is achieved by activation of carboxylic groups in the ECM to induce amide bond formation with primary amines in antibodies, which was found to increase endothelial cell adhesion under sheer conditions. Similarly, conjugation of other factors used for improvement of endothelial cell attachment include fibronectin (Ren 2015) and heparin-gelatin mixtures that both increased attachment and migration of endothelial cells, while also providing an antithrombotic coating to reduce blot clot formation (Bao 2015; Hussein 2016). The aforementioned study highlights an alternative approach to overcome the challenge of blood clot formation that relies on reduction of thrombogenicity independent of endothelial cells. One example is a recent study that explored layer-by-layer heparinization of decellularized organ matrices, resulting in decreased blood clot formation (Bruinsma 2015).

In terms of selection of cell source, the same alternatives previously mentioned for parenchymal cell source have been explored. In this section, we will focus on endothelial progenitor cells due to their numerous unique advantages. Endothelial progenitor cells are naturally occurring cells that participate in vessel formation, remodeling and repair. They can be isolated from a number of sources including peripheral blood, bone marrow and umbilical source, and selected by surface marker labeling methods. Finally, certain subsets of EPC have been found to be highly proliferative making them a potentially abundant source. Several groups have explored their use for endothelialization approaches, including a recent study where EPC were isolated and expanded from bone marrow and seeded into liver scaffolds through portal vein perfusion. The resulting scaffolds exhibited coverage of the lining of tubular structures by endothelial cell marker expressing cells, suggesting at the very least, maintenance of endothelial cells markers, however, further analysis is required to assess their maturation (Zhou 2016). EPC from cord blood have also been utilized for recellularization of decellularized rat lungs, although their viability after perfusion culture was lower compared to recellularization using other endothelial cell sources such as HUVEC (Ren 2015).

OTHER CONSIDERATIONS

Monitoring Decellularization

As previously mentioned, current methods for evaluating completion of decellurization consist of destructive methods that render the scaffolds unusable for further applications. This is acceptable in animal studies where homogeneity of the organs is higher, hence, the results obtained in one experiments are typically representative of subsequent experiments. However, due to variability of lifestyles in human subjects, variability of the organs is greater, and the possibility of developing a "one-size fits all" protocol is unfeasible. A great way to exemplify this is by mentioning dietary effects on variation of lipid contents in liver, which may increase difficulty of liver decellularization in humans, requiring the use of additional components that, while helping with removal of excess fat from fatty livers, may induce greater loss of important components in non-fatty organs. This highlights the need for creation of non-destructive and real-time monitoring methods that allow for the monitoring of decellularization progress, so that protocols can be modified to optimize decellularization in real time.

A limited number of studies have shown promise in using non-destructive techniques for monitoring various attributes of decellularized matrix scaffolds. This includes evaluation of perfusates, which have been used to determine appropriate removal of detergent from matrix through biochemical assays (Zvarova 2016). This has also been used to determine degree of removal of cellular components through rheological measurements (Jörn 2015). More sophisticated techniques such as phase-based X-ray tomography (Hagen 2015) which have been used to acquire high resolution images of the scaffolds, hence allowing for evaluation of their architectural integrity. Similarly, it has been shown that methods such as computer tomography can be used to estimate certain parameters such as Hounsfield unit of tissue, which was found to be correlated with DNA content in tissue, hence, in combination with other methods, such as perfusate analysis, could be an adequate method for non-destructive monitoring of decellularization (Geerts 2016).

Monitoring Recellularization

Equally important to the development of non-destructive methods for monitoring decellularization, it is essential to develop approaches to evaluate status of the engineered organs after recellularization. A number of these methods are in existence, as they rely on the same principles used to evaluate function or organs *in vivo*, such as measurement of electrical properties of heart, biochemical secretions from liver and pancreas that can be measured from perfusates (albumin, insulin, glucose levels). However, these are end points that are typically measured days after cell seeding to determine the function of the organs before implantation. Evaluation of additional parameter earlier in the process may prove beneficial, as they would provide information that can be used to change culture parameters that could aid optimize conditions for survival of the cells within the scaffolds.

Some novel techniques for monitoring recellularization include the evaluation of dynamic changes in physical parameters, such as hydrodynamic pressure, which increases with appropriate endothelialization (Uzarski 2015). Furthermore, methods such as perfusion with Resazurin has been found to be a non-cytotoxic method to assess metabolic activity of the grafts, hence can be used to determine cell engraftment, proliferation and survival (Ren 2015).

Immunogenicity

The ultimate goal of organ engineering is to develop fully functional tissue substitutes that will not elicit a host immune reaction, hence, bypassing the need for immunosuppression, which leaves patients vulnerable to infections and long-term complications such as cardiovascular diseases and increased risk for cancer. In addition to incomplete removal of cellular component, which has been extensively discussed in previous sections, immune response can be elicited both by the scaffold itself or cells used for recellularization. These issues have been addressed by a number of groups, and will be discussed in the following paragraphs.

The main activators of immune response from xenogeneic sources are DNA and Galα1-3Galβ1-4GlcNAc-R (alpha-Gal), a membrane epitope present in most mammals except primates (including humans). Theoretically, complete removal of cell and cellular components should render decellularized scaffold from other species usable for organ engineering applications for human use, however, other aspects should be considered such as differences in size and architecture of organ/tissues, and removal of pathogens. The possibility of using decellularized tissues from xenogeneic sources has most extensively been evaluated in heart valves, and it has been established that collagen and elastin from bovine and porcine sources does not elicit a response from human dendritic cells, B cells, or T cells, suggesting immunocompatibility (Bayrak 2013). Despite this, availability of human organs from cadaveric donors is abundant, hence, still remains the most desirable source for decellularized scaffolds.

As discussed earlier, cells from xenogeneic sources express a number of epitopes that elicit responses from the immune system of humans, making human sources the most viable alternative. Cells recovered from cadaveric donors would require HLA typing and possibly blood matching and cross matching and despite this, transplantation of these cells may still require immune therapy. From the sources mentioned earlier, iPS-derived cells, and some MSC-derived cells are perhaps the most non-immunogenic, as they can be patient-specific. A number of other stem cells, including ESC and some of the resident stem cells present in a number of tissues have been found to have little to no expression of HLA and elicit no immune responses, suggesting immune privileged status of these cells.

CONCLUSION

Engineering of functional organs through decellularization/recellularization of cadaveric organs is a field with great promise for the alleviation of current limitations to organ transplantation, including limited availability of donor organs. Decellularization can be achieved by a number of physical and chemical methods, all with several advantages and disadvantages, as well as success rates that depend on the specific characteristics of the organs themselves. Adequate recellularization is dictated by a number of parameters, including availability of a reliable and abundant cell source that needs to be successfully delivered into the scaffold, where it should remain both viable and functional. Recellularization also requires addition of non-parenchymal cells that support proper functioning of the organs. Particularly important is inclusion of endothelial cells that in addition to their supportive function, provide a functional vasculature, which is fundamental to the survival of the grafts. Other interactions yet to be investigated, include the incorporation of innervation into the engineered organs, however, most visceral organs function well without a nerve supply, and even in traditional transplantation approaches, innervations of the donor organ is not performed (Sanatani 2004). Finally, studies with several tissues including a recent work using decellularized liver scaffolds have shown some degree of inflammatory response in rats implanted with porcine liver matrices (Wang 2016). Crosslinking has been suggested as a possible method to overcome immunogenicity associated with use of xenogeneic scaffolds (Boer 2015, Wang 2016) and has led to promising results.

REFERENCES

Akhyari P, Aubin H, Gwanmesia P, Barth M, Hoffmann S, Huelsmann J, Preuss K, Lichtenberg A. The Quest for an Optimized Protocol for Whole-Heart Decellularization: A Comparison of Three Popular and a Novel Decellularization Technique and Their Diverse Effects on

Crucial Extracellular Matrix Qualities. *Tissue Eng. Part C: Methods* 2011; 17 (9): 915–926.

Azhim A, Ono T, Fukui Y, Morimoto Y, Furukawa K, Ushida T. Preparation of decellularized meniscal scaffolds using sonication treatment for tissue engineering. *Conf. Proc. IEEE Eng. Med. Biol. Soc.* 2013; 2013 6953–6.

Azhim A, Yamagami K, Muramatsu K, Morimoto Y, Tanaka M. The use of sonication treatment to completely decellularize blood arteries: a pilot study. *Conf. Proc. IEEE Eng. Med. Biol. Soc.* 2011; 2011: 2468–71.

Bao J, Wu Q, Sun J, Zhou Y, Wang Y, Jiang X, Li L, Shi Y, Bu H. Hemocompatibility improvement of perfusion-decellularized clinical-scale liver scaffold through heparin immobilization. *Sci. Rep.* 2015; 5: 10756.

Baptista PM, Orlando G, Mirmalek-Sani SH, Siddiqui M, Atala A, Soker S. Whole organ decellularization – a tool for bioscaffold fabrication and organ bioengineering. *Conf. Proc. IEEE Eng. Med. Biol. Soc.* 3–6 Sept. 2009; 2009: 6526–6529.

Barakat O, Abbasi S, Rodriguez G, Rios J, Wood RP, Ozaki C, Holley LS, Gauthier PK. Use of Decellularized Porcine Liver for Engineering Humanized Liver Organ. *J. Surg. Res.* 2012; 173 (1): e11–e25.

Bayrak A, Pruger P, Stock UA, Seifert M. Absence of immune responses with xenogeneic collagen and elastin. *Tissue Eng. Part A.* 2013; 19 (13–14): 1592–600.

Boer U, Schridde A, Anssar M, Klingenberg M, Sarikouch S, Dellmann A, Harringer W, Haverich A, Wilhelmi M. The immune response to crosslinked tissue is reduced in decellularized xenogeneic and absent in decellularized allogeneic heart valves. *Int. J. Artif. Organs.* 2015; 38 (4): 199–209.

Bonandrini B, Figliuzzi M, Papadimou E, Morigi M, Perico N, Casiraghi F, Dipl C, Sangalli F, Conti S, Benigni A, Remuzzi A, Remuzzi G. Recellularization of well-preserved acellular kidney scaffold using embryonic stem cells. *Tissue Eng. Part A.* 2014; 20 (9–10): 1486–98.

Bonandrini B, Figliuzzi M, Papadimou E, Morigi M, Perico N, Casiraghi F, Sangalli F, Conti S, Benigni A, Remuzzi A, Remuzzi G. Recellularization of Well-Preserved Acellular Kidney Scaffold Using Embryonic Stem Cells. *Tissue Eng. Part A.* 2014; 20 (9–10): 1486–1498.

Bonvillain RW, Danchuk S, Sullivan DE, Betancourt AM, Semon JA, Eagle ME, Mayeux JP, Gregory AN, Wang G, Townley IK, Borg ZD, Weiss DJ, Bunnell BA. A Nonhuman Primate Model of Lung Regeneration: Detergent-Mediated Decellularization and Initial *In Vitro* Recellularization with Mesenchymal Stem Cells. *Tissue Engineering. Part A.* 2012; 18 (23–24): 2437–2452.

Bonvillain RW, Scarritt ME, Pashos NC, Mayeux JP, Meshberger CL, Betancourt AM, Sullivan DE, Bunnell BA. Nonhuman Primate Lung Decellularization and Recellularization Using a Specialized Large-organ Bioreactor. *J. Vis. Exp.* 2013; (82): 50825.

Bronshtein T, Au-Yeung GCT, Sarig U, Nguyen EB-V, Mhaisalkar PS, Boey FYC, Venkatraman SS, Machluf M. A Mathematical Model for Analyzing the Elasticity, Viscosity, and Failure of Soft Tissue: Comparison of Native and Decellularized Porcine Cardiac Extracellular Matrix for Tissue Engineering. *Tissue Eng. Part A.* 2013; 19 (8): 620–630.

Bruinsma BG, Kim Y, Berendsen TA, Ozer S, Yarmush ML, Uygun BE. Layer-by-layer heparinization of decellularized liver matrices to reduce thrombogenicity of tissue engineered grafts. *J. Clin. Transl. Res.* 2015; 1 (1): 04.

Caralt M, Uzarski JS, Iacob S, Obergfell KP, Berg N, Bijonowski BM, Kiefer KM, Ward HH, Wandinger-Ness A, Miller WM, Zhang ZJ, Abecassis MM, Wertheim JA. Optimization and critical evaluation of decellularization strategies to develop renal extracellular matrix scaffolds as biological templates for organ engineering and transplantation. *Am. J. Transplant* 2015; 15 (1): 64–75.

Carvalho JL, de Carvalho PH, Gomes DA, Goes AM. Characterization of Decellularized Heart Matrices as Biomaterials for Regular and Whole Organ Tissue Engineering and Initial In-vitro Recellularization with Ips Cells. *J. Tissue Sci. Eng.* 2012; Suppl 11 002.

Crapo PM, Gilbert TW, Badylak SF. An overview of tissue and whole organ decellularization processes. *Biomaterials* 2011; 32 (12): 3233–3243.

Da Palma RK, Campillo N, Uriarte JJ, Oliveira LVF, Navajas D, Farré R. Pressure- and flow-controlled media perfusion differently modify vascular mechanics in lung decellularization. *J. Mech. Behav. Biomed. Mater.* 2015; 49 69–79.

Eitan Y, Sarig U, Dahan N, Machluf M. Acellular Cardiac Extracellular Matrix as a Scaffold for Tissue Engineering: *In Vitro* Cell Support, Remodeling, and Biocompatibility. *Tissue Eng. Part C: Methods.* 2009; 16 (4): 671–683.

Faulk DM, Wildemann JD, Badylak SF. Decellularization and Cell Seeding of Whole Liver Biologic Scaffolds Composed of Extracellular Matrix. *J. Clin. Exp. Hepatol.* 2015; 5 (1): 69–80.

Figueiredo C, Wedekind D, Müller T, Vahlsing S, Horn PA, Seltsam A, Blasczyk R. MHC Universal Cells Survive in an Allogeneic Environment after Incompatible Transplantation. *Biomed. Res. Int.* 2013; 2013 796046.

Garreta E, de Oñate L, Fernández-Santos ME, Oria R, Tarantino C, Climent AM, Marco A, Samitier M, Martínez E, Valls-Margarit M, Matesanz R, Taylor DA, Fernández-Avilés F, Izpisua Belmonte JC, Montserrat N. Myocardial commitment from human pluripotent stem cells: Rapid production of human heart grafts. *Biomaterials* 2016; 98 64–78.

Geerts S, Ozer S, Jaramillo M, Yarmush ML, Uygun BE. Nondestructive Methods for Monitoring Cell Removal During Rat Liver Decellularization. *Tissue Eng Part C: Methods.* 2016; 22 (7): 671–678.

Ghaedi M, Calle EA, Mendez JJ, Gard AL, Balestrini J, Booth A, Bove PF, Gui L, White ES, Niklason LE. Human iPS cell–derived alveolar epithelium repopulates lung extracellular matrix. *J. Clin. Invest.* 2013; 123 (11): 4950–4962.

Gilpin SE, Charest JM, Ren X, Tapias LF, Wu T, Evangelista-Leite D, Mathisen DJ, Ott HC. Regenerative potential of human airway stem cells in lung epithelial engineering. *Biomaterials* 2016; 108 111–119.

Gilpin SE, Guyette JP, Gonzalez G, Ren X, Asara JM, Mathisen DJ, Vacanti JP, Ott HC. Perfusion decellularization of human and porcine lungs: Bringing the matrix to clinical scale. *J. Heart Lung Transplant.* 2014; 33 (3): 298–308.

Goh SK, Bertera S, Olsen P, Candiello JE, Halfter W, Uechi G, Balasubramani M, Johnson SA, Sicari BM, Kollar E, Badylak SF, Banerjee I. Perfusion-decellularized pancreas as a natural 3D scaffold for pancreatic tissue and whole organ engineering. *Biomaterials* 2013; 34 (28): 6760–72.

Golberg A, Bruinsma BG, Jaramillo M, Yarmush ML, Uygun BE. Rat liver regeneration following ablation with irreversible electroporation. *Peer J.* 2016; 4 e1571.

Guan Y, Liu S, Sun C, Cheng G, Kong F, Luan Y, Xie X, Zhao S, Zhang D, Wang J, Li K, Liu Y. The effective bioengineering method of implantation decellularized renal extracellular matrix scaffolds. *Oncotarget* 2015; 6 (34): 36126–38.

Hagen CK, Maghsoudlou P, Totonelli G, Diemoz PC, Endrizzi M, Rigon L, Menk RH, Arfelli F, Dreossi D, Brun E, Coan P, Bravin A, De Coppi P, Olivo A. High contrast microstructural visualization of natural acellular matrices by means of phase-based x-ray tomography. *Sci. Rep.* 2015; 5: 18156.

He H, Liu X, Peng L, Gao Z, Ye Y, Su Y, Zhao Q, Wang K, Gong Y, He F. Promotion of Hepatic Differentiation of Bone Marrow Mesenchymal Stem Cells on Decellularized Cell-Deposited Extracellular Matrix. *Biomed. Res. Int.* 2013; 2013: 406871.

Hülsmann J, Aubin H, Kranz A, Godehardt E, Munakata H, Kamiya H, Barth M, Lichtenberg A, Akhyari P. A novel customizable modular bioreactor system for whole-heart cultivation under controlled 3D biomechanical stimulation. *J. Artif. Organs.* 2013; 16 (3): 294–304.

Hung SH, Su CH, Lee FP, Tseng H. Larynx decellularization: combining freeze-drying and sonication as an effective method. *J. Voice.* 2013; 27 (3): 289–94.

Hung SH, Su CH, Lin SE, Tseng H. Preliminary experiences in trachea scaffold tissue engineering with segmental organ decellularization. *Laryngoscope* 2016; 126 (11): 2520–2527.

Hussein KH, Park KM, Kang KS, Woo HM. Heparin-gelatin mixture improves vascular reconstruction efficiency and hepatic function in bioengineered livers. *Acta Biomater.* 2016; 38 82–93.

Izamis ML, Calhoun C, Uygun BE, Guzzardi MA, Price G, Luitje M, Saeidi N, Yarmush ML, Uygun K. Simple Machine Perfusion Significantly Enhances Hepatocyte Yields of Ischemic and Fresh Rat Livers. *Cell Med.* 2013; 4 (3): 109–123.

Izamis M-L, Perk S, Calhoun C, Uygun K, Yarmush ML, Berthiaume F. Machine Perfusion Enhances Hepatocyte Isolation Yields From Ischemic Livers. *Cryobiology* 2015; 71 (2): 244–255.

Jackson JR, Ko IK, Abolbashari M, Huling J, Zambon J, Kim C, Orlando G, Yoo J, Aboushwareb T, Atala A. CD31 Antibody Conjugation Improves Re-Endothelialization of Acellular Kidney Scaffolds for Whole Organ Engineering. *J. Am. Coll. Surg.* 2014; 219 (3): S141.

Jiang WC, Cheng YH, Yen MH, Chang Y, Yang VW, Lee OK. Cryo-chemical decellularization of the whole liver for mesenchymal stem cells-based functional hepatic tissue engineering. *Biomaterials* 2014; 35 (11): 3607–3617.

Jörn H, Hug A, Shahbaz TB, Alexander K, Volker RS, Artur L, Payam A. Rheology of perfusates and fluid dynamical effects during whole organ decellularization: A perspective to individualize decellularization protocols for single organs. *Biofabrication* 2015; 7 (3): 035008.

Kadota Y, Yagi H, Inomata K, Matsubara K, Hibi T, Abe Y, Kitago M, Shinoda M, Obara H, Itano O, Kitagawa Y. Mesenchymal stem cells support hepatocyte function in engineered liver grafts. *Organogenesis* 2014; 10 (2): 268–277.

Kajbafzadeh AM, Javan-Farazmand N, Monajemzadeh M, Baghayee A. Determining the Optimal Decellularization and Sterilization Protocol for Preparing a Tissue Scaffold of a Human-Sized Liver Tissue. *Tissue Eng Part C: Methods* 2012; 19 (8): 642–651.

Kawasaki T, Kirita Y, Kami D, Kitani T, Ozaki C, Itakura Y, Toyoda M, Gojo S. Novel detergent for whole organ tissue engineering. *J. Biomed. Mater. Res. A.* 2015; 103 (10): 3364−3373.

Khalpey Z, Qu N, Hemphill C, Louis AV, Ferng AS, Son TG, Stavoe K, Penick K, Tran PL, Konhilas J, Lagrand DS, Garcia JGN. Rapid Porcine Lung Decellularization Using a Novel Organ Regenerative Control Acquisition Bioreactor. *ASAIO J.* 2015; 61 (1): 71−77.

Kitahara H, Yagi H, Tajima K, Okamoto K, Yoshitake A, Aeba R, Kudo M, Kashima I, Kawaguchi S, Hirano A, Kasai M, Akamatsu Y, Oka H, Kitagawa Y, Shimizu H. Heterotopic transplantation of a decellularized and recellularized whole porcine heart. *Interact. Cardiovasc. Thorac. Surg.* 2016; 22 (5): 571−579.

Ko IK, Peng L, Peloso A, Smith CJ, Dhal A, Deegan DB, Zimmerman C, Clouse C, Zhao W, Shupe TD, Soker S, Yoo JJ, Atala A. Bioengineered transplantable porcine livers with re-endothelialized vasculature. *Biomaterials* 2015; 40 72−79.

Kobayashi N. Cell Therapy for Diabetes Mellitus. *Cell Transplant.* 2006; 15 (10): 849-854.

Korossis SA, Booth C, Wilcox HE, Watterson KG, Kearney JN, Fisher J, Ingham E. Tissue engineering of cardiac valve prostheses II: biomechanical characterization of decellularized porcine aortic heart valves. *J. Heart Valve Dis.* 2002; 11 (4): 463−71.

Levy G, Bomze D, Heinz S, Ramachandran SD, Noerenberg A, Cohen M, Shibolet O, Sklan E, Braspenning J, Nahmias Y. Long-term culture and expansion of primary human hepatocytes. *Nat. Biotech.* 2015; 33 (12): 1264−1271.

Maghsoudlou P, Georgiades F, Tyraskis A, Totonelli G, Loukogeorgakis SP, Orlando G, Shangaris P, Lange P, Delalande JM, Burns AJ, Cenedese A, Sebire NJ, Turmaine M, Guest BN, Alcorn JF, Atala A, Birchall MA, Elliott MJ, Eaton S, Pierro A, Gilbert TW, De Coppi P. Preservation of micro-architecture and angiogenic potential in a pulmonary acellular matrix obtained using intermittent intra-tracheal flow of detergent enzymatic treatment. *Biomaterials* 2013; 34 (28): 6638−6648.

Matsumoto S, Noguchi H, Naziruddin B, Onaca N, Jackson A, Nobuyo H, Teru O, Naoya K, Klintmalm G, Levy M. Improvement of pancreatic islet cell isolation for transplantation. *Proc. (Bayl. Univ. Med. Cent.).* 2007; 20 (4): 357−362.

Meyer SR, Chiu B, Churchill TA, Zhu L, Lakey JR, Ross DB. Comparison of aortic valve allograft decellularization techniques in the rat. *J. Biomed. Mater. Res A.* 2006; 79 (2): 254−62.

Mishra DK, Thrall MJ, Baird BN, Ott HC, Blackmon SH, Kurie JM, Kim MP. Human Lung Cancer Cells Grown on Acellular Rat Lung Matrix Create Perfusable Tumor Nodules. *Ann. Thorac. Surg.* 2012; 93 (4): 1075−1081.

Nagao RJ, Ouyang Y, Keller R, Lee C, Suggs LJ, Schmidt CE. Preservation of Capillary-beds in Rat Lung Tissue Using Optimized Chemical Decellularization. *J. Mater. Chem. B Mater. Biol. Med.* 2013; 1 (37): 4801−4808.

Nakayama KH, Batchelder CA, Lee CI, Tarantal AF. Decellularized Rhesus Monkey Kidney as a Three-Dimensional Scaffold for Renal Tissue Engineering. *Tissue Eng. Part A.* 2010; 16 (7): 2207−2216.

Nakayama KH, Lee CCI, Batchelder CA, Tarantal AF. Tissue Specificity of Decellularized Rhesus Monkey Kidney and Lung Scaffolds. *PLoS One* 2013; 8 (5): e64134.

Nari G, Cid M, Comín R, Reyna L, Juri G, Taborda R, Salvatierra N. Preparation of a three-dimensional extracellular matrix by decellularization of rabbit livers. *Rev. Esp. Enferm. Dig.* 2013; 105. (3): 6.

Oberwallner B, Brodarac A, Choi YH, Saric T, Anic P, Morawietz L, Stamm C. Preparation of cardiac extracellular matrix scaffolds by decellularization of human myocardium. *J. Biomed. Mater. Res. A.* 2014; 102 (9): 3263−72.

Oliveira AC, Garzon I, Ionescu AM, Carriel V, Cardona Jde L, Gonzalez-Andrades M, Perez Mdel M, Alaminos M, Campos A. Evaluation of small intestine grafts decellularization methods for corneal tissue engineering. *PLoS One* 2013; 8 (6): e66538.

Orlando G, Booth C, Wang Z, Totonelli G, Ross CL, Moran E, Salvatori M, Maghsoudlou P, Turmaine M, Delario G, Al-Shraideh Y, Farooq U, Farney AC, Rogers J, Iskandar SS, Burns A, Marini FC, De Coppi P, Stratta RJ, Soker S. Discarded human kidneys as a source of ECM scaffold for kidney regeneration technologies. *Biomaterials* 2013; 34 (24): 5915−25.

Orlando G, Farney AC, Iskandar SS, Mirmalek-Sani SH, Sullivan DC, Moran E, AbouShwareb T, De Coppi P, Wood KJ, Stratta RJ, Atala A, Yoo JJ, Soker S. Production and implantation of renal extracellular matrix scaffolds from porcine kidneys as a platform for renal bioengineering investigations. *Ann. Surg.* 2012; 256 (2): 363−70.

Ott HC, Clippinger B, Conrad C, Schuetz C, Pomerantseva I, Ikonomou L, Kotton D, Vacanti JP. Regeneration and orthotopic transplantation of a bioartificial lung. *Nat. Med.* 2010; 16 (8): 927−933.

Ott HC, Matthiesen TS, Goh S-K, Black LD, Kren SM, Netoff TI, Taylor DA. Perfusion-decellularized matrix: using nature's platform to engineer a bioartificial heart. *Nat. Med.* 2008; 14 (2): 213−221.

Pan J, Yan S, Gao JJ, Wang YY, Lu ZJ, Cui CW, Zhang YH, Wang Y, Meng XQ, Zhou L, Xie HY, Zheng J, Zheng MH, Zheng SS. In-vivo organ engineering: Perfusion of hepatocytes in a single liver lobe scaffold of living rats. *Int. J. Biochem. Cell Biol.* 2016; 80 124−131.

Peloso A, Petrosyan A, Da Sacco S, Booth C, Zambon JP, O'Brien T, Aardema C, Robertson J, De Filippo RE, Soker S, Stratta RJ, Perin L, Orlando G. Renal Extracellular Matrix Scaffolds From Discarded Kidneys Maintain Glomerular Morphometry and Vascular Resilience and Retains Critical Growth Factors. *Transplantation* 2015; 99 (9): 1807−16.

Peloso A, Urbani L, Cravedi P, Katari R, Maghsoudlou P, Fallas ME, Sordi V, Citro A, Purroy C, Niu G, McQuilling JP, Sittadjody S, Farney AC, Iskandar SS, Zambon JP, Rogers J, Stratta RJ, Opara EC, Piemonti L, Furdui CM, Soker S, De Coppi P, Orlando G. The Human Pancreas as a Source of Protolerogenic Extracellular Matrix Scaffold for a New-generation Bioartificial Endocrine Pancreas. *Ann. Surg.* 2016; 264 (1): 169−79.

Petersen TH, Calle EA, Colehour MB, Niklason LE. Matrix Composition and Mechanics of Decellularized Lung Scaffolds. *Cells Tissues Organs* 2012; 195 (3): 222−231.

Petersen TH, Calle EA, Zhao L, Lee EJ, Gui L, Raredon MB, Gavrilov K, Yi T, Zhuang ZW, Breuer C, Herzog E, Niklason LE. Tissue-engineered lungs for *in vivo* implantation. *Science* 2010; 329 (5991): 538−41.

Price AP, England KA, Matson AM, Blazar BR, Panoskaltsis-Mortari A. Development of a Decellularized Lung Bioreactor System for Bioengineering the Lung: The Matrix Reloaded. *Tissue Eng. Part A.* 2010; 16 (8): 2581−2591.

Rafighdoust A, Shahri NM, Baharara J. Decellularized kidney in the presence of chondroitin sulfate as a natural 3D scaffold for stem cells. *Iran. J. Basic Med. Sci.* 2015; 18 (8): 788−98.

Ren X, Moser PT, Gilpin SE, Okamoto T, Wu T, Tapias LF, Mercier FE, Xiong L, Ghawi R, Scadden DT, Mathisen DJ, Ott HC. Engineering pulmonary vasculature in decellularized rat and human lungs. *Nat. Biotech.* 2015; 33 (10): 1097−1102.

Ren X, Tapias LF, Jank BJ, Mathisen DJ, Lanuti M, Ott HC. Ex vivo Non-invasive Assessment of Cell Viability and Proliferation in Bio-engineered Whole Organ Constructs. *Biomaterials* 2015; 52 103−112.

Ross EA, Williams MJ, Hamazaki T, Terada N, Clapp WL, Adin C, Ellison GW, Jorgensen M, Batich CD. Embryonic Stem Cells Proliferate and Differentiate when Seeded into Kidney Scaffolds. *J. Am. Soc. Nephrol.* 2009; 20 (11): 2338−2347.

Sabetkish S, Kajbafzadeh A-M, Sabetkish N, Khorramirouz R, Akbarzadeh A, Seyedian SL, Pasalar P, Orangian S, Beigi RSH, Aryan Z, Akbari H, Tavangar SM. Whole-organ tissue engineering: Decellularization and recellularization of three-dimensional matrix liver scaffolds. *J. Biomed. Mater. Res. A.* 2015; 103 (4): 1498−1508.

Sanatani S, Chiu C, Nykanen D, Coles J, West L, Hamilton R. Evolution of heart rate control after transplantation: conduction versus autonomic innervation. *Pediatr. Cardiol.* 2004; 25 (2): 113−8.

Sanchez PL, Fernandez-Santos ME, Costanza S, Climent AM, Moscoso I, Gonzalez-Nicolas MA, Sanz-Ruiz R, Rodriguez H, Kren SM, Garrido G, Escalante JL, Bermejo J, Elizaga J, Menarguez J, Yotti R, Perez del Villar C, Espinosa MA, Guillem MS, Willerson JT, Bernad A, Matesanz R, Taylor DA, Fernandez-Aviles F. Acellular human heart matrix: A critical step toward whole heart grafts. *Biomaterials* 2015; 61 279−89.

Sano MB, Neal RE, Garcia PA, Gerber D, Robertson J, Davalos RV. Towards the creation of decellularized organ constructs using irreversible electroporation and active mechanical perfusion. *Biomed. Eng. Online* 2010; 9 (1): 83.

Sarig U, Au-Yeung GCT, Wang Y, Bronshtein T, Dahan N, Boey FYC, Venkatraman SS, Machluf M. Thick Acellular Heart Extracellular Matrix with Inherent Vasculature: A Potential Platform for Myocardial Tissue Regeneration. *Tissue Eng. Part A.* 2012; 18 (19−20): 2125−2137.

Schaner PJ, Martin ND, Tulenko TN, Shapiro IM, Tarola NA, Leichter RF, Carabasi RA, Dimuzio PJ. Decellularized vein as a potential scaffold for vascular tissue engineering. *J. Vasc. Surg.* 2004; 40 (1): 146−53.

Schneider C, Lehmann J, van Osch GP, Hildner F, Teuschl AH, Monforte X, Miosga D, Heimel P, Priglinger E, Redl H, Wolbank S, Nurnberger S. Systematic comparison of protocols for the preparation of human articular cartilage for use as scaffold material in cartilage tissue engineering. *Tissue engineering. Part C, Methods.* 2016.

Shamis Y, Hasson E, Soroker A, Bassat E, Shimoni Y, Ziv T, Sionov RV, Mitrani E. Organ-Specific Scaffolds for *In Vitro* Expansion, Differentiation, and Organization of Primary Lung Cells. *Tissue Eng Part C: Methods.* 2011; 17 (8): 861−870.

Silva AC, Rodrigues SC, Caldeira J, Nunes AM, Sampaio-Pinto V, Resende TP, Oliveira MJ, Barbosa MA, Thorsteinsdóttir S, Nascimento DS, Pinto-do-Ó P. Three-dimensional scaffolds of fetal decellularized hearts exhibit enhanced potential to support cardiac cells in comparison to the adult. *Biomaterials* 2016; 104 52−64.

Song JJ, Kim SS, Liu Z, Madsen JC, Mathisen DJ, Vacanti JP, Ott HC. Enhanced *In Vivo* Function of Bioartificial Lungs in Rats. *Ann. Thorac. Surg.* 2011; 92 (3): 998−1006.

Stabler CT, Caires LC, Mondrinos MJ, Marcinkiewicz C, Lazarovici P, Wolfson MR, Lelkes PI. Enhanced Re-Endothelialization of Decellularized Rat Lungs. *Tissue Eng. Part C: Methods.* 2016; 22 (5): 439−450.

Sullivan DC, Mirmalek-Sani S-H, Deegan DB, Baptista PM, Aboushwareb T, Atala A, Yoo JJ. Decellularization methods of porcine kidneys for whole organ engineering using a highthroughput system. *Biomaterials* 2012; 33 (31): 7756−7764.

Sun H, Calle E, Chen X, Mathur A, Zhu Y, Mendez J, Zhao L, Niklason L, Peng X, Peng H, Herzog EL. Fibroblast engraftment in the decellularized mouse lung occurs via a β1-integrin-dependent, FAK-dependent pathway that is mediated by ERK and opposed by AKT. *Am. J. Physiol. Lung Cell Mol. Physiol.* 2014; 306 (6): L463−L475.

Tsuchiya T, Mendez J, Calle EA, Hatachi G, Doi R, Zhao L, Suematsu T, Nagayasu T, Niklason LE. Ventilation-Based Decellularization System of the Lung. *Biores. Open Access.* 2016; 5 (1): 118−26.

Tsuchiya T, Mendez J, Calle EA, Hatachi G, Doi R, Zhao L, Suematsu T, Nagayasu T, Niklason LE. Ventilation-Based Decellularization System of the Lung. *Biores. Open Access.* 2016; 5 (1): 118−126.

Uygun BE, Izamis M-L, Jaramillo M, Chen Y, Price G, Ozer S, Yarmush ML. Discarded Livers Find a New Life: Engineered Liver Grafts Using Hepatocytes Recovered From Marginal Livers. *Artif. Organs.* 2016; n/a-n/a.

Uygun BE, Soto-Gutierrez A, Yagi H, Izamis M-L, Guzzardi MA, Shulman C, Milwid J, Kobayashi N, Tilles A, Berthiaume F, Hertl M, Nahmias Y, Yarmush ML, Uygun K. Organ reengineering through development of a transplantable recellularized liver graft using decellularized liver matrix. *Nature Med.* 2010; 16 (7): 814−820.

Uzarski JS, Bijonowski BM, Wang B, Ward HH, Wandinger-Ness A, Miller WM, Wertheim JA. Dual-Purpose Bioreactors to Monitor Noninvasive Physical and Biochemical Markers of Kidney and Liver Scaffold Recellularization. *Tissue Eng Part C: Methods.* 2015; 21 (10): 1032−1043.

Uzarski JS, Su J, Xie Y, Zhang ZJ, Ward HH, Wandinger-Ness A, Miller WM, Wertheim JA. Epithelial Cell Repopulation and Preparation of Rodent Extracellular Matrix Scaffolds for Renal Tissue Development. *J. Vis. Exp.* 2015; (102): e53271.

Vavken P, Joshi S, Murray MM. TRITON-X is most effective among three decellularization agents for ACL tissue engineering. *J. Orthop. Res.* 2009; 27 (12): 1612−8.

Vishwakarma SK, Bhavani PG, Bardia A, Abkari A, Murthy GS, Venkateshwarulu J, Khan AA. Preparation of natural three-dimensional goat kidney scaffold for the development of bioartificial organ. *Indian J. Nephrol.* 2014; 24 (6): 372−5.

Vossler JD, Ju YM, Williams JK, Goldstein S, Hamlin J, Lee SJ, Yoo JJ, Atala A. CD133 antibody conjugation to decellularized human heart valves intended for circulating cell capture. *Biomedical materials* 2015; 10 (5): 055001−055001.

Wainwright JM, Czajka CA, Patel UB, Freytes DO, Tobita K, Gilbert TW, Badylak SF. Preparation of Cardiac Extracellular Matrix from an Intact Porcine Heart. *Tissue Eng. Part C: Methods.* 2010; 16 (3): 525−532.

Wang Y, Bao J, Wu Q, Zhou Y, Li Y, Wu X, Shi Y, Li L, Bu H. Method for perfusion decellularization of porcine whole liver and kidney for use as a scaffold for clinical-scale bioengineering engrafts. *Xenotransplantation.* 2015; 22 (1): 48−61.

Wang Z, Wang Z, Yu Q, Xi H, Weng J, Du X, Chen D, Ma J, Mei J, Chen C. Comparative study of two perfusion routes with different flow in decellularization to harvest an optimal pulmonary scaffold for recellularization. *J. Biomed. Mater. Res. A.* 2016; 104 (10): 2567−2575.

Weymann A, Patil NP, Sabashnikov A, Jungebluth P, Korkmaz S, Li S, Veres G, Soos P, Ishtok R, Chaimow N, Pätzold I, Czerny N, Schies C, Schmack B, Popov AF, Simon AR, Karck M, Szabo G. Bioartificial Heart: A Human-Sized Porcine Model – The Way Ahead. *PLoS One* 2014; 9 (11): e111591.

Willenberg BJ, Oca-Cossio J, Cai Y, Brown AR, Clapp WL, Abrahamson DR, Terada N, Ellison GW, Mathews CE, Batich CD, Ross EA. Repurposed biological scaffolds: kidney to pancreas. *Organogenesis* 2015; 11 (2): 47−57.

Xu H, Xu B, Yang Q, Li X, Ma X, Xia Q, Zhang Y, Zhang C, Wu Y, Zhang Y. Comparison of decellularization protocols for preparing a decellularized porcine annulus fibrosus scaffold. *PLoS One* 2014; 9 (1): e86723.

Yam GH-F, Yusoff NZBM, Goh T-W, Setiawan M, Lee XW, Liu YC, Mehta JS. Decellularization of human stromal refractive lenticules for corneal tissue engineering. *Sci. Rep.* 2016; 6 26339.

Zhou P, Huang Y, Guo Y, Wang L, Ling C, Guo Q, Wang Y, Zhu S, Fan X, Zhu M, Huang H, Lu Y, Wang Z. Decellularization and Recellularization of Rat Livers With Hepatocytes and Endothelial Progenitor Cells. *Artif. Organs* 2016; 40 (3): E25−E38.

Zvarova B, Uhl FE, Uriarte JJ, Borg ZD, Coffey AL, Bonenfant NR, Weiss DJ, Wagner DE. Residual Detergent Detection Method for Nondestructive Cytocompatibility Evaluation of Decellularized Whole Lung Scaffolds. *Tissue Eng. Part C: Methods* 2016; 22 (5): 418−428.

In: Advances in Experimental Surgery. Volume 2
Editors: Huifang Chen and Paulo N. Martins
ISBN: 978-1-53612-773-7
© 2018 Nova Science Publishers, Inc.

Chapter 10

WOUND HEALING AND SCARRING

A. Samandar Dowlatshahi[*], *MD*
Plastic and Reconstructive Surgery,
Harvard Medical School, Boston, MA, US

ABSTRACT

Wounding is ubiquitous in clinical as well as experimental surgery. It is defined as any violation of tissue integrity in a live subject. The success of an experimental model in surgical research depends on control and predictability of the wounding as well as wound healing processes. Wounds typically are thought of in the context of skin wounds. In reality, even procedures deep within the torso, such as a model to study solid organ transplantation, rely on wound healing at every level: from the microvascular anastomosis, to the fascial layers that were obligatorily violated and to the skin at the site of the incision. In some circumstances, wound healing itself is the subject of study, such as in hernia or wound healing research. In experimental models, where it is not the subject matter in itself, any impaired tissue healing can contribute to morbidity and experiment failure. It is therefore critical for the surgical scientist to have a basic understanding of wound physiology and mechanisms of tissue regeneration and scarring, as well as animal-specific differences.

Keywords: wound healing, wound physiology, wounding, experimental wound models, surgical tissue handling, atraumatic technique, scarring, skin, tissue regeneration

ABBREVIATIONS

TF   Tissue Factor
ECM   Extracellular Matrix

---

[*] Corresponding author: A. Samandar Dowlatshahi, M.D., Plastic and Reconstructive Surgery, Harvard Medical School, Boston, MA161 S. Huntington Ave, #236, Jamaica Plain, MA 02130, drdowlat@gmail.com, Cell: +1 617 901 8131.

CD	Cluster of Differentiation
FGF	Fibroblast Growth Factor
VEGF	Vascular Endothelial Growth Factor
CCL	C-C Motif Chemokine Ligand
PDGF	Platelet Derived Growth Factor
IL	Interleukin
TGF	Transforming Growth Factor
MIP	Macrophage Infectivity Potentiator
MMP	Matrix Metalloproteinase
RNA	Ribonucleic Acid
DNA	Deoxyribonucleic Acid
siRNA	Small Interfering RNA
miRNA	Micro RNA

INTRODUCTION

From the beginning of recorded history, wound healing has been the subject of awe and fascination to healers, scientists, physicians, and even the layman in the form of "home remedies," throughout all cultures. The principles of primary and secondary intention healing were laid out by Galen in the first century A.D. Major advances occurred throughout the 19th and 20th centuries in particular with the advent of large-scale geopolitical conflicts, improving our understanding of the physiologic processes involved. The impetus underlying these advances was first and foremost the desire to save the lives of wounded warriors and civilian casualties, and decrease human suffering and physical morbidity.

Our advanced understanding of the physiologic processes involved has not only impacted clinical care but it also allowed for the development of more elaborate and sophisticated experimental models.

Every type of live tissue has, embedded within its genetic coding, mechanisms for tissue repair secondary to injury and wounding. Wounding does not only imply mechanical injury, but also includes tissue injury in a broader sense, such as chemical injury, radiation and reperfusion injury. It is critical to understand the difference between repair and regeneration. Regeneration refers to the reconstitution, or re-creation of the injured cells to result in an organ or tissue with its original integrity and architecture. It is a remarkable biochemical and physiologic pathway unique to select organs and animals and is the subject of regenerative medicine. Wound healing, on the other hand, leads to creation of repair tissue, which differs in varying degrees from the original tissue. In terms of skin, the resulting tissue is referred to as scar, which has a different cellular and extracellular composition as compared to native skin. In cartilage healing, the substrate is known as fibrocartilage. Virtually all types of human and animal tissue have a genetically programmed response to wounding.

Physiology of Wound Healing

Three Integrated Phases

Tissue wounding results in a series of physiologic processes that occur both consecutively and also simultaneously, traditionally defined as the phases of hemostasis and inflammation, proliferation, and remodeling (Childs 2017). They can also be referred to as the wound healing cascade, resulting in the formation of repair tissue, restoring the wounded organ's integrity and function.

Hemostasis and Inflammation

Immediately at wounding, the process of hemostasis begins. The key step which sets this process in motion is the exposure of blood components to the sub-endothelial layers of the vessel wall. This leads to vasoconstriction, as well as formation of a blood clot which in turn serves as a barrier against microbial invasion, at the same time minimizing blood loss. Our current understanding is that the blood clot is the epicenter that orchestrates wound chemotaxis, triggering the subsequent wound healing phases of inflammation and proliferation by attracting progenitor cells. It contains several growth factors and cytokines (Midwood 2004; Huntington 2005).

Hemostasis is initiated by the extrinsic pathway whereby Tissue Factor (TF) which is expressed by sub-endothelial tissues (vascular smooth muscle cells, pericytes and adventitial fibroblasts), comes in contact with circulating factor VII and creates the FVIIa-TF complex (Schecter 2000; Mackman 2007). This, activates FIX and FX. FXa and its cofactor FVa form the prothrombinase complex which leads to the activation of prothrombin to thrombin. The latter then converts the soluble plasma fibrinogen to fibrin which, in turn, is insoluble and leads to thrombocyte entrapment in the nascent clot. Thrombin also activates factors V and VIII, which both feed back into the cycle of factor X activation. Thrombin itself is also pro-inflammatory, leading to vasodilatation, edema, and a release of cytokines such as C-C Motif chemokine Ligand 2 (CCL2), Interleukin 8 (IL-8) and IL-6 (Levy 2016).

The role of fibrin in wound healing is substantial. It promotes stromal cell proliferation, binds to integrin CD11b/CD18 on monocytes and neutrophils, Fibroblast Growth Factor 2 (FGF-2) as well as Vascular Endothelial Growth Factor (VEGF) (Sahni 1998).

Degranulating platelets also release chemoattractants and growth factors such as Transforming Growth Factor β (TGF-β), Platelet Derived Growth Factor (PDGF), VEGF, CCL5, monocyte chemoattractant protein-1, CCL2, CCL3, Macrophage Inflammatory Protein 1α (MIP1α), TGF-α, C5a, C3a and nerve growth factor. (Maraganore 1993; Frank 2000).

Interferon-γ, IL-1β and TNF-α promote the transmigration of neutrophils across the capillary wall by means of adhesion and diapedesis. Current research indicates that macrophages within the wound require the guidance of neutrophils in the process of wound repair (Peters 2005). In the presence of infectious agents, as well as devitalized tissue, the neutrophil response appears to be enhanced. This is another reason why atraumatic technique is critical in controlling the amount of inflammation in the postoperative period; traumatic tissue handling can lead to tissue injury, necrosis, and inflammation.

Mast cells and macrophages also contribute to the inflammatory phase of wound healing. Once the monocyte leaves the blood vessel, it differentiates into a macrophage, now functioning as antigen presenting cell and phagocyte. It also secretes numerous growth factors such as TGF-β, TGF-α, PDGF, basic FGF (bFGF) and VEGF. Mast cells hereby modulate the inflammatory response and their influence extends throughout the entirety of the wound healing cascade. They have even been implicated in the pathogenesis of hypertrophic scarring as well as delayed healing (Noli 2001).

Proliferation

This phase has classically been described as taking place between two and 21 days post-injury. It overlaps with the inflammatory phase and begins with the gradual degradation of the blood clot which functions as a provisional matrix. During this phase, fibroblasts deposit extracellular matrix and proliferate. Within three to five days, they become the predominant cell type in the wound. They deposit collagen onto a fibronectin and glycosaminoglycan matrix resulting in scar tissue. In the skin, this collagen is initially histologically disorganized and is primarily of type III; it will eventually undergo remodeling and the ratio of type I to type III collagen reaches a ratio of 4:1, similar to native skin.

Granulation tissue refers to the beefy, dark red colored tissue which appears within days in open wounds. It consists of fibroblasts, macrophages, as well as sprouting blood vessels which explains its tendency to bleed, similar to a pyogenic granuloma. It is not only seen in cutaneous wounds. Even areas affected by chronic inflammation such as tendinitis, can often have an appearance and histopathologic similarity to granulation tissue.

In the case of skin healing, the proliferative phase is accompanied by epithelial resurfacing. This is clinically one of the most visible elements of wound healing and can be followed by visual inspection of the wound on a day-to-day basis. Within hours of injury, the keratinocytes at the margin of the wound undergo morphologic changes and migrate across the wound. Once the wound is resurfaced, a keratinocyte layering process takes place, increasing the thickness of the restored epidermal layer. This process is also visible when a thin skin graft thickens over time.

In conjunction with fibroblast and keratinocyte proliferation and migration of the latter, wound contraction can also contribute to wound closure. It is mediated by the presence of myofibroblasts, which are fibroblasts at the wound margin that differentiate into protomyofibroblasts and subsequently to myofibroblasts, when subjected to mechanical tension and PDGF. (Hermanns-Le 2015) The extent of wound contraction for non-cutaneous wounds remains to be determined. Interestingly, keratinocytes also appear to have a cytoskeleton allowing for contractility and may also contribute to skin wound contraction (Gniadecki 2001).

Remodeling

During this phase, the structural elements of the skin, and in particular the ECM, undergo changes. This is a balanced act of extracellular matrix (ECM) degradation and synthesis, partly modulated by matrix metalloproteinases (MMP). Collagen cross-linking also takes place, increasing wound tensile strength. Lysyl oxidase is the primary cross-linking enzyme.

(Kobayashi 1994) This phase of healing lasts at least one year and results in a mature scar. The initial erythema associated with ongoing inflammation and scar maturation eventually resolves and corresponds to regression of the dense capillary network.

Despite this length of time, the end-result of wound healing consists of repair tissue, and is different from unwounded skin. Its tensile strength can only reach a maximum of 80% of unwounded skin and the orientation and organization of sub-epithelial collagen is dissimilar to the reticular pattern in native dermis. In fetal wound healing on the other hand, the end-result is scarless tissue regeneration, with a restoration of normal epidermal and dermal architecture. (Beanes 2002, Buchanan 2009) It was once thought that scarless skin healing was associated with factors present in the amniotic fluid, but this hypothesis has been refuted (Buchanan 2009).

MODIFYING FACTORS IN WOUND HEALING

Colonization and Infection

Colonized wounds show no immune response, in contrast with infected tissue. Infection, in contrast to colonization, indicates that a threshold number of bacteria are present in the wound and have overcome host resistance, leading to slowing down fibroblast proliferation and ECM synthesis. Bacterial loads greater than 10^5 organisms per gram of tissue is the historically accepted threshold. (Robson 1990) In our clinical experience, however, this number is no longer of absolute relevance. Depending on the vascularity of the wound bed, the presence of ionizing radiation, level of oxygenation as well as tissue edema, the state of the immune system and the anatomical location, varying degrees of bacterial burden are tolerated and may or may not lead to an overwhelming immune response as seen in infected wounds. In consequence, the clinical presentation of an infected wound can vary, traditionally described as the presence of pus with associated tissue inflammation (tumor, calor, rubor, functio laesa), and be as subtle as increased drainage, or discolored appearing granulation tissue with increased friability. The virulence of the offending organism is another variable which is difficult to quantify.

The mechanisms by which bacteria affect the wound microenvironment are multiple. The organism's attempt at neutralizing the offending agent leads to release of proinflammatory cytokines, leading to inflammation and pain. Pain in itself has been shown to delay the immune response. (White 2009) Biofilm represents an accumulation of microorganisms within a matrix of extracellular material and has prompted interest in recent years because of its ability to shield itself from this host inflammatory response (Nouvong 2016).

Vascularization: Angiogenesis and Vasculogenesis

Wound healing requires blood supply, enabling tissue oxygenation, delivery of nutrients, and removal of waste products. Small wounds can heal by means of diffusion, as seen in the initial stages of free skin graft healing. Larger wounds require neovascularization. This process is divided into vasculogenesis and angiogenesis. The former refers to the formation of new blood vessels from marrow-derived stem cells, the latter is described as the sprouting of capillaries from already present blood vessels at the wound margins. In reality, these processes overlap. Their regulation is sophisticated and is primarily driven by proangiogenetic factors and cytokines originating from platelets, macrophages, leucocytes as well as local circumstances such as hypoxia. It is important to note that most of these key players are located within the hemostatic plug that eventually undergoes ECM and cellular changes during the proliferative and remodeling phases of healing.

Platelets induce migration of endothelial cells to the wound site. Macrophages secrete TGF-β, TGF-α, PDGF, bFGF and VEGF which drive angiogenesis. (Okizaki 2016) VEGF-A and IL-8 are proangiogenetic factors which originate from leucocytes. (Labler 2009) The VEGF mechanism of action consists of ligation with endothelial tyrosine kinase receptors, in particular VEGFR-2 and VEGFR-3. Many of the endothelial signal transmission pathways in vascularization involve tyrosine kinase receptors. The endothelial cell receptors Tie-1 and Tie-2, and VEGFR are the only known endothelial tyrosine kinases (Singh 2009; Savant 2015).

Once activated, endothelial cells proliferate and migrate. The ECM also contributes to this process of vascularization. (Sottile 2004) A significant element of the ECM, the basement membrane, is required in order to stabilize the tubular configuration of endothelial cell clusters. In addition to a structural and stabilizing role, the vessel basement membrane induces polarization of the endothelial cells.

The Role of Ischemia and Tissue Oxygenation

Ischemia and hypoxia designate different processes. Ischemia relates to hypoperfusion. Hypoxia will often be present in hypoperfused, ischemic tissues, but itself is defined by a lack of oxygen supply relative to oxygen demand. In consequence, tissue hypoxia can be induced by either increasing tissue oxygen demand (e.g., wound healing, wound infection with oxygen consumption to create reactive oxygen species such as oxygen free radicals), decreasing arterial oxygen supply (e.g., pulmonary fibrosis, anemia inefficient cardiac circulation, altitude), or increasing the resistance to oxygen diffusion (e.g., tissue fibrosis, radiation, edema). Tissue hypoxia will amplify angiogenetic pathways which, in turn, are linked into all three phases of wound healing. This has several implications for experimental surgery. One must keep in mind that within a wound, there may be local pockets of extreme hypoxia leading to focal apoptotic cell nests with a significantly different micro-environment and resulting cell behavior.

The Role of Micro RNA

In order to go from protein-coding gene to protein, the deoxyribonucleic acid (DNA) is transcribed to messenger ribonucleic acid (RNA), which is translated to protein. Micro RNAs (miRNAs) are 19–22 nucleotides long and are noncoding RNA which, in conjunction with small interfering RNAs (siRNAs) modulate both transcription and translation. 1048 miRNAs are encoded in the human genome. The role of miRNAs in wound healing is established, but poorly understood (Shilo 2007).

Endothelial cell capillary sprouting for instance can be inhibited by knockdown of the miRNAs Dicer and Drosha. (Kuehbacher 2007; Kuehbacher 2008) On the other hand, there exist antiangiogenic miRNAs such as miR-92a, miR-17, and miR-320, just to name a few.

Other proangiogenic miRNAs are miR-17-92, miR-126, miR-130a, miR-210, miR-296 and miR378 (Banerjee 2011).

miRNAs also play a role in the proliferative phase of wound healing (miR-184, miR-205, miR-210) as well as the inflammatory phase (miR-105 targets TLR2, miR-140 targets the PDGF receptor, miR-146a and miR-125b target TNF-α) (Banerjee 2011).

The purpose here is not to provide an exhaustive list, but to demonstrate that known chemokines have now been shown to have another layer of regulatory factors as seen in the miRNAs which adds another level of fine-control and complexity. It also offers a potential therapeutic strategy; modulating a group of functionally related genes in a pathway by targeting a single miRNA, as opposed to targeting a single gene at a time, as in conventional gene therapy.

In wound healing research, the most fascinating phenomenon is scarless wound healing as observed in mammalian fetal skin. (Beanes 2002) miRNA may explain some of these findings, as a number of these (miRNA-29b, miRNA-29c, miRNA-192) have been found to be differentially induced during different phases of gestation and may play a role in scarless cutaneous healing (Cheng 2010).

PRACTICAL IMPLICATIONS FOR EXPERIMENTAL SURGERY

Animal Models for Wound Healing

Role and Limitations of in Vitro Models
In vitro studies allow to study the effect of agents on specific cell types in a controlled environment. In particular, the presence or absence of confounding cell lines and chemokines can be controlled for, which is of particular interest in wound healing research because of the numerous cell-to-cell and cell-to-ECM interactions involved. They are however unable to completely reproduce biological conditions relevant to clinical wound healing. Furthermore, unlike many other physiologic processes, wound healing always involves biomechanical factors such as wound contraction as well as periodic changes in repair-tissue tensile strength that cannot be studied in an *ex vivo* construct, or even by computerized simulation. The animal study is therefore the logical next step. It should be noted that that the number of articles in Pubmed pertaining to animal wound healing models has exponentially increased since 1980.

Small Mammal Wound Healing Models

Rodents and small mammals find widespread use in wound healing models. They are inexpensive and require minimal space, food and water. They also exhibit accelerated wound healing as compared to humans, which shortens the duration of experiments. Small mammal anesthesia is relatively facile, and inexpensive. Due to their size, facilities with limited space are not an issue and animal transportation is easily accomplished, especially in studies with larger numbers. Wound healing experiments are typically carried out on the back of the animal, where partial and full thickness wounding can be reproducibly accomplished. Lastly, the availability of numerous knock out rodents allows the animal model to be more refined and specific to the needs of the study in question.

Limitations include the difficulty in securing dressings, wound care, a different hair growth cycle as compared with humans, the extremely thin skin (50 μm) and the presence of the subcutaneous panniculus carnosus muscle which aids in wound contraction. (Davidson 1998; Wong 2011). Furthermore, certain studies requiring larger numbers can be successfully accomplished with fewer animals of larger size. Murine models have been preferentially used for burn research but it has been shown that they have a physiologic response to injury that is dissimilar to what is seen in humans. (Seok 2013) Lastly, mice can only tolerate 30% Total Body Surface Area Burns, which in humans will only begin to induce a systemic inflammatory response (Pereira 2005).

Porcine Wound Healing Models

Of all animals, porcine skin is structurally as well as histologically the most similar to humans. (Lindblad 2008) Porcine collagen, cutaneous blood supply and follicular hair structure is similar to humans, as well as a similar physiologic response to wounding. The skin turnover time is 30 days, similar to human epidermis. The greatest downside is the cost compared to smaller animals, in terms of animal acquisition, as well as feeding, space requirement, dedicated vivarium and more complex anesthesia monitoring modalities. Miniature breeds are now available, weighing 12–45 kg as compared to the >100 kg domestic pig.

On the other hand, the swine model is much more convenient to use: partial thickness defects can be easily created using dermatomes or hydrodissection (salt split technique), ischemic wound models are easier to achieve by elevation of a skin flap and interposition of a barrier. Serial wound biopsies are easier to obtain because of the larger size and surface area. The thickness and architecture of the subcutaneous fat is also more similar to humans, whereas in a rodent model, a full thickness skin wound can often extend straight to muscle fascia. Lastly, wound healing is greatly dependent on wound hygiene as well as dressings utilized in wound care. Poorly applied dressings lead to contamination, shear, desiccation or maceration, and can affect the study outcome. Wound care is greatly facilitated in larger animal models.

With the increasing incidence of diabetes and diabetic wounds, studying the altered wound healing in the setting of diabetes is of particular interest. Streptozotocin can be utilized to induce a diabetic state in swine. (Sheets 2016) Hypertrophic scar models can be studied using Red Duroc pigs (Zhu 2003; Gallant 2004; Zhu 2004). Chronic, non-ischemic wounds can be created by irradiation and wounding. (Bernatchez 1998) Infected wound models are created by using different pathogens, most commonly Staph Aureus (Breuing 2003; Hirsch 2008).

Tissue Handling and Atraumatic Technique

As experimental models increase in complexity, it becomes more important to pay attention to adequate tissue handling, as this correlates directly with the ability of the tissues to heal. This is relevant for skin wound healing research, but also when the abdominal cavity or chest wall is entered and procedures on internal organs carried out. For microsurgeons this is obvious, as they have seen a vessel readily thrombose following a poorly placed stitch or aggressive grasping of the vessel wall during microvascular anastomosis. Meticulous technique is required when handling other tissues as well, and will determine outcome.

Instruments and Tissue Handling

All too often, instruments of poor quality, or even damaged instruments are made available to the experimental surgeon. Not only does this violate the core ethical values pertaining to animal research, in which animals are to be treated as living beings and respected as one would respect a human being (poor instruments are never acceptable in clinical surgery), but also, due to the more difficult circumstances in a laboratory, as well as smaller size of the anatomical structures, it becomes even more important to use clean and precisely engineered instruments that are in good shape.

Grasping instruments such as forceps and retractors should be utilized only when necessary, and for the shortest time possible. The most atraumatic instrument used for retraction is a sharp hook or double hook. Crushing of tissues must be prevented at all cost, as it will lead to obligatory tissue ischemia and injury. Therefore, when using forceps, preference is usually given to toothed forceps, except when handling nerves and blood vessels. Here, every effort is made to not grab the structure itself, but to use the vessel adventitia or the epineurium as a handle. Aggressive tissue handling will lead to perineurial scar formation, vessel thrombosis, skin injury and resulting wound dehiscence or delayed healing. In tendon surgery, careful handling will prevent adhesion formation and possibly failure of the experiment. Brutalization of bowel loops leads to bowel adhesions and possible serosal injury.

Bleeding and Hemostasis

The use of cautery and other hemostatic agents is fortunately less common today in the animal operating theatre than in the clinical setting where the monopolar electrocautery appears to be the only instrument able to cut tissue. The degree of thermal trauma caused by cautery has been well documented, and linked to poor wound healing, as well as adjacent organ injury. Most tissues will stop bleeding spontaneously or with gentle pressure. Visible vessels should be precisely cauterized or ligated. Thermal methods of cautery include the monopolar, bipolar and the handheld battery-powered cautery. The latter is the least traumatic and can be used as precisely as a knife. The only downside is the limited battery life. Surgifoam has been found to be very useful immediately post-anastomosis in microsurgical cases where it can be applied in a thinly cut sheet to cease bleeding from the anastomotic suture line.

Dissection and Desiccation

The most atraumatic dissection is carried out sharply with scissors or knife. The scalpel blade is the cheapest instrument in the operating room and fresh blades should therefore be used liberally. Atraumatic dissection is a largely acquired skill but obeys a few guiding principles. Tissue planes are always present and should be followed when possible. This allows for a rapid and precise dissection, following the naturally present tissue planes. When this plane is entered, it opens up and can be easily followed with good traction and counter-traction. Blood staining makes the identification of tissues more difficult and must be prevented. Blunt dissection can be considered an atraumatic technique when following the tissue planes. However, uncoordinated and aggressive spreading with scissors or a vascular clamp is usually indicative of lack of anatomical knowledge on the part of the surgeon, and leads to more bleeding and crush-avulsive tissue trauma.

Tissue desiccation must be prevented at all cost. Dry tissue is dead tissue. The operating room lights expedite this process because they act as a heat source. Lengthy procedures are at higher risk for tissue desiccation. Certain tissues such as tendon, nerves, blood vessels and bone are also at higher risk. The paratenon dries within seconds of air exposure. It is critical to moisten the tissues intermittently. The more practical solution for lengthy cases is the placement of saline-moistened sponges onto the tissues. This cannot be overemphasized.

Skin Closure

In animal surgery, skin closure is as important as it is in clinical surgery. If the skin edges are not precisely aligned at the end of the procedure, delayed wound healing can occur, with the high likelihood of wound separation, colonization and infection. Wound margin eversion will ensure uninterrupted healing and can be simply achieved with careful technique.

Planning

A well-conceived operation will ensure ease of execution. This pertains to all aspects of the procedure, including good lighting (which is often lacking), and operating theatre ergonomics (surgeon fatigue is directly correlated with the quality of the work delivered). Probably the most important point is not to compromise with any of the steps of the operation. When one compromises with the lighting for instance, then one compromises with a dull blade, poor instruments, uncomfortable posture, one thing after the next leading to fatigue, frustration and failure. Furthermore, in animal studies, often the same procedure is performed a number of times in repetition. Meticulous and standardized technique will provide reproducible and more consistent data.

CONCLUSION

Wound healing is a necessary prerequisite in all experimental surgery, whether or not it is wound healing itself that is being studied. Wound healing is broken down into various phases but in reality they overlap: hemostasis, inflammation, proliferation and remodeling. Each phase is characterized by up and down regulation of specific processes, in turn driven by chemokines that originate both from the repair tissue itself as well as the adjacent wound bed. Vascularization and oxygenation are rate-limiting factors which are at the core of all wound healing. Despite certain advantages of small mammalian animal models, the swine model is best suited for wound healing *in vivo* studies, albeit at higher cost and logistical effort.

Atraumatic tissue handling will ensure minimal tissue injury and uninterrupted healing in all experimental surgery procedures.

REFERENCES

Banerjee J, Chan YC, and Sen CK. MicroRNAs in skin and wound healing. *Physiol. Genomics* 2011; 43(10): 543−556.

Beanes SR, Hu FY, Soo C, Dang CM, Urata M, Ting K, Atkinson JB, Benhaim P, Hedrick MH, and Lorenz HP. Confocal microscopic analysis of scarless repair in the fetal rat: defining the transition. *Plast. Reconstr. Surg.* 2002; 109(1): 160−170.

Bernatchez SF, Parks PJ, Grussing DM, S. L. Matalas SL, and Nelson GS. Histological characterization of a delayed wound healing model in pig. *Wound Repair Regen.* 1998; 6(3): 223−233.

Breuing K, Kaplan S, Liu P, Onderdonk AB, and Eriksson E. Wound fluid bacterial levels exceed tissue bacterial counts in controlled porcine partial−thickness burn infections. *Plast. Reconstr. Surg.* 2003; 111(2): 781−788.

Buchanan EP, Longaker MT and Lorenz HP. Fetal skin wound healing. *Adv. Clin. Chem.* 2009; 48: 137−161.

Cheng J, Yu H, Deng S, and Shen G. MicroRNA profiling in mid- and late-gestational fetal skin: implication for scarless wound healing. *Tohoku. J. Exp. Med.* 2010; 221(3): 203−209.

Childs DR, and Murthy AS. Overview of Wound Healing and Management. *Surg. Clin. North Am.* 2017; 97(1): 189−207.

Davidson JM. Animal models for wound repair. *Arch. Dermatol. Res.* 1998; 290 Suppl: S1−11.

Frank S, Kampfer H, Wetzler C, Stallmeyer B, and Pfeilschifter J. Large induction of the chemotactic cytokine RANTES during cutaneous wound repair: a regulatory role for nitric oxide in keratinocyte-derived RANTES expression. *Biochem. J.* 2000, 347 Pt 1: 265−273.

Gallant CL, Olson ME, and Hart DA. Molecular, histologic, and gross phenotype of skin wound healing in red Duroc pigs reveals an abnormal healing phenotype of hypercontracted, hyperpigmented scarring. *Wound Repair Regen.* 2004; 12(3): 305−319.

Gniadecki R, Olszewska H, and Gajkowska B. Changes in the ultrastructure of cytoskeleton and nuclear matrix during HaCaT keratinocyte differentiation. *Exp. Dermatol.* 2001; 10(2): 71−79.

Hermanns−Le, T, Pierard GE, Jennes S, and Pierard−Franchimont C. Protomyofibroblast Pathway in Early Thermal Burn Healing. *Skin Pharmacol. Physiol.* 2015; 28(5): 250−254.

Hirsch T, Spielmann M, Zuhaili B, Koehler T, Fossum M, Steinau HU, Yao F, Steinstraesser L, Onderdonk AB, and Eriksson E. Enhanced susceptibility to infections in a diabetic wound healing model. *BMC Surg.* 2008; 8: 5.

Huntington J, Molecular A. recognition mechanisms of thrombin. *J. Thromb. Haemost.* 2005; 3(8): 1861−1872.

Kobayashi H, Ishii M, Chanoki M, Yashiro N, Fushida H, Fukai K, Kono T, Hamada T, Wakasaki H, and Ooshima A. Immunohistochemical localization of lysyl oxidase in normal human skin. *Br. J. Dermatol.* 1994; 131(3): 325−330.

Kuehbacher A, Urbich C, and Dimmeler S. Targeting microRNA expression to regulate angiogenesis. *Trends. Pharmacol. Sci.* 2008; 29(1): 12−15.

Kuehbacher A, Urbich C, Zeiher AM, and Dimmeler S. Role of Dicer and Drosha for endothelial microRNA expression and angiogenesis. *Circ. Res.* 2007; 101(1): 59−68.

Labler L, Rancan M, Mic L, Harter L, Mihic-Probst D, and Keel M. Vacuum−assisted closure therapy increases local interleukin-8 and vascular endothelial growth factor levels in traumatic wounds. *J. Trauma.* 2009; 66(3): 749−757.

Levy JH, Sniecinski RM, Welsby IJ, and Levi M. Antithrombin: anti-inflammatory properties and clinical applications. *Thromb.* 2016; 115(4): 712−728.

Lindblad WJ. Considerations for selecting the correct animal model for dermal wound-healing studies. *J. Biomater. Sci. Polym. Ed.* 2008; 19(8): 1087−1096.

Mackman N, Tilley RE, and Key NS. Role of the extrinsic pathway of blood coagulation in hemostasis and thrombosis. *Arterioscler. Thromb. Vasc. Biol.* 2007; 27(8): 1687−1693.

Maraganore JM. Thrombin, thrombin inhibitors, and the arterial thrombotic process. *Thromb. Haemost.* 1993; 70(1): 208−211.

Midwood KS, Williams LV, and Schwarzbauer JE. Tissue repair and the dynamics of the extracellular matrix. *Int. J. Biochem. Cell Biol.* 2004; 36(6): 1031−1037.

Noli C, and Miolo A. The mast cell in wound healing. *Vet. Dermatol.* 2001; 12(6): 303−313.

Nouvong A, Ambrus AM, Zhang FR, L. Hultman L, and Coller HA. Reactive oxygen species and bacterial biofilms in diabetic wound healing. Physiol Genomics: *physiol. Genomics* 00066 02016. 2016; 48: 889−896.

Okizaki S, Ito Y, Hosono K, Oba K, Ohkubo H, Kojo K, Nishizawa N, Shibuya M, Shichiri M, and Majima M. Vascular Endothelial Growth Factor Receptor Type 1 Signaling Prevents Delayed Wound Healing in Diabetes by Attenuating the Production of IL-1beta by Recruited Macrophages. *Am. J. Pathol.* 2016; 186(6): 1481−1498.

Pereira CT, and Herndon DN. The pharmacologic modulation of the hypermetabolic response to burns. *Adv. Surg.* 2005; 39: 245−261.

Peters T, Sindrilaru A, Hinz B, Hinrichs R, Menke A, Al-Azzeh EA, Holzwarth K, Oreshkova T, Wang H, Kess D, Walzog B, Sulyok S, Sunderkotter C, Friedrich W, Wlaschek M, Krieg T, and Scharffetter-Kochanek K. Wound-healing defect of CD18(-/-) mice due to a decrease in TGF-beta1 and myofibroblast differentiation. *EMBO J.* 2005; 24(19): 3400−3410.

Robson MC, Stenberg BD, and Heggers JP. Wound healing alterations caused by infection. *Clin. Plast. Surg.* 1990; 17(3): 485−492.

Sahni A, Odrljin T, and Francis CW. Binding of basic fibroblast growth factor to fibrinogen and fibrin. *J. Biol. Chem.* 1998; 273(13): 7554−7559.

Savant S, La Porta S, Budnik A, Busch K, Hu J, Tisch N, Korn C, Valls AF, Benest AV, Terhardt D, Qu X, Adams RH, Baldwin HS, Ruiz de Almodovar C, Rodewald HR, and Augustin HG. The Orphan Receptor Tie1 Controls Angiogenesis and Vascular Remodeling by Differentially Regulating Tie2 in Tip and Stalk Cells. *Cell. Rep.* 2015; 12(11): 1761−1773.

Schecter AD, Spirn B, Rossikhina M, Giesen PL, Bogdanov V, Fallon JT, Fisher EA, Schnapp LM, Y. Nemerson Y, and Taubman MB. Release of active tissue factor by human arterial smooth muscle cells. *Circ. Res.* 2000; 87(2): 126−132.

Seok J, Warren HS, Cuenca AG, Mindrinos MN, Baker HV, Xu W, Richards DR, McDonald-Smith GP, Gao H, Hennessy L, Finnerty CC, Lopez CM, Honari S, Moore EE, Minei JP, Cuschieri J, Bankey PE, Johnson JL, Sperry J, Nathens AB, Billiar TR, West MA, Jeschke MG, Klein MB, Gamelli RL, Gibran NS, Brownstein BH, Miller-Graziano C, Calvano SE,

Mason PH, Cobb JP, Rahme LG, Lowry SF, Maier RV, Moldawer LL, Herndon DN, Davis RW, Xiao W, Tompkins RG. Inflammation and L. S. C. R. P. Host Response to Injury. Genomic responses in mouse models poorly mimic human inflammatory diseases. *Proc. Natl. Acad. Sci. USA* 2013; 110(9): 3507–3512.

Sheets AR, Massey CJ, Cronk SM, Iafrati MD, and Herman IM. Matrix- and plasma-derived peptides promote tissue-specific injury responses and wound healing in diabetic swine. *J. Transl. Med.* 2016; 14(1): 197.

Shilo S, Roy S, Khanna S, and Sen CK. MicroRNA in cutaneous wound healing: a new paradigm. *DNA Cell Biol.* 2007; 26(4): 227–237.

Singh HCS, Milner CS, Aguilar MM, Hernandez NP, and Brindle NP. Vascular endothelial growth factor activates the Tie family of receptor tyrosine kinases. *Cell Signal.* 2009; 21(8): 1346–1350.

Sottile J. Regulation of angiogenesis by extracellular matrix. *Biochim. Biophys. Acta.* 2004; 1654(1): 13–22.

White RJ. Wound infection-associated pain. *J. Wound Care* 2009; 18(6): 245–249.

Wong VW, Sorkin M, Glotzbach JP, Longaker MT, and Gurtner GC. Surgical approaches to create murine models of human wound healing. *J. Biomed. Biotechnol.* 2011: 969618.

Zhu KQ, Engrav LH, Gibran NS, Cole JK, Matsumura H, Piepkorn M, Isik FF, Carrougher GJ, Muangman PM, Yunusov MY, and Yang TM. The female, red Duroc pig as an animal model of hypertrophic scarring and the potential role of the cones of skin. *Burns* 2003; 29(7): 649–664.

Zhu KQ, Engrav LH, Tamura RN, Cole JA, Muangman P, Carrougher GJ, and Gibran NS. Further similarities between cutaneous scarring in the female, red Duroc pig and human hypertrophic scarring. *Burns* 2004; 30(6): 518–530.

In: Advances in Experimental Surgery. Volume 2
Editors: Huifang Chen and Paulo N. Martins
ISBN: 978-1-53612-773-7
© 2018 Nova Science Publishers, Inc.

Chapter 11

ORGAN PRESERVATION

Cheng Yang[1], MD, PhD, Jiawei Li[1], MD and Ruiming Rong[1,2,], MD, PhD*

[1]Department of Urology, Zhongshan Hospital, Fudan University,
Shanghai Key Laboratory of Organ Transplantation; Shanghai, China
[2]Department of Transfusion, Zhongshan Hospital,
Fudan University, Shanghai, China

ABSTRACT

Organ transplantation has become a preferred clinical therapy for end-stage organ disease. Since the first kidney transplant was successfully performed in 1954, organ transplantation developed rapidly and more methods for transplantation have quickly emerged. Therefore, based on this background, the method with which to preserve organs for a long time and the ideal method for organ preservation could become meaningful problems that require discussion by specialists and doctors. In this chapter, we discuss the addition of materials in preservation solutions, list the main preservation solutions, and describe gene therapy in organ preservation and clinical trials. Some classic preservation solutions are still used in clinical works, such as University of Wisconsin solution and Histidine-tryptophan-ketoglutarate solution; however, others are mainly based on these classic solutions with the addition of some materials. Recent studies have found that new materials such as gas molecules added into a solution can provide better protection for organ preservation, and we are glad to see more studies about how to better preserve donor organs even while machine preservation appears to be most prominent.

Keywords: organ preservation, kidney transplantation, liver transplantation, heart transplantation, lung transplantation, pancreatic transplantation, RNA Interference

---

[*] Corresponding Author: Professor Ruiming Rong, Department of Urology, Zhongshan Hospital, Fudan University; Shanghai Key Laboratory of Organ Transplantation, Department of Transfusion, Zhongshan Hospital, Fudan University, 180 Fenglin Road, Shanghai, 200032, China. Tel.: +86-21-64041990, Fax: +86-21-64037269, E-mail: rong.ruiming@zs-hospital.sh.cn.

ABBREVIATIONS

ROS	reactive oxygen species
UW solution	University of Wisconsin solution
HTK	Histidine-tryptophan-ketoglutarate
IGL-1	Institute George-Lopez
EC	Euro-Collins
HOC	Hypertonic citrate
PBS	Phosphate-buffered sucrose
BNP-1	bovine neutrophil peptide-1
SP	substance P
NGF	nerve growth factor
EGF	epidermal growth factor
IGF-1	insulin-like growth factor-1
DGF	delayed graft function
siRNA	small interfering RNA
PEG	polyethylene glycol
CO-RMs	carbon monoxide release molecules
MDA	malondialdehyde
HES	hydroxy-ethyl starch
SCOT	Solution de conservation des organes et des tissus
SMO	Shanghai multi-organ preservation
HC-A	hyperosmolar citrate adenine
PGD	primary graft dysfunction
LPD	low-potassium dextran
PRRs	pattern recognition receptors
RIG1	retinoic acid inducible gene 1
PKR	protein kinase.

INTRODUCTION

With the development of organ transplantation, solid organ preservation has become a significant focus in the transplantation field. Considerable attention is given to the *ex vivo* period as this segment represents a vulnerable timeframe whereby organs are susceptible to ongoing cellular damage that is further compounded by reperfusion injury upon re-anastomosis (Korte 2016). In the late 1960s, two important studies demonstrated that kidneys could be safely preserved for 30 hours by cold storage and for as long as 72 hours by continuous perfusion. With this evidence, some experts considered hypothermia, which can be utilized to decrease the metabolic activity of donor organs during the *ex vivo* period. However, hypothermia is unable to abolish all cellular damage, as metabolism persists at approximately 5–10% of normal levels. In addition, hypothermia can lead to Na^+/K^+-ATPase alterations, ATP depletion, the dysregulation of Ca^{2+} homeostasis, mitochondrial perturbations, xanthine oxidase accumulation, and increased levels of reactive oxygen species (ROS), which may have deleterious effects on cellular viability. Therefore, preservation solutions have been implemented in conjunction with hypothermia for additional cellular protection. In 1988, Belzer et al. presented the opinions that proper solid organ storage solution should obey the following principles: (1) minimize hypothermic-induced cell swelling; (2) prevent intracellular acidosis; (3) prevent the expansion of the interstitial space during the flush-out period; (4) prevent injury from oxygen-free radicals (especially during reperfusion); and (5) provide substrates for regenerating high-energy phosphate compounds during reperfusion (Belzer and Southard 1988). According to these principles, numerous solutions are commercially available while others remain institutionally derived.

1. HISTORY OF PRESERVATION SOLUTIONS

Kidney transplantation remains limited by four problems: (1) a high rate of delayed graft function; (2) early loss of kidneys from chronic rejection; (3) donor kidney shortages; and (4) the need for immunomodulation treatments. However, improved cold storage methods can significantly impact the first 3 of these 4 major problems, so the development of new types of organ preservation solutions can be a new strategy for organ transplantation. After the introduction of static Collins solution by Collins in 1969, prolonged kidney preservation became feasible. Currently, the principle solutions for kidney preservation are University of Wisconsin (UW) solution, Histidine-tryptophan-ketoglutarate (HTK) solution, Celsior solution, Institute George-Lopez (IGL-1) solution, Polysol solution, Euro-Collins solution, hypertonic citrate (HOC) or Marshall solution, and Phosphate-buffered sucrose (PBS). Considering their electrolyte composition, these solutions are divided into intracellular-type and extracellular-type. Intracellular solutions are characterized by high potassium and low sodium concentrations, which is necessary to prevent cell swelling. Because the Na^+/K^+-ATPase is inactive during cold storage, a solution in the extracellular space with a Na^+/K^+ balance equal to the intracellular compartment reaches Donnan equilibrium, preventing sodium and chloride from entering the cell. Intracellular-type solutions such as UW are considered important to preserve cell viability. The extracellular-type of solution, such HTK, has low potassium and high sodium concentrations. Recent studies have suggested that this composition is equal to, or even better than, the intracellular type, as potassium can induce vasospasm.

2. THE IMPROVEMENT OF PRESERVATION SOLUTIONS BY ADDING MATERIALS

Growth Factors

Growth factors are cytokines that can stimulate cell growth. MeAnuhy et al. found that when a variety of growth factors were mixed into the UW solution, such as an antimicrobial peptide (bovine neutrophil peptide-1, BNP-1, also referred to as bactenecin), a neuropeptide (substance P, SP), a neurotrophin (nerve growth factor, NGF), and two polypeptide growth factors (epidermal growth factor (EGF) and insulin-like growth factor-1, IGF-1), dog kidneys were successfully preserved for 6 days. The serum creatinine level was lower in the normal UW solution group than in the normal group 3 days after storage for 4 days, and the canine kidney function for 6 days was the same as that of the normal group (McAnulty 2002). Another animal experiment showed that the addition of growth factor and FR167653 (a P38 mitogen-activated protein kinase inhibitor) to the UW solution significantly improved the preservation of a pig kidney, reduced ischemia-reperfusion injury, and reduced the incidence of long-term renal fibrosis and infection (Desurmont 2011). These studies suggest that the addition of growth factors to the organ preservation solution can improve the effect of simple cryopreservation of organs; further research is needed to explore potential applications.

Trimetazidine

Trimetazidine can enhance myocardial oxygen supplementation, maintain mitochondrial function and reduce vascular resistance and is mainly used in the clinical treatment of angina. In a study of acute coronary ischemia, trimetazidine was shown to protect mitochondrial structures and improve mitochondrial function via enhanced oxidative phosphorylation and a reduction in the production of reactive oxygen species. Faure et al. evaluated the mitochondrial protective effects of trimetazidine added to UW liquid and Celsior solution and showed that pig kidneys were saved at low temperature for more than 72 hours (Faure 2003). Belous et al. also found that hypothermia, especially combined with an elevated extracellular calcium concentration, would significantly increase mitochondrial calcium intake, and the increased calcium concentration would eventually lead to the irreversible damage of mitochondrial structure and function (Belous 2003). Mitochondrial damage is closely related to acute rejection, which is induced by ischemia reperfusion and could cause delayed graft function (DGF) and chronic graft rejection. Thus, the protective effect of trimetazidine in reducing mitochondrial damage might be the main mechanism by which ischemia reperfusion injuries are decreased. However, some studies found opposite results, suggesting that the role of trimetazidine in reducing ischemia reperfusion injury is not obvious (Abreu Lde 2011). Therefore, the use of trimetazidine in organ preservation solution still needs further study.

Thrombin Inhibitors

Recently, studies have shown that adding Melagatran, a type of thrombin inhibitor, to the UW solution can improve the recovery of renal function after ischemia reperfusion in porcine kidneys. Compared with the control group, the survival rate of the experimental group was significantly improved at 7 days after the operation, and kidney damage and the inflammatory response were significantly reduced (Giraud 2009). Moreover, the addition of a thrombin inhibitor to the preservation solution can prevent the occurrence of chronic diseases such as renal interstitial fibrosis, tubular atrophy and infection.

Small Interfering RNA (siRNA)

RNA interference is a way to down-regulate specific proteins by limiting gene expression and siRNA is one of the common tools. It has been demonstrated that cysteine-aspartate 3 (caspase-3) siRNA can be directly added to HOC solution for the preservation of porcine kidney, which can reduce the level of caspase-3 and cell death, improve kidney oxygenation and acid-base balance, thereby reducing ischemia-reperfusion injury (Yang 2011; Hosgood 2011; Nicholson 2011). The main challenge of applying siRNA to preservation solution is its safety, which includes the choice of vector, ectopic expression of the transgene, and the adverse effects of gene expression.

Polyethylene Glycol

Polyethylene glycol (PEG) was able to reduce the hypoxic ischemic injury of renal tubular cells. Hauet et al. added 30 g/L polyethylene glycol (20000 U) to UW solution and high sodium UW solution and found that the renal tubules in the PEG group were significantly smaller than renal tubules that had been maintained in the UW solution alone in porcine autologous kidney transplantation model 7 days after the operation (Hauet 2002).

Calcium Channel Blockers

Organ preservation can be regarded as a mitochondrial function protectant. Mitochondria produce ATP and maintain the intracellular calcium balance, and mitochondrial calcium overload is a characteristic change during ischemia reperfusion injury. Calcium channel blockers such as nitrendipine can inhibit ischemia reperfusion injury and improve the effect of cryopreservation (Sasaki 1999).

Fluorocarbon (Peflanca)

The capacity of Fluorocarbon dissolved oxygen is 20 to 25 times higher in the plasma, and the oxygen saturation curve also shows that low temperature is conducive to the release of oxygen. Studies found that the addition of fluorocarbon to UW solution can increase organ oxygen supplementation and improve the level of oxidative phosphorylation during cryopreservation. During pancreas preservation, the fully oxidized fluorocarbon can maintain the preservation solution at approximately 85% oxygen saturation for more than 18 hours. Compared with the UW solution, this method can increase the recovery of islet function and improve the effect of pancreas transplantation.

Gas Molecules

Recently, gas molecules have become a focus in organ preservation. In addition to traditional oxygen, the effects of gasses such as hydrogen, nitric oxide, hydrogen sulfide and carbon monoxide, on reducing ischemia reperfusion injury and the potential mechanisms involved have been explored. Among these findings, carbon monoxide release molecules (CO-RMs) have received more attention. The molecule is a transition metal carbonyl compound that can control the release of carbon monoxide into tissues. A recent study confirmed that the addition of CO-RMs to the preservation solutions can significantly reduce renal, liver and heart ischemia reperfusion injury. Gas molecules will have broad clinical prospects for the protection of transplanted organs (Wei 2010; Soni 2012; Jain 2012; Mehta 2012).

Chinese Medicine Ingredients

Recently, Chinese researchers added some traditional Chinese medicine ingredients to organ preservation solution and achieved encouraging results. Wang et al. used *Salvia miltiorrhiza* irrigation in a rat pancreas-duodenal kidney transplantation model and found that the levels of serum amylase, serum creatinine and serum malondialdehyde (MDA) in the treatment group were significantly lower than in the control group, and the pathological damage of the pancreas and kidney was also reduced after transplantation. That is because *Salvia miltiorrhiza* scavenges oxygen free radicals and protects against ischemia-reperfusion injury. Zhou et al. used ginseng extract in the HC-A kidney preservation solution for cryopreserved isolated canine kidneys, and the results showed that, compared with the control group, ultrastructural tissue damage was significantly reduced in the treatment group, and serum creatinine was significantly decreased, suggesting that ginseng extract can help reduce renal ischemia reperfusion injury. Another study also confirmed that Astragalus, dodder, oxymatrine and other traditional Chinese medicines can reduce of ischemia- reperfusion injury, suggesting that the addition of some traditional Chinese medicine ingredients to the organ preservation solution can improve the effect of existing preservation solutions. Chinese medicine has already shown advantages and is expected to become a field of study for organ preservation materials.

3. MAIN PRESERVATION SOLUTIONS

General without Organ Specificity

University of Wisconsin Solution
In 1988, Belzer et al. developed an excellent organ preservation solution at Wisconsin University named UW solution (University of Wisconsin), which has become the gold standard among organ preservation solutions (Belzer and Southard 1988). UW solution combines metabolically inert substrates, such as lactobionate and raffinose, with hydroxy-ethyl starch (HES) as a colloid, an ATP precursor (adenosine) and oxygen radical scavengers (glutathione and allopurinol). The principal benefit of this solution is that it is associated with good outcomes of short and long term kidney preservation. Its disadvantages are due to the high viscosity, which compromises the microcirculation, and the high potassium concentration that can produce vasoconstriction with hyperaggregation of HES. Two kinds of UW solution have been utilized for HMP and CS. In CS, UW-CSS is the main solution, while UW-G is used for HMP. Lactobionate is replaced by gluconate and the potassium level is reduced in UW-G, resulting in a consistency that more closely resembles an extracellular solution (Catena 2013).

Histidine-Tryptophan-Ketoglutarate Solution

HTK was introduced in 1980 by Bretschneider and was originally used as a cardioplegic solution (Yuan 2010). HTK contains histidine and tryptophan as membrane stabilizers as well as antioxidants and ketoglutarate for anaerobic metabolism. HTK studies have shown conflicting results. However, its low viscosity may improve microperfusion. Because of this characteristic, HTK is recommended in HMP at low pressures and high perfusion volumes (Yuan 2010; Catena 2013).

Celsior Solution

Celsior solution is a colloid that was developed in 1994 and was originally used in heart transplantation before being extended to other abdominal organs. It combines the osmotic efficacy of UW (lactobionate and mannitol) with the potent buffering ability of HTK (histidine) (Yuan 2010). Colloid solutions contain added macromolecules that do not pass the cellular membrane and thus prevent tissue edema caused by the hydrostatic pressure of HMP (Catena 2013).

Institute-George-Lopez

IGL-1, a fairly new preservation solution developed in France (Faure 2003), combines the advantages of UW and Celsior (Yuan 2010). Polyethylene glycol is bound to cell and tissue surfaces, thus stabilizing them from adverse interactions. Studies suggest that this feature modifies the inherent immunogenicity of donor tissue as a consequence of ischemia-reperfusion injury (Eugene 2004). Badet et al. demonstrated a reduced incidence of delayed graft function (DGF) compared with kidneys preserved with UW. However, a recently published multi-center study showed no significant difference in DGF when IGL-1 was compared with UW (Badet 2005; Catena 2013; Codas 2009).

Polysol

Polysol was recently introduced with the goal of facilitating the transplantation of ischemically damaged organs (Yuan 2010). Therefore, amino acids, vitamins, potent buffers, and antioxidants have been added to support metabolism under hypothermic conditions. The solution has also been tested during HMP (Bessems 2005). A case study by Schreinemachers et al. demonstrated superior graft survival with Polysol compared with UW in a porcine renal autotransplant model (Schreinemachers 2009; Doorschodt 2009; Florquin 2009; van den Bergh 2009; Weerman 2009). Further reports by the same group have shown beneficial effects of Polysol for kidneys damaged by warm ischemia (Schreinemachers, Doorschodt, Florquin, Idu, et al. 2009). Polysol is currently used in experimental trials only. While recent reports on Polysol appear to be promising, more clinical data are necessary to evaluate its efficacy and benefits (Bessems 2005; Catena 2013).

Hypertonic Citrate

HOC, or Marshall's solution, an intracellular-mimicking medium, is extensively used for clinical transplantation in the United Kingdom and Australia (Wilson 2007). HOC uses mannitol as the impermeable solute and citrate as its buffer to aid calcium extension from the cell while maintaining a physiologic pH. As a hypertonic solution, HOC prevents the entry of fluid into cells. Experimental trials using canine kidneys have demonstrated it to be effective for preservation periods of up to 72 hours (Kay 2009; Catena 2013).

Lifor Solution

Lifor solution is a type of anti-extracellular organ preservation solution developed on the basis of the comprehensive analysis of UW solution. It has low viscosity, low osmotic pressure, is rich in ATP and other nutrients, and the formula is simple and inexpensive. In 2007, Stowe et al. reported for the first time that Lifor preservation solution was used to preserve an isolated pig heart (Stowe 2007). Recently, a series of studies have shown that Lifor solution is superior to UW solution in reducing renal ischemia-reperfusion injury, alleviating cell apoptosis and improving renal blood flow and renal vascular resistance (Gage 2009; Regner 2010). In preserving small intestine, the effect is similar to UW solution, but the cost is low. However, Lifor solution is still in the experimental stage, and its effects need to be further evaluated.

Kyoto Solution

Kyoto solution is a type of extracorporeal multi-organ preservation solution that was developed by Kyoto University in Japan; it was initially used as a lung preservation solution (Chen 2004; Nakamura 2004; Wada 2004). The preservation solution uses trehalose and gluconic acid as non-permeable molecules, effectively reducing cell edema, which can replace the kapok and lactose acid in UW solution, but at a lower cost. Until now, the preservation solution has been used for clinical lung and kidney preservation and has shown benefits over UW solution (Chen 2004; Yoshida 2002). However, the use of Kyoto solution in liver, pancreas and small intestine preservation is still under research (Zhao 2008).

Solution De Conservation Des Organes Et Des Tissus

Solution de conservation des organes et des tissus (SCOT) is a multi-organ preservation solution developed by the University of Poitiers, France, with high sodium ion and low potassium ion concentration, which uses PEG 20 kDa (19 842 U, 30 g/L) as a colloidal component of the preservation solution. Animal experiments showed that the preservation effect in the kidney, liver and islet transplantation are better than with UW solution; therefore, it has been used in clinical kidney preservation (Billault 2006).

Shanghai Multi-Organ Preservation Solution

With the rapid development of organ transplantation in China, multiple organ transplantation has become increasingly common. Although simple solutions are still advantageous for domestic transplantations, high prices have become a huge problem. Some researchers invented a new kind of solution named shanghai multi-organ preservation (SMO) solution, which is based on UW solution. SMO solution uses Xylitol as energy and ligustrazine as an oxygen scavenger. In animal models, SMO showed significant protective function in the liver and kidney compared to HTK, and the effect was the same as UW.

Kidney Preservation Solutions

Collins Solution

Collins solution was designed in the 1960s and was considered the preservation solution of choice for more than 15 years until organ preservation was revolutionized by the introduction of UW solution in 1988 (Latchana 2014). Collins solution is a high potassium, high magnesium, low sodium intracellular liquid type solution. By maintaining glucose concentration at 420 mol/L, Collins used this liquid to successfully save the kidneys for 30 hours at 4°C, and after transplantation, the kidneys showed good function. In 1976, the European Transplantation Organization improved Collins solution and removed the negative effects of magnesium ions, forming the Euro-Collins (EC) solution. They recommended the solution as a standard preservation solution for clinical kidney transplantation. Thus, EC solution was widely used in Europe (de Boer 1999).

Hyperosmolar Citrate Adenine Solution

Hyperosmolar citrate adenine (HC-A) solution, also known as hypertonic citrate adenine solution, was jointly developed by the Second Military Medical University Changzheng Hospital and Shanghai Blood Center in 1979. Its main components are potassium, sodium, magnesium sulfate, citrate, mannitol and adenine. HC-A solution is the main irrigation and cryopreservation solution for organ transplantation in China. It has a simple preparation, good stability, and low price. Currently, the utility of HC-A solution has been widely affirmed after 20 years of use.

HCA-II Solution

HC-A solution has been used for more than 20 years. With the further study of preservation, the inadequacies in this solution have gradually appeared. In recent years, combined with the latest organ preservation theory, the HC-A preservation formula has undergone comprehensive improvement. In accordance with the preservation of the composition of the elements, a phosphate buffer system has been added, and a cell membrane protective agent and the antioxidant ligustrazine have been incorporated, which increased energy substrate content and osmotic pressure. HCA-II organ preservation solution was developed after animal experiments and a number of clinical applications in the transplant center confirmed that HCA-II preservation solution was significantly better than HC-A liquid for kidney preservation. Compared with the HTK solution, kidneys could be saved for 36 h, 48 h and 72 h. After 72 h, the apoptotic index was significantly lower in kidney tissue that had been stored in HCA-II solution compared to kidney tissue that had been stored in HTK solution. The results of an animal model of canine kidney transplantation showed that the preservation effect was better than that of HTK and was equivalent to that of UW preservation solution. HC is the upgraded liquid product. And the product has a national patent and is expected to officially enter production in 2007.

Heart Preservation Solutions

According to the systematic review of Demmy et al. as many as 167 HPSs were used for heart preservation in the USA in the middle of the 1990s. At present, the histidine-tryptophan-ketoglutarate (HTK) solution, the University of Wisconsin (UW) solution and the Celsior solution are most commonly used for heart preservation.

HTK (or Custodiol) was introduced by Bretschneider in the 1970s as a cardioplegic solution and has subsequently been used in organ preservation for the heart, liver and pancreas.

Its usage has been increasingly popular in cardiac surgery because a single administration of cold HTK in the coronary vascular bed provides reliable protection from IRI for at least 2 h.

The Euro-Collins solution is an intracellular HPS with high concentrations of glucose (194 mmol/l) and K^+ (115 mmol/l) that includes bicarbonate and phosphate buffer systems. The Stanford solution is similar to Euro-Collins with the exception of an even higher glucose level (250 mmol/l) and a lower K^+ concentration (27 mmol/l).

The UW solution, developed by Belzer et al., typically has a low Na^+ concentration, although an extracellular modification of this HPS that includes 125 mmol/l Na^+ also exists. Along with intracellular-type HPSs, there are several widely accepted extracellular solutions with high Na^+ and low K^+ concentrations.

The most common extracellular HPS is Celsior. Celsior is enriched with the reactive oxygen species scavengers lactobionate and glutathione, which ensures the prevention of oxidative stress during reperfusion. In contrast to other HPSs, Celsior contains 20 mmol/l glutamate, which has anti-ischemic activity and exerts cardio-protective effects. In addition, Celsior, HTK and the Stanford solution contain the polyatomic alcohol mannitol, which can prevent edema and quench reactive oxygen species (Minasian 2015).

However, the high molecular weight compounds within UW, such as hydroxyethyl starch (HES), result in a highly viscous solution that has been implicated, in part, in organ dysfunction, thereby supporting the development of less viscous alternatives, including Celsior (CEL) and histidine- tryptophan-ketoglutarate (HTK).

Many targeted approaches to cardiac organ preservation have been attempted, including the development of Plegisol, which arose from the initial St. Thomas solution used for cardioplegia, albeit with slight modifications, including the addition of a buffering system. In contrast to the aforementioned acellular approaches, Papworth solution was centered on the inclusion of donor blood in its composition. The different metabolic demand and physiology of the lung supported the construction of pulmonary specific solutions, including Perfadex (PER), which has been authorized to be used in pulmonary transplantations by the Food and Drug Administration (FDA) in the United States (Latchana 2014).

Liver Preservation Solutions

Preservation solutions for donor liver are required to preserve homeostasis, support liver metabolism and delay cell damage. Several solutions are currently available: University of Wisconsin (UW), Histidine-Tryptophan-Ketoglutarate (HTK), Celsior (CS) and the most recent Institute Georges Lopez-1 (IGL-1). They all differ in terms of composition, ion balance, viscosity, osmolality and cost.

UW is a high viscosity colloid solution due to the presence of hydroxyethyl starch (HES), high potassium and low sodium concentrations (125 mmol/l and 27 mmol/l, respectively). Despite its widespread use, UW carries some side effects: high viscosity might result in impaired flushing with microcirculatory disturbances; high potassium concentration might provoke cardiac arrest in the recipient upon liver reperfusion; and finally, ischemic-type biliary lesions are not rare.

HTK represents an alternative to UW and possesses advantages that can be summarized as lower viscosity, lower potassium content (10 mmol/l, thus avoiding the risk of hyperkalemia) and better buffering properties. HTK was believed equivalent to UW for SCS but less expensive; however, recent findings highlighted HTK-associated disadvantages. In a large single-center series and a retrospective analysis of the UNOS database, the survival of grafts from standard or ECD donors did not differ when grafts were preserved with HTK or UW; however, in subgroup analyses, HTK-preserved grafts achieved significantly inferior survival after exposure to long-lasting cold ischemia or procurement from DCD donors. Furthermore, two different clinical trials from Meine et al. and Gulsen et al. reported relevant increases in the incidence of NAS in patients receiving grafts from DCD donors preserved with HTK. The reason that HTK is associated with worse outcomes after LT is not fully understood; the lack of antioxidants and oncotic agents might be an explanation. To summarize, the available evidence points towards the avoidance of HTK as a preservation solution for livers.

Celsior solution has low viscosity, high sodium and low potassium concentration (100 mmol/l and 15 mmol/l, respectively) and combines the best aspects of both UW and HTK. It retains the buffering properties of HTK (histidine) and the presence of impermeants as in UW (lactobionic acid).

Sodium and potassium concentrations in IGL-1 are switched compared to UW ([Na$^+$] = 120 mmol/l, [K$^+$] = 25 mmol/l) and HES is replaced by polyethylene glycol, resulting in lower viscosity. These properties could improve liver wash-out during procurement and reduce IRI. IGL-1 has been previously tested in a rat model of isolated liver perfusion and in a pig model of auto-transplantation, showing better preservation of cell integrity. Dondero et al., in a recent randomized trial that included fatty livers, failed to demonstrate the superiority of IGL-1 and found that it is at least as effective as UW and is less expensive. However, the outcome of steatotic donor grafts was not the primary endpoint of this study, which was probably underpowered to draw solid conclusions. Randomized clinical trials comparing IGL-1 to other preservation solutions are still missing, but the recent large series analysis from Adam et al. confirmed good outcomes and postulated possible advantages for IGL-1. Further investigation is therefore needed to confirm this hypothesis.

Identifying the best preservation solution is a difficult task since randomized trials have shown conflicting results; however, some conclusions can be drawn from large studies or clustering data from different trials. In a recent meta-analysis, Zuluaga et al. reported no differences in LT outcomes when UW was compared to CS or HTK. In particular, no differences were observed in terms of EAD, 1-year patient survival and the occurrence of NAS. Adam et al. partly confirmed this observation in their recent retrospective analysis of the European Liver Transplant Registry that included more than 48,000 LTs. Grafts preserved with UW, IGL-1 or CS showed similar 3-year graft survival; however, IGL-1 was associated with a better preservation of partial liver grafts as shown by higher graft survival in this group. Notably, grafts preserved with HTK exhibited significantly inferior survival three years post-LT when compared to grafts preserved with other preservation solutions, and based on multivariate analysis, HTK was an independent risk factor for graft loss.

All available preservation solutions were developed with the purpose of preventing hepatocyte death during the ischemic storage phase. Other cell populations, including cholangiocytes, are probably not so well protected from IRI. Two recent studies that focused on the pathological aspects of the common bile duct have revealed that the bile duct epithelium is seriously injured at the end of SCS in up to 88% of cases. These findings indicate that the bile duct of almost all grafts suffers relevant injury, which might be responsible for NAS development. These complications add relevant morbidity and significantly reduce long-term graft survival, representing a rising concern due to the increased transplantation of DCD grafts, which is associated with markedly higher rates of biliary complications. Improved bile duct preservation might be offered by MP, which has been associated with better preservation of the bile duct in experimental settings (Gilbo 2016).

Pancreas Preservation Solutions

Islets are most often infused into the patient with an open laparotomy incision immediately after processing while the patient is still in the operating room. Alternatively, islets may be cultured and infused postoperatively via a percutaneous approach. Islets are infused into the portal system using a stump of the splenic vein, via direct puncture of the portal, or by cannulation of the umbilical vein. With a significant tissue volume infused into the portal vein, the elevation of portal pressure may lead to a reduction in blood flow and portal vein thrombosis. Because of this risk, heparin anticoagulation is recommended. Portal pressure is monitored closely during islet infusion and should not exceed 25–27 cm H_2O (18.4–20 mm Hg). When pellet volume is < 20 mL and the liver is healthy, portal pressure usually does not increase substantially. If portal pressure does increase during the infusion of a large volume of unpurified islets, portal infusion should be discontinued and the remaining islets should be dispersed into the peritoneal cavity or injected into the leaves of the mesentery or omentum, bowel subserosa, gastric submucosa, or intra-muscular space. Although islets transplanted into these alternative sites have been shown to survive in animal models, whether this approach is effective in the clinical setting is unknown (Witkowski 2014; Savari 2014; Matthews 2014).

Only a few studies have adequately evaluated lower temperature conditions in islet culture/preservation before our report. Frankel et al. reported the comparison of 8°C storage with 22°C storage or 37°C culture for 1 week using islets from obese (ob/ob) mice. They showed that the glucose-stimulated insulin release was better maintained by storage at 8°C in tissue culture medium with a high concentration (18 mM) of glucose and an additional pre-incubation period of 4 h at 37°C than by storage at 22°C or 37°C. In addition, 8°C storage in a high-potassium "intracellular medium" resulted in a better subsequent glucose-stimulated insulin release and islet morphology in comparison to a 37°C culture in traditional culture medium. Korbutt et al. reported the survival of rat pancreatic b-cells after 96 h of storage at 4°C. After 4°C storage in Collins solution with albumin and benzamidine, b-cells exhibited a higher insulin content than after culture in HAM's F10 at 20°C or 37°C, although their capacity for subsequent insulin synthesis and release was comparable. It was demonstrated that storage with UW solution plus pefabloc at 4°C was superior to culture at 20°C or 37°C; however, the experiments used unpurified islets (Noguchi 2015).

The first step after surgical dissection is to flush the extracted pancreas with a chilled preservation solution. This is usually done with University of Wisconsin (UW) solution. UW solution gives equivalent or superior results to other perfusations in many but not all studies by preventing the loss of amylase and inducing a slight shrinkage of the acinar cells, which in turn improves the density separation of islets and the viability of the cells. Other preservation solutions include Celsior, HTK, IGL-1 and others. The flushing step cools the pancreas and removes debris and thrombi.

Cold storage and transport of the pancreas is vital to islet yield and viability; warm ischemia has been found to damage tissue; however, cold ischemia time beyond 8 h also results in reduced yields and a lower quality of human islets. In most studies, shorter cold ischemic time is associated with better islet yields. Transport using a two-layer method where the pancreas rests on a substrate in the top layer of a perfluorocarbon "bath" appears to give slightly improved outcomes and showed promising results in pancreas tissues from humans (Deters 2011; Stokes 2011; Gunton 2011).

Lung Preservation Solutions

The procurement of lungs for transplantation is a challenging task since lung tissue is at a high risk of ischemic and hypoxic injuries, which can result in life-threatening primary graft dysfunction (PGD). During the first successful LTx surgeries, cooling was the only technique of preservation. The application of various organ preservation solutions emerged over the following decades. To extend the cold ischemic time, intracellular-type solutions such as Euro-Collins or University of Wisconsin solution were used when available. As understanding of the pathological and pharmaceutical pathways of lung preservation developed, practice shifted towards extracellular-type preservation solutions, primarily the low-potassium dextran (LPD) solution. The LPD solution is understood to work via the following two mechanisms: the low-potassium concentration maintains a low pulmonary artery (PA) pressure during perfusion and the dextran acts as an oncotic agent, increasing the intravascular pressure to prevent interstitial lung edema.

There are distinct advantages to using an extracellular-type LPD solution in lung procurement. LPD is the accepted standard pulmoplegic solution and shows superior preservation effects. In addition to potassium and dextran, other pharmaceutical agents are currently used in cold ischemic lung procurement, such as prostaglandins and/or methylprednisolone to prevent vasoconstriction (due to the cold flush) and inflammatory responses (Andreasson 2014; Dark 2014; Fisher 2014).

4. GENE THERAPY IN ORGAN PRESERVATION

RNA interference (RNAi) is a highly conserved biological phenomenon in all eukaryotes, including renal cells. In the late 1990s, due to the development of molecular biology and genetics, the biological understanding of RNA evolved from simply an intermediate between DNA and protein to a dynamic and versatile regulator that functions in genes and cells in all living organisms. In 1998, as a milestone, Fire et al. injected a few molecules of double-stranded RNA (dsRNA) into Caenorhabditis elegans and found that dsRNAs could specifically interfere with the protein expression of an endogenous gene. This molecule was named small interfering RNA (siRNA) and mediates RNAi. siRNA is able to recognize and degrade homologous host mRNA. Therefore, the gene from which the mRNA is transcribed is silenced, which is referred to post-transcriptional gene silencing.

Although RNAi exists naturally, synthetic artificial siRNA exerts similar effects as natural endogenous micro-RNA (miRNA). Both sense and antisense strands of siRNA can be synthesized separately and annealed to form double-stranded siRNA duplexes in vitro. After the siRNA is delivered into the cytoplasm, the artificial siRNA silences the target gene using similar biological processes as endogenous miRNA. Since the introduction of 21-nucleotide artificial siRNAs that can trigger gene silencing in mammalian cells, synthetic siRNA has generated much interest in biomedical research, including in the kidney. siRNA as a strategic molecule has been expected to impact the field of innovative therapy. Because siRNA is highly efficient at gene silencing, it is possible to develop specific siRNA-based drugs that could target any genes, including those that have no known pharmacological antagonists or inhibitors. Different types of synthetic siRNA have been tested for their efficacy in various disease models, including cancer, autoimmune disorders, cardiovascular injuries, and organ transplantation, including native and transplanted organ injuries.

In addition to the *in vitro* delivery of siRNA, ex vivo/in vivo siRNA delivery to target organs is an indispensable step before its clinical application. If it was directly delivered into the kidneys, siRNA could obtain higher local concentrations, which would result in improved gene silencing efficacy. During kidney transplantation, *ex vivo* local delivery of siRNA into the donor kidney is feasible because it could be facilitated by the unique structure of the kidney and the characteristics of kidney transplantation. Recently, we utilized an *ex vivo* isolated porcine kidney reperfusion system to assess the efficacy of naked caspase-3 siRNA. The caspase-3 siRNA was directly infused into the renal artery (locally) and autologous blood perfusate (mimic systemic delivery) before 24-hour cold storage (CS), followed by an additional reperfusion for 3 hours. The results demonstrated that the caspase-3 siRNA improved ischemic re-perfusion (IR) injury with reduced caspase-3 expression and apoptosis, better renal oxygenation and acid–base homeostasis (Yang 2013; Jia 2013). These promising proof-of-principle observations provide valuable guidance for the further development of siRNA in clinical practice.

Cold ischemia injury activates multiple signaling pathways and upregulates several genes, subsequently causing cell apoptosis and death and resulting in organ damage. In addition to single siRNA delivery, siRNA cocktails have been used for better efficacy to silence multiple genes. Recently, Min's group demonstrated that the perfusion and preservation of donor hearts with siRNA solution can attenuate cold I/R injury during heart transplantation, and an siRNA cocktail that contains 3 siRNAs that target C3, RelB, and TNFα showed a synergistic protective effect compared with single siRNAs (Zheng et al. 2009). Based on their previous study, the authors further reported that treatment with siRNA targeting the C3, Fas, and RelB genes successfully attenuated I/R injury and improved renal graft function in a murine kidney transplantation model (Zheng 2016). MMPs also play an important role in injury to the transplanted kidney. MMP expression is increased in patients with chronic antibody-mediated rejection, and because of the role of MMPs in fibrotic renal diseases, MMPs have been suggested as a possible common pathway for chronic allograft nephropathy in the transplanted kidney (Yan 2012). In a rat kidney cold perfusion model, the inhibition of MMP-2 during perfusion via MMP-2 siRNA led to a decrease in MMP-2 levels in the perfusate, as well as a decrease in LDH, NGAL, and CcO release after 22 hours of perfusion (Moser 2016).

Long-term pancreatic cold ischemia contributes to decreased islet number and viability after isolation and culture, leading to poor islet transplantation outcomes in patients with type 1 diabetes. Silencing Bbc3 by transfecting Bbc3 siRNA into islets *in vitro* prior to cold preservation improved post-preservation mitochondrial viability (Omori 2016). In a lung isolated preservation model, isolated lungs were exposed to 6 hours of cold ischemia (4°C), followed by 2 hours of warm (37°C) reperfusion with a solution that contained 10% of fresh whole blood and mechanical ventilation with constant low driving pressure. siRNA that targeted Fas was administered intratracheally, as was control small interfering RNA. The results revealed that silencing Fas gene expression reduced edema formation (bronchoalveolar lavage protein concentration and lung histology) and improved lung compliance (Del Sorbo 2016).

Although siRNA therapy for organ preservation is effective and promising, off-target effects are one of the major obstacles for further clinical translation. The induction of various side effects may be caused by unexpected perturbations between RNAi molecules and cellular components. The off-target effects of siRNA were first reported by Jackson and colleagues in 2003 (Baan 2016). Broadly speaking, off-target effects can be siRNA specific or non-specific. The former is caused by limited siRNA complementarity to non-targeted mRNAs. The latter, resulting in immune- and toxicity-related responses, is due to the construction of the siRNA sequence, its modification or the modification of the delivery vehicle. RNA-sensing pattern recognition receptors (PRRs), localized in endosomes, are the most important components of the innate immune system. The responses of PRRs to siRNAs are either TLR-mediated or non-TLR-mediated. The PRR responses are also associated with siRNA sequence specific side effects and have recently attracted lots of attention from researchers (Kabilova 2012). RNA-sensing TLRs (TLR3 and TLR7) are predominantly located intracellularly and recognize nucleic acids released from invading pathogens. The non-TLR-mediated innate immune responses triggered by siRNA binding are linked to the RNA-regulated expression of protein kinase (PKR) and retinoic acid inducible gene 1 (RIG1), which further induce caspase-3 and NF-κB expression, respectively. The activation of PRRs generates excessive cytokine release and subsequent inflammation (Robbins 2009; Judge 2009; MacLachlan 2009). Based on this second type of off-target RNAi effects, our group further investigated the mechanism of how short-acting caspase-3 siRNA impaired post-transplanted kidneys. The results suggested that the amplified inflammatory responses in caspase-3 siRNA preserved auto-transplant kidneys were associated with TLR3, TLR7 and PKR activation, which may be due to systemic compensative responses, although persistent actions initiated by short-acting caspase-3 siRNA cannot be completely excluded (Yang 2013; Li 2013). In the future, better siRNA designs will decrease these off-target effects to a minimum and acceptable level.

5. CURRENT CLINICAL TRIALS OF ORGAN PRESERVATION

Twenty-five current clinical trials of organ preservation solutions have already been registered on *clinicaltrials.gov*; 19 of them focus on solid organ transplantation. At the time of writing, 6 trials have been completed and relevant articles were published online. These trials have not focused on changing the recipes or inventing a kind of new solution but have addressed the use of new machines for the preservation of organs, especially marginal organs, which can be more complex. Thus, *clinicaltrials.gov* has published many trials mainly based on machine organ preservation, and several of them are still recruiting participants.

The Clinical Trial of Hydrogen-Rich Celsior Solution Applied in Aging DBD Liver/Kidney Transplantation (HRCSDBD) was sponsored by Renji Hospital, Shanghai, China, in 2015. This prospective, randomized clinical trial proposes to investigate whether hydrogen-rich Celsior solution improves the quality of aging grafts in liver/kidney transplantation. The study is based on the findings of the protective effects of hydrogen gas, which has been reported to display antioxidant properties and protective effects against organ dysfunction induced by various ischemia reperfusion injuries (Abe 2012; Buchholz 2011).

The Evaluation of a Marine OXYgen Carrier: HEMO2Life® for hypOthermic Kidney Graft preservation, Before Transplantation (OXYOP) study was received on December 22, 2015, provided by University Hospital, Brest. It was an interventional study that aimed to evaluate the use of an oxygen carrier HEMO2Life® as an additive in organ preservation solution in kidney transplantation for patients with end-stage renal disease.

The University of Bologna sponsored a trial about hypothermic oxygenated perfusion versus static cold storage for marginal graft (PIO) in 2017, and it is still recruiting participants. This trial aims to assess the impact of hypothermic oxygenated perfusion (PIO) of marginal human kidney and liver compared with static cold storage (SCS).

6. PERSPECTIVE

Although organ preservation solutions have become quite common, the method with which to protect donor organs can still be a valuable research topic in basic and clinical studies. To date, donor organs are different from those retrieved two decades ago, and new solutions and techniques have developed rapidly. However, due to the shortage of donor organs, just the consideration of new techniques is inadequate, and effective strategies to extend the donor pool are advocated.

DISCLOSURES

The authors declare that no conflicts of interest exist.

ACKNOWLEDGMENTS

This study was supported by the National Natural Science Foundation of China (81270832, 81400752).

REFERENCES

Abe T, Li XK, Yazawa K, Hatayama N, Xie L, Sato B, Kakuta Y, Tsutahara K, Okumi M, Tsuda H, Kaimori JY, Isaka Y, Natori M, Takahara S, Nonomura N. Hydrogen-rich University of Wisconsin solution attenuates renal cold ischemia-reperfusion injury. *Transplantation* 2012; 94(1): 14−21.

Abreu Lde A, Kawano PR, Yamamoto H, Damiao R, Fugita OE. Comparative study between trimetazidine and ice slush hypothermia in protection against renal ischemia/reperfusion injury in a porcine model. *Int. Braz. J. Urol.* 2011; 37(5): 649−656.

Andreasson AS, Dark JH, Fisher AJ. Ex vivo lung perfusion in clinical lung transplantation--state of the art. *Eur. J. Cardiothorac Surg.* 2014; 46(5): 779−788.

Baan CC. Basic sciences in development: What changes will we see in transplantation in the next five years? *Transplantation* 2016; 100(12): 2507−2511.

Badet L, Petruzzo P, Lefrancois N, McGregor B, Espa M, Berthillot C, Danjou F, Contu P, Aissa AH, Virieux SR, Colpart JJ, Martin X. Kidney preservation with IGL-1 solution: a preliminary report. *Transplant Proc.* 2005; 37(1): 308–311.

Belous A, Knox C, Nicoud IB, Pierce J, Anderson C, Pinson CW, Chari RS. Altered ATP-dependent mitochondrial Ca2+ uptake in cold ischemia is attenuated by ruthenium red. *J. Surg. Res.* 2003; 111(2): 284–289.

Belzer FO, Southard JH. Principles of solid-organ preservation by cold storage. *Transplantation* 1988; 45(4): 673–676.

Bessems M, Doorschodt BM, van Vliet AK, van Gulik TM. Machine perfusion preservation of the non-heart-beating donor rat livers using polysol, a new preservation solution. *Transplant Proc.* 2005; 37(1): 326–328.

Billault C, Vaessen C, Van Glabeke E, Rolland E, Ourahma S, Dimitru L, Richard F, Eugene M, Barrou B. Use of the SCOT solution in kidney transplantation: preliminary report. *Transplant Proc.* 2006; 38(7): 2281–2282.

Buchholz BM, Masutani K, Kawamura T, Peng X, Toyoda Y, Billiar TR, Bauer AJ, Nakao A. Hydrogen-enriched preservation protects the isogeneic intestinal graft and amends recipient gastric function during transplantation. *Transplantation* 2011; 92(9): 985–992.

Catena F, Coccolini F, Montori G, Vallicelli C, Amaduzzi A, Ercolani G, Ravaioli M, Del Gaudio M, Schiavina R, Brunocilla E, Liviano G, Feliciangeli G, Pinna AD. Kidney preservation: review of present and future perspective. *Transplant Proc.* 2013; 45(9): 3170–3177.

Chen F, Fukuse T, Hasegawa S, Bando T, Hanaoka N, Kawashima M, Sakai H, Hamakawa H, Fujinaga T, Nakamura T, Wada H. Effective application of ET-Kyoto solution for clinical lung transplantation. *Transplant Proc.* 2004; 36(9): 2812–2815.

Chen F, Nakamura T, Wada H. Development of new organ preservation solutions in Kyoto University. *Yonsei Med. J.* 2004; 45(6): 1107–1114.

Codas R, Petruzzo P, Morelon E, Lefrancois N, Danjou F, Berthillot C, Contu P, Espa M, Martin X, Badet L. IGL-1 solution in kidney transplantation: first multi-center study. *Clin. Transplant.* 2009; 23(3): 337–342.

de Boer J, De Meester J, Smits JM, Groenewoud AF, Bok A, van der Velde O, Doxiadis, II, Persijn GG. Eurotransplant randomized multicenter kidney graft preservation study comparing HTK with UW and Euro-Collins. *Transpl. Int.* 1999; 12(6): 447–453.

Del Sorbo L, Costamagna A, Muraca G, Rotondo G, Civiletti F, Vizio B, Bosco O, Martin Conte EL, Frati G, Delsedime L, Lupia E, Fanelli V, Ranieri VM. Intratracheal Administration of Small Interfering RNA Targeting Fas Reduces Lung Ischemia-Reperfusion Injury. *Crit. Care Med.* 2016; 44(8): e604–613.

Desurmont T, Giraud S, Cau J, Goujon JM, Scepi M, Roumy J, Chatauret N, Thuillier R, Hauet T. Trophic factor and FR167653 supplementation during cold storage rescue chronic renal injury. *J. Urol.* 2011; 185(3): 1139–1146.

Deters NA, Stokes RA, Gunton JE. Islet transplantation: factors in short-term islet survival. *Arch. Immunol. Ther. Exp. (Warsz).* 2011; 59(6): 421–429.

Eugene M. Polyethyleneglycols and immunocamouflage of the cells tissues and organs for transplantation. *Cell Mol. Biol. (Noisy-le-grand).* 2004; 50(3): 209–215.

Faure JP, Baumert H, Han Z, Goujon JM, Favreau F, Dutheil D, Petit I, Barriere M, Tallineau C, Tillement JP, Carretier M, Mauco G, Papadopoulos V, Hauet T. Evidence for a protective role of trimetazidine during cold ischemia: targeting inflammation and nephron mass. *Biochem. Pharmacol.* 2003; 66(11): 2241–2250.

Gage F, Leeser DB, Porterfield NK, Graybill JC, Gillern S, Hawksworth JS, Jindal RM, Thai N, Falta EM, Tadaki DK, Brown TS, Elster EA. Room temperature pulsatile perfusion of renal allografts with Lifor compared with hypothermic machine pump solution. *Transplant Proc.* 2009; 41(9): 3571–3574.

Gilbo N, Catalano G, Salizzoni M, Romagnoli R. Liver graft preconditioning, preservation and reconditioning. *Dig. Liver Dis.* 2016; 48(11): 1265–1274.

Giraud S, Thuillier R, Belliard A, Hebrard W, Nadeau C, Milin S, Goujon JM, Manguy E, Mauco G, Hauet T, Macchi L. Direct thrombin inhibitor prevents delayed graft function in a porcine model of renal transplantation. *Transplantation* 2009; 87(11): 1636–1644.

Hauet T, Goujon JM, Baumert H, Petit I, Carretier M, Eugene M, Vandewalle A. Polyethylene glycol reduces the inflammatory injury due to cold ischemia/reperfusion in autotransplanted pig kidneys. *Kidney Int.* 2002; 62(2): 654–667.

Kabilova TO, Meschaninova MI, Venyaminova AG, Nikolin VP, Zenkova MA, Vlassov VV, Chernolovskaya EL. Short double-stranded RNA with immunostimulatory activity: sequence dependence. *Nucleic. Acid Ther.* 2012; 22(3): 196–204.

Kay MD, Hosgood SA, Bagul A, Nicholson ML. Comparison of preservation solutions in an experimental model of organ cooling in kidney transplantation. *Br. J. Surg.* 2009; 96(10): 1215–1221.

Korte C, Garber JL, Descourouez JL, Richards KR, Hardinger K. Pharmacists' guide to the management of organ donors after brain death. *Am. J. Health Syst. Pharm.* 2016; 73(22): 1829–1839.

Latchana N, Peck JR, Whitson B, Black SM. Preservation solutions for cardiac and pulmonary donor grafts: a review of the current literature. *J. Thorac. Dis.* 2014; 6(8): 1143–1149.

McAnulty JF, Reid TW, Waller KR, Murphy CJ. Successful six-day kidney preservation using trophic factor supplemented media and simple cold storage. *Am. J. Transplant.* 2002; 2(8): 712–718.

Minasian SM, Galagudza MM, Dmitriev YV, Karpov AA, Vlasov TD. Preservation of the donor heart: from basic science to clinical studies. *Interact. Cardiovasc. Thorac. Surg.* 2015; 20(4): 510–519.

Moser MA, Arcand S, Lin HB, Wojnarowicz C, Sawicka J, Banerjee T, Luo Y, Beck GR, Luke PP, Sawicki G. Protection of the Transplant Kidney from Preservation Injury by Inhibition of Matrix Metalloproteinases. *PLoS One.* 2016; 11(6): e0157508.

Noguchi H, Miyagi-Shiohira C, Kurima K, Kobayashi N, Saitoh I, Watanabe M, Noguchi Y, Matsushita M. Islet Culture/Preservation Before Islet Transplantation. *Cell Medicine* 2015; 8(1): 25–29.

Omori K, Kobayashi E, Komatsu H, Rawson J, Agrawal G, Parimi M, Oancea AR, Valiente L, Ferreri K, Al-Abdullah IH, Kandeel F, Takahashi M, Mullen Y. Involvement of a proapoptotic gene (BBC3) in islet injury mediated by cold preservation and rewarming. *Am. J. Physiol. Endocrinol. Metab.* 2016; 310(11): E1016–1026.

Regner KR, Nilakantan V, Ryan RP, Mortensen J, White SM, Shames BD, Roman RJ. Protective effect of Lifor solution in experimental renal ischemia-reperfusion injury. *J. Surg. Res.* 2010; 164(2): e291–297.

Robbins M, Judge A, MacLachlan I. siRNA and innate immunity. *Oligonucleotides.* 2009; 19(2): 89–102.

Sasaki S, Yasuda K, McCully JD, LoCicero J, 3rd. Calcium channel blocker enhances lung preservation. *J. Heart Lung Transplant.* 1999; 18(2): 127–132.

Schreinemachers MC, Doorschodt BM, Florquin S, Idu MM, Tolba RH, van Gulik TM. Improved renal function of warm ischemically damaged kidneys using Polysol. *Transplant Proc.* 2009; 41(1): 32–35.

Schreinemachers MC, Doorschodt BM, Florquin S, van den Bergh Weerman MA, Reitsma JB, Lai W, Sitzia M, Minor TM, Tolba RH, van Gulik TM. Improved preservation and microcirculation with POLYSOL after transplantation in a porcine kidney autotransplantation model. *Nephrol. Dial. Transplant.* 2009; 24(3): 816–824.

Soni HM, Jain MR, Mehta AA. Mechanism(s) Involved in Carbon Monoxide-releasing Molecule-2-mediated Cardioprotection During Ischaemia-reperfusion Injury in Isolated Rat Heart. *Indian J. Pharm. Sci.* 2012; 74(4): 281–291.

Stowe DF, Camara AK, Heisner JS, Aldakkak M, Harder DR. Ten-hour preservation of guinea pig isolated hearts perfused at low flow with air-saturated Lifor solution at 26{degrees}C: comparison to ViaSpan solution. *Am. J. Physiol. Heart Circ. Physiol.* 2007; 293(1): H895-901.

Wei Y, Chen P, de Bruyn M, Zhang W, Bremer E, Helfrich W. Carbon monoxide-releasing molecule-2 (CORM-2) attenuates acute hepatic ischemia reperfusion injury in rats. *BMC Gastroenterol.* 2010; 10: 42–50.

Wilson CH, Asher JF, Gupta A, Vijayanand D, Wyrley-Birch H, Stamp S, Rix DA, Soomro N, Manas DM, Jaques BC, Peaston R, Talbot D. Comparison of HTK and hypertonic citrate to intraarterial cooling in human non-heart-beating kidney donors. *Transplant Proc.* 2007; 39(2): 351–352.

Witkowski P, Savari O, Matthews JB. Islet autotransplantation and total pancreatectomy. *Adv. Surg.* 2014; 48: 223–233.

Yan Q, Sui W, Wang B, Zou H, Zou G, Luo H. Expression of MMP-2 and TIMP-1 in renal tissue of patients with chronic active antibody-mediated renal graft rejection. *Diagn. Pathol.* 2012; 7: 141–146.

Yang B, Hosgood SA, Nicholson ML. Naked small interfering RNA of caspase-3 in preservation solution and autologous blood perfusate protects isolated ischemic porcine kidneys. *Transplantation* 2011; 91(5): 501–507.

Yang C, Jia Y, Zhao T, Xue Y, Zhao Z, Zhang J, Wang J, Wang X, Qiu Y, Lin M, Zhu D, Qi G, Qiu Y, Tang Q, Rong R, Xu M, Ni S, Lai B, Nicholson ML, Zhu T, Yang B. Naked caspase 3 small interfering RNA is effective in cold preservation but not in autotransplantation of porcine kidneys. *J. Surg. Res.* 2013; 181(2): 342–354.

Yang C, Li L, Xue Y, Zhao Z, Zhao T, Jia Y, Rong R, Xu M, Nicholson ML, Zhu T, Yang B. Innate immunity activation involved in unprotected porcine auto-transplant kidneys preserved by naked caspase-3 siRNA. *J. Transl. Med.* 2013; 11: 210–220.

Yoshida H, Okuno H, Kamoto T, Habuchi T, Toda Y, Hasegawa S, Nakamura T, Wada H, Ogawa O, Yamamoto S. Comparison of the effectiveness of ET-Kyoto with Euro-Collins and University of Wisconsin solutions in cold renal storage. *Transplantation* 2002; 74(9): 1231–1236.

Yuan X, Theruvath AJ, Ge X, Floerchinger B, Jurisch A, Garcia-Cardena G, Tullius SG. Machine perfusion or cold storage in organ transplantation: indication, mechanisms, and future perspectives. *Transpl. Int.* 2010; 23(6): 561–570.

Zhao X, Koshiba T, Nakamura T, Tsuruyama T, Li Y, Bando T, Wada H, Tanaka K. ET-Kyoto solution plus dibutyryl cyclic adenosine monophosphate is superior to University of Wisconsin solution in rat liver preservation. *Cell Transplant.* 2008; 17(1−2): 99−109.

Zheng X, Lian D, Wong A, Bygrave M, Ichim TE, Khoshniat M, Zhang X, Sun H, De Zordo T, Lacefield JC, Garcia B, Jevnikar AM, Min WP. Novel small interfering RNA-containing solution protecting donor organs in heart transplantation. *Circulation* 2009; 120(12): 1099−1107, 1091 p following 1107.

Zheng X, Zang G, Jiang J, He W, Johnston NJ, Ling H, Chen R, Zhang X, Liu Y, Haig A, Luke P, Jevnikar AM, Min WP. Attenuating Ischemia-Reperfusion Injury in Kidney Transplantation by Perfusing Donor Organs With siRNA Cocktail Solution. *Transplantation* 2016; 100(4): 743−752.

In: Advances in Experimental Surgery. Volume 2
Editors: Huifang Chen and Paulo N. Martins
ISBN: 978-1-53612-773-7
© 2018 Nova Science Publishers, Inc.

Chapter 12

MACHINE ORGAN PRESERVATION

Hazel L. Marecki, MD, Isabel Brüggenwirth and Paulo N. Martins, MD, PhD*

Department of Surgery, Division of Organ Transplantation
University of Massachusetts Medical School,
Worcester, Massachusetts, US

ABSTRACT

Ex-vivo machine perfusion is a promising way to better preserve organs prior to transplantation. Since the 1930s, researchers have explored machine perfusion as preservation method, but only recently has interest been renewed in this technology as a means to resuscitate extended criteria donor organs. Hypothermic machine perfusion has become the standard in kidney preservation and has been shown to be superior to simple cold storage in resuscitation of inferior quality organs. Now, new results show that normothermic machine perfusion of the kidney may be a yet more powerful tool in donor organ resuscitation. In livers as well, making machine perfusion technology clinically available holds the promise of expanding the donor pool through more effective preservation of extended criteria donor livers, showing potential in decreasing delayed graft function, primary non-function and biliary strictures, all common failure modes of transplanted extended criteria donor livers. However, the precise settings and clinical role for liver machine perfusion has not yet been established. In research, there are two schools of thought regarding both liver and heart perfusion: normothermic machine perfusion, closely mimicking physiologic conditions, and hypothermic machine perfusion, as a means of resuscitative cold storage. A new compromise has been introduced for liver preservation (and applied to kidney preservation as well) called subnormothermic or rewarming machine perfusion as a method to minimize the ischemia reperfusion injury following cold storage but also replenish energy stores prior to transplantation. In hearts, recent preclinical trials show hypothermic perfusion superior to simple cold storage, but normothermic perfusion has been used to extend the storage time and shows promise in resuscitating hearts donated after cardiac death (DCD). In lung allograft transplantation as well,

---

* Corresponding Author: Paulo Martins, MD, PhD, FAST, FACS, University of Massachusetts, Dept. of Surgery, Transplant Division. 55 Lake Ave North, Worcester, MA 01655, Tel: (508) 334-2023, Email: paulo.martins@umassmemorial.org.

normothermic machine perfusion offers to increase function of extended criteria donor grafts and provides a modality for pretransplantation assessment of function. The pancreas shows the highest rate of discard due to unsuitability of any transplanted organ and therefore perhaps stands the most to gain from experimentation in normothermic perfusion as means of extended criteria organ resuscitation.

Keywords: machine perfusion, liver transplantation, heart transplantation, kidney transplantation, lung transplantation, pancreatic transplantation, preservation

ABBREVIATIONS

ECD	extended criteria donor
NMP	Normothermic Machine Perfusion
HMP	Hypothermic Machine Perfusion
SNMP	Sub-Normothermic Machine perfusion
RMP	Rearming Machine Perfusion
IRI	Ischemia Reperfusion Injury
DGF	Delayed graft function
PNF	Primary non-function
DCD	donation after cardiac death
CS	cold storage
SCS	simple cold storage
ITBL	ischemic type biliary lesions
HOPE	hypothermic oxygenated perfusion
RV	right ventricle
WI	warm ischemia
LDH	lactate dehydrogenase
ATP	adenosine triphosphate

INTRODUCTION

The shortage of organ transplantation donors is a worldwide problem. For example, 1,410 patients on the liver transplant waiting list died in 2015. Because of the exponential discrepancy between organ demand and supply, more organs of inferior quality are used every year. However, many of these organs are still discarded. The use of extended criteria donors (ECD) is a promising way to expand the available donor pool. In particular, donation after cardiac death (DCD) liver grafts has become increasingly important as they have become a larger proportion of the donor pool; over 18% of the total donor pool in 2015 (UNOS 2016). DCD kidney grafts are used successfully for clinical transplantation, with outcomes very similar to brain-dead donor grafts, however poorer outcomes have delayed the use of other DCD organs. Due to warm ischemic damage, DCD liver grafts, carry higher risks for delayed graft function (DGF), primary non-function, and biliary complications following transplantation (Saidi 2013). Biliary complications in DCD organs are a major source of morbidity, graft loss, and even mortality long-term after liver transplantation. These complications are much more common in DCD grafts (20–40% compared to 5% in grafts from brain-dead donors) (Jay 2011). The most troublesome biliary complication is the ischemic-type biliary lesions (ITBL), also called ischemic cholangiopathy.

The risk of ischemic cholangiopathy in grafts from DCD donors is 10 times higher than for brain dead donors (Jay 2011). Eventually, up to 50–65% of the patients with ITBL will require a retransplantation or may die (Merion 2006; Verdonk 2006). Most of DCD organs are discarded because of prolonged warm ischemia time, with most centers declining when longer than 30min. Because of poor results with DCD liver grafts after conventional cold storage preservation, interest in liver machine preservation was renewed (Guarrera 2010). For similar reasoning, interest in lung, heart, and pancreatic machine perfusion has been renewed as well, with aim to expand the donor pool through the resuscitation of extended criteria donor grafts.

Machine perfusion allows the opportunity to repair the damage of warm ischemia and cold storage, reawakens metabolic functions and measures the viability of a graft *ex-vivo* prior to transplantation. However, the simplicity and low cost of cold storage (CS) have kept it the standard of care for transplantation centers. Growing data supports the use of liver machine perfusion preservation, but the variability of systems, techniques, settings, and costs have interfered with standardization and global use. Likewise, heart, lung and pancreatic machine perfusion preservation have a growing body of data demonstrating potential superiority, but the technology has not yet been widely commercialized (Tolboom 2016; Karcz 2010).

The main categorization of machine perfusion preservation has traditionally been by perfusion temperature. Hypothermic machine perfusion (HMP) has been an attractive option to avoid further warm ischemic time and minimize graft metabolic requirements for ease of transport, while still providing oxygenation and metabolic support. Contrarily, much research supports the use of normothermic machine preservation (NMP) to most closely mimic the physiologic environment with oxygenation, nutrition, and full metabolic support. In addition, NMP has the advantage of more thoroughly testing organ functionality (for example bile production and lactate clearance in liver) prior to transplantation, which cannot be tested during hypothermic perfusion preservation. Other researchers have advocated for temperature profiles somewhere in between. Subnormothermic (SNMP) or rewarming machine preservation (RMP) represent some of the newest approaches to both liver and now kidney perfusion in their attempts to maximally increase graft metabolism while minimizing reperfusion injury resulting after cold storage. Optimal temperature, mode of oxygenation, ideal perfusate, perfusion cannulation, and pressure and flow settings are debated, but with little consensus as to ideal perfusion settings, even in kidney where the technology is clinically available. This chapter compiles a summary of the history of machine organ preservation, its most promising research, successful clinical applications, and what the future may hold for kidney, liver, heart, lung and pancreatic machine perfusion preservation.

KIDNEY MACHINE PERFUSION PRESERVATION

History and Introduction

The stilted progression of machine preservation is perhaps best explained by the history of kidney machine preservation. In the 1960s, Belzer et al. started experiments studying hypothermic machine perfusion (HMP) in canine kidneys and the first successful human transplantation of a hypothermically machine perfused kidney took place in 1968 (Belzer

1967). The perfusion preservation of kidneys first became part of clinical practice in the late 1960s using a perfusate of blood and cryoprecipitated plasma. By the 1970s, HMP was used to preserve and transport kidneys, extending the time grafts could be stored prior to subsequent successful transplantation.

However, after the definition of irreversible coma in 1968, the term brain death became accepted in the early 1970s. Consequently, centers shifted to procure organs from heart beating instead of non-heart-beating (NHB) donors, with increased success rates. The majority of transplant centers abandoned the practice of donation after circulatory death (DCD) due to associated higher complication and failure rates. Additionally, in 1980, the development of UW Solution allowed for 72 hour kidney preservation by simple CS, and use of MP was largely discontinued. Only young trauma patients were considered suitable candidates for DCD donation and these pristine organs were preserved equally well by either static cold storage (SCS) or HMP (Belzer 1980).

Over the last few decades, more marginal donors, as well as DCD donors are accepted to overcome organ shortage which has re-sparked interest in machine perfusion worldwide. Substantial experimental work on machine organ preservation contributed to improved clinical results in extended criteria donor kidney preservation. An international multicenter trial of 672 paired kidneys found that HMP reduced the risk of DGF, and decreased serum creatinine (Moers 2009). Therefore, machine perfusion became the method of choice to obtain good long-term preservation and for the preservation of marginal kidneys.

By 2008, nearly half of U.S. kidney transplants from extended criteria donors (ECD) and 70% of those from DCD donors were machine perfused (Catena 2013). During perfusion, a recirculating perfusate is continuously pumped through the organ vasculature, which can be non-oxygenated or oxygenated. A heat exchanger regulates perfusate temperature at hypothermic (0–4°C), sub-normothermic (20–30°C) or normothermic (37°C) temperatures.

The machine itself generally consists of a circulatory pump (which perfuses the organ *ex vivo*, after procurement) and renal artery cannulation (Jochmans 2016). Continuous perfusion (from procurement to implantation) and pre-implantation perfusion (after a period of SCS and just before transplantation) are the two most commonly used modalities. During perfusion, the kidney is supplied with nutrients and oxygen, has waste products removed, and can be treated with therapeutic agents. Historical challenges which persist today include understanding the metabolic requirement of the *ex vivo* perfused organ, understanding the effect of simple cold storage and the capacity to alleviate reperfusion injury, the development of *ex vivo* viability biomarkers, maintenance of endothelial cell integrity, and the engineering the ideal perfusate delivery system and settings (Belzer 1980).

Hypothermic Kidney Perfusion

Our discussion begins with HMP modalities as these are currently the only widely clinically available machine perfusion technique. HMP places kidney grafts under continuous circulation of a cold perfusate (0–4°C) through the cannulated renal artery immediately after procurement. Circulation of the perfusate is achieved through a device that generates either a continuous or pulsatile flow by a roller pump. HMP maintains hemodynamic stimulation of the vasculature, known to play a critical role in renal function under normal physiologic conditions. HMP may reduce ischemia-reperfusion (I/R) injury as was suggested by decreased levels of genes that are correlated with I/R injury in HMP kidneys compared to SCS-treated kidneys (Wszola 2014). Zhang et al. observed increased apoptosis in cold stored kidneys versus HMP kidneys in a canine DCD model, with phospho-AKT and ezrin expression induced in the HMP group, implying that cell proliferation, turnover, and renewal are positively influenced by HMP (Zhang 2016). A meta-analysis conducted between 1971 and 2001 showed HMP to be associated with a decreased relative risk of DGF of 0.80 (95% CI = 0.67–0.96) compared to SCS (Jochmans 2015). In 2009, a large randomized controlled trial was conducted comparing continuous HMP with SCS of 336 kidney pairs using the LifePort™, which showed an overall reduced risk of DGF in HMP kidneys compared to SCS kidneys (20.8% vs. 26.5%, $p = 0.05$) with increased one-year graft survival from 90% in SCS kidneys to 94% in HMP kidneys ($p = 0.04$) (Moers 2009).

HMP is thought to be of particular benefit in more marginal ECD grafts, which are particularly prone to IRI, DGF and PNF. A study compared ECD kidneys that were subjected to CS followed by HMP to kidneys that were treated with SCS throughout and HMP-treated organs showed markedly reduced expression of cytokines and soluble intracellular adhesion molecule type 1 (Tozzi 2013). In a study on 91 randomized ECD kidney pairs, HMP compared to SCS significantly reduced the risk of DGF (adjusted odds ratio (OR) = 0.46; 95% CI = 0.21–0.99), reduced PNF (3% vs. 12%, $p = 0.04$) and increased 1-year graft survival (92.3% vs. 80.2%, $p = 0.02$) (Treckmann 2011).

One category of ECD donors is the DCD donor (previously referred to as non-heart-beating) whose cardiac arrest occurs before organ procurement, exposing kidneys to an unavoidable extra period of warm ischemia (WI). Warm ischemia makes DCD organs particularly prone to the development of DGF. The literature reveals conflicting data on HMP in DCD kidneys. Many studies suggest that HMP of DCD kidneys leads to better outcomes, but other studies are not able to show a significant difference in DGF or graft survival. In the multi-center Eurotransplant trial on 82 DCD kidney pairs, HMP showed a reduced risk of DGF compared to SCS kidneys (53.7% vs. 69.5% respectively, $p = 0.025$) (Jochmans 2010). In 2010, Watson et al. published results on a RCT comparing HMP with SCS for 45 DCD kidney pairs which showed no beneficial effect on 1- or 3-year graft survival or DGF for hypothermic machine perfused kidneys (Watson 2010). These contradicting outcomes of the world's currently largest RCTs may be related to timing of HMP throughout procurement and transplantation. Hosgood et al. showed in a porcine kidney transplant model that the beneficial effect of MP disappears when kidneys are not pumped immediately after procurement (Hosgood 2011). In the Eurotransplant trial, kidneys were pumped immediately after retrieval at the donor center, whereas in the U.K. trial, kidneys were cold stored during transfer and HMP was started subsequently. New data suggests that alternative temperature profiles besides hypothermic may be more clearly beneficial in DCD kidneys, particularly those treated with an unavoidable period of SCS (Bagul 2008; Hosgood 2013; Hosgood 2011).

HMP Preservation Solutions

Countless preservation solutions have been created and trialed, all with different compositions aimed to prevent IRI and maximize graft survival and function. Early preservation solutions consisted of diluted blood and ringers lactate solution. Currently, the most commonly used preservation solutions are University of Wisconsin (UW), histidine-tryptophan-ketoglurate (HTK), Celsior, Institute George-Lopez (IGL-1), Polysol, EuroCollins, hypertonic citrate or Marshall solution (HOC), and phosphate-buffered sucrose (PBS).

In 1987, Belzer and colleagues developed the University of Wisconsin (UW) solution (also known as KPS-1 or Belzer's solution) and this became the gold standard among organ preservation solutions. In the European Multicenter Trial, the use of UW versus EuroCollins solution significantly reduced the rate of DGF (10% vs. 23%) (Ploeg 1992). UW shows good outcome of short- and long-term kidney preservation, but the main disadvantage is its high viscosity mainly due to hydroxyl ethyl starch (HES) (Catena 2013). For HMP, UW-G is used, in which a more extracellular solution is achieved through replacing lactobionate by gluconate and reducing the potassium level (Catena 2013).

Some institutions favor low-viscosity HTK solution to preserve DCD kidneys. HTK was introduced in 1980 by Bretschneider and is recommended in HMP at low pressures and in high perfusion volumes. More recently, Rauen and De Groot developed Custodiol-N solution as improved modification of the former HTK solution with iron chelators to inhibit cold-induced free radical-mediated injury, shown to be efficacious in protecting rat livers during HMP (Stegemann 2010). Developed in 1994, Celsior solution is a colloid and combines the osmotic efficacy of UW (lactobionate and mannitol) with the potent buffering ability of HTK (histidine), with the benefit of reduced tissue edema from hydrostatic pressure since Celsior contains macromolecules that do not pass the cellular membrane (Catena 2013).

The fairly new preservation solution IGL-1 combines the advantages of UW and Celsior with high sodium concentration and polyethylene glycol (PEG, 35 kDa), substituting HES. A non-randomized prospective multi-center study showed the same effectiveness for IGL-1 versus UW solution, but lower costs favor the former (Codas 2009). Polysol, a new low-viscosity preservation solution, is introduced to facilitate transplantation of ischemically damaged organs. Amino acids, vitamins, potent buffers, and anti-oxidants have been added to support metabolism during HMP (Bessems 2005). One of the main components is PEG 35, a low-molecular-weight colloid that does not increase viscosity as seen with HES-containing solutions. Polysol is currently used in experimental settings only, but recent reports seem promising. A study in a porcine auto-transplant model reports better preservation of microcirculation and renal function after 20-h SCS preservation compared to UW (Schreinemachers 2009).

HOC, or Marshall's solution is extensively used for clinical transplantation in the U.K. and Australia. HOC is an intracellular solution with high potassium content, mannitol as the impermanent ion, and citrate as its buffer. The hypertonic character of HOC prevents entry of fluid into the cells and has shown to be effective for 72-h canine kidney preservation (Kay 2009).

Oxygenation during HMP

In HMP, oxygenation plays a central role of importance for reconditioning organs after ischemic time. Lack of oxygen leads to ATP decrease, which can be as large as 80% for kidneys (Jassem 2004). Continuous oxygenation during perfusion is thought to be useful to support the metabolic demand of the organ. However, high concentrations of oxygen are believed to favor the production of oxygen free radicals and promote adverse effects on tissue during long-term oxygenated preservation (Stegemann 2010; Rauen 2004). Many studies strongly suggest oxygen to be a constitutive adjunct in HMP, improving functional outcome of the graft. Hoyer and colleagues showed that HMP with 100% oxygen results in higher flow and lower renal resistance (RR) during perfusion and improved graft function as compared to oxygen-free HMP (Hoyer 2014). Positive results for oxygenated HMP were confirmed with a 3 month post-transplant follow-up by showing lower serum and peak creatinine levels and injury markers, which correlated with improved longer term outcomes of lower serum creatinine, less proteinuria and less chronic kidney fibrosis (Thuillier 2013). Kron et al. investigated the effects of 1 hour hypothermic oxygenated perfusion (HOPE) following a period of CS and immediately prior to transplantation, with dramatic improvements in graft function after transplantation as shown by decreased nuclear injury, macrophage activation, endothelium activation, tubular damage, and improved graft function (Kron 2016). Grafts exposed to warm ischemia, simulating DCD, seem to particularly benefit from oxygenated perfusion with restored ATP stores in DCD porcine kidneys, but no added benefit of oxygenation was found in kidneys without injury (Buchs 2011).

Commercial Hypothermic Machine Perfusion Devices

As HMP is gaining recognition, more perfusion machines are becoming available. (For more details see the chapter Isolated Kidney Perfusion Models). The most commonly used device in Europe and the USA is the pressure-driven LifePort Kidney Transporter (Organ Recovery Systems, Itasca, IL, USA). Another commercially available system is the flow-driven Waters Medical RM3 (Birmingham, AL, USA). In both systems, the operator can modify the systolic perfusion pressure, with flow and resistance recorded over time. Relevant differences between the systems are related to the way both devices generate and control flow and pressure. The RM3 uses a flow-driven system, which requires 50% higher systolic pressures (45 vs. 30 mm Hg) to obtain similar flow rates. A comparative study on both systems demonstrated minimal differences in early kidney recovery, but significantly higher levels of post-transplant fibrosis in kidneys preserved by RM3 compared to LifePort (Wszola 2013). Another study showed favorable results for the LifePort device compared to RM3 with shorter duration of DGF after transplant, lower incidences of interstitial fibrosis and tubular atrophy in biopsies taken within 1-year post transplant, and lower renal resistance during perfusion (Wszola 2013).

Sub-Normothermic Kidney Perfusion

The interest in sub-normothermic machine perfusion (SNMP) increased as an attempt to alleviate or prevent organ injury caused by a sometimes unavoidable period of SCS preservation, which seems to be especially damaging to DCD organs. In a porcine model of renal I/R injury, oxygenated SNMP demonstrated better protection of the organ compared to cold storage. Moreover, SNMP grafts showed nearly twofold better values of creatinine clearances compared to oxygenated HMP. SNMP also permits higher pressure perfusion with reduced risk of endothelial and vascular impairment, as higher temperatures increase vascular compliance (Hoyer 2014). Higher temperatures also lead to higher metabolic demands requiring active oxygenation and sufficient perfusion flow. The use of SNMP in clinical kidney transplantation has not yet been reported.

Gradual Rewarming

Another experimental machine perfusion temperature profile is gradual rewarming based on the hypothesis that ischemic damage results from the abrupt temperature shift from hypo- to normothermia, leading to mitochondrial dysfunction and proapoptotic signal transduction (Hoyer 2016). Recent studies have investigated the effect of the controlled oxygenated rewarming (COR), a concept that originated in liver perfusion due to logistical necessities of a period of SCS prior to machine perfusion. Schopp et al. reported a nearly twofold increase in renal clearances of creatinine and urea after COR of pig kidneys compared to controls. This was accompanied by significantly improved renal oxygen consumption and less cellular apoptosis (Schopp 2015). Similarly, Mahboub et al. demonstrated lower levels of transaminases, and heat shock protein 70, ICAM-1, VCAM-1 mRNA expressions were decreased in gradually rewarmed kidneys. Kidneys that underwent gradual rewarming suffered less renal parenchymal tubular injury and showed better endothelial preservation (Mahboub 2015). These data suggest that a gradual increase in temperature results in better energetic recovery, less cellular injury, and ultimately superior function of kidneys subjected to COR, however, there have been no clinical applications in kidney perfusion to date.

Normothermic Kidney Perfusion

In contrast to cold preservation, the concept of normothermic machine perfusion (NMP) is to closely replicate the physiological environment and maintain cellular metabolism during preservation. With aerobic metabolism restored, the kidney grafts regain function and minimize cold ischemic insult, thought to be preferred in the resuscitation of DCD and ECD kidneys. NMP has been shown to replenish ATP stores and up-regulate repair mechanisms such as heat shock protein 70, which aids repair due to oxidative damage (Hosgood 2013). However, the act of rewarming may aggravate inflammatory processes and increase graft injury, particularly without optimal perfusion settings, nutrients and oxygenation profiles. Proinflammatory cytokines, such as IL-6, are upregulated in response to ischemic injury and were released in the kidney during reperfusion after NMP (Hosgood 2013). Alternatively, IL-6 can also have anti-inflammatory properties in resolving tissue damage after an initial inflammatory response (Nechemia-Arbely 2008).

Ex vivo NMP should most ideally be used throughout the preservation interval, which is logistically difficult due to tenuous perfusion requirements. Alternatively, NMP can be implemented for a shorter period prior to transplantation as a form of graft resuscitation. One practical proposed approach is to use 1–2 hours of NMP as a restorative period prior to transplantation to allow graft function and replenish ATP stores (Bagul 2008; Hosgood 2013; Hosgood 2011). NMP-resuscitated kidneys had less tubular injury, improved blood flow and oxygenation and were metabolically more stable as compared to the cold stored kidneys. In 2011, Hosgood et al. reported the first case of successful kidney transplantation in man after the organ was cold stored for 11h, followed by 35 min of *ex vivo* NMP. The 55-year old recipient had slow graft function, but ultimately remained dialysis independent (Hosgood 2011). A pilot clinical study compared 18 ECD kidneys that received 1h of pre-implantation blood-based NMP with 47 matched SCS controls. Significantly lower DGF rates were observed with pre-implantation NMP (5.6% vs. 36.2%, $p = 0.014$) (Hosgood 2013).

Since DCD and ECD organs poorly tolerate the effects of hypothermia in SCS, a more novel approach of NMP totally avoids storage in hypothermic conditions. A study by Kaths et al. demonstrated that NMP with an erythrocyte-based solution could replace hypothermic storage techniques. NMP kidneys showed similar serum creatinine levels and creatinine clearance post-transplant compared to SCS grafts. After 10 days follow-up, NMP animals had serum creatinine and blood urea nitrogen values comparable to basal levels, whereas SCS grafts showed elevated values (Kaths 2016). Recently, Hosgood et al. reported the successful transplantation of a pair of human kidneys that were deemed unsuitable for transplantation due to inadequate perfusion, but subsequently were transplanted after perfusion and assessment using *ex vivo* NMP (Hosgood 2016).

Normothermic Preservation Solutions

Continuous perfusion with an oxygenated solution to support aerobic metabolism is key under normothermic conditions. During NMP, the perfusate can be based on either a natural oxygen carrier such as blood or an artificial-based medium. Early preservation solutions consisted of diluted blood and Ringers lactate solution. From 1985 until 1993 Collins or Euro-Collins solution was the commonly used solution, and from 1993 onwards, this shifted to UW, which is still the gold standard for abdominal organ preservation today (Wight 2003).

Brasile et al. were the first to develop an acellular normothermic solution based on perfluorocarbon (PFC) emulsion and enriched tissue culture-like medium containing essential and non-essential amino acids, lipids and carbohydrates (Brasile 1994). PFCs are inert solutions that have a high capacity for dissolving oxygen. New, more stable, PFCs are now being developed mainly as blood substitutes. Humphreys et al. recently used a commercially made PFC to provide oxygenation and reduce ischemic injury to the kidney during warm ischemia by retrograde infusion through the urinary system (Humphreys 2006). These new generation PFCs could potentially be developed as normothermic preservation solutions. However, due to complexity of manufacturing, they are very expensive. A more stable pyridoxalated haemoglobin polyoxyethylene (PHP) solution has proven to be more successful and Brasile et al. have since replaced the PFC with this solution (Stubenitsky 2000). Other solutions such as Lifor (an artificial preservation medium containing a non-protein oxygen carrier, nutrients and growth factors) have also been used during NMP. Some studies have shown higher flow rates in Lifor perfused kidneys compared to UW (Gage 2009; Olschewski 2010). The most newly reported acellular solution is Hemarina-M101, extracellular hemoglobin derived from a marine invertebrate. It has been formulated into an oxygen carrier mainly as a blood substitute. M101 has been used in SCS to deliver oxygen with favorable results and functions over a wide range of temperatures (4–37°C) (Thuillier 2011).

A blood-based solution during NMP was previously considered limited due to hemolysis, platelet activation, deterioration of red blood cell oxygen-carrying capacity, high intra-renal resistance and tissue edema (Thiara 2007). However, results of an isolated perfusion system with 1 unit of compatible packed red blood cells mixed with a priming solution and added protective agents are promising. In a series of 18 ECD kidneys, DGF was 5.6% compared to 36% in similarly matched recipients of a kidney undergoing SCS (Nicholson 2013).

Normothermic Machine Perfusion Viability Assessment

In contrast to HMP, kidney function can be evaluated during NMP by directly assessing functional measures such as blood perfusion, renal blood flow and urine output. Recently, Hosgood et al. used *ex vivo* NMP to develop a novel scoring system for pre-transplant assessment of marginal kidneys (Hosgood 2015). Based on assessment scores from their clinical series, it became clear that kidneys with a score of 1 to 4 could be transplanted successfully. Kidneys with a score of 5 would be considered very high-risk and unlikely to be suitable for transplantation. In their study on 36 kidneys, grafts with an assessment score of 3 had a significantly higher incidence of DGF (38%) compared to kidneys with a score of 1 (6%) or 2 (0%) ($p = 0.024$). The ability to assess organs adequately prior to transplantation is an especially important benefit of *ex vivo* machine perfusion and is an especially powerful use for NMP.

LIVER MACHINE PRESERVATION

History and Introduction

In 1935, Alexis Carrel and Charles Lindbergh designed the first liver perfusion machine using pressure-controlled, oxygenated normothermic perfusate in a glass device (Dutkowski 2008). In spite of significant technical advances, no system has been proven to clinically significantly extend the length of *ex vivo* organ viability as compared to CS in preservation solutions such as University of Wisconsin (UW), Histidine-Tryptophane-Ketoglutarate (HTK) and Celsior. After the first unsuccessful attempts of hypothermic perfusion of human livers by Starzl et al. in 1967, the clinical use and development of human liver perfusion devices did not move forward (Starzl 1967). Because of the success of cold storage preservation in UW solution, there was no need to use machine preservation until the use of marginal livers became necessary due to increased discrepancy between demand and supply. Several clinical trials now support the preferred use of machine perfusion in grafts which have been subjected to warm ischemic time, but the ideal machine perfusion set-up and settings are still very much debated. In 2010, Guarrera et al. reported the first successful human liver transplantations following hypothermic machine perfusion preservation (Guarrera 2010). More recently, Dutkowski has examined matched case analyses of HMP vs. cold storage with marked decrease of intrahepatic cholangiopathy, biliary complications and improved 1 year graft survival (Dutkowski 2015). In 2016, Bral et al. published the first clinical normothermic machine perfusion transplantation series, demonstrating feasibility and safety, but bringing to light the questions of ideal methodology (Bral 2016).

Liver Perfusion Route

Given the unique physiology of liver perfusion *in vivo*, several perfusion routes have been advocated for machine liver perfusion. Portal vein only perfusion is commonly used in rat liver perfusion for simplicity reasons, but is generally believed inferior for larger animal models and humans. Arguments for hepatic artery perfusion include perhaps superior oxygen supply to the peribiliary vascular plexus (Bruggenwirth 2016). Although it has been reported that the biliary ducts also have blood supply from the portal vein (Slieker 2012), the biliary tract is mainly supplied with arterial blood through the Peribiliary vascular plexus (PVP) and therefore, any injury to the PVP may contribute to the ischemic death of the biliary epithelial cells after transplantation (Nishida 2006). The importance of hepatic artery perfusion is illustrated by the high incidence of biliary necrosis and strictures after hepatic artery thrombosis (HAT) in patients after liver transplantation (Mourad 2014). Additionally, during early reperfusion, the O_2 delivery is heavily dependent on arterial flow and as a result, dual perfusion is superior to portal perfusion in bile production as well as output of phospholipid, cholesterol and bilirubin (Foley 1999, 2003). Combined arterial and portal machine perfusion of DCD porcine livers also results in a better preservation of the PVP and less arteriolonecrosis (Op den Dries 2014).

Hepatic artery perfusion alone seems to be less beneficial than portal vein or dual perfusion (Compagnon 2001). All trials of NMP, SNMP or rewarming machine perfusion (RMP) utilized dual perfusion circuits, as these methods attempt to approximate physiologic conditions and maximize oxygenation. Most HMP studies also utilized dual perfusion circuits with few studies demonstrating portal vein perfusion only. Portal vein only studies state goals such as simplifying machine perfusion or improving machine portability. No study argues portal vein only perfusion to be superior or even comparable to the benefits of a dual perfusion system (with the exception of Schlegel et al. in the setting of HMP (Shlegel 2015). Dual porcine machine perfusion through hepatic artery (HA) and portal vein (PV) appears to be more effective at alleviating reperfusion injury than either portal vein or hepatic artery alone (Foley 1999).

The physiology of liver perfusion is notably complex, and is an additional reason for dual perfusion that it most closely mimics *in vivo* mechanics. For example, one study showed the principle of *ex vivo* flow competition: arterial pressure alters portal flow (Monbaliu 2012). For reasons of functional rejuvenation of liver tissue as well as providing consistent physiology-mimicking perfusion, most researchers choose dual perfusion in porcine machine liver perfusion models, and this practice has transferred over to the first trials in human livers.

Normothermic Liver Perfusion

The tenant of NMP has long been the replication of physiologic parameters to minimize ischemia and maximize *ex vivo* metabolism. Hence, most NMP trials utilize modified heparinized blood solutions or Steen solution plus erythrocytes as the perfusate (Monbaliu 2012; St Peter 2002; Reddy 2005; Xu 2012; Knaak 2014; Liu 2014; Schon 2001). Other studies have utilized Celsior (Gringeri 2012), Steen (Boehnert 2013), Custodiol (Minor 2013), or UW gluconate (Obara 2013) or Modified nutritive Williams' medium E (Izamis 2014) as perfusate. Liu et al. directly compared Steen Solution vs. Steen with erythrocytes vs. whole blood with the result that aspartate aminotransferase (AST), alanine aminotransferase (ALT) and LDH production was decreased and bile production was increased with improved histology in the groups with erythrocytes or whole blood, emphasizing the importance of an oxygen carrier in NMP. All NMP studies utilized dual perfusion routes, mimicking physiology and perfused for a minimum of 3 hours up to as long as 24 hours (Liu 2014). Early studies were aimed to lengthen liver storage up to 72 hours (Butler 2002). Other proponents of NMP claimed that it decreased ischemia reperfusion injury and resulted in superior bile production (Imber 2002; St Peter 2002). All NMP studies utilize oxygenators. Perfusion was controlled by either pressure of flow with flow being less popular at 5 out of 16 studies and a few studies using flow for hepatic artery (HA) and pressure for portal vein (PV) or vice versa. Goal pressures ranged from 50–100 mm Hg for the hepatic artery and 3–10 mm Hg for the PV. Flows ranged from 150–700 mL/min for HA and 950–1750 mL/min for the PV, with a few studies reporting flow as a function of liver weight at HA 0.16–0.25 mL/min/g and PV as 0.22–0.8 mL/min/g.

The benefits of NMP are nearly undisputed in the literature, but the addition of NMP into clinical practice is logistically complicated. Now that CS is the established standard preservation, and most centers lack perfusion machines, some period of CS in clinical practice is unavoidable. Four hours of CS prior to NMP results in statistically significant reduction in bile and Factor V production, reduction of glucose stores, increased release of AST and ALT, and base excess and endothelial injury, as shown through increased hyaluronic acid as well as necrosis in histology, and none of these parameters were normalized if NMP was performed following CS (St Peter 2002).

Subnormothermic and Rewarming Liver Perfusion

The unavoidable period of CS has brought upon newer variations of NMP where the liver is perfused either at subnormothermic temperatures or the perfusate is gradually rewarmed from cold storage to normothermic temperatures. Initial perfusion at a cold temperature enables replenishment of cellular energy stores in order to reduce ischemia reperfusion injury upon rewarming. Subnormothermic Machine perfusion (SNMP) was shown to improve tissue energetics, peroxidation and increased bile production (Minor 2013) as well as better recover homeostasis, oxygen consumption, bile production and histology (Knaak 2014) However, others have found decreased bile production, increased AST/ALT and worse histology using SNMP (21C) versus NMP (38.5) (Nassar 2016). Temperature controlled rewarming has been found to result in decreased release of LDH and superior mechanistic properties of the livers such as pressure curves (Obara 2013). Gradually warming warm-ischemic treated livers to normothermic perfusion or subnormothermic perfusion was also shown to lower liver enzyme release, increase ATP stores, improve bile production and improve histology as compared to hypothermic or subnormothernic perfusions (Minor 2013; Furukori 2016). Most recently, rewarming perfusion was shown to improve international normalized ratio (INR) (marker of coagulation factor production), bile production as well as minimize sinusoidal endothelial cell injury and activation of Kupffer cells. However, extending the rewarming phase to 60 or 120 min rather than 20–30 min decreased synthetic liver functions perhaps by increasing anaerobic respiration time (Banan 2016). Preliminary studies also suggest a period of in situ subnormothermic extracorporeal membrane oxygenation (ECMO) prior to rewarming compounds the benefits of subnormothermic machine perfusion (SNMP) on resuscitation of livers after (warm ischemic time) WIT (Hagiwara 2016). Others found that gradual increase of perfusate flow and oxygen throughout the rewarming period minimized AST/ALT release (Morito 2016). Controlled oxygenated rewarming perfusion (COR) was also shown to be superior in recovering energy stores and minimizing hepatocellular and mitochondrial damage after 18 hours of CS as compared to NMP (Hoyer 2016). COR also resulted in lower mitochondrial caspase-9-activity. Significantly lower enzyme leakage and higher bile production were also observed during reperfusion. The first clinical application of COR has recently been successfully applied in liver transplantation (Hoyer 2016).

Hypothermic Liver Perfusion

In contrast to NMP settings, HMP settings are by definition, not particularly physiologic, with perfusate temperature most commonly defined as 4 C. Many porcine HMP studies used KPS-1 Solution (Jain 2004, Monbaliu 2007, Vekemans 2007), while many others used UW Solution or Belzer MP (Obara 2012; Schlegel 2013). Bessems at al. was unique in comparing Celsior perfusate versus Polysol with the result that Celsior solution was more damaging than Polysol, increasing AST/ALT and intravascular resistance to a greater extent (Bessems 2006). (For more detailed discussion of perfusion solutions see above where we discussed kidney perfusion). Most studies, besides the exceptions noted in section "perfusion routes," used a dual circuit (portal vein and hepatic artery perfusion) and most recent studies seem to agree that dual circuit HMP seems more beneficial. In many studies, the lengths of perfusion for HMP were much longer than NMP, up to 24 hours, as HMP is looked at as a potential means to extend the storage time of donated livers. Most studies since 2013 have focused on recovery of donor livers from warm ischemia time and have shorter perfusion times ranging from 1 to 4 hours. Most studies used pressure-controlled circuits with hepatic pressures 20–30 mm Hg (exception Monbaliu with increasing pressures to 55 then 70) and portal pressures 3–13mm Hg with the majority limited to less than 7 mm Hg.

Studies in 2005 through 2007 focused on defining the capabilities of HMP. HMP was shown to maintain superior oxygen consumption and decrease ALT when compared to cold storage (Jain 2004). A portable perfusion machine was shown to maintain a liver for 24 hours with no significant histological damage (van der Plaats 2006). The pattern of decreasing HA vascular resistance over the first 6 hours of perfusion was first noted by Monbaliu et al. Also noted in this study was the introduction of anoxic vacuoles by HMP, likely due to lack of oxygenation in this study, and inability of their HMP livers to produce bile *ex vivo*. Another study showed increased ATP stores after HMP, indicating better preservation of energy stores as well as use of an oxygenator directly protecting against anoxic vacuolization (Vekemans 2007).

Predicting Pretransplantation Viability

A strong argument for the use of machine preservation is the added ability to assess viability of donor liver grafts prior to transplantation. Proposed outcome measures include flow and pressure characteristics and perfusate enzymes such as AST and LDH. The assessment of liver grafts is complicated by its unique dual blood supply, and the wide ranged and low flow portal system. Obara et al. found that hepatic arterial pressure, AST and LDH correlated well with warm ischemia time (WIT) during HMP (Obara 2012). Logically, oxygen consumption, complement/factor V production, bile production, and hyaluronic acid (marker of endothelial injury) have been used as outcomes and their levels correlated to damage found in histology. Other recent studies suggest the use of microRNA profiles of perfusate samples as indicators of WI injury and prediction of PNF. One miRNA, miR-22, was correlated to transplantation survival outcome, but is believed to have low diagnostic potential (Khorsandi 2015). Further work must be done to establish the best *ex vivo* markers of WI injury and reperfusion injury to determine the best predictors of good transplantation outcomes.

When focusing on histologic changes caused by warm ischemia, it is important to perform reperfusion with whole blood because it magnifies ischemia reperfusion injury (IRI). Whole blood has all the key players of ischemia reperfusion injury, namely the complement system, white blood cells, and platelets. One cannot expect to see all the changes associated with IRI if the liver is not perfused with blood experimentally. Likewise, clinically it is difficult to assess the degree of IRI during HMP as the liver becomes metabolically less active and NMP allows for improved functional assessment *ex vivo* prior to transplantation. Despite many failed attempts to quantify in an experimental setting the impact of HMP using whole blood reperfusion, Op Den Dries et al. showed after 30 minutes WI and no CS, that HA flow and ATP content increased after HMP, while AST and LDH decreased significantly. HMP-treated livers also showed improved histology and lower caspase-3 levels. This study was also significant for the use of miRNA and the establishment of miRNA profiles in the porcine model which may be helpful in profiling livers damaged by WI (Op den Dries 2013). After 60 minutes WI and 5 hours CS, Schlegel et al. found that the effects of 1 hour of hypothermic oxygenated portal perfusion on NAD^+, CO_2, Cytochrome C, AST, HMGB1, histology, TNFα resulted in decreased cytochrome C, HMGB1, AST and better histology with reduced Kupffer cell activiation (decreased TNFα). This study also compared low perfusion pressures to high perfusion pressures, showing that low pressure perfusion (3 mm Hg) was superior to high (8 mm Hg) (Schlegel 2013). Liu et al. studied pH, AST, L-fatty acid binding protein (L-FABP), ATP and redox-activated iron after 0–120 minutes WI and no CS, attempting to create a damage index predictive of ischemia reperfusion injury. AST level and pH in the perfusate proved the most valuable predictors studied (Liu 2014).

Shifting attention to potential *ex vivo* assessment, a recent review by Verhoeven et al. showed that bile production during NMP correlated well with early graft survival, as did bilirubin and phospholipid concentration, which are increased by NMP (Verhoeven 2014). Impaired secretion of phospholipids after CS may result in a high bile salt/phospholipid ratio known to be toxic to cholangiocytes and associated with the development of ITBL. Hepatocyte injury is generally measured by release of AST, ALT, and LDH into the perfusate, and is correlated with both warm ischemia time and poorer survival post transplantation. Traditionally, energy status is recorded by ATP levels, hyaluronic acid and thrombomodulin have become established markers for endothelial injury. Inflammatory markers such as TNF-α levels are shown to correlate positively on histology with Kupffer cell activation. Peribiliary epithelial and vascular injury is represented by arteriolosclerosis and changes in the luminal size of the portal vein branch, but these changes were only present after reperfusion. Lastly, a particular profile of miRNA in the bile is associated with later development of ischemic type biliary injury (Khorsandi 2015).

Future of Clinical Liver Machine Perfusion

Nearly a century of experimental *ex vivo* machine perfusion of livers has left modern medical science in much the same place it started: What is the clinical role for *ex vivo* liver perfusion and how can it best be implemented? Recent breakthroughs finally may show what clinical liver machine perfusion may look like. Simple cold storage in UW Solution has become the gold standard worldwide such that any proposed perfusion must accept some period of interim cold storage prior to perfusion and that the perfusion must add some benefit beyond simple cold storage. At one point, the goal was to increase the length of the organ's viability as compared to cold storage, but with modern transportation and the organ donation system, machine perfusion has not been rigorously shown to be effective in this regard. Modern goals of machine perfusion look towards restoring organ damage, for example extending donor criteria by alleviating damaging effects of warm ischemia in DCD livers. Additionally, modern perfusion systems look to test viability and predict dysfunction of donated livers prior to transplantation. Reviewing the successes and pitfalls of various machine perfusion techniques can show us where the greatest successes have been and where future studies should focus their energies.

As early as 1970, Belzer et al. showed the promise of NMP in maintaining livers *ex-vivo* by showing equivalent outcomes after 8–10 hours NMP as compared to immediate transplantation. Schon et al. showed that 4 hours of NMP could reverse histology, bile production, alpha GST and AST levels after WI injury, and prevent the PNF seen within 24 hours of non-perfused livers (Schon 2001). However, many of these studies included no CS time. Brockmann et al. also showed improved survival with 5 or 20 hours of NMP, particularly in organs that had been severely ischemic (after 40 minutes of WI injury) (Brockmann 2009).

Of the porcine liver hypothermic machine preservation (HMP) studies, results have shown promising resuscitation of WI damaged livers, but the aspect of reperfusion injury remains largely untested. Obara et al. showed promise with the HA normalized pressure recovery to baseline with 2–3 hours of HMP. Li et al. were only able to show slightly delayed morphologic change, apoptosis and release of AST/ALT with cold storage as compared to CS (Li 2015). De Rougemont et al. showed HMP increased glutathione stores and arterial pressure and HMP liver recipients survived whereas CS recipients did not (de Rougemont 2009).

In trials of transplantation after HMP, no benefit is seen as compared to cold storage (Guarrera 2004) except in the resuscitation of unsalvageable livers after 60 min warm ischemia (de Rougemont 2009) where transplants were viable only after HMP, and had improved GSH stores and arterial pressure. Many pig liver transplant studies showed survival rates after WI and HMP as low as 33% (Vekemans 2009) and 20% (Fondevila 2011), speaking both to the technical difficulty of the porcine transplantation model and the livers sensitivity to warm ischemia. Most promising were livers with only 30 min warm ischemia for which HMP improved survival from 0% in CS to 75% in HMP with lower AST and LDH (Shigeta 2012). While histologically and biochemically HMP-treated porcine livers were better preserved as compared to CS, the liver viability is still less than excellent in these preclinical trials.

The clearest side by side demonstration of the effects of NMP, HMP, and rewarming machine perfusion (RMP) comes from a study by Shigeta et al. who studied porcine livers after 60 min WI and 2 hours CS and compared n = 3 orthotopic liver transplantations after 2 hours of either NMP, HMP, or RMP. In 24 hours, the study found that all NMP and HMP livers suffered PNF with 0% survival, with 75% survival and improved histology in the RMP group (Shigeta 2013). Others have been able to show 100% survival after no warm ischemia and preservation at 21°C RMP with total alleviation of post reperfusion syndrome, lower AST/ALT and less centrilobular necrosis. RMP transplants were perfused in UW gluconate solution with added branched chain amino acids, with the SNP livers perfused using cell-free bovine-derived hemoglobin with hetastarch colloid (Fontes 2015).

The porcine model has provided a stepping stone and a wealth of iterative learning about *ex vivo* liver machine perfusion preservation. With physiological, anatomical and immunological properties similar to humans, porcine livers have allowed the modeling of warm ischemia and ischemia reperfusion injury as well as establishing markers predictive of post-transplantation outcomes. With SNP and RMP, studies are showing clinically applicable methodology which is improving post-transplantation outcomes with modeled extended criteria donors. The potentials of SNP and RMP perfusions are clear to see, as more and more researchers are publishing results preferring these temperature settings. It has not been fully defined how slowly livers should be rewarmed, the critical temperature the liver must reach, and the length of warm perfusion needed to maximize metabolic parameters. Finally, researchers are producing clinically viable solutions to extending liver donation criteria to include DCD livers. Future studies should focus on essential requirements for limits of recoverable warm ischemic time, limits for length of CS prior to perfusion, in addition to perfusion settings, and upon ideal perfusion time to maximize liver viability. Additionally, studies which follow porcine perfusion transplantation models for three to six month would expand our understanding of the development of ischemic cholangiopathy and consequent biliary stenosis, and potentially protective role of machine perfusions. Before clinical implementation of machine perfusion preservation, *ex-vivo* markers which reliably predict major transplantation outcomes, such as primary non-function and early allograft dysfunction, must be established.

Lastly, we turn our attention towards machine preservation which has been implemented in human trials. Implementation of HMP after a period of CS for ECD human livers was shown to improve ATP stores and result in increased bile, bilirubin and bicarbonate production, but was not able to reduce hepatobiliary injury as measured by AST, ALT, LDH and gamma-glutamyl transferase as tested with NMP simulated transplantation (Westerkamp 2016). However, in a matched graft study of two European hospitals, DCD livers treated with oxygenated HMP prior to transplantation had reduced ALT, cholangiopathy, biliary complications and improved 1-year graft survival compared to SCS-treated DCD grafts, and decreased necessity of retransplantation (18% SCS to 0% HMP) (Dutowski 2015). The first ECD human liver was transplanted after resuscitation with NMP in 2015 (Perera 2016) with subsequent studies summarizing their results (Mergental 2016). Recently, a single-center study in Canada showed the feasibility of ten human DCD livers treated with NMP for a mean of 11.5 hours prior to transplantation, with a small decrease in six-month graft survival in NMP-treated livers (80%) versus SCS livers (100%), demonstrating the technical difficulty of implementing liver NMP clinically (Bral 2016). Additionally, the superiority of COR and SNMP in porcine livers sparked the first successful application of COR in liver transplantation (Hoyer 2016). Rewarming therapies, the newest methodology in machine preservation, may become the ultimate compromise with their ability to capture advantages of relative convenience as compared to NMP, longevity of storage comparable to HMP or SCS, optimal resuscitation in predictive animal models, and *ex vivo* assessment prior to transplantation. After nearly 60 years of experimental liver machine perfusion, we may soon see its role develop in clinical medicine. Now that trials are honing in on the particulars of a protocol for superior liver machine preservation, trials need to be thorough about reporting their perfusion results to allow for comparison and pooled analysis among clinical trials (Karangwa 2016).

Heart Machine Preservation

As with the liver, technical difficulty in cannulation and determination of perfusion settings has limited clinical applicability of machine perfusion. However, the heart is unique in that current preservation techniques and transplantation guidelines severely limit the number of usable grafts which can be matched with a recipient. Nearly 50% of discarded heart donations could have been used if a suitable recipient was available within the time constraints of modern heart transplantation (DiMaio 2013). Additionally, DCD heart donations are critically limited due to the unavoidable period of warm ischemia. HMP has produced encouraging results in porcine hearts subjected to warm ischemia, increasing energy stores, decreasing lactate levels and increasing contractility as compared to CS in simulated transplantation (Van Caenegem 2016). HMP has the capability to better preserve ultrastructure compared to CS as seen by electron microscopy with decreased muscle fiber and endothelial cell damage and less apoptosis (assessed by TUNEL) as compared to cold storage (Michel 2015). Most perfusion attempts have focused on perfusion via the aorta, which is limited by aortic valve incompetence. One recent study showed promising results of canine hearts treated with hypothermic retrograde perfusion via the coronary sinus, allowing for 14 hour preservation, increased pre-load recruitable stroke work and decreased creatinine kinase release as compared to SCS hearts, but unfortunately showing no differences in histological assessment of cell death (TUNEL) (Brant 2016.) Retrograde perfusion raises concerns over inferior right ventricle (RV) perfusion, and canine hearts did show decreased RV perfusion, with no RV dysfunction noted upon transplantation. The same retrograde system as applied to human hearts showed preservation of oxidative metabolism and low lactate-to-alanine ratios, suggesting superior RV tissue protection (Cobert 2014). Another concern with regards to machine perfusion of the heart in general is the resultant interstitial edema which results in graft weight increase prior to transplantation, but this edema has not been clearly proven to diminish graft function (Brant 2016).

Normothermic perfusion has also been trialed in heart resuscitation prior to transplantation, as a reconditioning method following cold storage and prior to transplantation. As found in the liver, NMP more closely mimics human physiology resulting in superior *ex vivo* assessment of organ functionality. Phase I Trials of the prospective multicenter European Trial to evaluate the safety and performance of the Organ Care System for heart transplants (PROTECT) and effectiveness evaluation (PROCEED) both showed promising results for heart NMP with whole blood perfusate, with 100% and 93% survival at 30 days, comparable to CS (McCurry 2008). It has since been found that functional parameters such as stroke work, ejection fraction and ventricular relaxation measured during NMP better predict myocardial performance as compared to metabolic parameters (White 2015). One study found rat hearts subjected to WI and CS time had improved contractility after normothermic reconditioning (Tolboom 2015). The same group recently compared normothermic resuscitation to subnormothermic (SNMP) at 20°C with superior preservation in the SNMP group with decreased troponin-t levels and higher ATP stores (Tolboom 2016). As has been found in liver perfusion, there may be a role for SNMP or rewarming perfusion as a compromise between the longevity benefits of hypothermic perfusion and the resuscitation and assessment capabilities of normothermic perfusion. As researchers learn more about heart machine preservation, many hope that clinical implementation of machine perfusion will increase the quality of DCD and ECD grafts and enable distant procurement for dramatic increase of the heart donor pool.

Lung Machine Preservation

As with DCD hearts, DCD lungs are fragile and often critically damaged by warm ischemia. Indeed, 80% of potential brain death donor lungs are injured in the intensive care unit and deemed unusable for transplantation (Cypel 2009.) Therefore, machine perfusion capable of reconditioning and repairing damaged grafts possesses the potential to drastically increase the donor pool. Lung machine preservation is unique among organ machine perfusion in that evaluation of high-risk graft function is a necessity rather than an improvement, and machine perfusion could additionally be used to treat and repair lung grafts. Preclinical trials have thus far focused on hyperoncotic perfusates to intentionally draw fluid from the intravascular space to decrease lung edema. A few early trials showed promising results with HMP. HMP was used as a delivery system for oxygen free radical scavengers in canine heart-lungs with improved histology and lower resulting creatinine phosphokinase in the treated heart-lungs (Hajjar 1986). HMP was also shown to ameliorate IRI in rat lungs subjected to WI, with replenished energy stores, decreased vascular resistance, increase pulmonary compliance and improved pulmonary oxygenation (Nakajima 2011). The same group showed similar promising results in canine hearts with 2 hour HMP (Steen perfusate) following WI and 12 hour SCS time with elimination of microthrombi histologically, improved energy stores and improved physiologic lung functions (Nakajima 2012).

Although only a small number of medical centers have begun to use lung machine preservation, early results show benefit in conditioning and resuscitation of lung grafts thought to be unsuitable for transplantation. In a study aimed to assess clinical feasibility, high risk lungs were treated with 4 hours of normothermic perfusion and then 20 of 23 high-risk lungs were transplanted, with no difference between these high risk grafts and regular lung grafts transplanted in the same time period (Cypel 2011). NMP was therefore useful in restoration of high risk graft function and a useful tool in the elimination of truly unsuitable grafts. Additionally, lung NMP has been found an effective delivery system for antibiotics and gene therapies to better optimize the fragile grafts for transplantation (Nakajima 2016). One anti-inflammatory cytokine, IL-10 was upregulated by an adenoviral vector delivered through 12 hours of NMP in discarded lung grafts, which resulted in superior arterial oxygen pressure and decreased pulmonary vascular resistance, suggestive of successful lung injury repair (Cypel 2009). Still in its early days, there is a long and promising road ahead for lung machine preservation, reconditioning, and therapeutics.

Pancreatic Machine Preservation

As in the organs mentioned previously, machine perfusion of the pancreas holds promise for decreasing IRI and expanding the donor pool through superior resuscitation of DCD and ECD organs. Historically, HMP of the pancreas has been shown to extend storage times to 24 to 48 hours as compared to SCS (Tersigni 1975). However, machine perfusion of the pancreas, particularly at normal to high pressures, has been associated with edema, congestion and ultimately early venous thrombosis and graft failure, due to the delicacy of the pancreatic vessels (Wright 1990; Karcz 2010). Further research delineated that tight control over arterial pressure in the range of 15–30 mm Hg with UW eliminated endothelial damage and improved graft function (Florack 1983). Difficulty with determining proper settings for pancreatic machine perfusion has been due to research optimizing the wrong endpoints: islet cell yield instead of whole-organ preservation (Barlow 2013). For example, high pressure perfusion resulting in endothelial damage and tissue edema actually improves islet cell yield (Taylor 2010), without improving transplantation outcomes. In addition to sensitivity to perfusion settings, pancreatic perfusion also faces a question of arterial cannulation: splenic or superior mesenteric separately or together.

Recently, pancreatic perfusions preservation has shifted interest from HMP to NMP due to promise in more thorough resuscitation of energy stores, warm ischemic damage, and pancreatic function prior to transplantation. Pancreatic NMP models began as early as 1926 by Babkin and Starling to assess exocrine and endocrine responses (Babkin 1926), and then later as a research model for transplantation following HMP preservation (Pegg 1982). Recent efforts have focused on NMP as a concept for preservation of DCD and ECD livers. However, despite potential benefits of pancreatic MP, the pancreas has proved to be a difficult organ to machine perfuse. Some researchers have attempted *ex vivo* co-perfusion of kidney and pancreas with the kidney functioning as a dialysis organ, hoping for tighter pH control and decreased pancreatic damage, but with limited success (Kuan 2016). The pancreas is particularly susceptible to ischemic damage, both increasing the necessity and relevance of an optimal preservation of DCD livers, but increasing the complexity and physiologic requirements of an *ex vivo* perfusion system. Insulin production and vascular resistance during NMP have both been shown to correlate well to pancreatic injury. While there are no current clinical applications, and relatively few animal studies in pancreatic machine perfusion, the technical limitations will likely be overcome in the future in order to expand the number of usable pancreatic allografts.

Conflict of Interest Statement

The authors of this chapter have no conflicts of interest to disclose.

REFERENCES

Babkin BP, Starling EH. A method for the study of the perfused pancreas. *J. Physiol.* 1926; 61: 245.

Bagul A, Hosgood SA, Kaushik M, Kay MD, Waller HL, Nicholson ML. Experimental renal preservation by normothermic resuscitation perfusion with autologous blood. *Br. J. Surg.* 2008; 95(1): 111–118.

Banan B, Xiao Z, Watson R, Xu M, Jia J, Upadhya GA, Mohanakumar T, Lin Y, Chapman W. Novel strategy to decrease reperfusion injuries and improve function of cold-preserved livers using normothermic *ex vivo* liver perfusion machine. *Liver Transpl.* 2016;22(3):333–343.

Barlow AD, Hosgood SA, Nicholson ML. Current state of pancreas preservation and implications for DCD pancreas transplantation. *Transplantation* 2013; 95(12):1419–1424.

Belzer FO & Southard JH. The future of kidney preservation. *Transplantation* 1980; 30(3):161–165.

Belzer FO, Ashby BS & Dunphy JE. 24-hour and 72-hour preservation of canine kidneys. *Lancet* 1967; 2(7515):536–538.

Bessems M, Doorschodt BM, Dinant S, de Graaf W, van Gulik TM. Machine perfusion preservation of the pig liver using a new preservation solution, polysol. *Transplant Proc.* 2006; 38(5):1238–1242.

Boehnert MU, Yeung JC, Bazerbachi F, Knaak JM, Selzner N, McGilvray ID, Rotstein OD, Adeyi OA, Kandel SM, Rogalla P, Yip PM, Levy GA, Keshavjee S, Grant DR, Selzner M. Normothermic acellular *ex vivo* liver perfusion reduces liver and bile duct injury of pig livers retrieved after cardiac death. *Am. J. Transplant.* 2013;13(6):1441–1449.

Bral M, Gala-Lopez B, Bigam D, Kneteman N, Malcom A, Livingstone S, Andres A, Emamaullee J, Russell L, Coussios C, West LJ, Friend PJ, Shapiro AMJ. Preliminary Single Centre Canadian Experience of Human Normothermic *Ex Vivo* Liver Perfusion: Results of a Clinical Trial. *Am. J. Transplant.* 2016; 17(4):1071–1080.

Brant S, Holmes C, Cobert M, Powell L, Shelton J, Jessen M, Peltz M. Successful transplantation in canines after long-term coronary sinus machine perfusion preservation of donor hearts. *J. Heart Lung Transplant.* 2016;35(8):1031–1036.

Brasile L, Delvecchio P, Amyot K, Haisch, Clarke J. Organ preservation without extreme hypothermia using an Oxygen supplemented perfusate. *ABB.* 1994; 22(4):1463–1468.

Brockmann J, Reddy S, Coussios C, Pigott D, Guirriero D, Hughes D, Morovat A, Debabrata R, Winter L, Friend PJ. Normothermic perfusion: a new paradigm for organ preservation. *Ann. Surg.* 2009; 250(1):1–6.

Brüggenwirth IMA, Burlage LC, Porte RJ, Martins PN. Is single portal vein perfusion the best approach for machine preservation of liver grafts? *J. Hepatol.* 2016; 64(5):1194–1195.

Buchs J, Lazeyras F, Ruttimann R, Nastasi A, Morel P. Oxygenated hypothermic pulsatile perfusion versus cold static storage for kidneys from non heart-beating donors tested by in-line ATP resynthesis to establish a strategy of preservation. *Perfusion* 2011; 26(2):159–165.

Butler AJ, Rees MA, Wight DG, Casey ND, Alexander G, White DJ, Friend PJ. Successful extracorporeal porcine liver perfusion for 72 hr. *Transplantation* 2002; 73(8):1212–1218.

Catena F, Coccolini F, Montori G, Vallicelli C, Amaduzzi A, Ercolani G, Ravaioli M, Gaudio MD, Schiavina R, Brunocilla E, Liviano G, Feliciangeli G, Pinna AD. Kidney preservation: review of present and future perspective. *Transplant Proc.* 2013;45(9):3170–3177.

Cobert ML, Merritt ME, West LSM, Ayers C, Jessen ME, Peltz M. Metabolic characteristics of human hearts preserved for 12 hours by static storage, antegrade perfusion, or retrograde coronary sinus perfusion. *J. Thorac. Cardiovasc.* 2014; 148(15): 2310–2315.

Codas, R. Petruzzo P, Morelon A, Lefrancois N, Danjou F, Berthillot C, Contu P, Espa M, Martin X, Badet L. IGL-1 solution in kidney transplantation: first multi-center study. *Clin. Transplant.* 2009;23(3):337–342.

Compagnon P, Clément B, Campion JP, Boudjema K. Effects of hypothermic machine perfusion on rat liver function depending on the route of perfusion. *Transplantation* 2001; 72(4):606–614.

Cypel M, Liu M, Rubacha M, Yeung J, Hirayama S, Ankaru M, Sato M, Medin J, Davidson B, Perrot M, Waddell T, Slutsky A, Keshavjee S. Functional repair of human donor lungs by IL-10 gene therapy. *Sci. Transl. Med.* 2009;1(4):4ra9.

Cypel M, Yeung JC, Liu M, Anraku M, Chen A, Karolak W, Sato M, Laratta J, Azad S, Madonik M, Chow CW, Chaparro C, Hutcheon M, Singer LG, Slutsky AS, Yasufuku K,

Perrot M, Pierre AF, Waddell TK, Keshavjee S. Normothermic *ex vivo* lung perfusion in clinical lung transplantation. *N. Engl. J. Med.* 2011; 364(15):1431–1440.

de Rougemont O, Breitenstein S, Leskosek B, Weber A, Graf R, Clavien PA, Dutowski P. One hour hypothermic oxygenated perfusion (HOPE) protects nonviable liver allografts donated after cardiac death. *Ann. Surg.* 2009; 250(5):674–683.

DiMaio JM, Morse M, Teeter WA, Cobert ML, West LM, Jessen ME, Peltz M. Donor hearts not offered or rejected for transplantation—a lost opportunity? *J. Heart Lung Transplant.* 2013;3: S156.

Dutkowski P, Polak WG, Muiesan P, Schlegel A, Verhoeven C, Scalera I, DeOliveira M, Kron P, Clavien PA. First Comparison of Hypothermic Oxygenated Perfusion Versus Static Cold Storage of Human Donation After Cardiac Death Liver Transplants: An International-matched Case Analysis. *Ann. Surg.* 2015; 262(5):764–771.

Dutkowski P, de Rougemont O, Clavien PA. Alexis Carrel: genius, innovator and ideologist. *Am. J. Transplant.* 2008; 8(10):1998–2003.

Florack G, Sutherland DE, Heil J, Squifflet JP, Najarian JS. Preservation of canine segmental pancreatic autografts: cold storage versus pulsatile machine perfusion. *J. Surg. Res.* 1983;34(5):493–504.

Foley DP, Ricciardi R, Traylor AN, McLaughlin TJ, Donohue SE, Wheeler SM, Meyers WC, Quarfordt SH. Effect of hepatic artery flow on bile secretory function after cold ischemia. *Am. J. Transplant.* 2003;3(2):148–155.

Foley DP, Vittimberga FJ, Quarfordt SH, Donohue SE, Traylor AN, MacPhee J, McLaughlin T, Ricciardi R, Callery MP, Meyers WC. Biliary secretion of extracorporeal porcine livers with single and dual vessel perfusion. *Transplantation* 1999; 68(3):362–368.

Fondevila C, Hessheimer AJ, Maathuis M-HJ, Munoz J, Taura P, Calatayud D, Leuvenik H, Rimola A, Ploeg RJ, Garcia-Valdecasas JC. Superior preservation of DCD livers with continuous normothermic perfusion. *Ann. Surg.* 2011; 254(6):1000–1007.

Fontes P, Lopez R, van der Plaats A, Vodovotz Y, Minervini M, Scott V, Soltys K, Shiva S, Paranjpe S, Sadowsky D, Barclay D, Zamora R, Stolz D, Demetris A, Michalopoulos G, Marsh JW. Liver preservation with machine perfusion and a newly developed cell-free oxygen carrier solution under subnormothermic conditions. *Am. J. Transplant.* 2015; 15(2):381–394.

Furukori M, Matsuno N, Meng LT, Shonaka T, Nishikawa Y, Imai K, Obara H, Furukawa H. Subnormothermic Machine Perfusion Preservation With Rewarming for Donation After Cardiac Death Liver Grafts in Pigs. *Transplant Proc.* 2016;48(4):1239–1243.

Gage F, Leeser DB, Porterfield NK, Graybill JC, Gillern JS, Hawksworth JS, Kindal RM, Thai N, Falta EM, Tadaki DK, Brown TS, Elster EA. Room temperature pulsatile perfusion of renal allografts with Lifor compared with hypothermic machine pump solution. *Transplant proc.* 2009; 41(9):3571–3574.

Gringeri E, Bonsignore P, Bassi D, D'Amico FE, Mescoli C, Polacco M, Buggio M, Luisetto R, Boetto R, Noaro G, Ferrigno A, Boncompagni E, Freitas I, Vairetti MP, Carraro A, Neri D, Cillo U. Subnormothermic machine perfusion for non-heart-beating donor liver grafts preservation in a Swine model: a new strategy to increase the donor pool? *Transplant Proc.* 2012; 44(7):2026–2028.

Guarrera JV, Estevez J, Boykin J, Boyce R, Rashid J, Sun S, Arrington B. Hypothermic machine perfusion of liver grafts for transplantation: technical development in human discard and miniature swine models. *Transplant Proc.* 2004:37(1):323–325.

Guarrera JV, Henry SD, Samstein B, Odeh-Ramadan R, Kinkhabwala M, Goldstein MJ, Ratner LE, Renz JF, Lee HT, Brown RS Jr., Emond JC. Hypothermic machine preservation in human liver transplantation: the first clinical series. *Am. J. Transplant.* 2010; 10(2):372–381.

Hagiwara M, Matsuno N, Meng LT, Furukori M, Watanabe K, Shonaka T, Imai K, Obara H, Nishikawa Y, Furukawa H. Applicability of Combined Use of Extracorporeal Support and Temperature-Controlled Machine Perfusion Preservation for Liver Procurement of Donors After Cardiac Death in Pigs. *Transplant Proc.* 2016; 48(4):1234–1238.

Hajjar G, Toledo-Pereyra LH, Mackenzie GH. Effect of 24-hour preservation with oxygen free radical scavengers on isolated-perfused canine heart-lungs. *P. R. Health Sci. J.* 1986; 5(1):19–25.

Hosgood SA & Nicholson ML. First in man renal transplantation after *ex vivo* normothermic perfusion. *Transplantation* 2011; 92(7):735–738.

Hosgood SA, Mohamed IH, Bagul A, Nicholson ML. Hypothermic machine perfusion after static cold storage does not improve the preservation condition in an experimental porcine kidney model. *Br. J. Surg.* 2011; 98(7): 943–950.

Hosgood SA, Barlow AD, Hunter JP, Nicholson ML. *Ex vivo* normothermic perfusion for quality assessment of marginal donor kidney transplants. *Br. J. Surg.* 2015;102(11):1433–1440.

Hosgood SA, Saeb-Parsy K, Hamed MO, Nicholson ML. Successful Transplantation of Human Kidneys Deemed Untransplantable but Resuscitated by *Ex Vivo* Normothermic Machine Perfusion. *Am. J. Transplant.* 2016; 16(11):3282–3285

Hosgood SA, Patel M. & Nicholson ML. The conditioning effect of *ex vivo* normothermic perfusion in an experimental kidney model. *J. Surg. Res.* 2013; 182(1):153–160.

Hoyer DP, Paul A, Luer S, Reis H, Efferz P, Minor T. End-ischemic reconditioning of liver allografts: Controlling the rewarming. *Liver Transpl.* 2016; 22(9):1223–1230.

Hoyer DP, Mathe Z, Gallinat A, Canbay A, Treckmann J, Rauen U, Paul A, Minor T. Controlled Oxygenated Rewarming of Cold Stored Livers Prior to Transplantation: First Clinical Application of a New Concept. *Transplantation* 2016; 100(1):147–152.

Hoyer DP, Gallinat A, Swoboda S, Wohlschläger J, Rauen U, Paul A, Minor T. Subnormothermic machine perfusion for preservation of porcine kidneys in a donation after circulatory death model. *Transpl. Int.* 2014; 27(10):1097–106.

Humphreys MR, Ereth MH, Sebo TJ, Slezak JM, Dong Y, Blute ML, Gettman MT. Can the kidney function as a lung? Systemic oxygenation and renal preservation during retrograde perfusion of the ischaemic kidney in rabbits. *BJU Int.* 2006;98(3):674–679.

Imber CJ, St Peter SD, Lopez de Cenarruzabeitia I, Pigott D, James T, Taylor R McGuire J, Hughes D, Butler A, Rees M, Friend PJ. Advantages of normothermic perfusion over cold storage in liver preservation. *Transplantation* 2002; 73:701–709.

Izamis ML, Efstathiades A, Keravnou C, Georgiadou S, Martins PN, Averkiou MA. Effects of Air Embolism Size and Location on Porcine Hepatic Microcirculation in Machine Perfusion. *Liver Transplant.* 2014; 20:601–611.

Jain S, Lee CY, Baicu S, Duncan H, Jones JW Jr., Clemens MG, Brassil J, Taylor MJ, Brockbank KGM. Hepatic function in hypothermically stored porcine livers: comparison of hypothermic machine perfusion vs cold storage. *Transplant Proc.* 2004; 37(1):340–341.

Jassem W & Heaton ND. The role of mitochondria in ischemia/reperfusion injury in organ transplantation. *Kidney Int.* 2004;66(2):514–7.

Jay CL, Lyuksemburg V, Ladner DP, Wang E, Caicedo J, Holl JL, Abecassis MM, Skaro AI. Ischemic cholangiopathy after controlled donation after cardiac death liver transplantation: a meta-analysis. *Ann. Surg.* 2011; 253(2):259– 264.

Jochmans I, Moers C, Smits J, Leuvenik HGD, Treckmann J, Paul A, Rahmel A, Squifflet J-P, van Heurn E, Monbaliu D, Ploeg RJ, Pirenne J. Machine perfusion versus cold storage for the preservation of kidneys donated after cardiac death: a multicenter, randomized, controlled trial. *Ann. Surg.* 2010; 252(5):756–64.

Jochmans I, O'Callaghan JM, Pirenne J, Ploeg RJ. Hypothermic machine perfusion of kidneys retrieved from standard and high-risk donors. *Transplant Int.* 2015; 28(6):665–676.

Jochmans I, Akhtar MZ, Nasralla D, Kocabayoglu P, Boffa C, Kaisar M, Brat A, O'Callaghan J, Pengel LHM, Knight S, Ploeg RJ. Past, present and future of dynamic kidney and liver preservation and resuscitation. *Am. J. Transplant.* 2016; 16(9)2545–2555.

Karangwa SA, Dutkowski P, Fontes P, Friend PJ, Guarrera JV, Markmann JF, Mergental H, Minot T, Quintini C, Selzner M, Uygun K, Watson CJ, Porte RJ. Machine Perfusion of Donor Livers for Transplantation: A Proposal for Standardized Nomenclature and Reporting Guidelines. *Am. J. Transplant.* 2016; 16(10) 2932–2942.

Karcz M, Cook HT, Sibbons P, Gray C, Dorling A, Papalois V. An ex-vivo model for hypothermic pulsatile perfusion of porcine pancreata: hemodynamic and morphologic characteristics. *Exp. Clin. Transplant.* 2010; 8(1):55– 60.

Kaths JM, Echeverri J, Goldaracena N, Louis KS, Chun Y-M, Linares I, Weibe A, Foltys DB, Yip PM, John R, Mucsi I, Ghaneker A, Bagli D, Grant DR, Robinson LA, Selzner M. Eight-Hour Continuous Normothermic *Ex Vivo* Kidney Perfusion Is a Safe Preservation Technique for Kidney Transplantation: A New Opportunity for the Storage, Assessment, and Repair of Kidney Grafts. *Transplantation* 2016; 100(9):1862–1870.

Kay MD, Hosgood SA, Bagul A, Nicholson ML. Comparison of preservation solutions in an experimental model of organ cooling in kidney transplantation. *Br. J. Surg.* 2009; 96(10):1215–21.

Khorsandi SE, Quaglia A, Salehi S, Jassem W, Vilca-Melendez H, Prachalias A, Srinivasan P, Heaton N. The microRNA Expression Profile in Donation after Cardiac Death (DCD) Livers and Its Ability to Identify Primary Non Function. *PLoS One.* 2015; 10(5):e0127073.

Knaak JM, Spetzler VN, Goldaracena N, Louis KS, Selzner N, Selzner M. Technique of subnormothermic *ex vivo* liver perfusion for the storage, assessment, and repair of marginal liver grafts. *J. Vis. Exp.* 2014(90):e51419.

Kron P, Schlegel A, de Rougemont O, Oberkofler CE, Clavien P-A, Dutowski P. Short, Cool, and Well Oxygenated - HOPE for Kidney Transplantation in a Rodent Model. *Ann. Surg.* 2016;264(5):815– 822.

Kuan KG, Wee MN, Chung WY Kumar R, Torge Mees S, Dennison A, Maddern G, Markus T. A Study of Normothermic Hemoperfusion of the Porcine Pancreas and Kidney. *Artif Organs.* 2017;41(5):490–495.

Li P, Liu Y-F, Yang L. Advantages of dual hypothermic oxygenated machine perfusion over simple cold storage in the preservation of liver from porcine donors after cardiac death. *Clin. Transplant.* 2015; 29(9):820–828.

Liu Q, Nassar A, Farias K, Buccini L, Baldwin W, Mangino M, Bennett A, O'Rourke C, Okamoto T, Diago Uso T, Fung J, Abu-Elmagd K, Miller C, Quintini C. Sanguineous normothermic machine perfusion improves hemodynamics and biliary epithelial regeneration in donation after cardiac death porcine livers. *Liver Transpl.* 2014; 20(8):987–999.

Liu Q, Vekemans K, Iania L, Komuta M, Parkkinen J, Heedfeld V, Wylin T. Assessing warm ischemic injury of pig livers at hypothermic machine perfusion. *J. Surg. Res.* 2014;186(1):379–389.

Mahboub P, Ottens P, Seelen M, Hart NT, Goor HV, Ploeg R, Martins PN, Leuvenink H. Gradual Rewarming with Gradual Increase in Pressure during Machine Perfusion after Cold Static Preservation Reduces Kidney Ischemia Reperfusion Injury. *PloS One.* 2015;10(12):e0143859.

McCurry K, Jeevanandam V, Mihaljevic T, Couper G, Elanwar M, Saleh H, Ardehali A. The 1-year follow-up results of the PROTECT patient population using the organ care system. *J. Heart Lung Transplant.* 2008; 27 (2 Supp):S166.

Mergental H, Perera MTPR, Laing RW, Muisan P, Issac JR, Smith A, Stephenson BTF, Cilliers H, Neil DAH, Hubscher. Transplantation SG, Afford SC, Mirza DF. Transplantation of Declined Liver Allografts Following Normothermic Ex-Situ Evaluation. *Am. J. Transplant.* 2016; 16(11):3235–3245

Merion RM, Pelletier SJ, Goodrich N, Englesbe MJ, Delmonico FL. Donation after cardiac death as a strategy to increase deceased donor liver availability. *Ann. Surg.* 2006; 244(4):555–562.

Michel S, La Muraglia GM II, Madariaga MLL, Titus JS, Selig MK, Farkash EA, Allan JS, Anderson LM, Madsen JC. Twelve-Hour Hypothermic Machine Perfusion for Donor Heart Preservation Leads to Improved Ultrastructural Characteristics Compared to Conventional Cold Storage. *Ann. Transplant.* 2015; 20:461–468.

Minor T, Efferz P, Fox M, Wohlschlaeger J, Lüer B. Controlled oxygenated rewarming of cold stored liver grafts by thermally graduated machine perfusion prior to reperfusion. *Am. J. Transplant.* 2013; 13(6):1450–1460.

Moers C, Smits JM, Maathuis M-HJ, Treckmann J, van Gelder F, Napieralski BP, van Kasterop-Kutz M, Homan van der Heide JJ, Squifflet J-P, van Heurn E, Kirste GR, Rahmel A, Leuvenink HGD, Paul A, Pirenne J, Ploeg RJ. Machine perfusion or cold storage in deceased-donor kidney transplantation. *N. Engl. J. Med.* 2009; 360(1):7–19.

Monbaliu D, Vekemans K, De Vos R, Brassil J, Heedfeld V, Qiang L, D'hollander M, Roskams T, Pirenne J. Hemodynamic, biochemical, and morphological characteristics during preservation of normal porcine livers by hypothermic machine perfusion. *Transplant Proc.* 2007; 39(8):2652–2658.

Monbaliu DR, Debbaut C, Hillewaert WJA, Brassil JM, Laleman WJC, Sainz-Barriga M, Kravitz D, Pirenne J, Segers P. Flow competition between hepatic arterial and portal venous flow during hypothermic machine perfusion preservation of porcine livers. *Int. J. Artif. Organs.* 2012; 35(2):119–131.

Morito N, Obara H, Matsuno N, Enosawa S, Watanabe K, Furukori M, Furukawa H. Regulated Oxygenation of Rewarming Machine Perfusion for Porcine Donation After Cardiac Death Liver Transplantation. *Transplant Proc.* 2016;48(4):1244–1246.

Mourad MM, Liossis C, Gunson BK, Mergental H, Isaac J, Muisan P, Mirza D, Perera TPR, Bramhall SR. Etiology and management of hepatic artery thrombosis after adult liver transplantation. *Liver Transpl.* 2014;20(6):713–723.

Nakajima D, Chen F, Okita K, Motoyama H, Hijiya K, Ohsumi A, Sakamoto J, Yamada T, Sato M, Aoyama A, Bando T, Date H. Reconditioning lungs donated after cardiac death using short-term hypothermic machine perfusion. *Transplantation* 2012; 94(10):999–1004.

Nakajima D, Chen F, Yamada T, Sakamoto J, Osumi A, Fujinaga T, Shoji T, Hiroaki S, Toru B, Date H. Hypothermic machine perfusion ameliorates ischemia-reperfusion injury in rat lungs from non-heart-beating donors. *Transplantation* 2011; 92(8):858–863.

Nakajima D, Cypel M, Bonato R, Muachuca TN, Iskender I, Hashimoto K, Linacre V, Chen M, Coutinho R, Azad S, Martinu T, Waddell TK, Hwang DM, Husain S, Liu M, Keshavjee S. Ex Vivo Perfusion Treatment of Infection in Human Donor Lungs. *Am. J. Transplant.* 2016; 16(4):1229–1237.

Nassar A, Liu Q, Farias K, D'Amico G, Tom C, Grady P, Bennett A, Diago Uso T, Eghtesad B, Kelly D, Fung J, Abu-Elmagd K, Miller C, Quintini C. *Ex vivo* normothermic machine perfusion is safe, simple, and reliable: results from a large animal model. *Surg. Innov.* 2015; 22(1):61–69.

Nassar A, Liu Q, Farias K, Buccini L, Baldwin W, Bennet A, Mangino M, Irefin S, Cywinski J, Okamoto T, Diago Uso T, Iuppa G, Soliman B, Miller C, Quintini C. Impact of Temperature on Porcine Liver Machine Perfusion From Donors After Cardiac Death. *Artif. Organs.* 2016; 40(10):999–1008.

Nechemia-Arbely Y, Barkan D, Pizov G, Shriki A, Rose-John S, Galun E, Axelrod JH. IL-6/IL-6R axis plays a critical role in acute kidney injury. *J. Am. Soc. Nephrol.* 2008;19(6):1106–1115.

Nishida S, Nakamura N, Kadono J, Komokata T, Sakata R, Madariaga JR, Tzakis AG. Intrahepatic biliary strictures after liver transplantation. *J. Hepatobiliary Pancreat. Surg.* 2006;13(6):511–516.

Obara H, Matsuno N, Enosawa S, Shigeta T, Huai-Che H, Hirano T, Muto M, Kasahara M, Uemoto S, Mizunuma H. Pretransplant screening and evaluation of liver graft viability using machine perfusion preservation in porcine transplantation. *Transplant Proc.* 2012; 44(4):959–961.

Obara H, Matsuno N, Shigeta T, Hirano T, Enosawa S, Mizunuma H. Temperature controlled machine perfusion system for liver. *Transplant Proc.* 2013; 45(5):1690–1692.

Olschewski P, GaB P, Ariyakhagorn V, Jasse K, Hunold G, Mensel M, Schoning W, Schmitz V, Neuhaus P, Puhl G. The influence of storage temperature during machine perfusion on preservation quality of marginal donor livers. *Cryobiology.* 2010; 60(3):337–343.

Op den Dries S, Sutton ME, Karimian N, de Boer MT, Wiersema-Buist J, Gouw ASH, Leuvenink HGD, Lisman T, Porte RJ. Hypothermic oxygenated machine perfusion prevents arteriolonecrosis of the peribiliary plexus in pig livers donated after circulatory death. *PLoS One.* 2014;9(2):e88521.

Pegg DE, Klempnauer J, Diaper MP, Taylor MJ. Assessment of hypothermic preservation of the pancreas in the rat by a normothermic perfusion assay. *J. Surg. Res.* 1982; 33(3): 194–200.

Perera T, Mergental H, Stephenson B, Roll GR, Cilliers H, Liang R, Angelico R, Hubscher S, Neil DA, Reynolds G, Isaac J, Adams DA, Afford S, Mirza DF, Muisan P. First human liver transplantation using a marginal allograft resuscitated by normothermic machine perfusion. *Liver Transpl.* 2016; 22(1):120–124.

Ploeg RJ, van Bockel JH, Langendijk PTH, Groenewegen M, van der Woude FJ, Persijn GG, Thorogood J, Hermans J. Effect of preservation solution on results of cadaveric kidney transplantation. *Lancet* 1992;340(8812):129–137.

Rauen U & de Groot H. New insights into the cellular and molecular mechanisms of cold storage injury. *J. Investig. Med.* 2004; 52(5):299–309.

Reddy S, Greenwood J, Maniakin N, Bhattacharjya S, Zilvetti M, Brockmann J, James T, Pigott D, Friend PJ. Non heart-beating donor porcine livers: the adverse effect of cooling. *Liver Transpl.* 2005;11: 35–38.

Saidi RF. Utilization of expanded criteria donors in liver transplantation. *Int. J. organ Transplant Med.* 2013; 4(2):46–59.

Schlegel A, Rougemont O de, Graf R, Clavien P-A, Dutkowski P. Protective mechanisms of end-ischemic cold machine perfusion in DCD liver grafts. *J Hepatol.* 2013; 58(2):278–286.

Schon MR, Kollmar O, Wolf S, Schrem H, Matthes M, Akkoc N, Schnoy NC, Neuhaus P. Liver transplantation after organ preservation with normothermic extracorporeal perfusion. *Ann. Surg.* 2001; 233:114–123.

Schopp I, Reissberg E, Luer B, Efferz P, Minor T. Controlled Rewarming after Hypothermia: Adding a New Principle to Renal Preservation. *Clini. Transl. Sci.* 2015; 8(5):475–478.

Schreinemachers MCJM, Doorschodt BM, Florquin S, Idu MM, Tolba RH, van Gulik TM. Improved renal function of warm ischemically damaged kidneys using Polysol. *Transplant proc.* 2009; 41(1):32–35.

Shigeta T, Matsuno N, Obara H, Mizunuma H, Kanazawa H, Tanaka H, Fukuda A, Sakamoto S, Kasahara M, Uemoto S, Enosawa S. Functional recovery of donation after cardiac death liver graft by continuous machine perfusion preservation in pigs. *Transplant Proc.* 2012; 44(4):946–947.

Shigeta T, Matsuno N, Obara H, Kanazawa H, Tanaka H, Fukuda A, Sakamoto S, Kasahara M, Mizunuma H, Enosawa S. Impact of rewarming preservation by continuous machine perfusion: improved post-transplant recovery in pigs. *Transplant Proc.* 2013;45(5):1684–1689.

Slieker JC, Farid WRR, van Eijck CHJ Lange JF, van Bommel J, Metselaar HJ, de Jonge J, Kazemier G. Significant contribution of the portal vein to blood flow through the common bile duct. *Ann. Surg.* 2012;255(3):523–527.

St Peter SD, Imber CJ, Lopez I, Hughes D, Friend PJ. Extended preservation of non-heart-beating donor livers with normothermic machine perfusion. *Br. J. Surg.* 2002;89(5):609–616.

Stegemann J, Hirner A, Rauen U, Minor T. Use of a new modified HTK solution for machine preservation of marginal liver grafts. *J. Surg. Res.* 2010; 160(1):155–162.

Stubenitsky BM, Booster M, Brasile L, Araneda D, Haisch C, Kootstra G. Exsanguinous metabolic support perfusion--a new strategy to improve graft function after kidney transplantation. *Transplantation* 2000;70(8):1254–1258.

Taylor MJ, Baicu SC. Current state of hypothermic machine perfusion preservation of organs: The clinical perspective. *Cryobiology* 2010;60(3 Suppl):S20–35.

Tersigni R, Toledo-Pereyra LH, Pinkham J, Najarian JS. Pancreaticoduodenal preservation by hypothermic pulsatile perfusion for twenty-four hours. *Ann. Surg.* 1975;182(6):743–748.

Thiara APS, Hoel TN, Kristiansen F, Karlsen HM, Fiane AE, Svennevig JL. Evaluation of oxygenators and centrifugal pumps for long-term pediatric extracorporeal membrane oxygenation. *Perfusion* 2007; 22(5):323–326.

Thuillier R, Dutheil D, Trieu MTN, Mallet V, Allain G, Rousselor M, Denizot M, Goujon J-M, Zal F, Hauet T. Supplementation with a new therapeutic oxygen carrier reduces chronic fibrosis and organ dysfunction in kidney static preservation. *Am. J. Transplant.* 2011;11(9):1845–1860.

Thuillier R, Allain G, Celhay O, Hebrard W, Barrou B, Badet L, Leuvenink HGD, Hauet T. Benefits of active oxygenation during hypothermic machine perfusion of kidneys in a preclinical model of deceased after cardiac death donors. *Journal Surg. Res.* 2013;184(2):1174–1181.

Tolboom H, Makhro A, Rosser BA, Wilhelm MJ, Bogdanova A, Falk V. Recovery of donor hearts after circulatory death with normothermic extracorporeal machine perfusion. *Eur. J. Cardiothorac. Surg.* 2015;47(1):173–9.

Tolboom H, Olejníčková V, Reser D, Rosser B, Wilhelm MJ, Gassmann M, Bogdanova A, Falk V. Moderate hypothermia during *ex vivo* machine perfusion promotes recovery of hearts donated after cardiocirculatory death. *Eur. J. Cardiothorac Surg.* 2016; 49(1):25–31.

Tozzi M, Franchin M, Soldini G, Ietto G, Chiappa C, Maritan E, Villa F, Carcano G, Dionigi R. Impact of static cold storage VS hypothermic machine preservation on ischemic kidney graft: inflammatory cytokines and adhesion molecules as markers of ischemia/reperfusion tissue damage. Our preliminary results. *Int. J. Surg.* 2013; 11(Suppl 1):S110–114.

Treckmann J, Moers C, Smits JM, Gallinat A, Maathuis M-HJ, van Kasterop-Kutz M, Jochmans I, Homan van der Heide JJH, Squifflet J-P, van Heurn E, Kirste GR, Rahmel A, Leuvenink HGD, Pirenne J, Ploeg RJ, Paul A. Machine perfusion versus cold storage for preservation of kidneys from expanded criteria donors after brain death. *Transplant Int.* 2011; 24(6):548–554.

United Network for Organ Sharing. Available at: http://www. unos.org/. Accessed March 17, 2016.

van Caenegem O, Beauloye C, Bertrand L, Horman S, Lepropre S, Sparavier G, Vercruysse J, Bethuyne N, Poncelet AJ, Gianello P, Demuylder P, Legrand E, Beaurin G, Bontemps F, Jacquet LM, Vanoverschelde J-L. Hypothermic continuous machine perfusion enables preservation of energy charge and functional recovery of heart grafts in an *ex vivo* model of donation following circulatory death. *Eur. J. Cardiothorac Surg.* 2016;49(5):1348–1353.

van der Plaats A, Maathuis MHJ, 't Hart NA, Bellekom AA, Hofker HS, van der Houwen EB, Verkerke GJ, Leuvenink HGD, Verdonck P, Ploeg RJ, Rakhorst G. The Groningen hypothermic liver perfusion pump: functional evaluation of a new machine perfusion system. *Ann. Biomed Eng.* 2006; 34(12):1924–1934.

Vekemans K, Liu Q, Brassil J, Komuta M, Pirenne J, Monbaliu D. Influence of flow and addition of oxygen during porcine liver hypothermic machine perfusion. *Transplant Proc.* 2007; 39(8):2647–2651.

Vekemans K, Liu Q, Heedfeld V, Van de Val K, Wylin T, Pirenne J, Monbaliu D. Hypothermic Liver Machine Perfusion With EKPS-1 Solution vs Aqix RS-I Solution: In Vivo Feasibility Study in a Pig Transplantation Model. *Transplant Proc.* 2009; 41(2):617–621.

Verdonk RC, Buis CI, Porte RJ, Haagsma EB. Biliary complications after liver transplantation: a review. *Scand. J. Gastroenterol Suppl.* 2006; (243):89–101.

Verhoeven CJ, Farid WRR, de Jonge J, Metselaar HJ, Kazemier G, van der Laan LJW. Biomarkers to assess graft quality during conventional and machine preservation in liver transplantation. *J. Hepatol.* 2014; 61(3):672–684.

Watson CJE, Wells AC, Roberts RJ, Akoh JA, Friend PJ, Akyol M, Calder FR, Allen JE, Jones MN, Collet D, Bradley JA. Cold machine perfusion versus static cold storage of kidneys donated after cardiac death: a UK multicenter randomized controlled trial. *Am. J. Tranplant.* 2010; 10(9):1991–1999.

Westerkamp AC, Karimian N, Matton APM, Mahboub P, van Rijn R, Wiersema-Buist J, de Boer MT, Leuvenink HGD, Gouw A, Lisman T, Porte RJ. Oxygenated Hypothermic Machine Perfusion After Static Cold Storage Improves Hepatobiliary Function of Extended Criteria Donor Livers. *Transplantation* 2016; 100(4):825–835.

White CW, Ambrose E, Müller A, Li Y, Le H, Hiebert B, Arora R, Lee TW, Dixon I, Tian G, Nagendran J, Hryshko L, Freed D. Assessment of donor heart viability during *ex vivo* heart perfusion. *Can J Physiol Pharmacol.* 2015; 93(10):893–901.

Wright FH, Wright C, Ames SA, Smith JL, Corry RJ. Pancreatic allograft thrombosis: donor and retrieval factors and early postperfusion graft function. *Transplant Proc.* 1990; 22(2):439–441.

Wszola M, Kwiatkowski A, Diuwe P, Domagala P, Gorski L, Kiesek R, Berman A, Perkowska-Ptasinska A, Durlik M, Paczek L, Chmura A. One-year results of a prospective, randomized trial comparing two machine perfusion devices used for kidney preservation. *Transplant Int.* 2013; 26(11):1088–1096.

Wszola M, Kwiatkowski A, Domagala P, Wirowska A, Bieniasz M, Diuwe P, Kiesek R, Durlik M, Chmura A. Preservation of kidneys by machine perfusion influences gene expression and may limit ischemia/reperfusion injury. *Prog. Transplant.* 2014;24(1):19–26.

Xu H, Berendsen T, Kim K, Soto-Gutierrez A, Bertheium F, Yarmush ML, Hertl M. Excorporeal normothermic machine perfusion resuscitates pig DCD livers with extended warm ischemia. *J. Surg. Res.* 2012; 173(2):e83–88.

Zhang Y, Fu Z, Zhong Z, Wang R, Hu L, Xiong Y, Wang Y, Ye Q. Hypothermic Machine Perfusion Decreases Renal Cell Apoptosis During Ischemia/Reperfusion Injury via the Ezrin/AKT Pathway. *Artificial organs.* 2016; 40(2):129–135.

In: Advances in Experimental Surgery. Volume 2
Editors: Huifang Chen and Paulo N. Martins
ISBN: 978-1-53612-773-7
© 2018 Nova Science Publishers, Inc.

Chapter 13

MICROCIRCULATION

Norbert Nemeth[1,*] and Andrea Szabo[2]

[1]Department of Operative Techniques and Surgical Research, Faculty of Medicine,
University of Debrecen, Debrecen, Hungary
[2]Institute of Surgical Research, Faculty of Medicine,
University of Szeged, Szeged, Hungary

ABSTRACT

In this chapter, we give a brief overview of the structural and functional aspects of the microcirculation with particular interest in the rheology of microcirculation. A summary of the up-to-date methodology for dynamic observation and quantification of microcirculatory characteristics and hemorheological changes is also given. A special emphasis is put on the applicability of the diverse methodological approaches in different experimental models and human diseases. Finally, we provide highlights of the key findings of vasoregulatory and inflammatory microcirculatory changes as well as rheological alterations seen in local and systemic circulatory disorders in clinically-relevant animal models of human diseases.

Keywords: microcirculatory perfusion, microcirculatory inflammation, hemorheology, methods, key findings

ABBREVIATIONS

CT	computed tomography
DIC	disseminated intravascular coagulation
EC	endothelial cells
EI	elongation index

---

[*] Corresponding author: Norbert Nemeth M.D., Ph.D., Department of Operative Techniques and Surgical Research, Faculty of Medicine, University of Debrecen, 22 Moricz Zs. krt., H-4032 Debrecen, Hungary, Tel: +36 52 416 915, E-mail: nemeth@med.unideb.hu.

ESR	erythrocyte sedimentation rate
FCD	functional capillary density
Htc	hematocrit
IDF	incident dark field
IVM	intravital microscopy
LORCA	laser-assisted optical rotational cell analyzer
MCHC	mean cell hemoglobin concentration
MCV	mean corpuscular volume
MFI	microvascular flow index
Micro-CT	Micro-computed tomography
MRI	magnetic resonance imaging
NIRS	near-infrared spectroscopy
NO	nitric oxide
OPS	orthogonal polarization spectral imaging
PMNs	polymorphonuclear neutrophil leukocytes
PPV	proportion of perfused vessels
SDF	sidestream dark-field imaging

INTRODUCTION

It is noteworthy that most of the cardinal clinical symptoms and signs of inflammation (redness/*rubor*, swelling/*tumor*, increased heat/*calor*, pain/*dolor*, and loss of function/*functio laesa*) can be linked to changes in microcirculation. Due to recent methodological improvements, assessment of the underlying contributory microcirculatory mechanisms has greatly improved in the last decades. Microcirculatory examinations provide not only excellent diagnostic opportunities, but have also been shown to predict clinical outcome and quantitatively express the therapeutic benefits of experimental and clinical interventions.

Microcirculation research is an extremely broad field in the aspects of physiology, pathophysiology, clinical medicine and methodology. Therefore it is challenging attempt to give a detailed outline of these topics. In this chapter, we aimed to overview briefly the morphological and functional aspects of microcirculation, including micro-rheology and a summary of the up-to-date methodology. We also depict some of the major findings and technical aspects of experimental surgical research.

A BRIEF OVERVIEW OF THE STRUCTURE AND FUNCTION OF MICROCIRCULATION

Structure and Function

The microcirculation represents the highest vascular surface of the cardiovascular system consisting of blood vessels with a diameter of <150 μm. The main function of the microcirculation is to deliver oxygen to the cells and maintain tissue oxygenation. Small arteries can give rise to several arterioles as its diameter decreases toward the periphery.

Arterioles have an external muscular coat with circumferentially arranged smooth muscle cells while the terminal (precapillary) arterioles (having an internal diameter of 15 to 20 µm) are surrounded by only one layer of smooth muscle cells. Arterioles show active changes in diameter, and account for a majority of total vascular resistance, therefore the smallest arterioles play a dominant role in the regulation of blood flow. At the level of vessels with the lowest diameter, parenchymal cell lay in close proximity to the capillaries, so that passive diffusion ensures an efficient supply of oxygen to the tissues. Because of the high permeability of the arteriolar and capillary wall to oxygen, the release of oxygen starts from oxyhemoglobin in the red blood cells, a further passaging across the capillary wall and the interstitium reaching the mitochondria where it is consumed by its reaction with cytochrome c oxidase. As the endothelial barrier is highly permeable to lipid-soluble and small water-soluble molecules, it ensures the exchange of not only gases, but also nutrients and waste products. In certain tissues such as the mesentery, precapillary sphincters (smooth muscle surrounding the entrance of a capillary) regulate the opening state of the capillary network according to the needs of the tissue segment. Capillaries drain into larger vessels, the postcapillary venules which are the most reactive sites of inflammation within the microvasculature and these veins contain intercellular endothelial junctions that allow transvascular protein exchange and trafficking of circulating cells including leukocytes into the interstitium. Indeed, venules represent the major site of leukocyte trafficking (leukocyte–endothelial cell adhesion). Larger venules that are draining the postcapillary venules, also possess smooth muscle in their media layer (Pries 2003; Pries 2008).

Regulatory Mechanisms in the Microvasculature

Arterioles show dramatic active changes in their diameter, and therefore arterioles account for a majority of total vascular resistance (capillaries and venules accounting for less than 25% of vascular resistance), therefore, the smallest arterioles are mostly liable for the regulation of blood flow under resting conditions. During intense vasodilation, however, this role is shifted toward the larger arterioles (Granger 1988).

Intact microcirculation is characterized by a high proportion of perfused capillaries with low level of flow heterogeneity. Open and closed states of the capillaries generally meet the metabolic needs of the surrounding tissues. Modulation of precapillary sphincters is partly under the influence of systemic factors (i.e., sympathetic stimulation, circulating factors and metabolites), being also dynamically regulated by local factors. In general, regional blood flow is regulated by myogenic, metabolic, and neurohumoral mechanisms. Myogenic autoregulation is the intrinsic ability of a blood vessel to constrict or dilate in response to a change in intraluminal pressure which is further modulated by shear stress-induced release of nitric oxide (NO) (Davis 2008; Davis 2012). According to the metabolic theory of autoregulation, local capillary blood flow meets the metabolic needs of the underlying tissue (Granger 1975).

It appears that there is an important interplay between vascular endothelial cells (EC) and smooth muscle cells. For instance during the phenomenon of endothelium-dependent vasodilation, ECs control the tone of adjacent vascular smooth muscle cells through the production and liberation of vasoactive substances (e.g., NO, prostaglandins, endothelin, … etc.) and the tone of the blood vessel wall has certain retroactive effect on the activity of ECs (Granger 2010).

Apart from being a selective barrier to fluids and solutes, EC regulate vasomotor tone and exhibit various anti-inflammatory and anti-thrombogenic properties. Intact EC functions are also secured by the endothelial glycocalyx layer which not only separates blood cells from the EC membrane, but also influences local hematocrit, flow, oxygen transport, and interactions between blood cells and the vessel wall (Reitsma 2007). EC activation can be evoked by a variety of chemical stimuli (e.g., cytokines) and physical/shear stress. ECs also play an active role in mediating an inflammatory response. Likewise, an endothelium-mediated vasodilation occurs in response to hypoxia which is mediated by the release of vasodilating prostaglandins and NO (Jackson 1983; Vallet 1994; Vallet 1998; Vallet 2002; Michiels 1993). Similar vasodilatory response is evoked by the release of metabolites (adenosine, lactate, H^+, and K^+) from the affected tissues (Nakhostine 1993). Neurohumoral modulation depends on vessel size and the distribution of adrenergic receptors within the particular tissue type (Watts 2008). During inflammation, EC activation leads to characteristic alterations in microvascular function (e.g., impaired vasomotor function, thrombus formation, leukocyte adhesion and increased microvascular permeability). During this process, reduction in endothelial glycocalyx thickness and mobilization of endothelium-derived P-selectin from Weibel-Palade bodies occur, causing a rapid initiation of leukocyte rolling, which is followed by a later release of E-selectin (Ley 2007; Langer 2009). These changes contribute to the propagation of the inflammatory response (Aird 2003). A balance between the production of reactive oxygen (superoxide) and nitrogen (NO) species has been implicated in the EC response to inflammation by influencing activating nuclear transcription factors for both pro-inflammatory and anti-inflammatory proteins.

Rheology in Microcirculation

Briefly, the main parameters determining blood viscosity are the plasma viscosity (as the characteristic of suspension fluid), the hematocrit (as the quantity of suspended corpuscle), the red blood cell deformability and aggregation. Main determinants of plasma viscosity are the state of hydration, concentration of large plasma proteins with elongated configuration (especially fibrinogen) and triglyceride level. Hematocrit derives from red blood cell count and mean corpuscular volume (MCV). Factors forming blood cell deformability are absolute cell volume, the surface-volume ratio, cell morphology, intracellular viscosity, cell membrane viscosity and elastic characteristics. Determinants of red blood cell aggregation include composition of plasma as suspension medium macromolecule (mainly fibrinogen concentration), surface features of red blood cells (glycocalyx composition), morphological and mechanical characteristics of the cell and shear rate (Chien 1975; Meiselman 1981; Cokelet 2007a, b; Mohandas 2008; Baskurt 2009; Saldanha 2013).

It is well known that the wall shear rate and the shear stress is the highest in the territory of the microcirculation (Table 13.1) (McDonald 1974; Lipowsky 1995; Lipowsky 2005; Chandran 2012).

Table 13.1. Quantitative and morphological data of various vessels types with flow velocity and wall shear rate distribution along the systemic circulatory system (McDonald 1974; Lipowsky 1995; Chandran 2012, Baskurt 2012)

Vessel	Mean diameter [mm]*	Number of vessels*	Mean length [mm]*	Total cross section [cm²]*	Total volume [mL]*	Percentage of total blood volume [%]*	Mean diameter [mm] #	Mean flow velocity [cm/s] #	Wall shear rate [s⁻¹] #
Aorta	19 – 45	1		2 – 16	60	11	16 – 32	6	150 – 300
Arteries	4	40	150	5	75		0.1 – 6	15 – 50	200 – 2 000
	1.3	500	45	6.6	30				
	0.45	6 000	13.5	9.5	13				
	0.15	110 000	4	19.4	8				
Arterioles	0.05	2.8 x 10⁶	1.2	55	7	5	0.04	0.5	1 000
Capillaries	0.008	2.7 x 10⁹	0.65	1 357	88		0.005 – 0.01	0.05 – 0.1	400 – 1 600
Venules	0.1	1 x 10⁷	1.6	785.4	126		0.02 – 0.1	0.2 – 0.5	800 – 400
Veins	0.28	660 000	4.8	406.4	196	67	0.2 – 10	15 – 20	120 – 320
	0.7	40 000	13.5	154	208				
	1.8	2 100	45	53.4	240				
	4.5	110	150	17.5	263				
Venae cavae	5 – 14	2		0.2 – 1.5	92		20	10.15	40 – 60

* in dogs (Chandran 2012), # estimated values in human (McDonald 1974; Lipowsky 1995; Baskurt 2012)

Blood and Plasma Viscosity

The blood is non-newtonian, thixotrop and viscoelastic fluid. Blood behaves as a non-newtonian fluid, i.e., its viscosity depends on the shear rate, and can be described by typical Casson-type curves. Non-newtonian characteristics of blood are hematocrit and shear rate dependent. At lower shear rate, the blood viscosity increases (thixotropic effect) due to the viscosity elevating effect of red blood cell aggregation. At higher flow velocity (i.e., higher shear rate), the cells disaggregate and elongate in the direction of the flow due to their deformability and elastic features. This makes the blood viscoelastic. The Maxwell-model serving for its characterization includes reversible elastic deformation and movement connected with the viscous energy (Cokelet 2007b; Chandran 2012).

The connection between *blood viscosity and hematocrit* (Htc) shows exponential rather than linear function ($\log\eta = k + k'Htc$, where k and k' are constants characteristic of the blood sample (Cokelet 2007a, b). The hematocrit/viscosity rate presented in the function of the hematocrit shows a connection reminding of a bell-shaped curve, with typical maximum value, which reflects the maximum of oxygen transporting capacity of blood ("optimal" hematocrit), i.e., the most red blood cells possible (the highest hematocrit possible) measured at speed gradient resulting from the lowest viscosity possible (Ernst 1983; Bogar 2005).

Main determining factors of *plasma viscosity* are its water content and the macromolecules with elongated configuration, as the fibrinogen concentration, globulin fractions and triglyceride level are important factors (Harkness 1971; Cokelet 2007b; Kesmarky 2008; Kwaan 2010). It is important to note, that while in several stages of circulation, the apparent viscosity of blood is not constant due to the intravascular interactions and distribution of different shear rate profile and the formed elements, mainly the red blood cells, the intravascular plasma viscosity can be considered constant. So the plasma viscosity maintains shear stress on the endothelium at the cell-poor or sometimes even cell-free zone in the direct vicinity of the ECs (Poiseuille-zone) due to the axial flow profile in vessels with diameter approximately under 300 μm. Moreover, the plasma viscosity provides the shear force in case of the so-called plasma-skimming, when at a certain point and at a certain site, there is no formed element and only plasma in the capillary (Cokelet 2007b; Kesmarky 2008).

Red Blood Cell Deformability

Red blood cell deformability is an ability of passive transformation appearing under the influence of shear stress, and it depends on the absolute volume, surface/volume ratio of the cells, morphological characteristics, viscoelastic properties of the cell membrane and intracellular viscosity (hemoglobin content) (Chien 1975; Meiselman 1981; Cokelet 2007a,b; de Oliveira 2010).

Mature red blood cells of mammals and humans are without nucleus, so the intracellular (cytoplasm) viscosity is mainly determined by the properties of hemoglobin solution. When the mean cell hemoglobin concentration (MCHC) increases above 37 g/dl, the intracellular viscosity increases precipitously, affecting the deformability of the whole cell, and thus also the tissue perfusion and the oxygenation due to impeded passage in the microcirculation. MCHC is regulated within a relatively narrow range (30–35 g/dl), where ATP-dependent Na^+, K^+ transporters participating in the cell volume regulation play the key roles (Chien 1975; Cokelet 2007b; Mohandas 2008; Baskurt 2012a).

Viscoelastic characteristics of red blood cells are complex (Thurston 2007). Viscosity property derives from membrane viscosity and cytoplasm viscosity. The elasticity feature consists of surface expansion, shearing and bending elements (Thurston 2007; Kim 2012). Surface area expansion (or compression) modulus (K) reflects the stored elastic energy, which develops through isotropic surface expansion or shrinkage of the membrane: $T_t = K\ (\Delta A/A_0)$, where T_t is the stress force, ΔA is the surface change, A_0 is the original surface. The shear module (μ) expresses the elastic energy which derives from membrane extension at same surface: $Ts = (\mu(\lambda^2 - \lambda^{-2}))/2$, where Ts is the shear stress, λ is the extension rate. Bending (fluxural) modulus (B) expresses the energy which is required for bending the membrane from one curve into another curve: $M = B\ (C_1 + C_2 - C_0)$, where M is the momentum of bending, C_1 and C_2 are the curves, C_0 is the curve of stress free state (Kim 2012).

Motion of red blood cells can be described in a complex way, depending on the flow conditions; rolling, rotation, swinging, elongation, elastic deformation due to collisions, the combination of all the above, in their hardly modellable complexity. When suspending the cells (such as in plasma) in a low viscosity medium, their motion is similar to that of solids. As the flow rate increases, most of the cells flow along the same path ($C = 0$), where they rotate around their symmetrical axis (perpendicular to the shear level) (Bitbol 1986). If the cells are suspended in a higher viscosity medium over a critical speed-gradient, their behavior is similar to that of fluid drops. The membrane transmits the momentum towards the cytoplasm, while maintaining the orientation of flow. At low and moderate speed gradient, the biconcave shape of cells remains stable, but at higher values they elongate and gain an ellipsoid shape. Under the effect of pulsatility and in the course of oscillation flow, the inclination angle of the cells is not equal and therefore it becomes chaotic. In smaller veins, especially in the capillaries, the friction has an increased role not only between the cells, but also in the relationship of endothelium and blood cells. The erythrocytes flow in a formation reminding of doughnuts flattened in their middle, where they are the thinnest (Goldsmith 1972; Pries 2003, 2008; Popel 2005; Dupire 2012).

Therefore, the deformability participates to a different extent in the different stages of circulation. Worsening deformability, i.e., the enhanced rigidity of red blood cells, in the mass flow zone of circulation (vessel diameter >300 μm) may lead to elevated blood viscosity. Red blood cells with reduced deformability can cause the most significant problem in the microcirculation (vessel diameter <100 μm), more precisely in the zone of so-called individual flow. Here, capillaries with diameter of 3–5 μm may also occur, not to mention the fenestration through the red pulp of the spleen to gaps of even smaller diameter. For passing through these capillaries, the appropriate deformability is essential.

Red Blood Cell Aggregation

Erythrocyte aggregation means the reversible connection of cells which happens at low shear rate or during stasis. Red blood cells initially arrange next to each other in a rouleaux formation, resembling a stack of coins. It takes place within few seconds: the simpler rouleaux form in 1–5 seconds. Over a period of further 10 to 60 seconds arranging in a two- then three-dimensional shape until the effects maintaining the aggregation are present (Baskurt 2012a). In anticoagulated blood samples, the aggregates coagulate into larger balls, then due to the gravity, start to sink. This provides the background of the erythrocyte sedimentation rate (ESR), since if the aggregation is fast and/or extensive, the erythrocyte sedimentation will also be more intensive (Hardeman 2007).

The process of red blood cell aggregation is not yet completely clear. At present there are two model theories to explain the aggregation development. (1) The aggregation of red blood cells approaching each other happens via non-covalent cross-connections of macromolecules (large proteins with elongated structure, such as fibrinogen, or *in vitro* with different polymers) (*bridging model*). This weak linkage dissolves as the disaggregation forces such as the electrostatic repulsion (due to negative charge, zeta potential: -15.7 mV), membrane tension, deformation and mechanical shear stress prevail (the aggregates can be completely dispersed at above 20–40 s^{-1} shear rate). This model supposes that the protein or polymer concentration is high on the cell surface. Absorbing macromolecules non-specifically binding to cell surface structures through their size and quantity may compensate the electrostatic repulsion, facilitating the aggregation. (2) According to the other explanation, the macromolecules are not able to penetrate as far as the membrane just because of the glycocalyx structure of cell surface (5–50 nm), therefore close to the cell surface, a layer deficient in macromolecules or depletion zone develops (*depletion model*). As two red blood cells approach each other, due to the osmotic gradient between the macromolecule concentration being in plasma phase and the depletion zone, a "pulling" force may develop, which makes the aggregation. The higher is the macromolecule concentration, the more intensive may this gradient be, causing enhanced aggregation (Baskurt 2012a; Saldanha 2013).

There is no unambiguous opinion pro or contra the absolute justification of the two theories, though most of the evidences promote the depletion model. However, the existence of direct intercellular or even cross-binding connections cannot be excluded. Carvalho et al. analyzed structures similar to $\alpha_{IIb}\beta_3$ glycoprotein complexes existing on platelets' surface, facilitating the direct binding of fibrinogen also in red blood cells by their spectroscopy techniques based on atomic-force microscopy. These receptors existing also in the erythrocytes, have lower affinity than that of platelets, the receptor-fibrinogen binding can be broken-up with less energy (Carvalho 2010). Is it possible that both models are true together? Depletion energies are essential for the "allurement" of the cells, and when in this situation, they are close to each other and real cross-binding may develop? No univocal explanation of this hypothesis exists so far.

It is a fact that various plasma proteins, and *in vitro* the polymers with different molecular size influence the development of aggregation process, and to a different degree. Red blood cell aggregability studies indicate that aggregation ability is influenced by cellular factors and is independent from the properties of the plasma (Baskurt 2012a). Aggregability can be measured comparatively *in vitro* in various macromolecule solutions. It has been proved that from the plasma proteins, fibrinogen, C-reactive protein and immunoglobulin M have the effects of facilitating and enhancing red blood cell aggregation. Further, immunoglobulin G and haptoglobin show rather increasing effect, while transferrin, coeruloplasmin and albumin do not influence erythrocyte aggregation (Baskurt 2012a; Saldanha 2013). *In vitro* the high molecular weight macromolecules and polymers such as 60 or 73 kDa dextran, or the 360 kDa polyvinylpyrrolidon (PVP), and the 36kDa polyethylen-glycol (PEG) promote/enable red blood cell aggregation, but their versions with lower kDa have no effect on the aggregation (e.g., PEG 10, 10.5 or 18.1 kDa dextran). Armstrong et al. stated that if hydrodynamic radius of macromolecules or polymers is more than 4 cm, they have an effect of enhancing the aggregation; if it is less than 4 cm, they do not influence the aggregation (Armstrong 2004).

When there are few red blood cells in a certain area, where other conditions of aggregation are normally available, they have less chance to get close to each other. Therefore, the aggregation depends on the hematocrit as well: the aggregation index (AI, which increases by the extent of aggregation) shows nearly linear connection, positive correlation between 20–40% Htc, between 40–50% Htc the curve is less precipitous, while between 50–60%, the AI does not change significantly by (adding) a unit of Htc (Baskurt 2012a).

For the aggregation to occur, the existence of biconcave cell form is crucial. Ovalocyte, spherocyte, echinocyte, sphero-echinocyte cell forms are not or less capable to aggregate. During the aggregation, according to the principle of the least energy loss, the process is going towards the binding on the maximal surface. That is why biconcave form is advantageous, and that is why rouleaux formation develops relatively quickly and then from these with the terminal and side connections geometrical shapes having smaller surface (Reinhart 1980; Meiselman 1981).

All in all, the process and extent of the aggregation depends on the shear rate, concentration of plasma fibrinogen, hematocrit and on cellular properties, like cell surface glycocalyx composition of red blood cells (type of depletion zone, glycoproteins enabling possible direct connections), and the formal characteristics of the cell (biconcave form). All these can vary in a very complex way in different diseases, pathological states, and it also provides a background to a great diversity in the comparison of mammalian species and the human.

Micro-Rheology and Microcirculation

Fåhræus observed in 1958, that by enhanced aggregation, the axial flow in the glass capillary (d = 95 μm, flow rate = 3.3 mm/s) i.e., the aggregation of red blood cells along the flow axis is more expressed and the cell-free side zone is wider. The parabolic flow rate profile developing due to the laminal flow and the presence of circulating particles (blood cells) dimming it to some extent, creates the phenomenon typically appearing in the range under 200–300 μm vein diameter, the axial migration of red blood cells (Figure 13.1). It means that within the vein's cross section, the distribution and velocity of red blood cells are not even, which leads to the dynamic reduction of hematocrit, to the Fåhræus-effect. Below approximately 30 μm diameter, down to about 10 μm, the apparent blood viscosity decreases with the diameter (Fåhræus-Lindqvist effect) (Fahraeus 1931). Along the vessel wall, a side plasma zone deficient of red blood cells develops or being even cell-free (Poiseuille-zone), which reduces the friction, hereby the hydrodynamic resistance between the vascular wall and the flowing fluid. If the flow rate is high enough, every formed element aggregates towards the flow axis. When the speed gradient and pressure conditions enable the development of red blood cell aggregation (typically in the area of postcapillary venules and venules), the size of particles (aggregates) flowing along the axis increases, the Poiseuille-zone widens, also facilitating the margination of white blood cells (Bishop 2001; Baskurt 2008; Nash 2008) (Figure 13.1).

In the microcirculation approaching the individual flow stage (capillaries) due to the extremely variable ramifications, connections, bends, endothelial surface features, red blood cell distribution, the tissue hematocrit is highly variable (Wells 1964; Lipowsky 2005; Popel 2005; Pries 2008).

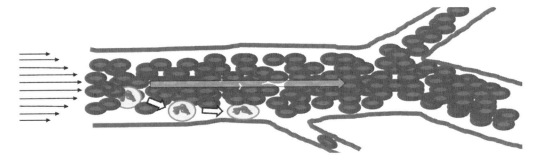

Figure 13.1. Schematic drawing of the circulatory pattern in vessels with diameter <100 μm. Due to the parabolic flow velocity profile (the flow speeds up along the axis of the vessel), the axial migration of red blood cells occur. In the vicinity of the endothelium, the cell-poor/cell-free plasma zone, the Poiseuille-zone is formed, allowing room for leukocytes. Increased red blood cell aggregation makes the axial flow more expressed with widening Poiseuille zone, driving the leukocyte tethering, margination, and also slowing down their rolling (based on Baskurt 2008; Nash 2008; Yalcin 2011).

Table 13.2. Brief overview of the available methodology for the detection of functional characteristics of the microvasculature

Method	Species/tissue	Parameters	Indications	Limitations	Reference
Nailfold videocapillaro-scopy	human/nailfold	Capillary distribution (density), morphological abnormalities, blood velocity,	chronic diseases (diabetes, vasculitis, arteritis)	Only human application	Awan 2010
Conventional fluorescence intravital microscopy	animal models/superficial tissue layers	FCD, red blood cell velocity, blood flow, microvascular permeability, PMN-endothelial interactions	ischemia-reperfusion, shock (hypovolemic, septic) wound healing, tumors	1) restricted imaging depths (~100–200 μm) dramatic depth- and tissue-dependent deterioration of spatial resolution 2) need of fluorescence labeling 3) light toxicity 4) motion artifacts (peristalsys, breathing) 5) difficult and time-consuming (off-line) analysis	Menger 1992
Confocal microscopy, two- and multiphoton microscopy	animal models/superficial tissue layers	(morphology), microvascular permeability, subcellular events	ischemia-reperfusion, shock (hypovolemic, septic) wound healing, tumors	See #1-5 at fluorescence IVM 6) photobleaching of chromophores 7) photodamage of the tissue at the focal plane 8) signal overlapping with tissue endogenous fluorescence 9) restricted range of applicable fluorescent proteins restricted range of applicable fluorescent proteins due to limited excitation wavelengths	Paramsothy 2010; Denk 1990; Zipfel 2003

Method	Species/tissue	Parameters	Indications	Limitations	Reference
OPS, SDF, IDF	human and animal models/superficial tissue layers	vascular density, vessel diameter, red blood cell velocity, heterogeneity of perfusion (microvascular blood flow)	ischemia-reperfusion, shock (hypovolemic, septic) wound healing, tumors	1) restricted imaging depths 2) motion artifacts (peristalsys, breathing) 3) difficult and time-consuming (off-line) analysis	Groner 1999; Goedhart 2007; Hernandez 2013; Gilbert-Kawai 2016
Laser Doppler perfusion monitoring	human and animal models/superficial tissue layers	flux, velocity and concentration of the moving blood cells	human: skin animals: perfusion deficit situations (ischemia-reperfusion, shock (hypovolemic, septic) wound healing, tumors	1) influence of tissue optical properties (on the perfusion signal) 2) motion artifact 3) lack of quantitative units for perfusion	Leahy 1999; Rajan 2009; Steenbergen 2012
Laser Doppler perfusion imaging, Laser speckle imaging	human and animal models/superficial tissue layers	perfusion (in arbitrary units), heterogeneity	human: skin animals: perfusion deficit situations (ischemia-reperfusion, shock (hypovolemic, septic) wound healing, tumors	4) lack of knowledge of the depth of measurement and the biological zero signal	Essex 1991; Boas 2010
Reflectance spectroscopy (in combination with Laser Doppler perfusion imaging)	human and animal models/superficial tissue layers	the oxygen saturation of hemoglobin, regional amount of hemoglobin, velocity and flow of the blood in microcirculation	Measurement of perfusion, oxygenation (in response to ischemia-reperfusion, septic shock, anemia, burn injury)		Sakr 2010; Menzebach 2008; Hölzle 2010; Merz 2010; Scheeren 2011,2016
NIRS	human and animal models/skeletal muscle, brain	microvascular reactivity, blood flow directly, vascular compliance	macro–microcirculatory uncoupling	low spatial resolution	De Blasi 1994, 2008
Protoporphyrin IX—Triplet State Lifetime Technique	human and animal models (skin)	mitochondrial oxygen tension (local treatment with 5-aminolevulinic acid; ALA)	sepsis	topical use, laser safety concerns	Harms 2015

OPS: orthogonal polarization spectral imaging, SDF: sidestream dark-field imaging, IDF: incident dark-field technology, NIRS: near-infrared spectroscopy

Several other factors should be considered to better understand circulation conditions in the field of microcirculation such as the extremely variable microvascular network geometry. The vesselcross section can almost never be described as a regular circle. Elasticity of vessel wall, hemodynamic features, flow profile and parameters (e.g., Reynolds number, Womersley number) have to be taken into consideration as well (Pries 2008; Chandran 2012). Thus, *in vivo* models have a great significance in further studying the connection of hemorheological factors and microcirculatory characteristics, which can provide simultaneous data on most of the above parameters.

So, the microcirculation possesses characteristic micro-hemodynamic features. Due to the decreasing size of the microvessels, the major pressure drop occurs in the first-order arterioles (based on the Hagen-Poiseuille equation), therefore constriction status of these vessels has the highest influence on the regional flow. Local capillary flow, however, is controlled by third-order, small-sized terminal arterioles. Efficacy of perfusion can be termed by a parameter called the "functional capillary density" (FCD) which reflects the length of perfused capillaries within a given area (Honig 1982). Reduced FCD results in a reduced surface area for capillary exchange and an increase in diffusion distance (Hepple 2000). Recruitment of capillaries depends on morphological features of vessels/endothelium of the given region and also on blood rheology factors (i.e., hematocrit, viscosity, blood cell deformability and aggregation), cellular factors, immune function, and coagulation function). Deterioration of microcirculatory perfusion is marker of severity for many forms of circulatory disorders such as hemorrhagic, cardiogenic, and septic shock, also reflecting the outcome of the disease (Sakr 2004; Fang 2006; den Uil 2010). Hence, microcirculation might be considered an important prognostic indicator in different clinical scenarios.

METHODS FOR DYNAMIC EXAMINATION OF MICROCIRCULATORY FUNCTIONS

There are numerous invasive and non-invasive methods for investigating the microcirculation. The limitation of this chapter does not allow to overview all the methods and their developments in details. Table 13.2 gives a brief overview of the currently available methodology for the detection of functional characteristics of the microvasculature.

Videomicroscopic Techniques

Direct visualization of the microcirculation with different types of *in vivo* microscopic methods (IVM) enables not only examination of the architecture of arterioles, capillaries and venules, but also provides an opportunity for continuous detection and quantification of dynamic functional changes. Apart from nailfold capillaroscopy, most organs can be reached via surgical exposure of the tissues for IVM examinations. Using meticulous microsurgical techniques, an access of the microscope objectives and the required tissue depth can be achieved by maintaining the proper physiological conditions without causing any disturbance of the patency of the microcirculation. Because of optical consideration (limited penetration of light into the tissue, scattering), limited depth for examination of the tissue is a characteristic feature of IVM methodology. For this reason, an appropriate imaging modality enabling examination of the required tissue depth should be chosen for all experimental studies. By these methods, the dynamics of microcirculatory environment can be assessed over time and space with the required resolution closely approximating the natural microcirculatory environment.

Nailfold Videocapillaroscopy

This non-invasive technique involves a conventional light microscope combined with a video camera and a recording system. It is suitable for the evaluation of capillary density, morphological abnormalities and blood flow in the nailfold area (Awan 2010). Main indications: chronic diseases such as diabetes, vasculitis and arteritis

Fluorescence Intravital Microscopy

In the earliest studies, bright-field transillumination of relatively translucent tissues was employed (Hoole 1800; Wagner 1839), but trans- and epi-illumination techniques (with microsurgical exposure of the tissue of interest) and the use of incident ultraviolet illumination and its combination with specific fluorescence tracers enabled observation of individual cells and cell-vessel wall interactions in later IVM studies (Ellinger 1929; Irwin 1953; Zweifach 1954; Reese 1960; Menger 1991). Epifluorescence microscopy has enabled detection of the dynamics of individual cells within the microcirculation (Endrich 1980). The spatial resolution has been further improved by the use of confocal microscopy (Villringer 1989), but these techniques still resolve structures 100–200 micrometers below the organ surface. By using the combination of IVM with high-resolution video recordings and an off-line analysis, dynamic microcirculatory processes could be analyzed in sufficient details (Menger 1991).

Due to atraumatic microsurgical techniques in experimental settings, almost all organs and tissues could be reached for IVM examinations (brain: Rovainen 1993; spine: Ishikawa 1999, heart: Tillmanns 1974, lung: Kuhnle 1993, liver: Menger 1991, pancreas: Klar 1990, intestine: Bohlen 1978, kidney: Steinhausen 1981, lymph nodes: von Andrian 1996, and bone marrow: Mazo 1998). A large range of vascular, cellular and molecular functions can be assessed by using specific fluorescent markers. Specifically, individual microvessels (from 3–5 µm in diameter), plasma, red blood cells, platelets and circulating immune cells can be visualized (Table 13.3, Figure 13.2).

The widefield fluorescence IVM methodology was advanced to the laser scanning confocal technology, two- and multiphoton and spinning disk microscopy, which made deep tissue imaging (at a single cell as well as subcellular level) also possible (Denk 1990; Zipfel 2003; for review see Pittet 2011 and Masedunskas 2012). Clinical applications of the new imaging technologies such as laser endomicroscopy have made *in vivo* real-time microscopic imaging and diagnostics also possible (Paramsothy 2010).

Table 13.3. Most common fluorescence labeling techniques used in fluorescence IVM studies

Targets	Fluorescence markers	Derived microcirculatory parameters	References
Red blood cells	FITC	red blood cell velocity, blood flow, functional capillary density	Ruh 1998
PMNs	Rhodamine 6G, Acridin orange	PMN-endothelial interactions	Saetzler 1997; Massberg 1998
Platelets	Rhodamine 6G (ex vivo)	platelet-PMN-endothelial interactions	Massberg 1998
Plasma (or plasma proteins)	FITC-dextrans (40-2000 kDa)	microvascular permeability	Persson 1985
	tetramethylrhodamine-labelled BSA	microvascular permeability	von Dobschuetz 2004
	FITC-albumin	microvascular permeability (two-photon IVM)	Egawa 2013
Hepatocytes	Rhodamine 123	mitochondrial membrane potential	Sun 2001
Hepatocytes	NADH autofluorescence	mitochondrial respiration	Roesner 2006
Kupffer cells	non-occluding fluorescent beads	Kupffer cell activation	Watanabe 2007

PMN: polymorphonuclear leukocytes, FITC (fluorescein-isothiocyanate),
BSA (bovine serum albumin),

OPS-SDF-IDF Techniques

Using these methods, microvessels can be observed via visualization of their hemoglobin-containing red blood cell content. By means of epi-illumination of superficial tissue layers (up to 2–3 mm in depth) with polarized light (Groner 1999) or incident light (Goedhart 2007), photons are reflected from the deeper tissue parts, providing illumination of the superficial layers. As the reflected-scattered light is absorbed by hemoglobin (at the isobestic point oxygenated and deoxygenated hemoglobin of 530 nm wavelength) within the red blood cells, they appear as black or grey points flowing along the vessels (Groner 1999; Goedhart 2007; Leahy 2012; Lehmann 2012).

The orthogonal polarization spectral (OPS) imaging device (Cytometrics, Philadelphia, PA, USA) uses linearly polarized green light source to illuminate the tissue. The reflected polarized light is blocked by an orthogonally polarized analyzer, while depolarized scattered light can pass through to the camera (providing a dark-field image). The OPS imaging was introduced by Groner et al. in 1999, which was followed by the more advanced Sidestream Dark-Field (SDF) imaging in 2007, introduced by Goedhart (produced by the Microvision Medical B.V., Amsterdam, the Netherlands; the device being called Microscan) (Goedhart 2007; Milstein 2012). Another SDF system (CapiScope HVCS) is produced by KK Technology (Honiton, UK) (reviewed by Massey 2016). Microscan and CapiScope HVCS have similar image size (720 × 480 and 752 × 480 pixels, respectively) and resolution (1.45 × 1.58 and 0.92 × 0.92 μm/pixel, respectively). An improved version of the latter one is the Capiscope HVCS-HR which has higher resolution (0.81 × 0.81 μm/pixel). The newest generation of videocapillaroscopy is based on the incident dark field (IDF) principle (Braedius Scientific™)

(Hernandez 2013). Recently, a new device based similarly on IDF imaging (Cytocam) was developed with improved optical lenses, a high-resolution (0.66 × 0.66 μm/pixel) computer-controlled image sensor, higher image size (2208 × 1648 pixels), and with an application for automatic data analysis (Aykut 2015; van Elteren 2015; Gilbert-Kawai 2016).

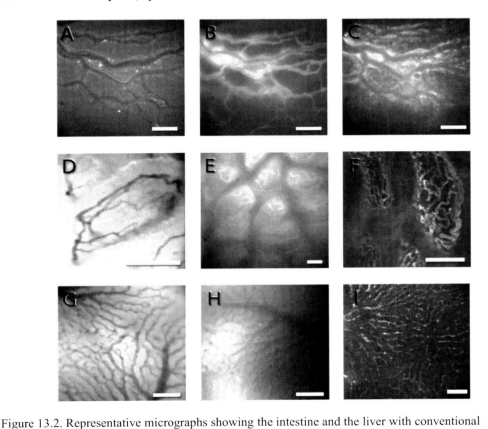

Figure 13.2. Representative micrographs showing the intestine and the liver with conventional fluorescence IVM (A-C, E, H), OPS (D, G) and laser scanning confocal microscopy (F, I). FITC-labeled red blood cells (A), plasma labeling (B) and rhodamine 6G-labeled leukocytes in the longitudinal muscle layer of the rat ileum (C); OPS images of the intestinal villi (D) and liver hepatic sinusoids (G) in Sprague-Dawley rats. FITC labeling of the microvessels in the intestinal villi in BALB/c mice as detected with fluorescence IVM (E) and in the intestinal villi (F) and the liver (I) in rats using laser scanning confocal microscopy. Bar denotes 100 μm.
The IVM images were taken by using a Zeiss Axiotech Vario 100HD IVM microscope, 100W HBO mercury lamp, Acroplan 20× water immersion objective, Carl Zeiss GmbH, Jena, Germany) and a CCD camera (Teli CS8320Bi, Toshiba Teli Corporation, Osaka, Japan). The OPS images were taken by the Cytoscan A/R device (Cytometrics, Philadelphia, PA, USA). (Original recordings of AS).

As these hand-held microscopes do not require any dye and allow for non-invasive visualization of the microcirculation in patients particularly in the oral cavity. For analysis of microcirculation with SDF/IDF devices, De Backer et al. have proposed the use of the following parameters: proportion of perfused vessels (PPV), perfused vessel density, microvascular flow index (MFI), and heterogeneity index (De Backer 2007). Further approaches together with those used in conventional fluorescence IVM are summarized in Table 13.4.

Table 13.4. Commonly used parameters for different IVM methods (partially based on ref. by Massey 2016)

Parameter	Definition	Method where the parameter is used	Reference
Red blood cell (or plasma) velocity (RBCV) (µm/s)	Velocity of red blood cells or plasma	conventional fluorescence IVM, OPS, SDF, IDF	Lehr 1993; Groner 1999
Total vessel density (mm/mm²)	Total length of vessels is divided by the total surface of the analyzed area	conventional fluorescence IVM, OPS, SDF, IDF	Donati 2013; Bezemer 2008
Functional capillary density (FCD) (mm/mm²)	Total length of capillaries with red blood cell flow referred to the observation area	conventional fluorescence IVM, OPS, SDF, IDF	Lehr 1993; Groner 1999
Functional vessel density #1 (mm/mm²)	Total length of perfused vessels (sluggish or continuous) referred to the observation area	OPS, SDF, IDF	Donati 2013
De Backer score (vessel density) (1/mm)	Calculated based on the line crossing method when the image is divided by three vertical and three horizontal lines. This score is calculated as the number of vessels crossing the lines divided by the total length of the lines.	SDF, IDF	De Backer 2007; Donati 2013, Bezemer 2008, Sakr 2010
Microvascular flow index (MFI) (arbitrary units)	Based on flow characterization (absent, intermittent, sluggish or normal) of vessels using the line crossing method (in four quadrants of the recorded images) An average of the scores is used.	SDF, IDF	De Backer 2007, Donati 2013, Bezemer 2008
Proportion of perfused vessels for large vessels (PPVl) (%)	100 × number of perfused vessels divided by the total number of vessels	IVM, OPS, SDF, IDF	Donati 2013, Bezemer 2008, Sakr 2010
Proportion of perfused vessels (length) (PPV) (%)	100 × length of perfused vessels divided by the total length of vessels	conventional fluorescence IVM, OPS, SDF, IDF	De Backer 2007
Perfused vessel density #2 (1/mm)	Vessel density x PPV	SDF, IDF	Bezemer 2008

Parameter	Definition	Method where the parameter is used	Reference
Flow heterogeneity index	The difference between highest and the lowest MFI is divided by the mean flow velocity	SDF, IDF	De Backer 2007, Donati 2013
PMN rolling (defined as rodamine 6G-labaled cells moving at a velocity less than 40% of that of the erythrocytes in the centerline of the microvessel) (1/mm/s or % of total PMNs)	The number of rolling cells devided by the vessel circumference	conventional fluorescence IVM	Lehr 1993, Bajory 2002
PMN adhesion (cells that did not move or detach from the endothelial lining within an observation period of 30 s) (1/mm^2)	The number of cells devided by mm^2 of endothelial surface	conventional fluorescence IVM	Lehr 1993

Laser Doppler Flowmetry

The background of laser Doppler monitoring is the "Doppler shift" phenomenon (Doppler 1942). When a monochromatic laser light enters the tissues and meets moving blood cells, it undergoes changes in wavelength (Doppler shift), but remains unchanged if the beam of light hits static tissue structures. Magnitude and frequency changes of wavelength correlate with the number of moving blood cells (Stern 1975). The Doppler technique provides "perfusion units" which cannot be transformed in terms of flow (e.g., ml/min), but rather a flux unit without dimension, since it is an integral over the velocity and the number of moving red blood cells in the tissue territory laying under the probe (Obeid 1990; Leahy 1999, 2012; Friedriksson 2012;).

There are two major approaches of perfusion measurements, the laser Doppler perfusion monitoring and laser Doppler perfusion imaging (Rajan 2009; Friedriksson 2012; Leahy 2012).

Laser Doppler Perfusion Monitoring

In this one-point measurement method, a fiber-optic probe is used to deliver the laser light to the tissue, and another fiber to detect the back-scattered photons recording the integrated perfusion in a sampling volume in real time. The measurement depth and sampling volume depend on the wavelength (usually 630, 780 and 830 nm are used) and the fiber separation used. In the skin, (using 780 nm wavelength), the measuring depth is 0.5–1 mm and the measurement volume is approximately 1 mm^3. The main manufacturers of laser Doppler instruments are Perimed AB (Stockholm, Sweden), Moor Instruments Ltd. (Axminster, UK), Transonic Systems Inc. (Ithaca, New York, USA), Oxford Optronix Ltd (Oxford, UK) and LEA Medizintechnik (Giessen, Germany).

Laser Doppler tissue flowmetry method can be widely applied both in the clinical and research work to study local or systemic effect of heat, reflex vasodilation, microcirculatory changes following occlusion, or the effects of vasoactive drugs, as well as endothelial reactivity using provocation tests (ischemia, heat) (Obeid 1990; Neviere 1996; Rajan 2009; Friedriksson 2012; Leahy 2012).

However, numerous factors may influence the results. This method considerably and sensitively indicates the changes occurring in microcirculation, but at the same time, several factors may influence the measurements. These factors on one hand include the thickness of the examined tissue, its anatomical structure, optical properties (pigmentation), possible morphological alteration and vascularity. On the other hand, from the patient's side, the gender, age, hormonal and neurological effects and drugs may affect the results of the measurement. From the side of the device, the displacement and contamination of the probe, kinking of fiber optics, distance of emission and receiving optical fibers, wavelength of laser light and biological zero signal may also be considered as influencing factors. Disturbing artifacts or "noises" may develop through the movement of optic fiber or from the affected tissue (e.g., breathing, intestinal peristalsis). External factors such as temperature, humidity, air movement also influence the measurement; therefore, it is very important to ensure standard circumstances. However, performing comparative studies (e.g., before and after intervention) is difficult, because to ensure the same conditions in all parameters is almost impossible (Obeid 1990; Neviere 1996; Nemeth 2003; Rajan 2009; Friedriksson 2012; Leahy 2012).

In pathophysiological processes, such as sepsis or ischemia-reperfusion, associated with acute changes of tissue microcirculation, laser Doppler technique is highly justified. In experimental models, probes available in various versions can be applied in several ways (Nemeth 2003; Rajan 2009; Friedriksson 2012; Leahy 2012):

- probe touched directly to the surface of skin or in open surgery of the organ (manual or preferred trestle fixing)
- probe fixed on the surface of the organ (stitches)
- in laparoscopy introduced via trocar and touched to the surface of examined intraperitoneal organ or the peritoneum
- introduced in endoscopy and touched to the surface of mucosa (multichannel endoscopy, fiber optic probe)
- implanted between tissue layers or bone mortise for monitoring

Depending on the wavelength of the applied laser, the depth of the tissue area that can be examined may range from 0.1 to 0.8 mm, e.g., by applying laser with 780 mm wavelength and probe with 0.5 mm diameter, this tissue depth is 0.73 mm in muscles, 0.52 mm in the liver and 0.5 mm in the skin. The duration of the examination and positioning of probe should be taken into consideration. The 0.5 mW energy derives from laser light, and in the examined tissue, it may also influence the state of capillaries after some time (Friedriksson 2012).

The probe stabilization is essential. Overpressure of the tissues may cause local microcirculatory disturbance; if too loose, displacing or fixing may lead to inaccurate measurements and several artifacts.

Several solutions are known for the right interpretation of the recorded signal in the literature. For instance, the native values measured and assessed at a certain interval by the device can be used. Within this interval (e.g., data of stable signal over 10 or 20 seconds), the values can be averaged. Relative changes compared to initial values, moving average, Fourier transformation and various timeline analysis methods can also be used for analyzing laser Doppler recordings (Obeid 1990; Nemeth 2003, 2014b; Rajan 2009; Friedriksson 2012; Leahy 2012).

An organ may show different laser Doppler signals with different recorded patterns depending on the functional and morphological state of microvasculature. Therefore, it is important to observe the characteristics of the recorded signal and decide how to analyze and interpret the data. Signals recorded in skin, liver, kidney and muscles vary within a relatively small range, but they are never consistent. In other organs such as bowel, omentum or pancreas, the signals oscillate between wider ranges, so the averaging is difficult in these cases; it may even be misleading if we analyze a data set of t an inadequate period with their extremes (Nemeth 2003, 2014b).

During a prolonged monitoring, when the probe of the device is fixed in a steady, permanent position and the microcirculation is being monitored for half an hour or even longer, the extent and dynamics of changes can be analyzed separately. This point of view is of particular importance in examinations which aim to follow organic microcirculatory effects of different materials and surgical maneuvers.

Regarding the several factors which influence the measured values, examining the changes in correlation with the baseline values is an extremely useful data analyzing method. Thus it can be expressed as a percentage to what extent a certain tissue area changes during a surgery. It is a very important point to indicate baseline value, as it was mentioned, intensity of laser Doppler signal is not constant in any of the tissue areas, more or less irregularities, periodicity and artifacts appear. Should we use any data analysis and interpretation method, it has to beconsistent and standardized.

Laser Doppler Perfusion Imaging (Laser Doppler Scanner Technology)

A laser Doppler perfusion imaging technology maps the perfusion from a larger area by scanning the laser beam over the area of interest without having any direct contact with the tissues (Essex 1991; Fredriksson 2012; Steenbergen 2012 a, b). These instruments provide perfusion map of an area with a (normally) heterogeneous perfusion and also gives the average of perfusion of the examined area in a single measurement. The main manufacturers of laser Doppler perfusion imagers are Perimed AB and Moor Instruments Ltd. Using stepwise changes in the illuminating laser beam wavelength or different wavelength simultaneously, the spatial resolution can be increased up to 0.1 mm.

Laser Doppler Flowmetry Combined with Reflectance Spectrometry

The more recent technology (the O2C device, Lea, Giessen, Germany) combines the laser Doppler technique and reflection spectroscopy. Using specific probes, white light (wavelengths 500–800 nm) and laser light (wavelength 830 nm) are introduced simultaneously. The absorbed portion of the light spectrum is absorbed on erythrocytes assuming the color of the hemoglobin as measured by oxygen saturation, while laser light reflects perfusion (based on the Doppler shift). The sum of all erythrocytes and their velocity provides a measure of blood flow (volume flow). The following parameters can be measured simultaneously with this technology: oxygen saturation of hemoglobin at the venous end of the capillaries, regional amount of hemoglobin as a measure of blood volume and capillary density, velocity and flow of the blood within the microcirculation. This method has been employed to assess the microvascular response in patients with septic shock (Sakr 2004; Sakr 2010) and in anemia (Menzebach 2008), to estimate flap viability (Hölzle 2010) and wound healing in burn injury (Merz 2010).

Laser Speckle Imaging

A speckle image is created when an object is illuminated by laser light. The backscattered light will forms a random interference pattern consisting of dark and bright areas (speckle pattern). In case of a moving object (e.g., red blood cells) in the underlying tissue, the speckle pattern changes over time depending on the extent of movements within the examined area. As a result, the level of blurring differs resulting in various extent of speckle contrast (Briers 1999; Briers 2012; Boas 2010; Steenbergen 2012b). Consequently, changes in microcirculatory perfusion characteristics under a surface (within a typical depth range of 1–5 mm, max. 15 mm) can be analyzed. The resolution depends on the characteristics of detector as well as the size of examined surface and the distance of the detector. Using this method, preclinical and clinical detection of the skin (Choi 2004; Rege 2011; Sandker 2014) and even cerebral blood flow (Parthasarathy 2010; Qin 2012) could be performed.

It was recently demonstrated that the distribution of blood flow within tissue beds can noninvasively be visualized also by the motion-contrast laser speckle imaging which leads to enhanced visibility of distinct vascular beds, including capillaries (Liu 2013).

Near-Infrared Spectroscopy

Near-infrared spectroscopy (NIRS) is a non-invasive technique that assesses the redox state of microcirculatory hemoglobin by measuring oxyhemoglobin, deoxyhemoglobin, total hemoglobin and other chromophores (myoglobin, cytochrome aa3) in mostly the venous system (De Blasi 1994; Pareznik 2006). Vascular occlusion tests allow quantification of the rate of decay of microcirculatory oxygen saturation thus representing the metabolic status of the underlying tissue (muscle) (De Blasi 2008).

Measurements of O₂ Tension and Saturation

Conventional oximetry (hemoglobin oxygen saturation measurement) is widely used in the clinical practice and is based on the assessment of differences in the absorption spectra of oxy- and deoxy-hemoglobin. Interestingly, it was first applied *in vivo* within the microcirculation to obtain oxygen saturation in single vessels using IVM (Pittman 1975; Pittman 2013). Transcutaneous arterial oxygen pressures can simultaneously be measured using standard pulsoximetry, whereas transcutaneous venous carbon monoxide tensions with CO_2-sensitive electrodes (Fromy 1997).

Phosphorescence quenching microscopy is based on the collisional quenching phenomenon which occurs when excited phosphor decays back to the ground state by emitting a photon (phosphorescence) or by transferring energy to nearby oxygen molecules. This enables measurements of the O_2 tensions (Vinogradov 2002). The energy transfer to oxygen results in the formation of the reactive species singlet oxygen, which can then react with nearby organic molecules, thereby resulting in the consumption of the original oxygen molecule.

Oxygen tensions in the microcirculation can be measured using oxygen-sensitive polarographic microcathodes (Buerk 2004). Oxygen saturation can also be non-invasively measured using the Resonance Raman microspectroscopy (Ward 2006). The phosphorescence quenching approach (Vinogradov 2002) and oxygen electrodes (Buerk 2004) can also measure oxygen tensions in the interstitium.

In Vivo Measurements of Mitochondrial Functions and Oxygen Tensions

The "Protoporphyrin IX–Triplet State Lifetime Technique" is a new approach developed for the measurement of mitochondrial function and oxygen tension (mitoPO2) *in vivo* (Mik 2006, Harms 2015). A recently developed non-invasive technique is able to measure a decline in mitoPO2 after pressure-induced cessation of blood supply (called oxygen disappearance rate), also providing estimates of mitochondrial oxygen consumption. The oxygenation data was validated in a sepsis study in rats with the use of reflectance spectroscopy (combined laser Doppler) in the skin. They also demonstrated the feasibility of the non-invasive technology to assess mitochondrial function in the human skin.

Further Methods

Due to the limitations of the chapter, further special methods are just briefly summarized, referring to detailed handbooks (e.g., Leahy 2012).

Subsurface Spectroscopy (Tissue Viability Imaging)

For tissue viability imaging (TiVi), further possibilities are based on wideband spectroscopy of backscattered light (subsurface spectroscopy) for mapping local red blood cell concentration. The sequential photo recordings are being analyzed by a software package, allowing studies of dynamic skin reactions (using agent or effects that cause vasodilatation or vasoconstriction) (O'Doherty 2012).

Optical Microangiography

Because of the high spatiotemporal resolution and the small dimension, microvasculature imaging is technologically challenging. Optical microangiography (OMAG) is capable of resolving three-dimensional distribution of dynamic blood perfusion by imaging the endogenous light scattering from moving red blood cells. The technique is based on Fourier domain optical coherence tomography (FDOCT) (Wang 2012).

Photoacoustic Tomography

Photoacoustic tomography (PAT) detects endogenous or exogenous optical absorption contrast acoustically. When red blood cells are irradiated by a short-pulsed laser beam, a transient thermoelastic expansion occurs that induces high-frequency ultrasonic (photoacoustic) waves. The device encodes the red blood cell distribution and makes a reconstruction of a three-dimensional microvascular image. Using multi-wavelength measurements, differentiation of oxyhemoglobin and deoxyhemoglobin is also possible. Based on PAT, photoacoustic microscopy (PAM) and photoacoustic computed tomography (PACT) methods are known (Hu 2012).

High Frequency Ultrasound Imaging

Maximal imaging frequency of clinical ultrasound systems are typically 12–15 MHz, providing resolution on structures of > 300 µm. The micro-ultrasound devices (preclinical imaging) have been developed for the range of 15–80 MHz (Foster 2012).

Micro-CT, Nano-SPECT-CT, NMR

Micro-computed tomography (Micro-CT) is a powerful tool to study small animals, corrosion specimens or biopsies. The resolution of Micro-CT is about 1–100 µm in rotating state, ~50–100 µm in rotating scanner in plane. Micro-SPECT and micro-PET resolution is about 1–2 mm, while micro-magnetic resonance imaging (MRI) provides a resolution about 100–200 µm in plane and ~0.5–10 mm slice thickness (Kline 2012). Boundaries of the nuclear magnetic response imaging (NMRI) techniques and applications (MR angiography, MR perfusion imaging, functional MRI) widen, providing more possibilities to investigate structural and functional state of the vasculature as well (Kerskens 2012).

BRIEF OVERVIEW ON METHODS FOR ASSESSMENT OF RHEOLOGICAL PARAMETERS

Methods for Measuring Blood and Plasma Viscosity

For the determination of blood viscosity, only those measuring devices are suitable, which can determine viscosity at different shear rates (Cokelet 2007a, b). The shearing tension or speed gradient profile may be generated under the effect of gravitational force (e.g., in capillary viscometers), or through rotational motion with a certain angular velocity, produced by a built-in mechanism (rotational viscometers) (Baskurt 2009).

Most of the viscometers were the capillary type until the 1960s, rotational viscometers appeared later. In the capillary-type ones, the flow rate profile can be determined from the position-time data of fluid column, and the shearing tension can be calculated from the geometry of tube. The geometry of rotational viscometers can be various: cone-plate, cone-in-cone or coaxial cylinder (or Couette-system) in speed-gradient controlled or shearing tension controlled form. The fluid to be measured can be filled in between the two elements (e.g., 'bob' and 'cup'). One element can be rotated by adjusted angular velocity. The torque relocated to the non-rotated element to an extent is depending on the viscosity of the fluid. The torque is tested by laser reflection, and the viscosity can be calculated at a certain shear rate-gradient. Oscillation flow viscometers are also known, which are suitable for the investigation of viscous and elastic components. The viscous component can be calculated from the amplitude of speed gradient, and the elastic component is calculated from phase delay of shearing tension in relation to the speed gradient (Rosencranz 2006; Hardeman 2007).

For the measurement of plasma viscosity-based on the newtonian characteristics-viscometers, whose method does not depend on shear rate gradient, are suitable. The dynamic viscosity of the fluid can be calculated from fluid flow rate in a system with a certain geometry, from position-time data (U-tube or capillary viscometers: e.g., Ostwald, Coulter-Harkness, Rheomed, Luckham viscometers), or in the falling ball viscometers (e.g., Haake-type) from the effect of drag force applying the Navier-Stokes equation: $F = 6\pi r \eta v$, where F is the frictional force, r is the radius of the spherical object, η is the fluid viscosity, v is the particle's velocity. With a simpler method: $\eta = k(\rho_1-\rho_2)t$, where k is constant, ρ_1 is the density of the particles, ρ_2 is the density of the fluid, t is the duration of ball falling (Rosencranz 2006; Hardeman 2007; Baskurt 2009).

Methods for Testing red Blood Cell Deformability

For the determination of red blood cell deformability, several methods and various approaches are known. The best-known and still in use techniques are based on the filtration method, the micropipette aspiration technique, microchannel methods and the ektacytometry (Hardeman 2007; Baskurt 2009).

Filtration technique has been used since the 1960s: measuring the passage of blood cell suspension through a filter with a certain pore diameter/size (~200 000 pores), the cells' deformability can be concluded; due to the clogging of pores, the permeability of the filtering membrane gradually decreases. The initially used classical paper filters were replaced by polycarbonate filter membranes containing cylindrical channels (diameter: 3, 5 or 8 µm, length: 10 µm). The Reid-Dormandy type filtration method utilized the filtration of red blood cell aggregation through the filter with 5 µm in diameter. Improving the principle, Dormandy and his colleagues prepared the St. George's filtrometer. The oligopore (23–30 pores) and the single pore technique (Single Erythrocyte Rigidometer, SER) are more sophisticated methods; here mainly the time of change in conductivity between the two sides of the filter correlate with presence of red blood cells just passing through the pore, where the process is analyzed by the attached computer according to the pores transit time histogram (Cell Transit Analyzer, CTA) (Hardeman 2007; Baskurt 2009; Musielak 2009).

With the *micropipette aspiration method*, a single cell can be examined, which is wholly or partly aspirated into a glass capillary with 1–5 µm diameter. From the measurement of the negative pressure and the length of the aspirated membrane phase provides shearing elastic module, while the aspiration of the whole cell gives the deformability. It requires serious technical skills (Hardeman 2007; Baskurt 2009; Musielak 2009).

The basic principle of the *microchannel method* is that the cell suspension is flowing through one or two parallel channels, or through an artificial microchannel network, while the movement of red blood cells, the transit time, and position of the cells can be visually analyzed (Baskurt 2009; Musielak 2009; Reinhart 2015).

The *ektacytometry* is based on the diffraction analysis of laser beam (wavelength: 670 nm) reflected from red blood cells suspended in high-viscosity (preferably ~30 mPas) macromolecule solution (e.g., 70 kDa dextran or 350 kPa polyvinylpyrrolidone isotonic solution) and elongated due to the shear stress, providing the elongation index (EI) in the function of shear stress (Chien 1975; Chasis 1986; Hardeman 2007). The shear stress on the sample is generated by the motor or vacuum device, while the laser diffraction pattern is captured by a CCD camera and projected on a screen. The EI can be calculated from the analyzed picture by the software diffractrogram: EI = (L-W) / (L + W), where L is the length and W is the width of the diffractogram. Different shearing geometries are used in ektacytometer devices: plane-plane rotational system in the Rheodyn device, Couette-system in laser-assisted optical rotational cell analyzer (LORCA), or vacuum-driven slit-flow technique in the Rheoscan device (Hardeman 2007; Baskurt 2009; Musielak 2009). Besides the classical deformability measurements, some modern ektacytometers are capable of testing osmotic gradient deformability (i.e., deformability test at constant shear stress over an osmotic gradient range) and membrane mechanical stability (deformability test before and after a period pf mechanical shearing at definitive magnitude and duration) (Hardeman 2007; Baskurt 2009).

Further deformability measurement methods are the rheoscope technique (a combination of ektacytometry and microscopy), atomic-force microscopy, the laser optical tweezers and magnetic twisting cytometry (Hardeman 2007; Musielak 2009).

Methods for Testing Red Blood Cell Aggregation

Several indirect and direct methods are known for the determination of red blood cell aggregation. The classical and modern methods (Westergren, Seditainer, Automatic ESR) based on the already mentioned measurement of erythrocyte sedimentation rate (ESR) are widely used and well standardized methods. Also known is the determination of zeta sedimentation rate (by centrifugation) and the determination of indirect aggregation parameters (aggregation index = $(\eta_{low} - \eta_{high}) / \eta_{high}$, where η is the blood viscosity determined at a certain low and a higher speed gradient) from the results of blood viscosity measured at low speed gradient (e.g., 1 s^{-1}). By microscopy techniques or rheoscope the morphology of aggregates can also be examined and their size and red blood cell count per aggregate can be determined. By this method, the heteroaggregates (white blood cell, platelet, red blood cell) can also be separated. Ultrasound techniques enable non-invasive *in vivo* examinations (mainly B-mode echography) of aggregation developing in a certain vascular region (Hardeman 2007; Baskurt 2009, 2012b).

In clinical and experimental hemorheological studies, the most commonly used methods are based on the principles of photometry. The presence of aggregates increases the light transmission of blood sample related to a certain wavelength, as in this case the width of plasma phase (or other suspending medium) between the particles increases. In the course of disaggregation, the cells dispersed on a larger surface decreasing the plasma phase width and so the light-transmittance. When cells start to aggregate during stasis or at low shear rate, the plasma phase width and the light-transmittance increase. Furthermore, red blood cell aggregates reflect light differently compared to the individual cells. Based on these principles, different devices are available to analyze the light transmission (e.g., Myrenne MA-1 erythrocyte aggregometer), or the reflection of light (laser) from the aggregating cells (syllectometry, e.g., LORCA). Using these methods, both the extent and the dynamics of aggregation can be examined (Hardeman 2007; Baskurt 2009, 2012b).

Thoughts on the Link between Microcirculatory and Micro-Rheological Investigations

The examination of rheological conditions of microcirculation and their interaction cannot be simplified to the correlation of Poiseuille's law related to the rigid-walled, straight regular pipes. The large region of microcirculation is not even homogenous from rheological point of view. In addition to the vein diameter and vascular geometry, the viscosity cannot be considered constant due to axial migration of red blood cells (Fåhræus and Fåhræus-Lindqvist effect), phase separation, very diverse and changeable, unsteady distribution of tissue hematocrit (microvascular hematocrit), and the particularities of the zone of individual flow (Fahreus 1931, 1958; Wells 1964; Lipowsky 2005; Pries 2008).

Therefore, in the isolated organs, in perfusion *ex vivo* models, the solutions ensuring the stability of vessel diameter (maximal dilatation or maximal constriction) could only show a thorough picture if we hypothesized and presumed that the viscosity is constant at every stage of the circulation. This is however, obviously not true. That is why a more detailed investigation of the role of micro-rheological parameters in the microcirculation is required (Wells 1964; Lipowsky 2005; Popel 2005).

Parallel investigations of hemodynamic, microcirculatory, hemorheological, acid-base parameters, hematological and hemostaseological factors may provide enough information to evaluate and understand the dynamics of these changes and their interactions (Baskurt 2007; Nemeth 2014b).

MAIN MICROCIRCULATORY AND MICRO-RHEOLOGICAL FINDINGS IN VARIOUS PATHOPHYSIOLOGICAL PROCESSES

Ischemia/Reperfusion

Ischemia/reperfusion injury causes all of the microcirculatory symptoms which can develop during local or systemic circulatory disorders (Ames 1968; Menger 1992; Anaya-Prado 2002; Eltzschig 2011). It appears that the ECs are primary targets during the pathogenesis of ischemia/reperfusion-induced reactions (including inflammation). Being a major source of the xanthine oxidase-derived radicals (Granger 1981; Granger 1986; McCord 1985), a microvascular dysfunction (increased capillary permeability) develops. The xanthine oxidase-derived radicals further attract neutrophils (PMNs), thus augmenting tissue injury (Hernandez 1987). The endothelium-derived oxidants promote neutrophil adhesion to ECs via endothelial production of chemotactic factors (Yoshida 1992) as well as by activation of transcription factors (e.g., NFκB), causing an increased expression of adhesion molecules on ECs (Ichikawa 1997). Bioavailability of NO (an endogenous inhibitor of PMN adhesion) is reduced via its interaction with superoxide (Grisham 1998). This is accompanied by an activation of interstitial immune cells (macrophages and mast cells) with resultant generation of inflammatory mediators causing a chemotactic gradient which facilitates neutrophil emigration into the interstitium (Kanwar 1998). Lymphocytes may also be involved in the modulation of PMN-related reactions by releasing soluble factors, such as TNF–α or INF–γ (Osman 2009).

Micro-rheological parameters can be altered during ischemia and reperfusion by several pathways (Baskurt 2007). Impaired red blood cell deformability may contribute to an increased blood viscosity and cause perfusion problems in the capillaries (Wells 1964; Maeda 1996; Lipowsky 2005; Popel 2005). The enhanced red blood cell aggregation elevates blood viscosity and increases the flow resistance in the microcirculation (Baskurt 2007; Baskurt 2008). When erythrocyte aggregation is enhanced, the axial migration of the red blood cells in the vessel becomes more expressed, resulting in a widening cell-poor zone at the vicinity of the endothelium (Poiseuille-zone) (Fahraeus 1958). Widening Poiseuille-zone facilitates leukocyte tethering and margination; furthermore, the wide cell-poor zone slows down the rolling (Nash 2008; Yalcin 2011) (Figure 13.1). Additionally, altered blood rheology has an impact on the shear stress profile on the endothelial surface, thus modulating numerous vascular functions (Gori 2007, 2011; Pober 2008; Chandran 2012).

During ischemia, the local metabolic changes such as decrease in pH, increase of H^+ and lactate, affects blood cells (Weed 1969; Johnson 1985; Reinhart 2002). The pH of stagnant blood decreases in the area excluded from the circulation during the ischemia, which turns the red bloods cells' discocyte shape into a stomacyte or sphero-stomacyte form (Reinhart 1980). The echinocyte and sphero-echinocyte forms may appear when the ATP depletion and calcium accumulation are dominant (Reinhart 1980). Both morphological transformations result in worsened micro-rheological characteristics: impairment of red blood cells' deformability and disturbed aggregation (Meiselman 1981; Mohandas 2008).

During stasis, hematocrit increases locally and the altered fluid distribution results in elevated protein concentration, leading to increased plasma viscosity. These factors together with the less deformable erythrocytes and aggregates formation result in an increased local blood viscosity (Koppensteiner 1996; Baskurt 2007; Nemeth 2014a). Furthermore, the mechanical trauma to red blood cells has to be taken into consideration (Kameneva 2007). The hypoxia leads to impaired EC barrier function (Gori 2007, 2011). By revascularization, the metabolites flushing into the systemic circulation together with the damaged erythrocytes may cause further changes in the microcirculation and even in remote organs (Anaya-Prado 2002; Eltzschig 2011; Nemeth 2015b).

During reperfusion, the nascent oxygen-centered free radicals initiate harmful chain reactions in the erythrocytes: damaging the cell membrane (lipid peroxidation), the transmembrane and structural proteins (receptors, ion pumps) by sulfhydryl cross-links and transforming the hemoglobin molecules (methemoglobin, Heinz-body formation) (McCord 1985; Baskurt 1997, 2007). Red blood cells are rich in iron, which catalyzes the free radical reactions through the Fenton-reaction; making these cells highly sensitive to oxidative stress (Baskurt 1997; Kayar 2001). The "second" assault of free-radicals happens by the activated PMNs during the inflammatory process that is triggered by an ischemic injury of the tissues.

NO plays an important role in the local flow regulation over the complex hemodynamic changes during ischemia-reperfusion (Anaya-Prado 2002; Eltzschig 2011). The NO has a beneficial effect on red blood cells, improving their deformability, and erythrocytes also act as an enzymatic source of NO (Bor-Kucukatay 2003; Baskurt 2007). However, in the presence of NO and O_2^-, peroxynitrite anion formation can jeopardize the red blood cells (Baskurt 2007).

The macro-hemorheological changes are also non-specific and are related to the acute phase reactions: increase of plasma viscosity by elevated fibrinogen concentration and α_2-macroglobulin, increase in immunoglobulin levels, decrease in albumin level, rise in leukocyte count, increase or decrease of platelet count, as well as hemoconcentration and erythrocytes' micro-rheological changes (Koppensteiner1996; Baskurt 2007; Nemeth 2014a).

In the microcirculatory bed, the "no-reflow" phenomenon is characteristic for tissue ischemia-reperfusion. Despite of restarting the circulation in large-caliber vessels, there is a significant slow-down or total arrest in the microcirculatory flow (Ames 1968). In the background of this paradoxical phenomenon, numerous factors can be listed: microvascular spasm, swelling of ECs, bleb formation on the endothelial surface, increased capillary permeability, interstitial edema, micro-thrombi, neutrophil adhesion and plugging, and local acidosis (Menger 1992; Reffelmann 2002; Granger 2010; Vollmar 2011). The presence of red blood cells with impaired deformability and enhanced aggregation contributes further to the microcirculatory disturbance (Pries 2003, 2008; Lipowsky 2005; Popel 2005).

Systemic Circulatory Disorders

Hypovolemia-induced microcirculatory (arteriolar) vasoconstriction develops on the basis of an increased sympathetic activation causing A1 vasoconstriction and inverse A4 vasodilation with resultant reduction of capillary cross-sectional area and endothelial swelling (Mazzoni 1992; Szopinski 2011). Furthermore, an arteriolar hypo-responsiveness develops via up-regulation of inducible NO synthase and endothelin-1 (Liu 2005; van Meurs 2008). Widening gap junctions of the capillary endothelium is typical reaction seen also at sepsis causing tissue infiltration of PMNs (Czabanka 2007), which creates a positive feedback loop of microcirculatory derangement and obstruction of the capillary lumen (Ivanov 2006). Furthermore, red blood cell deformability is diminished (Baskurt 1998; Baskurt 2007). As a result, FCD is reduced and the oxygen delivery and removal of waste products are impaired. Similar reactions are seen in cardiogenic shock (Mazzoni 1992; Moore 2015).

Sepsis

The pathophysiology of sepsis includes several points which link it to the rheology of blood, since it is a disorder of the microcirculation (Levy 2003; Spronk 2004; Ince 2005; Trzeciak 2007, 2008; Lundy 2009; Nduka 2011; Hernandez 2013). The microcirculatory deterioration in sepsis is multifactorial. Septic process affects the entire microcirculation, disturbing micro-vascular blood flow and vascular resistance. The amount of blood entering the capillaries is affected by hemodynamic changes, redistribution of organ flow, vasodilatation and vasoplegia, as well as by opening arterio-venous shunts. Rigid blood cells may easily plug the capillaries. As result of dysfunction of the huge endothelial surface along the microcirculation, the perfusion further decreases due to increased adhesiveness for platelets, leukocytes and even erythrocytes. Microvascular thrombosis (as part of DIC) increased capillary permeability, edema and enhanced red blood cell aggregation also contributes to perfusion problems (Spronk 2004; Ince 2005; Moutzouri 2007; Trzeciak 2007; Lundy 2009; Ostergaard 2015). In a developed manifest sepsis, fibrinogen concentration increases (Baskurt 1997; Baskurt 2007; Reggiori 2009). However, in early stage, due to the fibrinogen consumption and other direct effects on blood cells, a decrease in erythrocyte aggregation might be also observed (Nemeth 2015a). Since several endothelial functions are controlled by the shear stress via mechanotransducers, any changes in the rheology of circulating blood, and consequently in shear forces and flow profile on the vascular wall, may influence the endothelial functions (Gori 2007; Chiu 2011; Chandran 2012). Altered rheology can cause further progression in the pathophysiological process that may result in rheological changes again, as a part of a vicious circle (Baskurt 2007).

EXPERIMENTAL SURGICAL CONSIDERATIONS INVESTIGATING MICROCIRCULATION AND MICRO-RHEOLOGY

Most of the surgical investigations, by their nature, involve animal models. Using the well-defined, animal protection and laboratory animal science considerations (van Zutphen 2001), correctly designed animal experimentation is still important nowadays. Several questions exist that cannot be examined by *in vitro* methods or in tissue cultures: sufficient information can only be obtained by complex investigation in organ systems or in organs *in vivo*. Extrapolatability of the questions, i.e., their extrapolation to the original clinical issue in human references, is a further determining factor.

In view of factors determining the blood and plasma viscosity, red blood cell deformability and aggregation, and microcirculation, it is clear, that with respect to laboratory animal species, we have to expect significant interspecies and gender differences (Usami 1969; Chien 1971; Chen 1994; Popel 1994; Windberger 2003, 2007; Szabo 2006; Nemeth 2010). We have to carefully consider all these aspects when deciding on the necessity of adaptation and methodological standardization of measuring methods.

For humans the currently known hemorheological measuring methods or a measurement technique guideline is available (Baskurt 2009). This guideline covers the sampling and sample handling instructions and recommendations beside the special measurement technique details. With respect to animal experimentation, no such guideline is available; therefore, in addition to exploring the interspecies and gender hemorheological differences, we have to examine the handling and preparation details of blood samples required during the experiments, where considerable interspecies differences can also be anticipated. They can seriously influence the results, their evaluation, assessment and extrapolatability.

Another question is the way and location of blood sampling. In addition to the animal welfare considerations, such as the quantity of blood sample and the repeatability (van Zutphen 2001), we have to consider the possible arterio-venous micro-rheological differences (Nemeth 2014b).

In the detectability of the alterations, the different sensitivity and specifications of hemorheological measuring instruments and devices, such as cell size/pore size ratio during filtrometry or the orientation of cells and the viscosity of suspending medium in the ektacytometry examinations of EI need to be considered (Hardeman 2007; Baskurt 2009; Nemeth 2014a). A detailed analysis of these issues, the standardization and comparative hemorheological tests may contribute to the safe planning, performing of the experimental surgical models and to the evaluability of the obtained results with objective data.

In microcirculatory and micro-rheological investigations of animal experiments, several issues have to be taken into consideration (Nemeth 2014a):

- *Concerns a priori:* planning of experiments and techniques; counting on inter-species and gender differences (additionally: the estrus cycle of animals); careful planning of blood sampling and handling (site of sampling, required blood sample volume versus available sample volume, anticoagulant, storage); sample preparation protocols (centrifugation, buffers, etc.); standardized measurement conditions depending on the method/device.
- *Concerns a posteriori:* extrapolation, reliability.

All of these issues are important for critical revision and correct evaluation of the results, so they could be comparable and may provide useful information for the clinical medicine.

CONCLUSION

Adequate microcirculation and restored micro-rheology strikingly influence tissue oxygenation and overall tissue survival during experimental and clinical surgical interventions. Dynamic assessment of the microcirculatory functions can be conducted by numerous methods. The required spatial resolution and tissue depth as well as the type of tissue/organ of interest critically necessitate the use of appropriate microcirculatory methodology when visualization is concerned. Vascular and circulatory (cellular and micro-rheological) elements of the microcirculation have dynamic interactions and these usually show parallel changes in different surgical models. By using appropriate and up-to-date methodology, these changes can be dynamically assessed and the effect of alleviating therapies be accurately judged by using proper quantification. These findings provide a rational basis for tailoring future life-saving interventions.

REFERENCES

Aird, WC. The role of the endothelium in severe sepsis and multiple organ dysfunction syndrome. *Blood,* 2003, 101(10), 3765–3777.

Ames, A; 3rd, Wright, RL; Kowada, M; Thurston, JM; Majno, G. Cerebral ischemia. II. The no reflow phenomenon. *Am. J. Pathol.*, 1968, 52(2), 437–453.

Anaya-Prado R, Toledo-Pereyra LH, Lentsch AB, Ward PA. Ischemia/reperfusion injury. *J. Surg. Res.*, 2002, 105(2), 248–258.

Armstrong, JK; Wenby, RB; Meiselman, HJ; Fisher, TC. The hydrodynamic radii of macromolecules and their effect on red blood cell aggregation. *Biophys. J.*, 2004, 87(6), 4259–4270.

Awan, ZA; Wester, T; Kvernebo, K. Human microvascular imaging, a review of skin and tongue videomicroscopy techniques and analysing variables. *Clin. Physiol. Funct. Imaging*, 2010, 30(2), 79–88.

Aykut, G; Veenstra, G; Scorcella, C; Ince, C; Boerma, C. Cytocam-IDF (incident dark field illumination) imaging for bedside monitoring of the microcirculation. *Intensive Care Med. Exp.*, 2015, 3(1), 4. http: //icm-experimental.springeropen.com/articles/ 10.1186/s40635-015-0040-7.

Bajory, Z; Hutter, J; Krombach, F; Messmer, K. The role of endothelin-1 in ischemia-reperfusion induced acute inflammation of the bladder in rats. *J. Urol.*, 2002, 168(3), 1222–1225.

Baskurt, OK; Boynard, M; Cokelet, GC; Connes, P; Cooke, BM; Forconi, S; Hardeman, MR; Jung, F; Liao, F; Meiselman, HJ; Nash, G; Nemeth, N; Neu, B; Sandhagen, B; Shin, S; Thurston, G; Wautier, JL. International Expert Panel for Standardization of Hemorheological Methods, New guidelines for hemorheological laboratory techniques. *Clin. Hemorheol. Microcirc.*, 2009, 42(2), 75–97.

Baskurt, OK; Gelmont, D; Meiselman, HJ. Red blood cell deformability in sepsis. *Am. J. Respir. Crit. Care Med.*, 1998, 157(2), 421–427.

Baskurt, OK; Neu, B; Meiselman, HJ. Determinants of red blood cell aggregation. In, Baskurt OK, Neu B, Meiselman HJ, editors. *Red Blood Cell Aggregation.* Boca Raton, CRC Press, 2012. pp. 9–29.

Baskurt, OK; Neu, B; Meiselman, HJ. Measurement of red blood cell aggregation. In, Baskurt OK, Neu B, Meiselman HJ, editors. *Red Blood Cell Aggregation.* Boca Raton, CRC Press, 2012. pp. 63–132.

Baskurt, OK; Temiz, A; Meiselman, HJ. Red blood cell aggregation in experimental sepsis. *J. Lab. Clin. Med.*, 1997, 130(2), 183–190.

Baskurt, OK. *In vivo* correlates of altered blood rheology. *Biorheology*, 2008, 45(6), 629–638.

Baskurt, OK. Mechanisms of blood rheology alterations. In: Baskurt OK, Hardeman MR, Rampling MW, Meiselman HJ, editors. *Handbook of Hemorheology and Hemodynamics.* Amsterdam, IOS Press, 2007. pp. 170–190.

Bezemer, R; Khalilzada, M; Ince, C. Recent advancements in microcirculatory image acquisition and analysis. In, *Yearbook of intensive care and emergency medicine*. Berlin, Springer, 2008. p. 677–690.

Bishop, JJ; Popel, AS; Intaglietta, M; Johnson, PC. Rheological effects of red blood cell aggregation in the venous network, a review of recent studies. *Biorheology*, 2001, 38, 263–274.

Bitbol, M. Red blood cell orientation in orbit C = 0. *Biophys. J.*, 1986, 49(5), 1055–1068.

Boas, DA; Dunn, AK. Laser speckle contrast imaging in biomedical optics. *J. Biomed. Opt.*, 2010, 15(1), 011109.

Bogar, L; Juricskay, I; Kesmarky, G; Kenyeres, P; Toth, K. Erythrocyte transport efficacy of human blood, a rheological point of view. *Eur. J. Clin. Invest.*, 2005, 35(11), 687–690.

Bohlen, HG; Henrich, H; Gore, RW; Johnson PC. Intestinal muscle and mucosal blood flow during direct sympathetic stimulation. *Am. J. Physiol.*, 1978, 235, H40–H45.

Bor-Kucukatay, M; Wenby, RB; Meiselman, HJ; Baskurt, OK. Effects of nitric oxide on red blood cell deformability. *Am. J. Physiol. Heart Circ. Physiol.*, 2003, 284(5), H1577–H1584.

Briers, JD; McNamara, PM; O'Connell, ML; Leahy MJ. Laser Speckle Contrast Analysis (LASCA) for measuring blood flow. In: Leahy MJ, editor. *Microcirculation imaging*. Weinheim, Wiley-Blackwell, 2012. pp. 147−164.

Briers, JD; Richards, G; He XW. Capillary Blood Flow Monitoring Using Laser Speckle Contrast Analysis (LASCA). *J. Biomed. Opt.*, 1999, 4(1), 164−175.

Buerk, DG. Measuring tissue PO2 with microelectrodes. *Methods Enzymol.*, 2004, 381, 665−690.

Carvalho, FA; Connell, S; Miltenberger-Miltenyi, G; Pereira, SV; Tavares, A; Ariëns, RA; Santos NC. Atomic force microscopy-based molecular recognition of a fibrinogen receptor on human erythrocytes. *ACS Nano*, 2010, 4(8), 4609–4620.

Chandran, KB; Rittgers, SE; Yoganathan AP. Rheology of blood and vascular mechanics. In, Chandran KB, Rittgers SE, Yoganathan AP, editors. *Biofluid Mechanics*. CRC Boca Raton, Press, 2012. pp. 109–154.

Chasis, JA; Mohandas N. Erythrocyte membrane deformability and stability, two distinct membrane properties that are independently regulated by skeletal protein associations. *J. Cell Biol.*, 1986, 103(2), 343–350.

Chen, D; Kaul DK. Rheologic and hemodynamic characteristics of red cells of mouse, rat and human. *Biorheology*, 1994, 31(1), 103–113.

Chien, S; Usami, S; Dellenback, RJ; Bryant CA. Comparative hemorheology – hematological implications of species differences in blood viscosity. *Biorheology*, 1971, 8(1), 35–57.

Chien, S. Biophysical behavior of red cells in suspension. In: Surgenor DM, editor. *The red blood cell*. New York, Academic Press, 1975. pp. 1031–1133.

Chiu, JJ; Chen S. Effects of disturbed flow on vascular endothelium, pathophysiological basis and clinical perspectives. *Physiol. Rev.*, 2011, 91(1), 327–387.

Choi, B; Kang, NM; Nelson JS. Laser speckle imaging for monitoring blood flow dynamics in the in vivo rodent dorsal skin fold model. *Microvasc. Res.*, 2004, 68(2), 143−146.

Cokelet, GR; Meiselman HJ. Basic aspects of hemorheology. In: Baskurt OK, Hardeman MR, Rampling MW, Meiselman HJ, editors. *Handbook of Hemorheology and Hemodynamics*. Amsterdam, IOS Press, 2007a pp. 21–33.

Cokelet, GR; Meiselman HJ. Macro- and micro-rheological properties of blood. In, Baskurt OK, Hardeman MR, Rampling MW, Meiselman HJ, editors. *Handbook of Hemorheology and Hemodynamics.* Amsterdam, IOS Press, 2007b pp. 45–71.

Czabanka, M; Peter, C; Martin, E; Walther A. Microcirculatory endothelial dysfunction during endotoxemia –insights into pathophysiology, pathologic mechanisms and clinical relevance. *Curr. Vasc. Pharmacol.*, 2007, 5(4), 266–275.

Davis, MJ; Hill, MA; Kuo L. Local regulation of microvascular perfusion. In, Tuma RF, Duran WN, Ley K, editors. *Handbook of Physiology, Microcirculation.* 2nd edition. Amsterdam, Elsevier Academic Press, 2008. pp. 161–284.

Davis, MJ. Perspective, physiological role(s) of the vascular myogenic response. *Microcirculation*, 2012, 19(2), 99–114.

De, Backer, D; Hollenberg, S; Boerma, C; Goedhart, P; Büchele, G; Ospina-Tascon, G; Dobbe, I; Ince C. How to evaluate the microcirculation, report of a round table conference. *Crit. Care.* 2007, 11(5), R101. http, //ccforum.com/content/11/5/R101.

De, Blasi, RA; Ferrari, M; Natali, A; Conti, G; Mega, A; Gasparetto A. Noninvasive measurement of forearm blood flow and oxygen consumption by near-infrared spectroscopy. *J. Appl. Physiol., (1985)* 1994, 76(3), 1388–1393.

De Blasi, RA. Is muscle StO2 an appropriate variable for investigating early compensatory tissue mechanisms under physiological and pathological conditions? *Intensive Care Med.*, 2008, 34(9), 1557–1559.

de Oliveira, S; Saldanha, C. An overview about erythrocyte membrane. *Clin. Hemorheol. Microcirc.*, 2010, 44(1), 63–74.

den Uil, CA; Lagrand, WK; van der Ent, M; Jewbali, LS; Cheng, JM; Spronk, PE; Simoons, ML. Impaired microcirculation predicts poor outcome of patients with acute myocardial infarction complicated by cardiogenic shock. *Eur. Heart J.*, 2010, 31(24), 3032–3039.

Denk, W; Strickler, JH; Webb WW. Two-photon laser scanning fluorescence microscopy. *Science*, 1990, 248(4951), 73–76.

Donati, A; Domizi, R; Damiani, E; Adrario, E; Pelaia, P; Ince C. From macrohemodynamic to the microcirculation. *Crit. Care. Res. Pract.*, 2013, 2013, 892710.

Doppler, JC. Uber das farbige Licht der Doppelsterne und einiger anderer Gestirne des Himmels. [About the colored light of the double stars and some other stars of the sky.] In: *Versuch einer das Bradley'sche berrations-theorem als integrirrenden Theil in sich schlissenden allgemeineren Theorie.* Prag, In Commission bei Borrosch & Andre, 1842.

Dupire, J; Socol, M; Viallat A. Full dynamics of a red blood cell in shear flow. *Proc. Natl. Acad. Sci. USA*, 2012, 109(51), 20808–20813.

Egawa, G; Nakamizo, S; Natsuaki, Y; Doi, H; Miyachi, Y; Kabashima K. Intravital analysis of vascular permeability in mice using two-photon microscopy. *Sci. Rep.*, 2013, 3, 1932.

Ellinger, P; Hirt A. Mikroscopische Untersuchungen an lebenden Organen. [Mikroscopische Untersuchungen an lebenden Organen. I. Mitt. Metodik, Intravitalmikroskopie.] I. Mitt. Metodik, Intravitalmikroskopie. *Zeitschrift für Anatomie und Entwicklungs-Geschichte*, 1929, 80, 791–802.

Eltzschig, H; Eckle T. Ischemia and reperfusion – from mechanism to translation. *Nature Medicine*, 2011, 17(11), 1391–1401.

Endrich, B; Asaishi, K; Götz, A; Messmer K. Technical report--a new chamber technique for microvascular studies in unanesthetized hamsters. *Res. Exp. Med. (Berl).*, 1980, 177(2), 125–134.

Ernst, E; Matrai A. Zum Thema 'optimaler Hämatocrit' – Rationale der Hämodilutionstherapie. [On the subject of 'optimal hematocrit' - Rationale of hemodilution therapy.] *Herz Kreislauf.*, 1983, 9, 409–415.

Essex, TJ; Byrne PO. A laser Doppler scanner for imaging blood flow in skin. *J. Biomed. Eng.*, 1991, 13(3), 189−194.

Fåhraeus, R; Lindqvist T, The viscosity of the blood in narrow capillary tubes. *Am. J. Physiol.* 1931, 96, 562–568.

Fåhraeus, R. The influence of the rouleau formation of the erythrocytes on the rheology of the blood. *Acta Med. Scand.*, 1958, 161(2), 151–165.

Fang, X; TangW; Sun, S; Huang, L; Chang, YT; Castillo, C; Weil MH. Comparison of buccal microcirculation between septic and hemorrhagic shock. *Crit. Care Med.*, 2006, 34 (12 Suppl), S447–S453.

Foster, FS. High frequency ultrasound for the visualization and quantification of the microcirculation. In, Leahy MJ, editor. *Microcirculation imaging.* Weinheim, Wiley-Blackwell, 2012. pp. 293−312.

Fredriksson, I; Larsson, M; Strömberg T. Laser Doppler flowmetry. In, Leahy MJ, editor. *Microcirculation imaging.* Weinheim, Wiley-Blackwell, 2012. pp. 67−86.

Fromy, B; Legrand, MS; Abraham, P; Leftheriotis, G; Cales, P; Saumet JL. Effects of positive pressure on both femoral venous and arterial blood velocities and the cutaneous microcirculation of the forefoot. *Cardiovasc. Res.*, 1997, 36(3), 372−376.

Gilbert-Kawai, E; Coppel, J; Bountziouka, V; Ince, C; Martin D. A comparison of the quality of image acquisition between the incident dark field and sidestream dark field videomicroscopes. *BMC Med. Imaging* 2016, 16, 10.http, //bmcmedimaging.biomedcentral.com/articles/10.1186/ s12880-015-0078-8

Goedhart, PT; Khalilzada, M; Bezemer, R; Merza, J; Ince C. Sidestream Dark Field (SDF) imaging, a novel stroboscopic LED ring-based imaging modality for clinical assessment of the microcirculation. *Opt. Express.*, 2007, 15(23), 15101–15114.

Goldsmith, HL; Marlow J. Flow behavior of erythrocytes, I. Rotation and deformation in dilute suspensions. *Proc. R. Soc. Lond.*, B 1972, 182, 351–384.

Gori, T; Forconi S. Endothelium and hemorheology. In: Baskurt OK, Hardeman MR, Rampling MW, Meiselman HJ, editors. *Handbook of Hemorheology and Hemodynamics.* Amsterdam, IOS Press, 2007. pp. 339–350.

Gori, T; Münzel T. Oxidative stress and endothelial dysfunction, therapeutic implications. *Ann. Med.*, 2011, 43(4), 259−272.

Granger, DN; Höllwarth, ME; Parks DA. Ischemia-reperfusion injury, role of oxygen-derived free radicals. *Acta Physiol. Scand Suppl.*, 1986, 548, 47–63.

Granger, DN; Rutili, G; McCord JM. Superoxide radicals in feline intestinal ischemia. *Gastroenterology*, 1981, 81(1), 22−29.

Granger, DN; Senchenkova E. *Inflammation and the Microcirculation.* San Rafael, Morgan & Claypool Life Sciences, 2010.

Granger, DN. Physiology and pathophysiology of the microcirculation. *Dialogues Cardiovasc Med.*, 1988, 3, 123–140.

Granger, HJ; Goodman, AH; Cook BH. Metabolic models of microcirculatory regulation. *Fed. Proc.*, 1975, 34(11), 2025−2030.

Grisham, MB; Granger, DN; Lefer DJ. Modulation of leukocyte–endothelial interactions by reactive metabolites of oxygen and nitrogen, relevance to ischemic heart disease. *Free Radic. Biol. Med.*, 1998, 25(4-5), 404−433.

Groner, W; Winkelman, JW; Harris, AG; Ince, C; Bouma, GJ; Messmer, K; Nadeau RG. Orthogonal polarization spectral imaging, a new method for study of the microcirculation. *Nat. Med.*, 1999, 5(10), 1209−1212.

Hardeman, MR; Goedhart, PT; Shin S. Methods in hemorheology. In, Baskurt OK, Hardeman MR, Rampling MW, Meiselman HJ, editors. *Handbook of Hemorheology and Hemodynamics.* Amsterdam, IOS Press, 2007. pp. 242–266.

Harkness, J. The viscosity of human blood plasma, its measurement in health and disease. *Biorheology*, 1971, 8(3), 171−193.

Harms, FA; Bodmer, SI; Raat, NJ; Mik EG. Cutaneous mitochondrial respirometry, non-invasive monitoring of mitochondrial function. *J. Clin. Monit. Comput.*, 2015, 29(4), 509−519.

Hepple, RT; Hogan, MC; Stary, C; Bebout, DE; Mathieu-Costello, O; Wagner PD. Structural basis of muscle O2 diffusing capacity, evidence from muscle function in situ. *J. Appl. Physiol.*, 2000, 88(2), 560–566.

Hernandez, G; Bruhn, A; Ince C. Microcirculation in sepsis, new perspectives. *Curr. Vasc. Pharmacol.*, 2013, 11(2), 161−169.

Hernandez, LA; Grisham, MB; Twohig, B; Arfors, KE; Harlan, JM; Granger DN. Role of neutrophils in ischemia–reperfusion-induced microvascular injury. *Am. J. Physiol.*, 1987, 253(3 Pt 2), H699−H703.

Hölzle, F; Rau, A; Loeffelbein, DJ; Mücke, T; Kesting, MR; Wolff KD. Results of monitoring fasciocutaneous, myocutaneous, osteocutaneous and perforator flaps, 4-year experience with 166 cases. *Int. J. Oral Maxillofac. Surg.*, 2010, 39(1), 21−28.

Honig, CR; Odoroff, CL; Frierson JL. Active and passive capillary control in red muscle at rest and in exercise. *Am. J. Physiol.*, 1982, 243(2), H196−H206.

Hoole, S. *The select works of Antony van Leeuwenhoek, containing his microscopical discoveries in many of the works of nature.* Fleet-Street, Black-Horse Court, 1800.

Hu, S; Wang LV. Photoacoustic tomography of microcirculation. In, Leahy MJ, editor. *Microcirculation imaging.* Weinheim, Wiley-Blackwell, 2012. pp. 259−278.

Ichikawa, H; Flores, S; Kvietys, PR; Wolf, RE; Yoshikawa, T; Granger, DN; Aw TY. Molecular mechanisms of anoxia/reoxygenation-induced neutrophil adherence to cultured endothelial cells. *Circ. Res.*, 1997, 81(6), 922−931.

Ince, C. The microcirculation is the motor of sepsis. *Crit. Care.*, 2005, 9(Suppl 4), S13–S19.

Irwin, JW; Macdonald, J; 3rd. Microscopic observations of the intrahepatic circulation of living guinea pigs. *Anat. Rec.*, 1953, 117(1), 1−15.

Ishikawa, M; Sekizuka, E; Sato, S; Yamaguchi, N; Shimizu, K; Kobayashi, K; Bertalanffy, H; Kawase T. *In vivo* rat closed spinal window for spinal microcirculation, observation of pial vessels, leukocyte adhesion, and red blood cell velocity. *Neurosurgery.*, 1999, 44, 156–161.

Ivanov, KP; Mel'nikova NN. Leukocytes as a cause of microcirculatory dysfunction. *Bull. Exp. Biol. Med.*, 2006, 141(6), 666–668.

Jackson, WF; Duling BR. The oxygen sensitivity of hamster cheek pouch arterioles. *In vitro* and in situ studies. *Circ. Res.*, 1983, 53(4), 515−525.

Johnson, RM. pH effects on red blood cell deformability. *Blood Cells*, 1985, 11(2), 317–321.

Kameneva, MV; Antaki JF. Mechanical trauma to blood. In, Baskurt OK, Hardeman MR, Rampling MW, Meiselman HJ, editors. *Handbook of Hemorheology and Hemodynamics.* Amsterdam, IOS Press, 2007. pp. 206–227.

Kanwar, S; Hickey, MJ; Kubes P. Postischemic inflammation, a role for mast cells in intestine but not in skeletal muscle. *Am. J. Physiol.*, 1998, 275(2 Pt 1), G212–G218.

Kayar, E; Mat, F; Meiselman, HJ; Baskurt OK. Red blood cell rheological alterations in a rat model of ischemia-reperfusion injury. *Biorheology*, 2001, 38(5-6), 405–414.

Kerskens, CM; Piech, RM; Meaney JFM. Imaging blood circulation using Nuclear Magnetic Resonance. In: Leahy MJ, editor. *Microcirculation imaging.* Weinheim, Wiley-Blackwell, 2012. pp. 349–385.

Kesmarky, G; Kenyeres, P; Rabai, M; Toth K. Plasma viscosity, a forgotten variable. *Clin. Hemorheol. Microcirc.,* 2008, 39(1-4), 243–246.

Kim, Y; Kim, K; Park YK. Measurement techniques for red blood cell deformability, recent advances. In, *Blood Cell – An Overview of Studies in Hematology.* Moschandreou TE, ed. InTech, 2012. pp. 167–194.

Klar, E; Endrich, B; Messmer K. Microcirculation of the pancreas. A quantitative study of physiology and changes in pancreatitis. *Int. J. Microcirc. Clin. Exp.*, 1990, 9, 85–101.

Kline, TL; Ritman EL. Studying microcirculation with Micro-CT. In, Leahy MJ, editor. *Microcirculation imaging.* Weinheim, Wiley-Blackwell, 2012. pp. 313–348.

Koppensteiner, R. Blood rheology in emergency medicine. *Semin. Thromb. Hemost.*, 1996, 22(1), 89–91.

Kuhnle, GE; Leipfinger, FH; Goetz AE. Measurement of microhemodynamics in the ventilated rabbit lung by intravital fluorescence microscopy. *J. Appl. Physiol.*, 1993, 74, 1462–1471.

Kvietys, PR. *The Gastrointestinal Circulation.* San Rafael, Morgan & Claypool Life Sciences, 2010.

Kwaan, HC. Role of plasma proteins in whole blood viscosity, a brief clinical review. *Clin. Hemorheol. Microcirc.*, 2010, 44(3), 167–176.

Langer, HF; Chavakis T. Leukocyte-endothelial interactions in inflammation. *J Cell Mol Med.*, 2009, 13(7), 1211–1220.

Leahy, MJ; de, Mul, FF; Nilsson, GE; Maniewski R. Principles and practice of the laser-Doppler perfusion technique. *Technol. Health Care*, 1999, 7(2-3), 143–162.

Leahy, MJ. editor. *Microcirculation imaging.* Weinheim, Wiley-Blackwell, 2012.

Lehmann, C. editor. *Intravital microcirculation imaging.* Lengerich, Pabst Science Publishers, 2012.

Lehr, HA; Leunig, M; Menger, MD; Nolte, D; Messmer K. Dorsal skinfold chamber technique for intravital microscopy in nude mice. *Am. J. Pathol.*, 1993, 143(4), 1055–1062.

Levy, MM; Fink, MP; Marshall, JC; Abraham, E; Angus, D; Cook, D; Cohen, J; Opal, SM; Vincent, JL; Ramsay G, International Sepsis Definitions Conference. 2001 SCCM/ESICM/ACCP/ATS/SIS International Sepsis Definitions Conference. *Intensive Care Med.*, 2003, 29(4), 530–538.

Ley, K; Laudanna, C; Cybulsky, MI; Nourshargh S. Getting to the site of inflammation, the leukocyte adhesion cascade updated. *Nat Rev Immunol.*, 2007, 7(9), 678–689.

Lipowsky, HH. Microvascular rheology and hemodynamics. *Microcirculation*, 2005,12(1), 5–15.

Lipowsky, HH. Shear stress in the circulation. In, Bevan J, Kaley G, editors. *Flow Dependent Regulation of Vascular Function.* Clinical Physiology Series. New York, Oxford University Press, 1995. pp. 28–45.

Liu, LM; Dubick MA. Hemorrhagic shock-induced vascular hyporeactivity in the rat, relationship to gene expression of nitric oxide synthase, endothelin-1, and select cytokines in corresponding organs. *J. Surg. Res.*, 2005, 125(2), 128–136.

Liu, R; Qin, J; Wang RK. Motion-contrast laser speckle imaging of microcirculation within tissue beds *in vivo*. *J. Biomed. Opt.*, 2013, 18(6), 060508.

Lundy, DJ; Trzeciak S. Microcirculatory dysfunction in sepsis. *Crit. Care Clin.*, 2009, 25(4), 721–731.

Maeda, N. Erythrocyte rheology in microcirculation. *Jpn. J. Physiol.*, 1996, 46(1), 1–14.

Masedunskas, A; Milberg, O; Porat-Shliom, N; Sramkova, M; Wigand, T; Amornphimoltham, P; Weigert R. Intravital microscopy, a practical guide on imaging intracellular structures in live animals. *Bioarchitecture*, 2012, 2(5), 143–157.

Massberg, S; Enders, G; Leiderer, R; Eisenmenger, S; Vestweber, D; Krombach, F; Messmer K. Platelet-endothelial cell interactions during ischemia/reperfusion, the role of P-selectin. *Blood*, 1998, 92, 507–515.

Massey, MJ; Shapiro NI. A guide to human *in vivo* microcirculatory flow image analysis. *Crit. Care*, 2016, 20, 35. http://ccforum.biomedcentral.com/articles/10.1186/s13054-016-1213-9

Mazo, IB; Gutierrez-Ramos, JC; Frenette, PS; Hynes, RO; Wagner, DD; von, Andrian UH. Hematopoietic progenitor cell rolling in bone marrow microvessels, parallel contributions by endothelial selectins and vascular cell adhesion molecule 1. *J. Exp. Med.*, 1998, 188, 465–474.

Mazzoni, MC; Intaglietta, M; Cragoe, EJ; Jr. Arfors, KE. Amiloride-sensitive Na+ pathways in capillary endothelial cell swelling during hemorrhagic shock. *J. Appl. Physiol.*, 1992, 73(4), 1467–1473.

McCord, JM; Roy RS; Schaffer SW. Free radicals and myocardial ischemia. The role of xanthine oxidase. *Adv. Myocardiol.*, 1985, 5, 183–189.

McCord, JM. Oxygen-derived free radicals in post-ischemic tissue injury. *N. Engl. J. Med.*, 1985, 312, 159–163.

McDonald. *Blood Flow in Arteries.* Baltimore, The Williams and Wilksin Co, 1974. pp. 356–378.

Meiselman, HJ. Morphological determinants of red blood cell deformability. *Scand. J. Clin. Lab. Invest.*, 1981, 41(Suppl. 156), 27–34.

Menger, MD; Marzi, I; Messmer K. *In vivo* fluorescence microscopy for quantitative analysis of the hepatic microcirculation in hamsters and rats. *Eur. Surg. Res.*, 1991, 23, 158–169.

Menger, MD; Steiner, D; Messmer K. Microvascular ischemia-reperfusion injury in striated muscle, significance of 'no-reflow'. *Am. J. Physiol.*, 1992, 263(6 Pt 2), H1892–H1900.

Menzebach, A; Mutz, C; Scheeren TW. Microcirculatory monitoring of a Jehovah's Witness suffering from haemorrhagic shock. *Eur. J. Anaesthesiol.*, 2008, 25(1), 81–83.

Merz, KM; Pfau, M; Blumenstock, G; Tenenhaus, M; Schaller HE, Rennekampff HO. Cutaneous microcirculatory assessment of the burn wound is associated with depth of injury and predicts healing time. *Burns.*, 2010, 36(4), 477–482.

Michiels, C; Arnould, T; Knott, I; Dieu, M; Remacle, J. Stimulation of prostaglandin synthesis by human endothelial cells exposed to hypoxia. *Am. J. Physiol. Cell Physiol.*, 1993, 264(4 Pt 1), C866–C874.

Mik, EG; Stap, J; Sinaasappel, M; Beek, JF; Aten, JA; van, Leeuwen, TG; Ince C. Mitochondrial PO2 measured by delayed fluorescence of endogenous protoporphyrin IX. *Nat. Methods*, 2006, 3(11), 939–945.

Milstein, DMJ; Bezemer, R; Ince C. Sidestream Dark-Filed (SDF) video microscopy for clinical imaging of the microcirculation. In, Leahy MJ, editor. *Microcirculation imaging*. Weinheim, Wiley-Blackwell, 2012. pp. 37–52.

Mohandas, N; Gallagher PG. Red cell membrane, past, present, and future. *Blood*, 2008, 112(10), 3939–3948.

Moore, JP; Dyson, A; Singer, M; Fraser J. Microcirculatory dysfunction and resuscitation, why, when, and how. *Br. J. Anaesth.*, 2015, 115(3), 366–375.

Moutzouri, AG; Skoutelis, AT; Gogos, CA; Missirlis, YF; Athanassiou GM. Red blood cell deformability in patients with sepsis, a marker for prognosis and monitoring of severity. *Clin. Hemorheol. Microcirc.*, 2007, 36(4), 291–299.

Musielak, M. Red blood cell-deformability measurement, review of techniques. *Clin. Hemorheol. Microcirc.*, 2009, 42(1), 47–64.

Nakhostine, N; Lamontagne D. Adenosine contributes to hypoxia-induced vasodilation through ATP-sensitive K+ channel activation. *Am. J. Physiol.*, 1993, 265(4 Pt 2), H1289–H1293.

Nash, GB; Watts, T; Thornton, C; Barigou M. Red cell aggregation as a factor influencing margination and adhesion of leukocytes and platelets. *Clin. Hemorheol. Microcirc.*, 2008, 39(1-4), 303–310.

Nduka, OO; Parrillo JE. The pathophysiology of septic shock. *Crit. Care Nurs. Clin. North Am.*, 2011, 23(1), 41–66.

Nemeth, N; Berhes, M; Kiss, F; Hajdu, E; Deak, A; Molnar, A; Szabo, J; Fulesdi B. Early hemorheological changes in a porcine model of intravenously given E. coli induced fulminant sepsis. *Clin. Hemorheol. Microcirc.*, 2015a, 61(3), 479–496.

Nemeth, N; Furka, I; Miko I. Hemorheological changes in ischemia-reperfusion, an overview on our experimental surgical data. *Clin. Hemorheol. Microcirc.*, 2014a, 57(3), 215–225.

Nemeth, N; Kiss, F; Furka, I; Miko I. Gender differences of blood rheological parameters in laboratory animals. *Clin. Hemorheol. Microcirc.*, 2010, 45(2-4), 263–272.

Nemeth, N; Kiss, F; Klárik, Z; Tóth, E; Mester, A; Furka, I; Miko I. Simultaneous investigation of hemodynamic, microcirculatory and arterio-venous micro-rheological parameters in infrarenal or suprarenal aortic cross-campling model in the rat. *Clin. Hemorheol. Microcirc.*, 2014b, 57(4), 339–353.

Nemeth, N; Lesznyak, T; Brath, E; Acs, G; Nagy, A; Pap-Szekeres, J; Furka, I; Miko I. Changes in microcirculation after ischemic process in rat skeletal muscle. *Microsurgery*, 2003, 23(5), 419–423.

Nemeth, N; Toth, E; Nemes B. Agents targeting ischemia-reperfusion injury. In, Huifang C, Shiguang Q, editors. *Current Immunosuppressive Therapy in Organ Transplantation*. Hauppauge, New York, Nova Science Publishers, 2015b pp. 487–533.

Neviere, R; Mathieu, D; Chagnon, JL; Lebleu, N; Millien, JP; Wattel, F. Skeletal muscle microvascular blood flow and oxygen transport in patients with severe sepsis. *Am. J. Respir. Crit. Care Med.*, 1996, 153(1), 191–195.

O'Doherty, J; Leahy, MJ; Nilsson GE. Tissue viability imaging. In, Leahy MJ, editor. *Microcirculation imaging.* Weinheim, Wiley-Blackwell, 2012. pp. 165−196.

Obeid, AN; Barnett, NJ; Dougherty, G; Ward G. A critical review of laser Doppler flowmetry. *J. Med. Eng. Technol.*, 1990, 14(5), 178−181. 37, 43−69.

Pries, AR; Secomb TW. Blood flow in microvascular networks. In, Tuma RF, Duran WN, Ley K, editors. *Handbook of Physiology, Microcirculation.* 2nd edition. Amsterdam, Elsevier Academic Press, 2008. pp. 3−36.

Pries, AR; Secomb TW. Rheology of the microcirculation. *Clin. Hemorheol. Microcirc.*, 2003, 29(3-4), 143–148.

Qin, J; Shi, L; Dziennis, S; Reif, R; Wang RK. Fast synchronized dual-wavelength laser speckle imaging system for monitoring hemodynamic changes in a stroke mouse model. *Opt. Lett.*, 2012, 37(19), 4005−4007.

Rajan, V; Varghese, B; van, Leeuwen, TG; Steenbergen W. Review of methodological developments in laser Doppler flowmetry. *Lasers Med. Sci.*, 2009, 24(2), 269–283.

Reese, AJ. The effect of hypoxia on liver secretion studied by intravital fluorescence microscopy. *Br. J. Exp. Pathol.*, 1960, 41, 527−535.

Reffelmann, T; Kloner RA. The "no-reflow" phenomenon, basic science and clinical correlates. *Heart*, 2002, 87(2), 162–168.

Rege, A; Murari, K; Seifert, A; Pathak, AP; Thakor NV. Multiexposure laser speckle contrast imaging of the angiogenic microenvironment. *J. Biomed. Opt.*, 2011, 16(5), 056006.

Reggiori, G; Occhipinti, G; De, Gasperi, A; Vincent, JL; Piagnerelli M. Early alterations of red blood cell rheology in critically ill patients. *Crit. Care Med.*, 2009, 37(12), 3041–3046.

Reinhart, WH; Chien S. Red cell rheology in stomatocyte-echinocyte transformation, roles of cell geometry and cell shape. *Blood*, 1980, 67(4), 1110–1118.

Reinhart, WH; Gaudenz, R; Walter R. Acidosis induced by lactate, pyruvate, or HCl increases blood viscosity. *J. Crit. Care*, 2002, 17(1), 38–42.

Reinhart, WH; Piety, NZ; Goede, JS; Shevkoplyas SS. Effect of osmolality on erythrocyte rheology and perfusion of an artificial microvascular network. *Microvasc. Res.*, 2015, 98, 102–107.

Reitsma, S; Slaaf, DW; Vink, H; van, Zandvoort, MA; oude, Egbrink MG. The endothelial glycocalyx, composition, functions, and visualization. *Pflugers Arch.*, 2007, 454(3), 345–359.

Roesner, JP; Vagts, DA; Iber, T; Eipel, C; Vollmar, B; Nöldge-Schomburg GF. Protective effects of PARP inhibition on liver microcirculation and function after haemorrhagic shock and resuscitation in male rats. *Intensive Care Med.*, 2006, 32(10), 1649−1657.

Rosencranz, R; Bogen SA. Clinical laboratory measurement of serum, plasma, and blood viscosity. *Am. J. Clin. Pathol.*, 2006, 125(Suppl), S78 –S86.

Rovainen, CM; Woolsey, TA; Blocher, NC; Wang, DB; Robinson OF. Blood flow in single surface arterioles and venules on the mouse somatosensory cortex measured with videomicroscopy, fluorescent dextrans, nonoccluding fluorescent beads, and computer-assisted image analysis. *J. Cereb. Blood Flow. Metab.*, 1993, 13(3), 359–371.

Ruh, J; Ryschich, E; Secchi, A; Gebhard, MM; Glaser, F; Klar, E; Herfarth C. Measurement of blood flow in the main arteriole of the villi in rat small intestine with FITC-labeled erythrocytes. *Microvasc. Res.*, 1998, 56(1), 62−69.

Saetzler, RK; Jallo, J; Lehr, HA; Philips, CM; Vasthare, U; Arfors, KE; Tuma RF. Intravital fluorescence microscopy, impact of light-induced phototoxicity on adhesion of fluorescently labeled leukocytes. *J. Histochem. Cytochem.*, 1997, 45, 505–513.

Sakr, Y; Dubois, MJ; De, Backer, D; Creteur, J; Vincent JL. Persistent microcirculatory alterations are associated with organ failure and death in patients with septic shock. *Crit. Care Med.*, 2004, 32(9), 1825–1831.

Sakr, Y; Gath, V; Oishi, J; Klinzing, S; Simon, TP; Reinhart, K; Marx G. Characterization of buccal microvascular response in patients with septic shock. *Eur. J. Anaesthesiol.*, 2010, 27(4), 388−394.

Saldanha, C. Fibrinogen interaction with the red blood cell membrane. *Clin. Hemorheol. Microcirc.*, 2013, 53(1-2), 39–44.

Sandker, SC; Hondebrink, E; Grandjean, JG; Steenbergen W. Laser speckle contrast analysis for quantifying the Allen test, a feasibility study. *Lasers Surg. Med.*, 2014, 46(3), 186−192.

Scheeren, TW. Journal of Clinical Monitoring and Computing 2015 end of year summary, tissue oxygenation and microcirculation. *J. Clin. Monit. Comput.*, 2016, 30(2), 141−146.

Scheeren, TW. Monitoring the microcirculation in the critically ill patient, reflectance spectroscopy. *Intensive Care Med.*, 2011, 37(6), 1045−1046.

Spronk, PE; Zandstra, DF; Ince C. Bench-to-bedside review, Sepsis is a disease of the microcirculation. *Crit. Care*, 2004, 8(6), 462–468.

Steenbergen, W. Fast Full-Field Laser Doppler Perfusion Imaging. In, Leahy MJ, editor. *Microcirculation imaging*. Weinheim, Wiley-Blackwell, 2012. pp. 113−134.

Steenbergen, W. Speckle effects in Laser Doppler Perfusion Imaging. In, Leahy MJ, editor. *Microcirculation imaging*. Weinheim, Wiley-Blackwell, 2012. pp. 135−146.

Steinhausen, M; Zimmerhackl, B; Thederan, H; Dussel, R; Parekh, N; Esslinger, HU; von, Hagens, G; Komitowski, D; Dallenbach FD. Intraglomerular microcirculation, measurements of single glomerular loop flow in rats. *Kidney Int.*, 1981, 20, 230–239.

Stern, MD. *In vivo* evaluation of microcirculation by coherent light scattering. *Nature*, 1975, 254(5495), 56–58.

Sun, CK; Zhang, XY; Zimmermann, A; Davis, G; Wheatley AM. Effect of ischemia-reperfusion injury on the microcirculation of the steatotic liver of the Zucker rat. *Transplantation.*, 2001, 72(10), 1625−1631.

Szabo, A; Vollmar, B; Boros, M; Menger MD. Gender differences in ischemia-reperfusion-induced microcirculatory and epithelial dysfunction in the small intestine. *Life Sci.*, 2006, 78(26), 3058–3065.

Szopinski, J; Kusza, K; Semionow M. Microcirculatory responses to hypovolemic shock. *J. Trauma*, 2011, 71(6), 1779–1788.

Thurston, GB; Henderson NM. Viscoelasticity of human blood. In, Baskurt OK, Hardeman MR, Rampling MW, Meiselman HJ, editors. *Handbook of Hemorheology and Hemodynamics*. Amsterdam, IOS Press, 2007. pp. 72–90.

Tillmanns, H; Ikeda, S; Bing RJ. The effects of nicotine on the coronary microcirculation in the cat heart. *J. Clin. Pharmacol.*, 1974, 14, 426–433.

Trzeciak, S; Cinel, I; Dellinger, PR; Shapiro, NI; Arnold, RC; Parrillo, JE; Hollenberg SM. Microcirculatory Alterations in Resuscitation and Shock (MARS) Investigators. Resuscitating the microcirculation in sepsis, the central role of nitric oxide, emerging concepts for novel therapies, and challenges for clinical trials. *Acad. Emerg. Med.*, 2008, 15(5), 399–413.

Trzeciak, S; Dellinger, RP; Parrillo, JE; Guglielmi, M; Bajaj, J; Abate, NL; Arnold, RC; Colilla, S; Zanotti, S; Hollenberg SM. Early microcirculatory perfusion derangements in patients with severe sepsis and septic shock, relationship to hemodynamics, oxygen transport, and survival. *Ann. Emerg. Med.*, 2007, 49(1), 88–98.

Usami, S; Chien, S; Gregersen MI. Viscometric characteristic of blood of the elephant, man, dog, sheep, and goat. *Am. J. Physiol.*, 1969, 217(3), 884–890.

Vallet, B; Winn, MJ; Asante, NK; Cain SM. Influence of oxygen on endothelium-derived relaxing factor/nitric oxide and K(+)-dependent regulation of vascular tone. *J. Cardiovasc. Pharmacol.*, 1994, 24(4), 595–602.

Vallet, B. Endothelial cell dysfunction and abnormal tissue perfusion. *Crit. Care Med.*, 2002, 30(5 Suppl), S229–S234.

Vallet, B. Vascular reactivity and tissue oxygenation. *Intensive Care Med.*, 1998, 24(1), 3–11.

van, Elteren, HA; Ince, C; Tibboel, D; Reiss IK; de Jonge, RC. Cutaneous microcirculation in preterm neonates, comparison between sidestream dark field (SDF) and incident dark field (IDF) imaging. *J. Clin. Monit. Comput.*, 2015, 29(5), 543–548.

van Meurs, M; Wulfert, FM; Knol, AJ; De Haes, A; Houwertjes, M; Aarts, LP; Molema, G. Early organ-specific endothelial activation during hemorrhagic shock and resuscitation. *Shock*, 2008, 29(2), 291–299.

van Zutphen, LFM; Baumans, V; Beynen, AC; editors. *Principles of Laboratory Animal Science.* Amsterdam, Elsevier, 2001.

Villringer, A; Haberl, RL; Dirnagl, U; Anneser, F; Verst, M; Einhäupl KM. Confocal laser microscopy to study microcirculation on the rat brain surface *in vivo*. *Brain Res.*, 1989, 504(1), 159–160.

Vinogradov, SA; Fernandez-Seara, MA; Dupan, BW; Wilson DF. A method for measuring oxygen distributions in tissue using frequency domain phosphorometry. *Comp. Biochem. Physiol. A Mol. Integr. Physiol.*, 2002, 132(1), 147–152.

Vollmar, B; Menger M. Intestinal ischemia/reperfusion, microcirculatory pathology and functional consequences. *Langenbecks Arch. Surg.*, 2011, 396(1), 13–29.

von Andrian, UH. Intravital microscopy of the peripheral lymph node microcirculation in mice. *Microcirculation*, 1996, 3(3), 287–300.

von Dobschuetz, E; Pahernik, S; Hoffmann, T; Kiefmann, R; Heckel, K; Messmer, K; Mueller-Hoecker, J; Dellian M. Dynamic intravital fluorescence microscopy--a novel method for the assessment of microvascular permeability in acute pancreatitis. *Microvasc. Res.*, 2004, 67(1), 55–63.

Wagner, Z. Erlauterungstaflen zur Physiologie und Entwicklungsgeschichte. Leipzig, Leopold Voss, 1839.

Wang, RK; Subhash HM. Optical microangiography, theory and application. In, Leahy MJ, editor. *Microcirculation imaging.* Weinheim, Wiley-Blackwell, 2012. pp. 197–258.

Ward, KR; Torres, Filho, I; Barbee, RW; Torres, L; Tiba, MH; Reynolds, PS; Pittman, RN; Ivatury, RR; Terner J. Resonance Raman spectroscopy, a new technology for tissue oxygenation monitoring. *Crit. Care Med.*, 2006, 34(3), 792–799.

Watanabe, R; Munemasa, T; Matsumura, M; Fujimaki M. Fluorescent liposomes for intravital staining of Kupffer cells to aid *in vivo* microscopy in rats. *Methods Find. Exp. Clin. Pharmacol.*, 2007, 29(5), 321–327.

Watts, SW; Kanagy, NL; Lombard JH. Receptor-mediated events in the microcirculation. In, Tuma RF, Duran WN, Ley K, editors. *Handbook of Physiology, Microcirculation.* 2nd edition. Amsterdam, Elsevier Academic Press, 2008. pp. 285–348.

Weed, RI; LaCelle, PL; Merrill EW. Metabolic dependence of red cell deformability. *J. Clin. Invest.*, 1969, 48(5), 795–809.

Wells, RE. Jr. Rheology of blood in the microvasculature. *N. Engl. J. Med.*, 1964, 270, 832–839.

Windberger, U; Bartholovitsch, A; Plasenzotti, R; Korak, KJ; Heinze G. Whole blood viscosity, plasma viscosity and erythrocyte aggregation in nine mammalian species, reference values and comparison of data. *Exp. Physiol.*, 2003, 88(3), 431–440.

Windberger, U; Baskurt OK. Comparative hemorheology. In, Baskurt OK, Hardeman MR, Rampling MW, Meiselman HJ, editors. *Handbook of Hemorheology and Hemodynamics.* Amsterdam, IOS Press, 2007. pp. 267–285.

Yalcin, O; Wang, Q; Johnson, PC; Palmer, AE, Cabrales P. Plasma expander viscosity effects on red cell-free layer thickness after moderate hemodilution. *Biorheology*, 2011, 48(5), 277–291.

Yoshida, N; Granger, DN; Anderson, DC; Rothlein, R; Lane, C; Kvietys PR. Anoxia/reoxygenation-induced neutrophil adherence to cultured endothelial cells. *Am. J. Physiol.*, 1992, 262(6 Pt 2), H1891–H1898.

Zipfel, WR; Williams, RM; Webb WW. Nonlinear magic, multiphoton microscopy in the biosciences. *Nat. Biotechnol.*, 2003, 21(11), 1369–1377.

Zweifach, BW. Direct observation of the mesenteric circulation in experimental animals. *Anat. Rec.*, 1954, 120(1), 277–291.

In: Advances in Experimental Surgery. Volume 2
Editors: Huifang Chen and Paulo N. Martins
ISBN: 978-1-53612-773-7
© 2018 Nova Science Publishers, Inc.

Chapter 14

EXPERIMENTAL GENE THERAPY USING NAKED DNA

Eiji Kobayashi[*]*, MD, PhD*
Department of Organ Fabrication, Keio University School of Medicine, Tokyo, Japan

ABSTRACT

Experimental surgery using animal models is indispensable for applying new science developments to human clinical surgery. In recent years, attempts have been made to apply gene transfer technology in the surgical field as well as various naked genes.

In this chapter, we first introduced non-viral *in vivo* gene transfer techniques that we have applied thus far. In addition to describing the historical background of the development of the gene gun, we showed cancer treatment research and organ transplant research models implemented in small animals. We also introduced the hydrodynamic approach, which involves using catheter techniques via the arteries and veins of the target organ. We used a rat model to demonstrate that gene transfer can be effectively performed on the liver and muscles due to the characteristics of this organ and tissue. This approach was then extended to pig models. Finally, we introduced DVA vaccine in pigs via electroporation, which is a technique that is already clinically used in the veterinary field.

These advanced surgical technologies and models are expected to contribute to future research.

Keywords: gene therapy, naked DNA, pig, gene gun, hydrodynamic method, DNA vaccine

ABBREVIATIONS

AAV	Adeno-associated vector
ALT	Auxiliary liver transplantation

---

[*] Corresponding author: Eiji Kobayashi, M.D., Ph.D., Department of Organ Fabrication, Keio University School of Medicine, 35 Shinanomachi, Shinjuku-ku, Tokyo, Japan, TEL: +81-3-5315-4090, FAX: +81-3-5315-4089, Email: organfabri@keio.jp.

APC	Antigen presenting cell
CAT	Chloramphenicol acetyltransferase
CTLA4Ig	Cytotoxic T-lymphocyte antigen 4-immunoglobulin
GFP	Green fluorescent protein
HBs	Hepatitis B virus surface
IVIS	*In vivo* imaging system
LacZ	Beta-galactosidase
OLT	Orthotopic liver transplantation
Tg	Transgenic

GENE GUN TECHNOLOGY IN LIVING ANIMALS

The gene gun was developed as a device to physically deliver genes to the target cell by accelerating the delivery of small particles coated with DNA using blasts from gunpowder or high-pressure gas (Figure 14.1). The process should be of value for studying transient and stable gene expression within intact cells and tissues (Klein 1988).

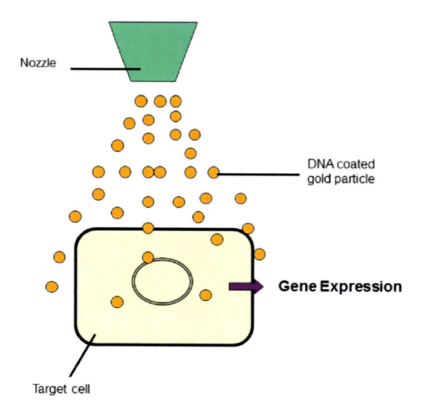

Figure 14.1. Theoretical schema of high-velocity microprojectiles for delivering nucleic acids into living cells. Small gold particles coated with naked DNA were acetated by blast wind of gunpowder or high-pressure gas. Transient expression of external genes was observed in the living cells of animals and plants.

The historical background of this technological development has been summarized previously (Belyantseva 2016). A process was developed for delivering foreign genes into maize cells that did not require the removal of cell walls and was capable of delivering DNA into embryogenic and nonembryogenic tissues. A plasmid harboring a chloramphenicol acetyltransferase (CAT) gene was adsorbed into the surface of microscopic tungsten particles (microprojectiles). These microprojectiles were then accelerated to velocities sufficient for penetrating the cell walls and membranes of maize cells in a suspension culture. High levels of CAT activity were consistently observed after the bombardment of cell cultures into the cultivars of black Mexican sweet corn, and these levels were comparable to the CAT levels observed after the electroporation of protoplasts. Measurable increases in CAT levels were also observed in two embryogenic cell lines after bombardment. Because this process circumvents the difficulties associated with regenerating whole plants from protoplasts, the particle bombardment process provides significant advantages over existing DNA delivery methods for the production of transgenic maize plants.

In the 1900s, modifications were made to substitute gunpowder with high-pressure helium gas for injection and to allow its delivery while holding the gene gun in the hand instead of within a chamber. The gene gun is now commercialized and is commonly used in experiments. The following is also a summary of the Helios® Gene Gun, which is a representative gene gun (Belyantseva 2016). The mechanical energy of compressed helium gas is used for the biolistic delivery of exogenous DNA, mRNA, or siRNA to bombard tissue with micron- or submicron-sized DNA- or RNA-coated gold particles, which can penetrate and transfect cells *in vitro* or *in vivo*. Helios Gene Gun-mediated transfection has several advantages: (1) It is simple and can be learned in a short time; (2) it is designed to overcome cell barriers, even those as tough as the plant cell membrane or stratum corneum in the epidermis; (3) it can transfect cells deep inside a tissue such as specific neurons within a brain slice; (4) it can deliver practically of any size of mRNA, siRNA, or DNA; and (5) it works well with various cell types, including non-dividing, terminally differentiated cells that are difficult to transfect such as neurons or mammalian inner ear sensory hair cells, which is particularly important for inner ear research.

We have made attempts at *in vivo* gene transfer (Yoshida 1997). For the first time anywhere in the world, we attempted to introduce marker genes *in vivo* into the liver of a rat that was directly exposed under general anesthesia. DNA-coated Au particles were accelerated by pressurized He gas to supersonic velocities to introduce a gene into the cells. Experimental and theoretical analyses both revealed a heterogeneous distribution of the particles in each shot (1 mg Au = 2.4×10^7 particles with 2 μg [32P] DNA = 2.5×10^{11} moles). To introduce genes into the liver of living rats, the best results were obtained with a newly developed handheld gene delivery system. The beta-galactosidase gene was introduced into the rat liver with Au particles using He at 250 psi and was expressed (1.2 μunits/μg protein) in a limited area of the liver surface (8×8 mm, depth 0.5 mm). When the same gene gun was used on a monolayer of cultured COS7 cells (about 5 μm thick), the cells in the central area of heavy bombardment were killed. Cell death caused by the influx of Ca^{2+} was prevented by the use of a cytosol-type culture medium. This method is extremely useful because genes can be easily introduced into living plants and animals without using viral vectors (Figure 14.2). We introduced experimental gene therapies that we have performed to date using mice, rats (Figure 14.3), and hamsters. Later, the possible use of this technique for the *in vivo* topical introduction of anticarcinogenic cytokines, among other genes, was examined, and the research area of this technique was expanded (Yang 1995).

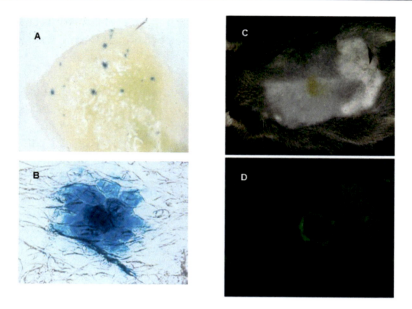

Figure 14.2. Expression of marker genes in a plant and mouse by Helios Gene Gun. LacZ Expression (A and B) in lemon. GFP gene was applied on the surface of mouse back skin (C) and a circular fluorescent intensity was observed under excitation light (D).

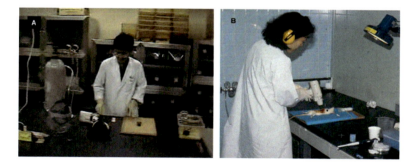

Figure 14.3. Application of gene gun in mice and rats. Eye protector and ear plugs were prepared. Gene gun was applied on a mouse which received it with sufficient anesthesia (A). Under inhalation anesthesia, the rat liver was exposed (B).

APPLICATION FOR ORGAN TRANSPLANTATION

We have conducted experiments to determine whether this technique could be used to introduce genes into the liver. Genes can be easily introduced into the surface of the rat liver with a gene gun while also introducing the green fluorescent protein (GFP) gene as a marker gene (Figure 14.4). This direct introduction of DNA into liver allografts before transplantation has been considered an effective strategy for inducing protective immunity against infections and malignancies (Nakamura 2003). We examined the feasibility of the gene gun-mediated vaccination of liver grafts. Using plasmids expressing luciferase and GFP, the expression of introduced genes was tested in a graft liver. The protein expression was observed in the graft liver of hepatectomized rats and was significantly enhanced. A short course of tacrolimus (FK506) also evoked the expression of these proteins. The effects of primary immunization of the liver on the humoral response were then tested using an expression plasmid encoding the hepatitis B virus surface (HBs) antigen and were compared to those of skin immunization alone. The results showed that local immunization of the liver strongly induced antibody formation. Furthermore, the combination of an immunized partial liver graft with tacrolimus significantly enhanced antibody production against HBs antigen. A DNA vaccine delivered to the liver is a possible strategy for preventing infectious diseases associated with liver transplantation under tacrolimus treatment.

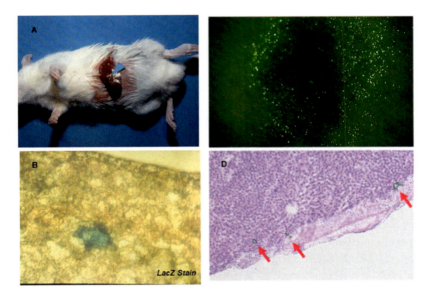

Figure 14.4. *In vivo* gene transfer with a marker gene in the rat liver. LacZ gene was applied on the rat liver (A &B). Circle GFP expression was observed on the surface of the rat liver (C & D). Reproduced from: Nakamura M, Wang J, Murakami T, Ajiki T, Hakamata Y, Kaneko T, Takahashi M, Okamoto H, Mayumi M, Kobayashi E. DNA immunization of the grafted liver by particle-mediated gene gun. *Transplantation* 2003; 76(9):1369−1375. Copyright ©2003 by Wolters Kluwer Health, Inc. Reproduced with permission. http://journals.lww.com/transplantjournal/pages/default.aspx.

APPLICATION FOR CANCER THERAPY

In addition, we have conducted research in the field of cancer research by expressing anticarcinogenic cytokines in the oral mucosa (Wang 2001) and muscle (Ajiki 2003). We examined the immunological effects of topical introduction into the oral mucosa by targeting the antigen presenting cell (APC) of macrophages.

Malignant melanoma in the oral cavity has a highly metastatic potential. Curative surgery is required to resect an extensive amount of oral tissue and often results in dysfunction as well as a severe cosmetic deformity in patients with the disease. An alternative technology for the local and sustained delivery of cytokines for cancer immunotherapy has been shown to induce tumor regression, suppress metastasis, and lead to the development of systemic antitumor immunity. However, local immunization of the oral cavity has not previously been studied. We examined the efficacy of particle-mediated oral gene transfer on luciferase and GFP production (Wang 2001). The results showed that these proteins were expressed as significantly higher in the oral mucosa than in the skin, stomach, liver, and muscle. Using an established hamster oral melanoma model, particle-mediated oral gene gun therapy with interleukin (IL)-12 cDNA was then evaluated. The results indicated that the direct bombardment with mouse IL-12 cDNA suppressed tumor formation and improved the survival rate. A skin tumor model created by inoculation with melanoma cells was also significantly inhibited by the oral bombardment of IL-12 cDNA coupled with an irradiated melanoma vaccine administrated to the oral mucosa compared with a treatment of a percutaneous vaccine. IL-12 gene gun therapy, combined with an oral mucosal vaccine, induced interferon-gamma mRNA expression in the host spleen for an extended period. These results suggest that immunization of the oral mucosa may induce systemic antitumor immunity more efficiently than immunization of the skin and that the oral mucosa may be one of the most suitable tissues for cancer gene therapy using particle-mediated gene transfer. To characterize the effects of the oral mucosa-mediated genetic vaccination, we also compared the antigen-specific immune responses of the oral mucosal DNA vaccine with those of flank skin vaccination against the influenza virus and the malaria parasite (Wang 2003). DNA vaccines against the influenza A/WSN/33 (H1N1) hemagglutinin and the malaria *Plasmodium berghei* circumsporozoite protein were each administered three times at 3-week intervals into the oral mucosa, skin, or liver of hamsters. The effects of the vaccines were evaluated by assessing antigen-specific antibody production and cell-mediated killing activity. Furthermore, the *in vivo* malaria challenge test was also performed after the vaccination. No significant specific antibody production was observed in any case, but interferon-gamma production and cell-mediated killing activity were strongly induced in splenic lymphocytes from hamsters given the oral vaccination. In the *in vivo* malaria experiment after the vaccination, the oral mucosal vaccination significantly delayed the blood appearance on the day that the parasites were compared with the other immunization sites ($p < 0.05$). These results suggest that gene immunization via the oral mucosa may induce cell-mediated immunity more efficiently than immunization via the skin or liver and that the oral mucosa may be one of the most suitable tissues for gene gun-based DNA vaccination against infectious diseases.

In evaluations of *in vivo* gene transfer using a gene gun, the muscle showed lasting effects (Figure 14.5). We then performed the following experiment. The immune response was modulated by genetic adjuvants using plasmid vectors expressing cytokines. Skeletal muscle can express a foreign gene intramuscularly administered via a needle injection, and the potential of muscle as a target tissue for somatic gene therapy in treating cancer has been explored. We investigated the efficacy of particle-mediated intramuscular transfection modified with a local anesthetic agent, bupivacaine, for luciferase and GFP expression. The results indicated that these proteins were more efficiently expressed and persisted longer in muscle modified in this way compared with the needle-injection method. Using an established rat sarcoma model, particle-mediated intramuscular gene gun therapy combined with IL-12 and IL-18 cDNA was evaluated. The growth of the distant sarcoma was significantly inhibited by particle-mediated intramuscular combination gene therapy, and the survival rate was also improved (Figure 14.6). Furthermore, after the combination gene gun therapy, significant levels of interferon-gamma were maintained, and a high activity level of tumor-specific cytotoxic T lymphocytes was induced. These results suggest that the sustained local delivery of IL-12 and IL-18 cDNA using intramuscular gene gun therapy modified with bupivacaine can induce long-term antitumor immunity and has the great advantage of inhibiting the disseminated tumor (Ajiki 2003).

However, it became evident that this method is not quite as effective as a long-term immunosuppressive therapy, as the expression of the genes is temporary and its effects are not expected to last for a long period of time (Ajiki, Transplantation 2003).

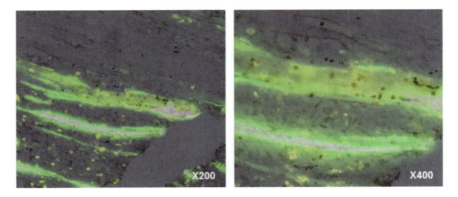

Figure 14.5. GFP expression in the regenerative muscle fibers in rats. Efficacy of gene transfection by a gene gun is independent of the cell cycle, but acts more effectively in BrdU positive myofibers.

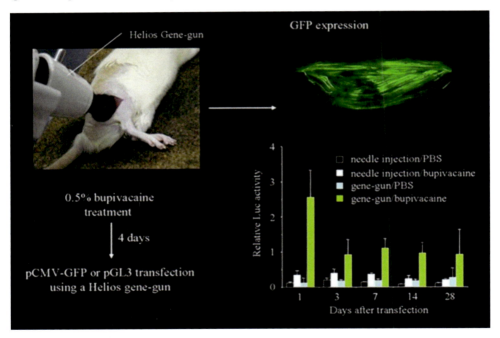

Figure 14.6. Long-term GFP gene expression in the rat muscle treated by a gene gun. Adapted from: Ajiki T, Murakami T, Kobayashi Y, Hakamata Y, Wang J, Inoue S, Ohtsuki M, Nakagawa H, Kariya Y, Hoshino Y, Kobayashi E. Long-lasting gene expression by particle-mediated intramuscular transfection modified with bupivacaine: combinatorial gene therapy with IL-12 and IL-18 cDNA against rat sarcoma at a distant site. *Cancer Gene Ther.* 2003; 10(4):318-329. Copyright ©2003 by Nature Publishing Group. Adapted with permission. http://www.nature.com/cgt/index.html.

Experiments have recently been conducted to introduce genes into the muscle using this technique (Tsai 2016). Tsai et al. investigated the possible underlying mechanisms associated with myostatin propeptide gene delivery via a gene gun in a rat denervation muscle atrophy model and evaluated the gene expression patterns. In a rat botulinum toxin-induced nerve denervation muscle atrophy model, we evaluated the effects of wild-type (MSPP) and mutant-type (MSPPD75A) myostatin propeptide gene delivery and observed changes in gene activation associated with the neuromuscular junction, muscle, and nerve. Muscle mass and muscle fiber size were moderately increased in myostatin propeptide-treated muscles ($p < 0.05$). Moreover, the enhanced gene expression of muscle regulatory factors, neurite outgrowth factors (IGF-1, GAP43), and acetylcholine receptors was observed. Their results demonstrated that myostatin propeptide gene delivery, especially the mutant-type of MSPPD75A, attenuates muscle atrophy through myogenic regulatory factors and acetylcholine receptor regulation. Their data showed that myostatin propeptide gene therapy might be a promising treatment for nerve denervation-induced muscle atrophy.

HYDRODYNAMIC APPROACH FROM RATS TO PIGS

The hydrodynamic approach was developed as a method for injecting DNA with a large amount of solvent via blood vessels (Figure 14.7). This technique is similar to the aforementioned gene gun method in that it enables *in vivo* gene transfer without using viral vectors. Liu et al. described this technique as follows (Liu 2001). The need for a safe and efficient method for gene delivery has stimulated the recent emergence of vectorless methods (e.g., naked DNA) as promising alternatives to the available viral- and non-viral-based systems. Among these methods, hydrodynamic-based gene delivery through the systemic injection of DNA offers a convenient, efficient, and powerful means for high-level gene expression in mice. This new gene delivery method, as well as the potential mechanism underlying the hydrodynamic-based DNA transfer into cells, has potential applications for gene function analysis, protein expression, and gene therapy in whole animals.

We have conducted studies focusing on the superior characteristics of the liver and muscles as target organs and tissues for gene expression (Sato 2003). We applied a non-viral gene transfer method using the rapid injection of naked DNA into the graft limb in rats. Naked DNA (beta-galactosidase-, luciferase-, or GFP-expressing plasmid) was used to test an intravascular gene transfer approach under various conditions on the Lewis rat limb. Then, in a rat limb transplantation model, these marker genes were administered preoperatively (Day 2) or perioperatively (Day 0) to the graft limb using the authors' "venous protocol." The expression level of luciferase was observed over a long period using a noninvasive living image acquisition IVIS system. The effective intravascular delivery of a gene to the rat limb was achieved using a rapid bolus injection of naked DNA through the femoral caudal epigastric vein. Using this procedure, the limb graft with the marker gene perioperatively in place was safely transplanted. After limb transplantation, sustained marker gene expression was observed for more than 2 months. This was the first report showing that the method of the rapid injection of naked DNA into a limb can be applied to gene modification for organ transplantation.

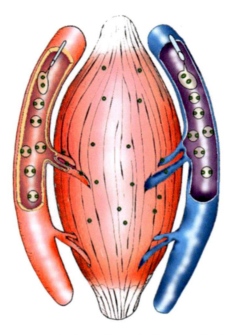

Figure 14.7. Theoretical schema of a hydrodynamic method by use of naked DNA. A large volume of saline with naked DNA was injected through either an artery or vein in rats.

APPLICATION OF A CATHETER-BASED TECHNIQUE IN RAT MODELS

We examined a non-viral gene transfer method using the rapid injection of naked DNA targeting the liver and applied it in a rat model of liver transplantation (Inoue 2004). Inbred Dark Agouti and Lewis rats were used. To test the efficacy and adverse effects of systemic or local (catheter-based) injection, different volumes of phosphate-buffered saline containing naked DNA encoding beta-galactosidase (LacZ) were injected. Luciferase expression was followed over time with non-invasive imaging, and the cytotoxic T-lymphocyte antigen 4-immunoglobulin (CTLA4Ig) protein was tested functionally via allogenic heart transplantation. Gene transfer was then tested in rat auxiliary liver transplantation (ALT) and orthotopic liver transplantation (OLT). The timing of gene transfer was evaluated in the ALT model, and OLT was performed using a liver graft to which luciferase or the CTLA4Ig gene was transferred two days before. LacZ was expressed extensively in a volume-dependent manner; however, a large volume often induced recipient death. After the local delivery of CTLA4Ig cDNA to the liver, the survival time of Dark Agouti heart grafts increased with increases in CTLA4Ig serum levels. Liver grafts injected with naked DNA at the time of donation did not survive, but livers grafted two days after gene transfer survived. Successful expression of luciferase and production of CTLA4Ig were finally confirmed in the rat that underwent OLT. We successfully applied a non-viral hydrodynamic gene transfer method to the rat liver and showed its potential in liver grafting. The high incidence of graft failure when this procedure is performed on the day of organ donation is a potential limitation that needs to be overcome prior to clinical application.

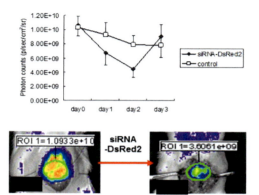

Figure 14.8. Liver targeting gene therapy in transplantation research. Reproduced from: Sato Y, Ajiki T, Inoue S, Fujishiro J, Yoshino H, Igarashi Y, Hakamata Y, Kaneko T, MurakamidT, Kobayashi E. Gene silencing in rat liver and limb grafts by rapid injection of small interference RNA. *Transplantation*, 2005; 79(2):240–243. Copyright ©2005 by Wolters Kluwer Health, Inc. Reproduced with permission. http://journals.lww.com/transplantjournal/pages/default.aspx. Also reproduced from: Inoue S, Hakamata Y, Kaneko M, Kobayashi E. *Transplantation*, 2004; 77(7):997–1003. Copyright ©2004 by Wolters Kluwer Health, Inc. Reproduced with permission. http://journals.lww.com/transplantjournal/pages/default.aspx.

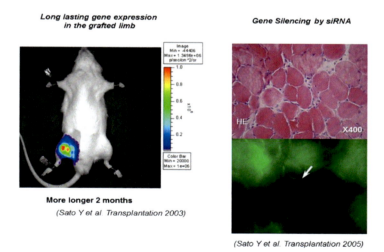

Figure 14.9. Limb targeting gene therapy in a rat model. Reproduced from: Sato Y, Ajiki T, Inoue S, Fujishiro J, Yoshino H, Igarashi Y, Hakamata Y, Kaneko T, Murakamid T, Kobayashi E. Gene silencing in rat liver and limb grafts by rapid injection of small interference RNA. *Transplantation*. 2005; 79(2):240–243. Copyright ©2005 by Wolters Kluwer Health, Inc. Reproduced with permission. http://journals.lww.com/transplantjournal/pages/default.aspx. Also reproduced from: Sato Y, Ajiki T, Inoue S, Hakamata Y, Murakami T, Kaneko T, Takahashi M, Kobayashi E. A novel gene therapy to the graft organ by a rapid injection of naked DNA I: long-lasting gene expression in a rat model of limb transplantation. *Transplantation* 2003 (Nov 15); 76(9):1294–1298. Copyright ©2003 by Wolters Kluwer Health, Inc. Reproduced with permission. http://journals.lww.com/transplantjournal/pages/default.aspx.

We introduced a non-viral method of gene transfer to donor grafts using an organ-selective injection technique to up-regulate gene expression. Based on the attractive methodology of RNA interference for silencing the expression of a particular gene, we also applied our catheter-based injection method to transfer small interference RNA (siRNA)-GFP into the liver and limb grafts (Figures 14.8 and 14.9) (Sato 2005). We quantified the interfering activity after the systemic delivery of siRNA into the liver of Alb-DsRed2 transgenic (Tg) rats using an *in vivo* bioimaging system. Then, using GFP Tg Lewis rats as donors, the preoperative rapid injection of siRNA resulted in the transient down regulation of GFP expression in both the liver and limb transplantation models. Genetic modification by siRNA may provide new therapeutic options for the down regulation of endogenous antigenicity.

APPLICATION IN LARGE ANIMAL MODELS

For the first time worldwide, we successfully performed gene transferance with a pig liver as the target using this technique (Yoshino 2006). We attempted to transfect naked plasmid DNA into the porcine liver using a modified hydrodynamic method. We transferred plasmid DNA to a part of the liver using an angio-catheter to reduce damage to the liver. To discern the injection conditions, naked plasmid DNA encoding GFP was transferred for use as a marker gene. The GFP gene was markedly expressed in the gene-transferred pig livers (Figure 14.10). In large animals, in addition to the naked gene quantity, the solution volume containing the plasmid DNA, and the injection speed, the additional treatments for the portal vein and the preparation of the hepatic artery are crucial. We found that the following injection conditions were needed: 3 mg of plasmid DNA, a solution volume of 150 ml, and an injection speed of 5 ml/s. The portal vein and the hepatic artery were clamped during gene delivery, and the blood flow of the portal vein was flushed out using normal saline. The CTLA4-Ig gene was used to test for the secretory protein. The CTLA4-Ig gene was injected with a large volume of solution via the hepatic vein specifically into the left outer lobe of the liver. CTLA4-Ig was detected in the blood of the pigs at a maximum serum level of 161.7 ng/ml 1 day after gene transfer, and CTLA4-Ig was detected for several weeks. This new technique of inserting a catheter into only a selected portion of the liver reduces liver toxicity and increased gene transfer efficiency.

With this method, gene transfer efficiency is increased by washing out the blood in the liver using a balloon catheter. This catheter technique was also applied to monkeys using AAV vector therapy (Mimuro 2013). This method results in high transfer efficiency in the liver, and studies using rats (Kobayashi 2016) and pigs (Sendra 2016) are currently underway to develop the technique for use in clinical practice.

DVA VACCINATION BY ELECTROPORATION IN PIGS

The development of a safe DNA vaccination strategy is underway following advances concerning the *in vivo* electroporation technique (Liu 2011). Advances have been made in research using pigs in particular for preclinical application (Ramanathan 2009, Luo 2016). We also evaluated universal influenza vaccines on pigs using the electroporation technique (Figure 14.11). A conduction needle was inserted into the medial thigh area of a pig under general anesthesia, and the naked target DNA was injected into the central region. Gene transfer was completed by immediate conduction.

This technique has already been used in clinical practice and has been tested on hepatitis B (Yang 2017) and HIV (Huang 2017), and its effects are being revealed.

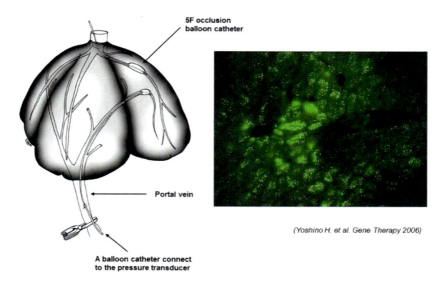

Figure 14.10. Naked plasmid DNA transfer to the porcine liver. Reproduced from: Yoshino H, Hashizume K, Kobayashi E. Naked plasmid DNA transfer to the porcine liver using rapid injection with large volume. *Gene Ther.* 2006; 13(24):1696–1702. Copyright ©2006 by Nature Publishing Group. http://www.nature.com/gt/index.html.

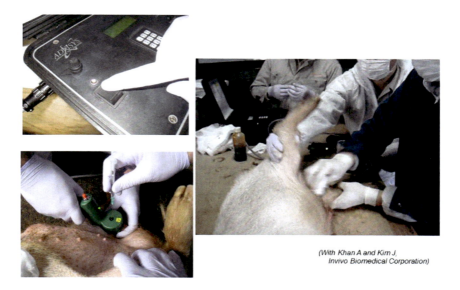

Figure 14.11. DNA vaccine by electroporation in pigs.

CONCLUSION

We have described the gene gun, catheter-based hydrodynamic approaches, and the electroporation technique as experimental *in vivo* gene transfer methods that do not use viral vectors while also presenting the data from our experiments via a historical background.

REFERENCES

Ajiki T, Murakami T, Kobayashi Y, Hakamata Y, Wang J, Inoue S, Ohtsuki M, Nakagawa H, Kariya Y, Hoshino Y, Kobayashi E. Long-lasting gene expression by particle-mediated intramuscular transfection modified with bupivacaine: combinatorial gene therapy with IL-12 and IL-18 cDNA against rat sarcoma at a distant site. *Cancer Gene Ther.* 2003; 10(4): 318−329.

Ajiki T, Takahashi M, Hakamata Y, Murakami T, Kariya Y, Hoshino Y, Kobayashi E. Difficulty of achieving long-term graft survival of MHC-disparate composite graft using CTLA4IG. *Transplantation* 2003; 76(2): 438; author reply 438−439. No abstract available.

Belyantseva IA. Helios (®) Gene Gun-Mediated Transfection of the Inner Ear Sensory Epithelium: Recent Updates. *Methods Mol. Biol.* 2016; 1427: 3−26.

Huang Y, Zhang L, Janes H, Frahm N, Isaacs A, Kim JH, Montefiori D, McElrath MJ, Tomaras GD, Gilbert PB Predictors of durable immune responses six months after the last vaccination in preventive HIV vaccine trials. *Vaccine* 2017 Jan 25. pii: S0264-410X(16)30879-9. doi: 10.1016/j.vaccine.2016.09.053. [Epub ahead of print].

Inoue S, Hakamata Y, Kaneko M, Kobayashi E. Gene therapy for organ grafts using rapid injection of naked DNA: application to the rat liver. *Transplantation* 2004; 77(7): 997−1003.

Klein TM, Fromm M, Weissinger A, Tomes D, Schaaf S, Sletten M, Sanford JC. Transfer of foreign genes into intact maize cells with high-velocity microprojectiles. *Proc. Natl. Acad. Sci. U S A.* 1988; 85(12): 4305−4309.

Kobayashi Y, Kamimura K, Abe H, Yokoo T, Ogawa K, Shinagawa-Kobayashi Y, Goto R, Inoue R, Ohtsuka M, Miura H, Kanefuji T, Suda T, Tsuchida M, Aoyagi Y, Zhang G, Liu D, Terai S. Effects of fibrotic tissue on liver-targeted hydrodynamic gene delivery. *Mol. Ther. Nucleic Acids.* 2016; 5:e359. doi: 10.1038/mtna.2016.63.

Liu D, Knapp JE. Hydrodynamics-based gene delivery. *Curr. Opin. Mol. Ther.* 2001; 3(2): 192−197. Review.

Liu MA. DNA vaccines: an historical perspective and view to the future. *Immunol. Rev.* 2011; 239(1): 62−84. doi: 10.1111/j.1600-065X.2010.00980.x. Review.

Luo X, Liang X, Li J, Shi J, Zhang W, Chai W, Wu J, Guo S, Fang G, Zhou X, Zhang J, Xu K, Zeng J, Niu L. The effects of irreversible electroporation on the colon in a porcine model. *PLoS One* 2016; 11(12):e0167275. doi: 10.1371/journal.pone.0167275.

Mimuro J, Mizukami H, Hishikawa S, Ikemoto T, Ishiwata A, Sakata A, Ohmori T, Madoiwa S, Ono F, Ozawa K, Sakata Y. Minimizing the inhibitory effect of neutralizing antibody for efficient gene expression in the liver with adeno-associated virus 8 vectors. *Mol. Ther.* 2013; 21(2): 318−323. doi: 10.1038/mt.2012.258.

Nakamura M, Wang J, Murakami T, Ajiki T, Hakamata Y, Kaneko T, Takahashi M, Okamoto H, Mayumi M, Kobayashi E. DNA immunization of the grafted liver by particle-mediated gene gun. *Transplantation* 2003; 76(9): 1369−1375.

Ramanathan MP, Kuo YC, Selling BH, Li Q, Sardesai NY, Kim JJ, Weiner DB. Development of a novel DNA SynCon tetravalent dengue vaccine that elicits immune responses against four serotypes. *Vaccine* 2009; 27(46): 6444−53. doi: 10.1016/j.vaccine.2009.06.061.

Sato Y, Ajiki T, Inoue S, Fujishiro J, Yoshino H, Igarashi Y, Hakamata Y, Kaneko T, Murakamid T, Kobayashi E. Gene silencing in rat-liver and limb grafts by rapid injection of small interference RNA. *Transplantation* 2005; 79(2): 240−243.

Sato Y, Ajiki T, Inoue S, Hakamata Y, Murakami T, Kaneko T, Takahashi M, Kobayashi E. A novel gene therapy to the graft organ by a rapid injection of naked DNA I: long-lasting gene expression in a rat model of limb transplantation. *Transplantation* 2003; 76(9): 1294−1298.

Sendra L, Miguel A, Pérez-Enguix D, Herrero MJ, Montalvá E, García-Gimeno MA, Noguera I, Díaz A, Pérez J, Sanz P, López-Andújar R, Martí-Bonmatí L, Aliño SF. Studying closed hydrodynamic models of "in vivo" DNA perfusion in pig liver for gene therapy translation to humans. *PLoS One* 2016 3; 11(10): e0163898. doi: 10.1371/ journal.pone.0163898.

Tsai SW, Tung YT, Chen HL, Yang SH, Liu CY, Lu M, Pai HJ, Lin CC, Chen CM. Myostatin propeptide gene delivery by gene gun ameliorates muscle atrophy in a rat model of botulinum toxin-induced nerve denervation. *Life Sci.* 2016; 146: 15−23. doi: 10.1016/j.lfs.2015.12.056.

Wang J, Murakami T, Hakamata Y, Ajiki T, Jinbu Y, Akasaka Y, Ohtsuki M, Nakagawa H, Kobayashi E. Gene gun-mediated oral mucosal transfer of interleukin 12 cDNA coupled with an irradiated melanoma vaccine in a hamster model: successful treatment of oral melanoma and distant skin lesion. *Cancer Gene Ther.* 2001; 8(10): 705−712.

Wang J, Murakami T, Yoshida S, Matsuoka H, Ishii A, Tanaka T, Tobita K, Ohtsuki M, Nakagawa H, Kusama M, Kobayashi E. Predominant cell-mediated immunity in the oral mucosa: gene gun-based vaccination against infectious diseases. *J. Dermatol. Sci.* 2003; 31(3): 203−210.

Yang FQ, Rao GR, Wang GQ, Li YQ, Xie Y, Zhang ZQ, Deng CL, Mao Q, Li J, Zhao W, Wang MR, Han T, Chen SJ, Pan C, Tan DM, Shang J, Zhang MX, Zhang YX, Yang JM, Chen GM. Phase IIb trial of in vivo electroporation mediated dual-plasmid hepatitis B virus DNA vaccine in chronic hepatitis B patients under lamivudine therapy. *World J. Gastroenterol.* 2017; 23(2): 306−317. doi: 10.3748/wjg.v23.i2.306.

Yang NS, Sun WH. Gene gun and other non-viral approaches for cancer gene therapy. *Nat. Med.* 1995; 1(5): 481−483. No abstract available.

Yoshida Y, Kobayashi E, Endo H, Hamamoto T, Yamanaka T, Fujimura A, Kagawa Y. Introduction of DNA into rat liver with a hand-held gene gun: distribution of the expressed enzyme, [32P] DNA, and Ca2+ flux. *Biochem. Biophys Res. Commun.* 1997; 234(3): 695−700.

Yoshino H, Hashizume K, Kobayashi E. Naked plasmid DNA transfer to the porcine liver using rapid injection with large volume. *Gene Ther.* 2006; 13(24):1696−1702.

Chapter 15

ROBOTIC SURGERY IN EXPERIMENTAL MEDICINE

Sandra S. Y. Kim, B.Sc., David Ian Harriman, MD
and Christopher Nguan[*]*, MD, FRCPSC*
Department of Urologic Sciences
University of British Columbia, Vancouver, British Columbia

ABSTRACT

Robotic assisted surgery has become a vitally important surgical modality developed through experimentation, innovation and collaboration between engineers, scientists, and surgeons. Digitalization of the surgeon-patient interaction allows for previously unheard of feats of engineering in procedural medicine including increased degrees of freedom of dexterity beyond human capability, telesurgery across great distances, and augmented reality. Animal models for training and testing these robotic platforms have been developed along the way which have helped the field progress. There remains a lack of randomized control trials comparing robot-assisted surgery versus other surgical modalities, however preliminary studies are promising. Despite initial upfront costs, the appeal of robot-assisted surgery continues to increase and its use will continue to expand as knowledge of how best to implement the technology continues to advance.

Keywords: robotic surgery, telesurgery, daVinci, Zeus

ABBREVIATIONS

BMI	Body Mass Index
CI	Confidence Interval
FDA	Federal Drug and Administration

---

[*] Corresponding author: Christopher Nguan M.D., FRCPSC. Department of Urological Sciences, Gordon & Leslie Diamond Health Care Centre, Level 6, 2775 Laurel Street, Vancouver, BC Canada V5Z 1M9, Tel: 604-875-5003. E-mail: chris.nguan@ubcurology.com.

LOS   Length of Stay
MIS   Minimally invasive surgery
NASA   National Aeronautics and Space Administration

HISTORY OF ROBOTIC SURGERY

Robotic technology was originally developed so manufacturing industries could perform precise, repetitive and potentially dangerous jobs with intent on improving quality, efficiency and safety. The progression of robotics into the operating theatre seemed pre-ordained as there are many parallels in the ongoing challenges to improve accuracy and precision of surgical techniques to optimize patient outcomes.

Minimally invasive surgery (MIS) has a long history, as Georg Kelling first developed and performed laparoscopic surgery using a Nitze cystoscope in a dog in 1901 Germany (Hatzinger 2006). Hans Christian Jacobaeus from Sweden went on to perform the first clinical laparoscopic operation and since then, MIS adoption has steadily increased with both hand-assisted and pure laparoscopic techniques having been validated and successfully incorporated into many surgical fields around the world (Hatzinger 2006). The advantages of laparoscopic surgery over open surgery are well described and include: smaller incisions, shorter postoperative hospital stays, quicker return to normal function, decreased risk of wound infection and better cosmesis (Lanfranco 2004; Kim 2002; Fuchs 2002). Drawbacks of MIS are also recognized, specifically: loss of 3D vision, reduction of tactile feedback, amplification of tremor through rigid laparoscopic instruments, range of motion limitation, and poor ergonomics that put additional stress on the operating surgeon. In fact, these issues in MIS are thought to contribute to the steep learning curve to master complex MIS procedures (Lanfranco 2004; Prasad 2001). Robotic surgical systems were envisioned to overcome the limitations of standard laparoscopy and to further bolster the penetration of MIS procedures in more complex and restrictive scenarios.

The first surgical robots used computer interfaces and an effector arm to carry out surgical procedures. In 1985, the PUMA 560 (Programmable Universal Manipulation Arm), an industrial robot, became one of the earliest robots to be used in a clinical setting for stereotactic CT-guided brain biopsy (Kwoh 1988). ROBODOC (Integrated Surgical Systems) is comprised of a preoperative planning computer workstation and a five-axis robotic arm with a high speed milling device to more precisely core out the femur for improved placement of orthopedic implants (Bargar 1998).

In the early 1990s, NASA, the US military and researchers at Stanford combined efforts to develop telepresence robotic systems (Satava 2002). The initial impetus of telepresence robotic surgery was to provide surgical care to people over great distances per a battlefield situation, or in remote locations such as in space or deep sea scenarios (Lanfranco 2004). The first robot to incorporate telepresence technology was AESOP (Automated Endoscopic System for Optimal Positioning; Computer Motion Inc.) and approved by the FDA in December 1993. The Zeus robotic system complemented the AESOP robot and further extended its capabilities, representing the first 'master-slave' system with a separate surgeon console and robotic system (Lanfranco 2004). In a master-slave configuration, a human operator manipulates control interfaces which translate those movements to instruments manipulating the patient's anatomy;

no autonomous motions are made by the robot itself. Intuitive Surgical Systems developed their own telepresence robot during the late 1990s, the daVinci robotic surgical system. These rival companies eventually elected to merge together to promote the daVinci system, resulting in the discontinuation of the Zeus platform.

The daVinci surgical system has become the de facto standard in medical robotics, and is currently the dominant surgical robotic system in clinical practice. The coincidental miniaturization and evolution of stereoscopic imaging, instrumentation, hardware and software engineering combined to make surgical robotics possible. Operations that were previously thought to be impossible without resorting to traditional open methods of surgery can now often be tackled in a minimally invasive fashion with robotic assistance. Robotic surgery remains at the frontier of surgical innovation and continues to advance the limits of conventional thinking in minimally invasive surgery.

TYPES OF TELEPRESENCE ROBOTS

There has been rapid progress in surgical robotics and their applications, and robotic MIS systems are now widely available with uses ranging from endoluminal, laparoscopic, single port to natural orifice based procedures (Barbash 2010; Lanfranco 2004; Davies 2000). The development and technology of each telesurgical system is reviewed here.

AESOP: Automated Endoscopic System for Optimal Positioning

AESOP was the first telesurgical robotic device. It was originally developed from a research grant from NASA for the development of a robotic arm to be used in the US space program (Ballantye 2002). The current iteration of AESOP is voice controlled and commands a robotic endoscope holder with 7 degrees of freedom. Urologists at John Hopkins demonstrated the success of AESOP as a surgical assistant in 17 different urological procedures (Partin 1995). The success of AESOP led to further developments in surgical robots and an influx of interest from medical technology companies.

ARTEMIS: Advanced Robotics and Telemanipulator System for Minimally Invasive Surgery

ARTEMIS was developed by scientists experienced in the nuclear and industrial applications fields, at the Karlsruhe Research Centre (Rininsland 1993). ARTEMIS is a master-slave robotic system comprised of 2 robotic arms that are controlled by a surgeon through a control console and a 3-D endoscopic system (Schurr 2000). ARTEMIS also gave the surgeon six degrees of freedom with a flexible distal robotic arm, allowing for precise motion in surgery (Rininsland 1999).

Zeus Surgical System

The Zeus robot was developed in 1999 and is a comprehensive surgical robotic system in which the surgeon controls two robotic arms attached to the bed rails of the operating table. The third arm is an AESOP for visualization, which is voice controlled. The surgeon sits upright in a cockpit-like console facing a 2-dimensional viewing system of the operating field (Maseo 2010).

daVinci Surgical System

The daVinci Surgical System consists of 3 separate parts; 1) a master console consisting of a work station, computer and 3D display system; 2) a control tower which houses the 3D video capture equipment and synchronizers; and 3) a patient side cart comprised of a motorized wheeled platform and a vertical post with four robotic arms suspended from it. The master console translates a full 7 degrees of freedom to the instruments of the patient side cart, while the high definition stereoendoscopic cameras are mixed to provide true 3D stereoscopic views of the operative field back to the surgeon console. By converting the standard "analog" interaction of the surgeon with the patient to a digital process, the system allows for adjunctive benefits to the operator: tremor filtration, motion scaling, swapping of controls and arms, control of additional robotic arms greater than the number of master controllers through hot swapping, and all the while providing a seated, ergonomic approach to surgery which promotes the efficient and effective conduct of a potentially prolonged operation. Finally, research conducted at Intuitive and academic centers worldwide can provide surgical platform "plugins" to add novel functionality to the standard robotic system.

Typically, major operations require the assistance of an additional person at the bedside, but with the latest versions of the daVinci robot, the patient side cart's four arms are able to be controlled by two concurrent master controller units controlled by one primary surgeon and one assistant. Although telesurgery across distances is possible with the daVinci surgical system, in North America, the FDA does not allow the use of this functionality and requires the patient and surgeon always be in the same room (Maseo 2010).

The daVinci system has evolved over time where in 1999, the original daVinci system ("Standard") had a 2-dimensional viewing screen and 3 robotic arms, a 4th arm was added in 2003. In 2006, the daVinci S was released that had 3-dimensional high definition vision. In 2009, the daVinci Si was produced with a dual console option to aid with operative teaching and assistance, the Firefly Fluorescence Imaging System to aid in real-time visualization of tissue perfusion, the option for single site surgery, system integration with complex imaging modalities and advanced instrumentation for finer tasks. The most recent model was produced in 2014 and is termed the daVinci Xi. This model is the first major overhaul since 1999 and has redesigned instrument arm architecture to facilitate anatomical access from any position, increased flexibility of visualization through repositioning of the endoscope through any port, and a smaller footprint.

SPORT Surgical System

Titan Medical Incorporation based in Toronto, Ontario is currently developing the Single Port Orifice Robotic Technology (SPORT) surgical system, unveiled in early 2016, with the aim to expand the field of robotics surgery by lowering the cost barrier to allow for pervasive use in all surgical specialties. The SPORT is a single-incision surgical system with multi-articulated instruments, camera with 3D high definition view of the surgical field, ergonomic work station, single-arm mobile patient cart, with single-use replaceable tips. This surgical system is not yet available for sale.

CURRENT ROBOTIC APPLICATIONS

Cardiac Surgery (Table 15.1)

MIS cardiac surgery became reality with advances in perfusion strategies, myocardial protection and access techniques (Bush 2013). Robotic cardiac valve and bypass surgery have become a mainstay of the discipline with use cases including: atrial septal defect closure on a beating heart, atrial fibrillation ablation and cardiac tumor resections (Gao 2010; Schilling 2012). Advantages of robotic assistance include improved cosmesis, shorter recovery and comparable outcomes to traditional techniques with the main disadvantage being prolonged operative times (Bush 2013).

Mitral valve surgery is the most common robotic assisted cardiac procedure performed, the first case performed in 1998 with an early prototype of the daVinci surgical system (Carpentier 1998). Within a week after the first robot-assisted mitral valve repair, Mohr et al. performed 5 more robotic mitral valve repairs as well as a coronary revascularization procedure (Mohr 1999). Between 2006 and 2009, Mihaljevic et al. compared key outcomes grouped by surgical technique for 759 patients undergoing mitral valve repair (Mihaljevic 2011). On average, the robot-assisted procedures took 42 minutes longer than complete sternotomy, 39 minutes longer than partial sternotomy, and 11 minutes longer than right mini-anterolateral thoracotomy ($p < 0.05$). The increased robot operative time was offset by decreased blood transfusion rates as well as lower rates of pleural effusion and atrial fibrillation compared to standard open or MIS methods, leading to significantly reduced hospital stay (median 4.2 days vs. 5.2, 5.8 and 5.1 days respectively; $p < 0.05$).

As briefly alluded to above, robotic assisted surgery has also been employed for total endoscopic coronary artery bypass grafting (TECAB). A multicenter, prospective study by Argenziano et al. assessed the safety and efficacy of TECAB surgery (Argenziano 2006). Of 85 patients undergoing TECAB surgery, 5 were converted to open procedures, 1 required reintervention for bleeding and 1 experienced myocardial infarction. Mean hospital length of stay was 5.1 ± 3.4 days. Angiographic success, defined as patient anastomosis, was 91% and the authors concluded non-inferiority to traditional techniques. More recently, robotic surgical techniques in the absence of cardiac bypass have been performed with encouraging results (Bush 2013). From these studies, it has been demonstrated that the use of robot-assisted CABG can be successful in properly chosen operative candidates.

Table 15.1. Compilation of procedures performed by surgical robots as reported in humans

Cardiac	Atrial fibrillation ablation
	Coronary artery bypass graft
	Cardiac septal defect repair: Atrial septal defect
	Coronary revascularization
	Intracardiac tumor resections
	Left lead implantation for pacemaker
	Lobectomy
	Mammary artery harvest
	Valve surgery: Mitral valve repair
General Surgery	Acid reflux surgery
	Bariatric surgery: gastric bypass, gastrectomy, fundoplication
	Cholecystectomy
	Colorectal resections: colectomy, low anterior resection, rectopexy, rectal resections
	Esophageal surgery
	Heller myotomy
	Hernia repair
	Pancreatectomy
	Splenectomy
Gynecology	Adnexal surgery
	Endometrial ablation
	Hysterectomy
	Lymphadenectomy
	Myomectomy
	Oophorectomy
	Sacrocolpopexy
	Tubal re-anastomosis
Neurosurgery	Image guided surgery: tumor resection, biopsy, endoscopic fenestration, ventriculostomy
	Myelomeningocele repair
	Pedicle screw placement under image guidance
	Transoral odontoidectomy
Orthopedic Surgery	Knee arthroplasty
	Image guided intra-articular injection
	Spine surgery
	Total hip arthroplasty: femur preparation/coring, acetabular cup placement
Otolaryngology	Marsupialization of a vallecular cyst
	Obstructive sleep apnea hypopnea syndrome treatment
	Parathyroidectomy
	Resection of head and neck tumors: laryngeal, oropharyngeal, hypopharyngeal, oral cavity
	Thyroidectomy
	Transoral robotic surgery
Urology	Cystectomy
	Nephrectomy: partial, radical, donor
	Dismembered Pyeloplasty
	Radical prostatectomy
	Ureteral Reconstruction
	Vasovasostomy

General Surgery

Contemporary results in the field of General Surgery show modest benefit of surgical robotics over traditional laparoscopic methods across a range of operations (Maseo 2010). Additionally, it has been estimated that per-procedure cost increases of up to $1500 are incurred as a result of robot assistance (Barbash 2010). As such, adoption of robotic laparoscopic techniques in General Surgery have been variable and limited with an eye towards gaining further evidence and ongoing cost containment.

A large study out of the University of Illinois at Chicago assessed outcomes for 676 robotic cholecystectomies compared to 289 laparoscopic cholecystectomies (Gangemi 2016). Statistically significant differences were identified favoring robotic cholecystectomy with decreased minor biliary injuries ($p = 0.049$), decreased open conversion ($p < 0.001$) and reduced blood loss ($p < 0.001$). Mean hospital stay and number of biliary anomalies identified intraoperatively were comparable across groups. Overall, this study indicates benefit of robotic versus laparoscopic cholecystectomy. Robotic multi-port (n = 4) and single site cholecystectomy (n = 5) has been safely performed in a pediatric population (mean age 14) (Ahn 2015). Median console time was 47 minutes (range, 44–58) for multi-port cholecystectomy and 69 minutes (range, 66–86) for single site cholecystectomy. Eight of 9 patients were discharged home on day 0 with no complications. Both techniques were deemed safe in a pediatric population with possibly increased anesthetic time with single-site surgery for the trade-off of potential improved cosmesis and functional recovery.

Robotic colorectal surgery has also garnered increasing interest and a recent meta-analysis composed of data from 2 randomized controlled trials and 22 non-randomized controlled trials (5 prospective and 17 retrospective) representing 3318 patients (robotic n = 1852; laparoscopic n = 1466) compared outcomes for robotic assisted versus laparoscopic colorectal surgery (Zhang 2016). Length of hospital stay, conversion rates and blood loss were significantly reduced in the robotic group ($p < 0.05$) while the operation times (SMD = 0.78, 95% CI 0.54 – 1.02) and total costs (SMD = 1.23, 95% CI 1.01–1.45) trended in favor of laparoscopic surgery while not reaching statistical significance between groups. A separate study by Shiomi et al. assessed the advantages of robotic assisted surgery (n^{tot} = 127; n^{obese} = 52) compared to laparoscopic surgery (n^{tot} = 109; n^{obese} = 30) for lower rectal cancer and visceral obesity cases, defined as visceral fat area ≥ 130 cm^2 (Shiomi 2016). Robotic assisted surgery had lower overall complication rate (9.4% vs. 23.9%; $p = 0.007$), less blood loss ($p = 0.007$), shorter length of stay ($p < 0.01$) with comparable operative time and pathological results. Visceral obesity cases displayed decreased blood loss, length of stay and complication rate in favor of the robotic group (all $p < 0.05$). These results suggest that robotic assisted surgery may have advantages for challenging surgical locations and patient factors.

Gynecology

Multiple studies have compared the daVinci surgical system to standard laparoscopic myomectomy. These are technically challenging operations and many surgeons prefer open surgical approaches compared to MIS for this reason. Advincula et al., demonstrated that the use of surgical robots was associated with fewer intraoperative complications and decreased blood loss with a mean of 196 mL 95% CI [50, 700] compared to 365 mL 95% CI [75, 1550] ($p < 0.05$), increased operative time with a mean of 231 minutes 95% CI [199, 263] for the robot-assisted surgery compared to mean of 154 minutes 95% CI [138,170] ($p < 0.05$), decreased mean hospital stay (1.5 days 95% CR [1, 3] compared to 3.6 days 95% CR [3, 8] ($p < 0.05$), and increased cost compared to traditional laparoscopic methods. The largest study comparing the daVinci surgical system to laparoscopic and open myomectomy approaches demonstrated the ability to resect larger masses with the robot (223g 95% CI [85.2, 391.5]) compared to laparoscopy (96.65 g 95% CI [49.5, 227.3]) ($p < 0.001$). Additionally, robotic surgical time was 181 minutes 95% CI [151, 265] compared to laparoscopy (115 minutes 95% CI [98, 200]) compared to open procedure time of 126 minutes 95% CI [95, 177] ($p < 0.010$) (Barakat 2011). Patients undergoing the open procedure had increased LOS of 3 days, 1 day for laparoscopic, compared to 1 day for robot-assisted surgery ($p < 0.001$) (Barakat 2011). The findings of these studies suggest that the use of surgical robots may benefit patients with complex, multiple myomas who would traditionally not be considered candidates for a minimally invasive approach.

Uterine cancer is one of the most common cancers in women, and surgical treatment consists of combination of a hysterectomy, bilateral salpingo-oophorectomy, and pelvic and para-aortic lymphadenectomy (Weinberg 2011). The largest study to date comparing 377 robot-assisted surgeries to historical data of 131 patients undergoing open surgery for staging of endometrial cancer demonstrated that the conversion rate from robotic surgery to open surgery was 2.9% (Paley 2011). The robotic surgery group had a decreased blood loss of 46.9 mL compared to 197.6 mL ($p < 0.0001$) for open procedures, decreased intraoperative and postoperative complications (6.4% compared to 20.6% $p < 0.0001$), a higher lymph node count of 15.5 compared to 13.1 ($p = 0.007$) as well as a shorter LOS (1.4 days compared to 5.3 days for open procedure, ($p < 0.0001$) (Paley 2011).

The utility of the daVinci robot treating early stage cervical cancer with radical hysterectomy has been evaluated, given the complexity of performing laparoscopic radical hysterectomy. A study done by Nam et al. compared 32 cases each of robot-assisted as well as open hysterectomy with similar patient and tumor demographics. There was no significant difference between the operative time between the robotic and open procedures (218.8 ± 78.3 minutes, 209.9 ± 87.8 minutes respectively, $p = 0.654$), with similar number of lymph nodes sampled (20.2 ± 9.4, 24.2 ± 11.1 respectively, $p = 0.121$), and decreased blood loss (220.0 ± 134.7 mL, 531.5 ± 435.5 mL respectively, $p = 0.002$) (Nam 2010).

Ovarian cancer requires operative staging including: exploratory laparotomy with hysterectomy, adenectomy, abdominal-pelvic washing, omentectomy, pelvic and paraaortic lymphadenectomy, and peritoneal biopsies, as well as debulking of resectable metastatic tumor (Weinberg 2011). One study done by Magrina et al., compared 25 cases of daVinci-assisted robotic surgery for staging of endothelial ovarian cancer compared to 27 laparoscopic surgery and 119 open surgery cases over 3 years (Magrina 2011). Despite confounding variables in this study, the authors demonstrated that the robotic, laparoscopic and open treatment arms were associated with: mean operative times of 314.8 minutes, 253.8 minutes, and 260.7 minutes respectively ($p < 0.05$), decreased blood loss of 164.0 mL, 266.7 mL, and 1307.0 mL respectively ($p = 0.001$), and mean length of hospital stay of 4.2, 3.2, and 9.2 days respectively ($p = 0.08$) (Magrina 2011).

Currently there are no substantial randomized trials with long-term outcomes comparing robotic surgery efficacy and safety in Gynecology compared to traditional surgical approaches to definitively change pattern of practice, but studies remain ongoing and robotics in Gynecology remains an emerging field.

Neurosurgery

The field of neurosurgery has undergone monumental changes as a result of revolutions in stereotactic and minimally invasive surgery (Nathoo 2005) NOT IN LIST. MIS Neurosurgery has directly led to improved patient outcomes and new surgical options for tumors that were previously thought to be unresectable, all the while improving safety for patients in these critical operations.

The initial types of robots helped surgeons perform basic stereotactic tasks, the first one of which was the PUMA 560 used to predetermine the trajectory of a brain biopsy procedure (Kwoh 1988). NeuroMate (Integrated Surgical Systems, 1987, Sacramento, California) was the first surgical robot to be approved by FDA comprises a system with 6 degrees of freedom that can be used for biopsy procedures, stereoencephalography, endoscopy, as well as deep brain stimulation with its ability to properly and accurately orient, position, hold, and manipulate tools in a 3D space with high precision and accuracy (Nathoo 2005; Haegelen 2010). NeuroArm, developed at the University of Calgary in 2001, is an ambidextrous robot designed to work within an MRI which allows the neurosurgeon to perform operations while leveraging real-time MRI scans throughout the procedure (Sutherland 2013). NeuroArm was used in 2008 to remove a brain tumor from a 21 year old patient, and since then has shown positive clinical results in other cranial neoplasia cases (Sutherland 2013; Pandya 2009).

Spine surgery saw the development of SpineAssist (Mazor Robotics, Caeserea, Israel), the predecessor to the Renaissance surgical system from the same company, which was FDA approved in 2011. Both of these surgical systems consist of a miniature robot securely attached to the operating table coordinated with real-time fluoroscopy to assist in accurate placement of spinal pedicle screws (Devito 2010). A retrospective study comparing the use of SpineAssist showed that 3204 of 3271 (97.9%) pedicle screws were appropriately placed on targeted positions by the robot (Devito 2010).

The daVinci surgical system has also been used in Neurosurgery for spinal schwannoma removal, transoral odontoidectomy, and intrauterine repair of myelomeningocele, with inconclusive outcome reports comparing robot-assisted to conventional open methodologies (Perez-Cruet 2012). However, daVinci is limited in this capacity due to reduced instrumentation availability and need for multiple access ports (Doulgeris 2015).

Current studies of robotics in Neurosurgery draw inconclusive results due to lack of good quality clinical trials and current evidence is comprised primarily of case reports or on *in vivo* models. However the increasing number of case reports from institutions illustrates the desire of surgeons to investigate this emerging technology in the context of Neurosurgery.

Orthopedics

Although the field of Orthopedic surgery pioneered surgical robotics, their use has not gained the widespread popularity and growth as seen in other surgical specialties. The external fixation of limbs in optimal position presents fewer challenges to accessing the operative field and providing adequate exposure compared to other surgical specialties which work with mobile viscera and soft tissues (Yen 2010).

Traditional knee replacement surgery (TKR) involves intraoperative sizing guides to assist the surgeon determine the appropriate implant size to ensure a tight fit between the bone and prosthetic. Intraoperative cutting errors and resulting gaps can lead to delays in bone growth and increased use of bone cement in such cases. Many surgical robots were developed for the purposes of knee arthroplasty, with only few of them having clinical success throughout the world. These robots include the CASPAR system (URS Ortho Rastatt, Germany), RGA system (formerly known as ACROBOT), ROBODOC system (Curexo Technology Corporation, Fremont, California, USA), and the Robotic Arm Interactive Orthopedic System (RIO; MAKO Surgical Corporation, Fort Lauderdale, Florida, USA), with the most commonly used orthopedic surgical robots being the ACROBOT and ROBODOC systems (Netravali 2013).

The Active Constraint ROBOT (ACROBOT) was first developed in Imperial College in London, United Kingdom (Jakopec 2003) and is now known as the Stanmore Sculptor Robotic Guidance Arm (RGA) system (Stanmore Implants, Elstree, UK) (Netravali 2013). Its main parts include a high-speed cutter mounted on a robotic device that uses 3D reconstruction and visual guidance to precisely target and core out long bones for implants (Cobb 2006). The ACROBOT allows free movement inside a predetermined safe region, however, motion at the boundaries becomes progressively more stiff, preventing inadvertent errors (Jakopec 2003). A prospective double-blind randomized control trial by Cobb et al., compared conventional and robot-assisted unicompartmental knee arthroplasty in 27 patients using the ACROBOT system showed increased operating time but significantly better alignment that achieved near normal coronal plane alignment within 2 degrees of the targeted position with the ACROBOT, while only 40% (6/15) of the conventional method resulted in this degree of accuracy (Cobb 2006). Likewise, the difference between tibiofemoral angles planned and achieved favored ACROBOT assistance (0.65 ± 0.59 degrees vs. -0.84 ± 2.75 degrees respectively, $p = 0.001$). Three other studies done by Coon, Pearle et al., and Plate et al., also evaluated the use of robot-assisted unicompartmental knee arthroplasty, which all demonstrated more accurate implant placement, improvements in restoration of natural knee kinematics, and positive outcomes for implant survival as a result of accurate placement of implants (Coon 2009; Pearle 2010; Plate 2013).

ROBODOC is one of the first clinically successful robots, and is the first robot to be approved by the FDA to be used in orthopedic surgery (Karthik 2015).

Robot-assisted total hip arthroplasty (THR) was originally performed with ROBODOC in 1992 and has been used in over 24,000 surgeries worldwide with data showing improved patient outcomes, with more precise implant positioning and elimination of intraoperative femoral fractures (Bargar 1998). A study done by Harris et al., compared the surgical outcomes of hip replacements performed in three different centers with 69 ROBODOC-assisted total hip replacement compared to 65 control cases. As with knee replacement surgery, the robot-assisted procedure was associated with longer operative times (258 minutes, which was later reduced to 90 minutes with surgeon experience, compared to 134 minutes for the control group, $p < 0.0001$) (Bargar 1998). Blood loss was reported to be higher in the robot-assisted group (1189 mL compared to 644 mL compared to the conventional open surgical method, $p < 0.0001$), and average length of stay was not significantly different between the two groups (8.2 days for the ROBODOC and 7.5 days vs. control) (Barger 1998). Postoperative complications including intraoperative fractures, dislocations, partial sciatic nerve palsy, deep vein thrombosis and pulmonary embolism were evaluated with no significant differences in complication rates between the two treatment groups, other than no intraoperative femoral fractures in the ROBODOC group compared to three in the control group ($p < 0.01$) (Barger 1998). The modified Harris hip scores postoperatively showed no difference in the first year favoring the robotic group (89.4 for the ROBODOC vs. 86.6 for the control group), and two years (88.5 for the ROBODOC vs. 91.1 for the control group) (Bargar 1998).

The innovative motion (INNOMOTION, Innomedic, Herxheim & FZK Karlsruhe Germany & TH Gelsenkir, Germany) allows for robot-guided intraarticular injections into the many joint articulations of the foot under CT or MRI guidance, including: calcaneocuboid, subtalar, tarsometatarsal, talonavicular, and tibiotalar joints. INNOMOTION was successful in infiltrating all 16 joints of patients (n = 16) with no intra or postinterventional complications. Small case studies to date have shown that patients had relief of pain following injections with a preinterventional pain measurement visual analogue scale (VAS) 5.3 ± 2.33 to a score of 1.1 ± 1.45 postinterventionally (Wiewiorski 2009).

Surgical robotics in Orthopedic surgery has a long and storied history, and remains an active area of research and development. Given the current widespread use of mechanical instruments in the field of Orthopedic surgery, lends the specialty especially well transition into the world of robotics surgery.

Otolaryngology

The field of Otolaryngology has traditionally performed procedures involving large incisions and extensive surgical dissections to adequately perform head, neck and airway surgeries to minimize damage to vital structures (Oliveira 2012). Thus the nature of these surgical procedures can lead to significant tissue damage, extended time to functional recovery, decreased cosmesis, and decreased quality of life (Garg 2010). Robotic assisted surgery is well poised to positively affect these negative patient outcomes (Oliveira 2012).

The daVinci robot is currently used for Transoral Robotic Surgery (TORS) and was FDA approved in 2009 (Moore 2009). TORS surgery involves the use of the oral cavity as an entry site, and was first carried out by McLeod and Melder for marsupialization of a vallecular cyst in 2005 (McLeod 2005). This technique was further adapted and developed by Weinstein and O'Malley in 2006 on three human patients with tongue base cancers (O'Malley 2006).

There are few studies to date looking into the functional surgical outcomes associated with patients undergoing TORS for oncologic resection in the head and neck. Case reports of a variety of different surgical procedures performed in head and neck regions from the oropharynx, laryngopharynx, oral cavity, skull base surgery (infratemporal and parapharyngeal fossae), thyroid glands, and in pediatric airways have been documented (Garg 2010). The most comprehensive study thus far was done by Boudreaux et al. in 2009 with 36 patients with laryngeal, oropharyngeal, hypopharyngeal, and oral cavity tumors. Although 36 patients were recruited for the study, only 29 (81%) underwent successful robotic resections with negative surgical margins reported in all 29 patients (Boudreaux 2009). Of the 7 patients who failed to undergo successful robotic resection of their tumors, the biggest factor was adequate and appropriate exposure of the surgical site, extensive infiltrative tumor requiring free-flap reconstruction, or patients opting for chemotherapy or chemoradiotherapy treatments instead (Boudreaux 2009). The mean robotic operative time was 99 ± 32.6 minutes, mean estimated blood loss was 51 ± 42 mL and no transfusion was required for any cases (Boudreaux 2009). The mean hospital stay was 2.9 ± 2.9 days, and 16 of the 29 patients (55%) were able to return to oral nutrition prior to discharge. Postoperative complications were limited to bleeding in 4 patients, one whom required cautery and another as a result of coumadin therapy several days postoperatively. 21 patients (21/29, 72%) undergoing TORS were safely extubated prior to exiting the operating room, and 7 patients required postoperative intubation with only one patient requiring a planned short term tracheotomy tube placement. This study demonstrated that TORS is a safe surgical alternative for patients with suitable airway anatomy and limited tumor disease pathology, however, further studies comparing TORS to conventional open procedures will need to be carried out to further elucidate the benefits of using the daVinci robot in these procedures.

The use of TORS has also been extended to non-malignant lesions in the head and neck. Vicini et al., in 2012 assessed the utility of TORS in treating obstructive sleep apnea hypopnea syndrome in 20 patients. The mean operative time was 42.5 ± 15.2 minutes, with a mean setup time of 31.2 ± 18.2 minutes and estimated blood loss was at 27.7 ± 13.6 mL (Vicini 2012). There were no serious intraoperative or postoperative complications in this study other than minor bleeding managed non-surgically in three patients (Vicini 2012). Evaluation of the surgical outcome was done through the apnea hypopnea index (AHI) score and Epworth sleepiness scale (ESS) with improvements of 24.6 ± 22.2 for AHI and 5.9 ± 4.4 for ESS, and using cutoff values of AHI, ESS, and oxygen saturation levels postoperatively, 12 (60%) of the patients were considered to be cured (Vicini 2012).

The use of the daVinci has been evaluated more extensively in the case of thyroidectomies, comparing it to the conventional open method. The first case was performed by Lobe et al., in 2005 who used a transaxillary robotic technique to resect a thyroid nodule in one patient and placement of a vagal nerve stimulator for intractable seizures in another (Lobe 2005). A recent systematic review and meta-analysis looked at 11 articles comparing robot-assisted thyroidectomy to conventional open procedures. The mean operative time for robot-assisted thyroidectomy was increased compared to conventional open methods by 48.1 minutes 95% CI [33.6, 62.7] in total thyroidectomies and by 37.3 minutes 95% CI [12, 62.5] in subtotal thyroidectomies (Sun 2014). Conversion from robot-assisted to open cases was required in 2 out of 243 cases (0.8% cases). Length of hospital stay was decreased in the robot-assisted thyroidectomy group by -0.006 days 95% CI [-0.25, 0.24]. There was no significant difference between the two patient groups in terms of postoperative complications including hematoma or seroma formation, recurrent laryngeal nerve injury, hypocalcemia, or chyle leak, (Sun 2014). Postoperatively, the conventionally open procedure treated patients had increased severity of voice symptoms at postoperative day 1 ($p = 0.008$), first month postoperatively ($p = 0.049$), 3 months postoperatively ($p = 0.043$), but not at 6 months (Tae 2012).

The feasibility of skull base surgery was first demonstrated by O'Malley and Weinstein in humans in a patient who underwent parapharyngeal cystic neoplasm resection in the infratemporal fossa with no adverse surgical events such as damage to many vital structures (carotid artery, jugular vein, cranial nerves) (Oliveira 2012). Further development of appropriate instruments for Otolaryngology in terms of size, function, and flexibility will be needed prior to execution of more robot-assisted skull base surgery in Otolaryngology patients (Oliveira 2012).

Urology

The field of Urology has been a frontrunner in exploring surgical robots use in a spectrum of operations. The first reports of the use of the daVinci robot in surgery were described by Partin et al. in 1995 who utilized robotic assistance as surgical assistant substitutes during 17 laparoscopic procedures (Burch bladder suspension (n = 2), nephrectomy (n = 4), nephropexy (n = 1), orchiopexy (n = 1), pelvic lymph node dissection (n = 1), pyeloplasty (n = 3), retroperitoneal lymph node sampling (n = 2), varix ligation (n = 2), and ureterolysis (n = 1) (Partin 1995). The study reported no increase in total operative time when the robotic arms were used, and no difference between the set up and take down times for the robot-assisted surgeries compared to the conventional laparoscopic surgical assists ($p > 0.05$) (Partin 1995). DaVinci robot-assisted prostatectomy (DVP) is the most frequently performed robotic procedure worldwide, and has supplanted both laparoscopic and open approaches at many centers (Barbash 2010). There remains insufficient data to determine if robotic prostatectomy can decrease the long term rates of impotence and incontinence which are potential complications of this operation. However, introduction of robotic Urology has changed the landscape of radical prostatectomy operations as a whole, as it has leveled the steep learning curve of laparoscopic prostatectomy and allowed an entire population of MIS-naive surgeons seemingly the ability to offer an MIS approach to this procedure overnight (Barbash 2010).

The literature supports the fact that DVP leads to significantly less blood loss secondary to improved visualization of the dorsal venous complex coupled with the tamponade effect of the pneumoperitoneum compared to conventional open or laparoscopic methods (Jain 2015; Skolarus 2010; Krambeck 2009).

Comparing robot-assisted radical prostatectomy to traditional open procedures, the current studies show longer operative time for robot-assisted laparoscopic prostatectomy (2.3 hours for open and 4.8 hours for robot-assisted, $p < 0.001$) in the early phases of the learning curve with decreased operative time with increased robot-assisted surgical cases (N = 200) (163 minutes for open and 160 minutes for robot-assisted) (Menon 2002; Tewari 2003). Transfusion rates were lower in the robot-assisted group compared to the open surgical treatment group with a relative ratio of 4.51 95% CI [1.35, 15.03] ($p = 0.01$) (Ficarra 2009). Only a single study by Tewari et al., looked into mean catheterization time which demonstrated a lower catheterization time in robot-assisted treatment group of 15.8 days for open compared to 7 days ($p < 0.05$) (Tewari 2003). The current studies comparing the various surgical modalities show similar rates of complication in prostatectomies in the different treatment groups, with the exception of the study done by Tewari et al., which demonstrated a 20% intraoperative complication rate for open surgical group (N = 100) compared to 5% in the robot-assisted surgical group (n = 200) ($p < 0.05$) (Tewari 2003).

Comparison of laparoscopic prostatectomy to robot-assisted prostatectomy showed similar mean operative time after 20 robot cases (Ficarra 2007). The cumulative weighted mean difference for the mean operative time were overlapping in laparoscopic compared to robot-assisted treatment groups with a faster operative time in the laparoscopic group of -19.39 minutes 95% CI [-49.34, 88.13] ($p = 0.58$) and an increased weighted mean difference blood loss in the laparoscopic group of 19.45 mL 95% CI [-112.53, 106.73] compared to robot-assisted prostatectomy (Ficarra 2009). Robot-assisted prostatectomy did not have significant differences with regards to transfusion rate, in-hospital stay, or catheterization time, with conflicting results with regards to overall complication rates (Ficarra 2009). The cumulative analysis of very limited data looking into urinary incontinence after robot-assisted or laparoscopic prostatectomy shows a similar relative risk of 0.87 95% CI [0.54, 1.39] ($p = 0.56$) for the two groups, and one study looking into recovery of erectile function demonstrated a median time to erectile function recovery of 440 days for open prostatectomy compared to 180 days for robot-assisted prostatectomy ($p < 0.5$) and median time to intercourse of 700 days for open compared to 340 days for robot-assisted procedures ($p < 0.05$) (Ficarra 2009; Tewari 2003).

The oncologic outcomes following DVP (biochemical recurrence, positive surgical margins) appear similar between robot-assisted and conventional open radical prostatectomy (Masterson 2013; Barocas 2010). A cumulative analysis of studies found similar reports of positive surgical margins amongst robot-assisted and laparoscopic prostatectomy with a relative risk of 1.08 95% CI [0.97, 1.19] ($p = 0.17$) (Ficarra 2009). Recent systematic review and meta-analysis looking into the current studies of oncological outcomes associated with robot-assisted prostatectomy showed positive surgical margins with a mean of 15% in all cases and 9% in localized cancers (Novara 2012). Only very few studies reported follow up over 5 years with a 7 year biochemical recurrence-free survival being 80% for robot-assisted prostatectomy (Novara 2012). Cumulative analysis comparing robot-assisted prostatectomy to open prostatectomy showed similar positive surgical margins with an odds ratio of 1.25 ($p = 0.19$) and similar biochemical recurrence survival estimate hazard ratio of 0.9 ($p = 0.526$) (Novara 2012). Looking into robot-assisted prostatectomy compared to laparoscopic prostatectomy, the studies also demonstrate similar positive surgical margins with an odds ratio of 1.12 ($p = 0.47$) and similar biochemical recurrence survival estimate hazard ratio of 0.5 ($p = 0.141$) (Novara 2012).

The promising results of DVP and the demonstration of technical success of the platform in a restricted space performing complex reconstruction, paved the way for expansion of daVinci applications to other urological procedures. MIS radical nephrectomy procedures for renal cell carcinoma is a prime example of the benefits of minimally invasive surgery as there are well documented reductions in (LOS), pain, improved cosmesis and earlier return to activity. However, MIS partial nephrectomy, in which only a portion of the kidney is removed which harbors a tumor, followed by reconstruction of the remaining kidney, is a much more technically challenging operation and one for which daVinci has proven effective (Fergany 2000). The operation is often stressful as the renal hilum is clamped, depriving the kidney of blood during the resection, but also instituting a time limit to complete the procedure within 30 minutes. A retrospective review of daVinci partial nephrectomies performed at four large centers in Europe and United States by Benway et al. (n = 183), reported a mean ischemic time of 23.9 minutes (range: 10–51 minutes), a mean total operative time of 210 minutes (range: 86–370 minutes) with the robot, and a mean estimated blood loss of 131.5 mL (range: 10–900 mL), the tumor size was positively correlated with both the operative time ($p = 0.003$) and warm ischemic time ($p = 0.005$), with a mean tumor size of 2.87 cm (range: 1.0–7.9 cm). Two cases (1%) were converted to open partial nephrectomies due to failure to progress (extensive perinephric scarring in one patient and another failure to identify tumor in intraoperative ultrasounds). A total of 18 (9.8%) complications were reported in the study with 15 (8.2%) being major in nature, such as two postoperative bleeds requiring transfusion, two postoperative urine leaks (stent placement and drainage), hepatic laceration in one patient and splenic laceration in another, two chylous leaks, three pseudoaneurysms requiring embolization, one subscapsular renal hematoma, and two patients suffering from postoperative stroke and one myocardial infarction, with no fatalities. There were 3 (1.6%) minor complications such as incisional cellulitis and self-resolving gross hematuria, with no reported disease-specific mortalities. However, continued investigation of the efficacy of daVinci partial nephrectomy is required to document long term outcomes (Wu 2014).

The current gold standard treatment for muscle invasive bladder cancer is radical cystectomy. Laparoscopic radical cystectomy leads to lower morbidity and comparable oncological outcomes compared to open radical cystectomy (Haber 2007). The familiar benefits and MIS approach including: decreased hospital stay and blood loss, and early recovery from ileus are also reported benefits of daVinci robot-assisted radical cystectomy (Nix 2010). Staging pelvic lymph node dissection during these operations can be challenging via laparoscopy, but robot approaches yield numbers similar to that of the open procedure (Hellenthal 2011). It should also be noted that currently the preference is to complete the urinary diversion step of radical cystectomy via extracorporeal technique, although methods have recently been developed to facilitate a completely intracorporeal reconstruction (Pruthi 2010). A study evaluating the learning curve for robot-assisted radical cystectomy was appraised at 14 different institutions (N = 496) (Hayn 2010). Mean operative time for daVinci cystectomy was 441 minutes, 368 minutes, and 307 minutes for surgeons who had performed < 30, 30–50, or > 50 cases respectively ($p < 0.0001$) The median lymph node yield increased by 73% amongst surgeons who had done < 30 or > 50 cases ($p < 0.0001$), with lymph node yields of 13, 18, or 20 for surgeons who had performed < 30, 30–50, or > 50 cases respectively ($p < 0.0001$) The mean estimated blood loss was 477 mL (n = 476), 283 mL (n = 193), and 451 mL (n = 419) with surgeons who had performed < 30, 30–50, or > 50 cases respectively ($p < 0.0001$). The mean length of hospital stay was found to be 12 days, 10 days, and 12 days in the groups with surgeons who had performed < 30, 30–50, or > 50 cases respectively ($p = 0.4889$) and 21%, 27%, and 26% of cases performed by surgeons who had performed < 30, 30–50, or > 50 cases respectively required transfusions ($p = 0.2923$). Positive margins were found in 12%, 10%, and 6% of cases performed by surgeons who had performed < 30, 30–50, or > 50 cases respectively ($p = 0.6054$).

Benefits

Surgical robotics originally had foundations in the US military's desire to deliver specialized care in forward hospitals without risking these specialized human assets' lives. Following the advent of telesurgical robotics, refinement in the platform followed parallel developments in the fields of computational power and complexity, hardware miniaturization, and videoendoscopy. While traditional open surgery allows for wide operative field visualization and manipulation and the recruitment of surgical assistants, traditional laparoscopy suddenly handcuffed the surgeon, limiting their range of motion, degrees of freedom and taking away depth perception during conduct of the operation. For these reasons, surgeons wishing to implement laparoscopy into their practice must undertake specific training in MIS techniques as there is a steep learning curve to relearn how to conduct procedures under such restrictive conditions. Surgeons were willing to continue to push MIS procedures over traditional open procedures despite the difficulties inherent in the surgical modality as there quickly became obvious benefits to patient postoperative recovery and return to normal function. At this point, surgical robotics fortuitously matured into a viable entity and quickly gained popularity as it severely flattened the learning curve to deliver MIS style surgical approaches. The robot added back increased dexterity and range of motion, improved visualization and depth perception, motion scaling and tremor filtration, and did away with the fulcrum effect; all factors which made minimally invasive surgery distinctly foreign, now made entirely intuitive (Prajapati 2012; Lanfranco 2004; Davies 2000).

Incorporation of robotic MIS has promoted the undertaking of surgical procedures previously thought to be too technically challenging or complex using laparoscopic methods. The development of "endowrist" technology which places an additional joint next to the tip of the instrument allows for fine, dextrous movements and a full 6 degrees of freedom, further increased the impression of deploying and controlling miniaturized virtual "hands" in the operative field. To many, it was essentially inconceivable to perform complex MIS procedures on the brain or spine, or pelvis, and the field of robotics has shown that these are not only feasible, but also often with improved patient outcomes.

Limitations

Despite its accelerating popularity and traction in the health care delivery landscape, there remain some disadvantages to surgical robotics, and there are currently no definitive high quality clinical trials comparing robotics to other MIS procedures. Furthermore, compared to other surgical methods such as their laparoscopic counterparts, there are very little long-term follow-up studies on patients of robotics-assisted surgery (Lafranco 2004; Maseo 2010; Weinberg 2011; Karthik 2015).

With any new technology comes additional cost, and robotic surgery is no exception. The capital cost of acquiring the daVinci surgical system is on the order of $3–5 million dollars (Turchetti 2012; Barbash 2010). The robotic instruments are the principal driver in incremental cost as they are disposable consumables which may be used a maximum of 10 cases before being decommissioned through an internal mechanism (Maseo 2010). A study published in the New England Journal of Medicine by Barbash and Sherry showed that on average across 20 different types of surgeries, the incorporation of robots into the procedure adds about $1600, or 6% to the cost (Barbash 2010). Intuitive Surgical is the sole provider of commercially available surgical robots and enjoys a monopoly in the market to date. The prohibitive cost of implementing a robotic surgery program can prevent more widespread adoption outside of large, academic centers (Kim 2002). Contemporary surgical training programs in North America particularly in the USA often teach trainees operations via robotics approaches first, and thus this generation of surgeons and those following are destined to accept these technologies as just a part of the standard armamentarium in the delivery of patient care. Even still, it is important to recognize that like any surgical procedure, it is estimated that one would need to perform 150 to 250 procedures prior to becoming proficient, and anywhere between 8 to 150 cases to reach a plateau on the learning curve (Barbash 2010; Jain 2015).

Another limitation of surgical robots is their physical presence in the operating rooms (Lafranco 2004). These machines are large, and take up valuable operating room real estate, particularly in already crowded operating rooms with other essential equipment and personnel. Questions have been raised as to safe conduct of procedures in these cramped quarters, however, these concerns may be circumvented with future development of smaller robots, or larger operating rooms built with these technologies in mind (Savata 2001). Already, between the daVinci Standard and the most recently released version, the daVinci Xi, there has been a significant reduction in footprint and resources required for the robotics platform in the OR.

The primary limitation in preventing widespread use of surgical robots is the prohibitive cost of purchasing and maintaining the robot, prolonged operative time which can further prolong surgical wait lists, and the need for specially trained operating staff and surgeons. It is predicted that with time, these limitations will be overcome; some through market competition, and some through "network effects" in that the more robots are in use, the more robotic operations are integrated, the more robots are purchased, and so on.

Training Models

Intuitive surgical has developed the daVinci Skills Simulator™ which consists of various modules designed to gain comfort in basic robotic skills such as endowrist manipulation, camera and clutching, fourth arm integration, system setting, needle and control driving and energy and dissection (Intuitive Surgical 2016). Cho et al. prospectively assessed if this trainer could improve performance (Cho 2013). 12 subjects were randomized into 2 groups, virtual reality plus standard training (n = 6) versus standard training alone (n = 6), to assess needle control and suturing. Participants were evaluated across two time points with the intervention group undergoing virtual reality training in between. Those subjects in the virtual reality group displayed significantly improved performance skills ($p = 0.028$) and suturing time (7.1 ± 1.54 minutes versus 10.55 ± 1.93 minutes, respectively; $P = .018$). Improved performance following robotic virtual reality simulation training has also been verified by other investigators (Foell 2013).

Robotic training on inanimate objects has gained popularity. Finan et al. created a dry lab in which the procedure for robotic hysterectomy was broken down into critical steps of the operation (i.e., identification of ureter, suturing vaginal cuff, etc.) (Finan 2010). They used objects such as balloons, rubber bands, nails, a 'beer huggie', foley catheters and plywood to model female anatomy. 16 residents were put through the dry lab training and graduated to live surgery if they showed proficiency at the critical steps as judged subjectively by an expert. 10 of 16 residents were granted permission to move onto live surgery performing key parts or the entire robotic hysterectomy with no complications to date.

Animal models are another mainstay of robotic surgical training. Mehrabi et al. used a small (rat) and large (porcine) animal model to evaluate performance improvement over time for visceral and vascular robotic surgical procedures (Mehrabi 2006). 4 trainees with different experience level underwent a baseline evaluation in a porcine model for cholecystectomy, gastrotomy, anastomosis of small intestine and aorta. Following this, training on a rat model performing 4 procedures each of gastrotomy and anastomosis of colon, aorta and small intestine was performed. Finally, re-evaluation on the porcine procedures occurred to conclude the study. Operative times significantly improved for everything except cholecystectomy (11 min and 8 min for cholecystectomies; $p = 0.24$, 18 and 10 min for gastrotomies; $p = 0.002$, 28 and 18 min for anastomosis of small intestine; $p = 0.007$, and 25 and 12 min for anastomosis of the aorta; $p = 0.049$). Also, complication rates and performance quality significantly improved for all procedures across time points as gauged by expert evaluators ($p < 0.05$). In the field of Urology, a novel robot-assisted partial nephrectomy model consisting of an ex vivo porcine kidney with an implanted Styrofoam ball mimicking the tumor was developed and tested by

Hung et al. (Hung 2012). This study divided participants into 3 groups based on number of robotic cases completed: expert (>100 cases; n = 13), intermediate (1–100 cases; n = 9), and novice (0 cases; n = 24). Partial nephrectomy using the daVinci Si was performed by each group, with each procedures being judged by 3 blinded expert reviewers using the validated Global Operative Assessment of Laparoscopic Skills tool (Vassiliou 2005). Expert surgeons outperformed the other groups in all performance metrics ($p < 0.05$) and felt the model may be beneficial for residents and fellows, but they were unsure how useful it would be for more experienced surgeons.

Hung et al. designed a study to gauge the relative performance of three standardized robotic training methods: virtual reality using the da Vinci Skills Simulator™, structured inanimate tasks and a live porcine model (Hung 2013). Two groups were identified consisting of urology residents (novice) with median (range) of 0 (0–20) robotic cases (n = 38) and faculty surgeons (expert) with median (range) of 300 (30–2000) robotic cases (n = 11). Blinded experts graded performance using the Global Evaluative Assessment of Robotic Skills tool (Goh 2012). As expected, experts received higher scores than novices over all three training methods ($p < 0.001$). Performance on all three methods was found to be strongly correlated ($p < 0.001$) indicating cross method validity, thus signifying the training value of each of these training methods.

Telesurgery

The master-slave configuration of the daVinci robotic surgical system has the primary surgeon sitting at a console that is connected to robotic effector arms via a series of cables. A logical extension of this set up is to increase the distance between the console and the robot to allow greater access to expert robotic surgical therapy. Telesurgery over great distances has the potential to deliver quality surgical care to people of remote areas without the added costs of travel and logistics. Additional benefits are quite intuitive, as clearly identified by two of the original collaborators of the technology; NASA and the USA army. Both of these groups hope to be able to deliver surgical care to their personnel either in space or on the battlefield (Satava 2002). Additional advantages include surgeon safety, as there are reports of surgeon morbidity when travel is required (Cazac 2014), and telementoring whereby novice surgeons can receive active feedback from expert surgeons across the world (Ballantyne 2002).

Pre-surgical telesurgery trials have been performed with encouraging results. Nguan et al. used an Internet-based virtual private network (VPN) with data transfer speeds of 17 Mb/s to assess robot-assisted laparoscopic pyeloplasty in a porcine model over a distance of 2848 km with the daVinci system (Nguan 2008). Surgical anastomotic times for the 6 porcine pyeloplasties were evaluated. Despite connection latency of 370 ms, the procedure was feasible with average anastomosis of 20.7 ± 4.7 min. In a separate study, Nguan et al. performed 18 total robotic-assisted pyeloplasties with the Zeus system on a porcine model using real-time (n = 6), Internet-based VPN (n = 6) and satellite network connections (n = 6) (Nguan 2008). Latency and operative time did not reach statistical significance between groups and were as follows: real time (0 ms; 41.3 ± 15.0 min), VPN (66.3 ms; 47.0 ± 24.1 min) and satellite (560.7 ms; 51.8 ± 4.7 min). Both the landline and satellite groups had 2 of 6 anastomoses display mild leak with pressure test of 100 cmH$_2$O whereas the real time procedures had no such leak. Finally, despite no statistically significant results between groups, surgeons subjectively reported that pyeloplasty was more difficult with delays between actions and response in the landline and satellite groups.

Innovative communication systems are necessary to achieve more widespread accessibility to telesurgery while also minimizing latency of data transfer. Sterbis et al. have shown that telesurgery is feasible over public Internet (Sterbis 2008). Using a combination of telementoring and telesurgical approaches, 4 robotic assisted porcine nephrectomies were carried out with the primary surgeon greater than 1200 miles away. Data transfer delays were between 450 to 900 ms, however blood loss was minimal, there were no inter-operative complications and all surgeries were successfully performed. A group from the University of Washington, in collaboration with the US military is attempting to develop a fully mobile, wireless robotic telesurgery system (Lum 2007). This group implemented a study in which a surgical robot was deployed in the Simi Valley desert of California for experiments on an inanimate model with communication facilitated via an Unmanned Aerial Vehicle in the HAPs/MRT (High Altitude Platform/Mobile Robotic Telesurgery) project. Time delay between console and robot was 200 ms for video stream and 20 ms for robotic control signals with no loss of signal. This communication system, along with the development of deployable surgical robot systems such as "The Trauma Pod" with the purpose of being a rapidly deployable robotic system with no human personnel that can be telesurgically controlled to perform critical life-saving procedures on wounded soldiers on the battlefield, could be used to perform complex care to people in disaster areas, on the battlefield or in other remote areas (Garcia 2009).

In 2001, a surgeon in New York performed the first long distance telesurgical operation by performing a laparoscopic cholecystectomy on a patient in Strasbourg, France over 14000 km away (Marescaux 2001). This was accomplished with the Zeus robotic system and a dedicated fiber optic line, known as Asynchronous Transfer Mode (ATM), with a rate of data transfer of 10 Mb/s. The 68 year old patient who was operated on recovered well from the surgery without complication. In Canada, telesurgery has been practiced between McMaster University in Hamilton, Ontario and North Bay, Ontario located 400 km apart, also with the Zeus robotic system (Anvari 2005). Between 2003 and 2005, Dr. Anvari and colleagues were able to perform 21 robot-assisted laparoscopic telesurgeries using an internet protocol virtual private network with 15 Mb/s of bandwidth which included 13 fundoplications, 3 sigmoid resections, 2 right hemicolectomies, 2 inguinal hernia repairs and 1 anterior resection. Latency experienced by the telerobotic surgeon was 135–140 ms. Surgeries were performed in a comparable time to on-site laparoscopic surgery with no significant surgical complications or increases in post-operative stay.

Despite the excitement, there are several concerns regarding telesurgery that has limited widespread acceptance. First, remote locations that may benefit from telesurgery may not currently have skilled individuals to set up the robot platform required for surgery or take control of the operation should a complication arise. Second, hospital and communication infrastructure in non-urban centers may be insufficient to accommodate the data quality and bandwidth required in a mission critical telesurgery setup where unreliable data transfer could be catastrophic (Korte 2014). Third, the financial cost of robotic surgery is prohibitive in many remote locations. Finally, latency in communication speeds does present technical challenges. Perez et al. used the robotic daVinci Trainer to determine impact of communication latency on telesurgical performance (Perez 2016). As latency of data transfer increases, this appears to have an expanding effect on performance. Deterioration in performance was initially identified with delays in data transfer of 300 ms with many surgeons being unable to perform complex tasks with delays greater than 700 ms. Ultimately, a dedicated, reliable, rapid connection with appropriate resources and personnel on the other end is required to ensure a safe procedure.

CONCLUSION AND FUTURE DEVELOPMENTS

Robotic surgery has become widely available throughout major cities globally. Initial costs of acquiring, setting up and training personnel in a surgical robotics program remain prohibitive in many areas of the world. Despite this, robotic assisted laparoscopic surgical platforms will continue to evolve and further penetrate surgical specialties, driven by a desire to conduct ever more complex operations at no incremental morbidity to the patient.

Surgical robots are unique in that they have the capacity to integrate and interface between other technologies widely used in the operating rooms. Preoperative imaging results (computed tomography or magnetic resonance imaging) can be integrated with the daVinci surgeon console to help surgeons more accurately target pathologies. Simulated complex procedures could also potentially be practiced prior to live surgery to improve outcomes (Lanfranco 2004). Furthermore, the original goal of long-distance surgeries might eventually become possible to bring care to remote areas with limited access to skilled surgeons.

The continued growth and development of new technological advances in medicine, coupled with the efforts of surgeons and researchers to further improve patient care will continue to fuel the development of new approaches to tackle procedures thought to be inaccessible. The expansion of the surgical robotics market with additional manufacturers will help lower the cost of entry for many institutions. Robotic surgery has demonstrated promising results thus far with respect to patient outcomes despite formal clinical trials and is likely to take its place in the standard armamentarium of patient care.

REFERENCES

Advincula AP, Xu X, Goudeau S 4th, Ransom SB. Robot-assisted laparoscopic myomectomy versus abdominal myomectomy: a comparison of short-term surgical outcomes and immediate costs. *J. Minim. Invasive Gynecol.* 2007; 14(6):698–705.

Ahn N, Signor G, Singh TP, Stain S, Whyte C.Robotic single- and Multisite Cholecystectomy in Children. *J. Laparendosc. Adv. Surg. Tech. A* 2015; 25:1033–1035.

Amr AN, Giese A, Kantelhardt SR. Navigation and robot-aided surgery in the spine: historical review and state of the art. *Dove Press* 2014; 2014(1):19–26.

Anvari M, McKinley C, Stein H. Establishment of the world's first telerobotic remote surgical service for provision of advanced laparoscopic surgery in a rural community. *Ann. Surg.* 2005; 241(3):460–464.

Anvari M, Birch D, Bamehriz F, Gryfe, R, Chapman T. Robotic-assisted laparoscopic colorectal surgery. *Surg. Laparosc. Endosoc. Percutan. Tech.* 2004; 14(6):311–315.

Argenziano M, Katz M, Bonatti J, Srivastava S, Murphy D, Poirier R, Loulmet D, Siwek L, Kreaden U, Ligon D; TECABResults of the prospective multicenter trial of robotically assisted totally endoscopic coronary artery bypass grafting. *Ann. Thorac. Surg.* 2006; 81(5):1666–74.

Ballantyne, GH. Robotic surgery, telerobotic surgery, telepresence, and telementoring. Review of early clinical results. *Surg. Endosc.* 2012; 16(10):1389−1402.

Barbash GI and Glied SA. New technology and health care costs - the case of robot-assisted surgery. *N. Engl. J. Med.* 2010; 363(8): 701−704.

Bargar WL, Bauer A, Börner M. Primary and revision total hip replacement using the Robodoc system. *Clin. Orthop. Relat. Res.* 1998(354); 354:82−91.

Barakat EE, Bedaiwy MA, Zimberg S, Nutter B, Nosseir M, Falcone T. Robot-assisted, laparoscopic, and abdominal myomectomy a comparison of surgical outcomes. *Obstet. Gynecol.* 2011; 117(2 pt 1):256−265.

Barocas DA, Salem S, Kordan Y, Herrell SD, Chang SS, Clark PE, David R, Baumgartner R, Phillips S, Cookson MS, Smith JA Jr. Robotic assisted laparoscopic prostatectomy versus radical retropubic prostatectomy for clinically localized prostate cancer: Comparison of short-term biochemical recurrence-free survival. *J. Urol.* 2010; 183(3):990−996.

Benway BM, Bhayani SB, Rogers CG, Porter JR, Buffi NM, Figenshau RS, Mottrie A. Robot-assisted partial nephrectomy: an international experience. *Eur. Urol.* 2010; 57(5):815−820.

Bodner J, Kafka-Ritsch R, Lucciarini P, Fish JH, Schmid T. A critical comparison of robotic versus conventional laparoscopic splenectomies. *World J. Surg.* 2005; 29(8):982−985.

Bodner J, Prommegger R, Profanter C, Schmid T. Thoracoscopic resection of mediastinal parathyroids: current status and future perspectives. *Minim. Invasive Ther. Allied. Technol.* 2004; 13(3):199−204.

Bozkurt M, Apaydin N, Isik C, Bilgetekin YG, Acar HI, Elhan A. Robotic arthroscopic surgery: a new challenge in arthroscopic surgery part-I: robotic shoulder arthroscopy: a cadaveric feasibility study. *Int. J. Med. Robot.* 2011; 7(4):496−500.

Bush B, Nifong WL, Chitwood, RW. Robotics in Cardiac Surgery: Past, Present, and Future. *Rambam. Maimonides Med. J.* 2013; 4(3):1−8.

Cadierre GB, Himpens J. Feasibility of robotic laparoscopic surgery: 146 cases. *World J. Surg.* 2001; 25(11):1467−1477.

Carpentier A, Loulmet D, Aupecle B, Kieffer JP, Tournay D, Guibort P, Fiemeyer A, Méléard D, Richomme P, Cardon C. Computer assisted open heart surgery. First case operated on with success. *C. R. Acad. Sci. III.* 1998; 321(5):427−442.

Cazac C and Radu G. Telesurgery - an efficient interdisciplinary approach used to improve the health care system. *J. Med. Life.* 2014; 7(3):137−141.

Chammas MF Jr, Kim FJ, Barbarino A, Hubert N, Feuiliu B, Coissard A, Hubert J. Asymptomatic rectal and bladder endometriosis: a case for robotic-assisted surgery. *Can. J. Urol.* 2008; 15(3):4097−4100.

Chitwood WR Jr, Nifong LW, Elbeery JE, Chapman WH, Albrecht R, Kim V, Young JA. Robotic mitral valve repair: trapezoidal resection and prosthetic annuloplasty with the da vinci surgical system. *J. Thorac. Cardiovasc. Surg.* 2000; 120(6):1171−1172.

Cho JS, Hahn KY, Kwak JM, Kim J, Baek SJ, Shin JW, Kim SH. Virtual reality training improves da Vinci performance: a prospective trial. *J. Laparoendosc. Adv. Surg. Tech. A* 2013; 23(12):992−998.

Cobb J, Henckel J, Gomes P, Harris S, Jakopec M, Rodriguez F, Barrett A, Davies B. Hands-on robotic unicompartmental knee replacement: a prospective, randomised controlled study of the acrobot system. *J. Bone. Joint. Surg. Br.* 2006; 88(2):188−197.

Coon TM. Integrating robotic technology into the operating room. *Am. J. Orthop.* 2009; 38(2):7−9.

Davies B. A review of robotics in surgery. *Proc. Inst. Mech. Eng.* 2000; 214(1):129–140.

Deane LA, Lee JH, Box GN, Melamud O, Yee DS, Abraham JB, Finley DS, Borin JF, McDougall EM, Clayman RV, Ornstein DK. Robotic versus standard laparoscopic partial/wedge nephrectomy: a comparision of intraoperative and perioperative results from a single institution. *J. Endourol.* 2008; 22(5):947–952.

Devito DP, Kaplan L, Dietl R, Pfeiffer M, Horne D, Siberstein B, Hardenbrook M, Kiriyanthan G, Barzilay Y, Bruskin A, Sackerer D, Alexandrovsky V, Stüter C, Burger R, Maeurer J, Donald GD, Schoenmayr R, Friedlander A, Knoller N, Schmieder K, Pechlivanis I, Kim IS, Meyer B, Shoham M. Clinical acceptance and accuracy assessment of spinal implants guided with SpineAssist surgical robot: retrospective study. *Spine.* (Phila Pa 1976). 1010; 35(24):2109–2015.

Dharia P SP, Steinkampf MP, Witten SJ, Malizia BA. Robotic tubal anastomosis: surgical technique and cost effectiveness. *Fertil. Steril.* 2008; 90(4):1175–1179.

Doulgeris JJ, Gonzalez-Blohm SA, Filis AK, Shea ™, Aghayev K, Vironis FD. Robotics in Neurosurgery: Evolution, Current Challenges, and Compromises. *Cancer Control.* 2015; 22(3):352–359.

Gao C, Yang M, Wang G, Wang J, Xiao C, Wu Y, Li J. Totally endoscopic robotic atrial septal defect repair on the beating heart. *Heart Surg. Forum* 2010; 13(3):e155–158.

Gao C, Yang M, Wang G, Wang J, Xiao C, Wu Y, Li J. Excision of atrial myxoma using robotic technology. *J. Thorac. Cardiovasc. Surg.* 2010; 139(5):1282–1285.

Gangemi A, Danilkowicz R, et al. Could ICG-aided robotic cholecystectomy reduce the rate of open conversion reported with laparoscopic approach? A head to head comparison of the largest single institution studies. *J. Robot. Surg.* 2016; Epub; PMID: 27435700.

Ganpule A, Chhabra JS, Desai M. Chicken and porcine models for training in laparoscopy and robotics. *Curr. Opin. Urol.* 2015; 25(2):158–162.

Garcia P, Rosen J, Kapoor C, Noakes M, Elbert G, Treat M, Ganous T, Hanson M, Manak J, Hasser C, Rohler D, Satava R. Trauma Pod: a semi-automated telerobtoic surgical system. *Int. J. Med. Robot.* 2009; 5(2):136–146.

Geller EJ, Siddiqui NY, Wu JM, Visco AG. Short-term outcomes of robotic sacrocolpopexy compared with abdominal sacrocolpopexy. *Obstet. Gynecol.* 2008; 112(6):1201–1206.

Giep BN, Giep HN, Hubert HB. Comparison of minimally invasive surgical approaches for hysterectomy at a community hospital: robotic-assisted laparoscopic hysterectomy, laparoscopic-assisted vaginal hysterectomy and laparoscopic supracervical hysterectomy. *J. Robot. Surg.* 2010; 4(3):167–175.

Fergany AF, Hafez KS, Novick AC. Long-term results of nephron sparing surgery for localized renal cell carcinoma: 10-year followup. *J. Urol.* 2000; 163(2):442–445.

Ficarra V, Cavalleri S, Novara G, Aragona M, Artibani W. Evidence from robot-assisted laparoscopic radical prostatectomy: a systematic review. *Eur. Urol.* 2007; 51(1): 9–11.

Ficarra V, Novara G, Artibani W, Cestari A, Galfano A, Graefen M, Guazzoni G, Guillonneau B, Menon M, Montorsi F, Patel V, Rassweiler J, Van Poppel H. Retropubic, laparoscopic, and robot-assisted radical prostatectomy: a systematic review and cumulative analysis of comparative studies. *Eur. Urol.* 2009; 55(5): 1037–1063.

Finan MA, Clark ME, Rocconi RP. A novel method for training residents in robotic hysterectomy. *J. Robot. Surg.* 2010; 4:33–39.

Foell K, Finelli A, Yasufuki K, Bernardini MQ, Waddell TK, Pace KT, Honey RJ, Lee JY. Robotic surgery basic skills training: Evaluation of a pilot multidisciplinary simulation-based curriculum. *Can. Urol. Assoc. J.* 2013; 7(11–12):430–434.

Fuchs KH. Minimally invasive surgery. Endoscopy. 2002; 34:154–159.

Ganpule A, Chhabra JS, Desai M. Chicken and porcine models for training in laparoscopy and robotics. *Curr. Opin. Urol.* 2015; 25(2):158–162.

Garg A, Dwivedi RC, Sayed S, Katna R, Komorowski A, Pathak KA, Rhys-Evans P, Kazi R. Robotic surgery in head and neck cancer: a review. *Oral Oncol.* 2010; 46(8):571–576.

Goh AC, Goldfarb DW, Sander JC, et al. Global evaluative assessment of robotic skills: validation of a clinical assessment tool to measure robotic surgical skills. *J. Urol.* 2012; 187:247–252.

Haber GP, Crouzet S, Kamoi K, Berger A, Aron M, Goel R, Desai M, Gill IS, Kaouk JH. Robotic NOTES (Natural Orifice Translumenal Endoscopic Surgery) in reconstructive urology: initial laboratory experience. *Urology* 2008; 71(6): 996–1000.

Haber GP and Gill IS. Laparoscopic radical cystectomy for cancer: oncological outcomes at up to 5 years. *BJU Int.* 2007; 100(1):137–142.

Haegelen C, Touzet G, Reyns N, Maurage CA, Ayachi M, Blond S. Stereotactic robot-guided biopsies of brain stem lesions: Experience with 15 cases. *Neurochirurgie* 2010; 56(5):363–367.

Hanley EJ, Marohn MR, Bachman SL, Talamini MA, Hacker SO, Howard RS, Schenkman NS. Multiservice laparoscopic surgical training using the daVinci surgical system. *Am. J. Surg.* 2004; 187(2):309–315.

Hanna EY, Holsinger C, DeMonte F, Kupferman M. Robotic endoscopic surgery of the skull base: a novel surgical approach. Arch Otolaryngol. *Head Neck Surg.* 2007; 133(12):1209–1214.

Hatzinger M, Häcker A, Langbein S, Kwon S, Hoang-Böhm J, Alken P. Hans-Christian Jacobaeus (1879-1937): The inventor of human laparoscopy and thoracoscopy. *Urologe A* 2006; 45(9):1184–1186.

Hayn MH, Hussain A, Mansour AM, Andrews PE, Carpentier P, Castle E, Dasgupta P, Rimington P, Thomas R, Khan S, Kibel A, Kim H, Manoharan M, Menon M, Mottrie A, Omstein D, Peabody J, Pruthi R, Palou Redorta J, Richstone L, Schanne F, Stricker H, Wiklund P, Chandrasekhar R, Wilding GE, Guru KA. The learning curve of robot-assisted radical cystectomy: results from the international robotic cystectomy consortium. *Eur. Urol.* 2010; 58(2):197–202.

Heemskerk J, de Hoog DE, van Gemert WG, Baeten CG, Greve JW, Bouvy ND. Robot-assisted vs. conventional laparoscopic rectopexy for rectal prolapse: a comparative study on costs and time. *Dis. Colon Rectum.* 2007; 50(11):1825–1830.

Hellenthal NJ, Hussain A, Andrews PE, Carpentier P, Castle E, Dasgupta P, Kaouk J, Khan S, Kibel A, Kim H, Manoharan M, Menon M, Mottrie A, Omstein D, Palou J, Peabody J, Pruthi R, Richstone L, Schanne F, Stricker H, Thomas R, Wiklund P, Wilding G, Guru KA. Lymphadenectomy at the time of robot-assisted radical cystectomy: results from the international robotic cystectomy consortium. *BJU Int.* 2011; 107(4):642–646.

Honl M, Dierk O, Gauck C, Carrero V, Lampe F, Dries S, Quante M, Schwieger K, Hille E, Morlock MM. Comparison of robotic-assisted and manual implantation of a primary total hip replacement. A prospective study. *J. Bone Joint Surg.* 2003; 85-A (8):1470–1478.

Hung AJ, Jayaratna IS, Teruya K,Desai MM, Gill IS, Goh AC. Comparative assessment of three standardized robotic surgery training methods. *BJU Int.* 2013; 112:864–871.

Hung AJ, Ng CK, Patil MB, Zehnder P, Huang E, Aron M, Gill IS, Desai MM. Validation of novel robotic-assisted partial nephrectomy surgical training model. *BJU Int.* 2012; 110(6):870–874.

Intuitive Surgical [Internet]. California; 2016 [cited 2016 Sept 26]. Available from: http://www.intuitivesurgical.com/products/

Jain S, and Gautam G. Robotics in urologic oncology. *J. Minim. Access. Surg.* 2015; 11(4):40–44.

Jakopec M, Rodriguez y Baena F, Harris SH, Gomes P, Cobb J, Davies BL. The hands-on Orthopaedic robot "Acrobot": Early clinical trials of total knee replacement surgery. *IEEE Trans. Rob. Autom.* 2003; 19(5):902–911.

Kakeji Y, Konishi K, Leiri S, Yasunaga T, Nakamoto M, Tanoue K, Baba H, Maehara Y, Hashizume M. Robotic laparoscopic distal gastrectomy: a comparison of the da Vinci and Zeus systems. *Int. J. Med. Robot.* 2006; 2(4):299–304.

Kamath GS, Balaram S, Choi A, Kuteyeva O, Garikipati NV, Steinberg JS, Mittal S. Long-term outcome of leads and patients following robotic epicardial left ventricular lead placement for cardiac resynchronization therapy. *Pacing. Clin. Electrophysiol.* 2011; 34(2):235–240.

Karthik K, Colegate-Stone T, Dasgupta P, Tavakkolizadeh A, Sinha J. Robotic surgery in trauma and orthopaedics: a systematic review. *Bone Joint J.* 2015; 97-B (3):292–299.

Kerr B, O'Leary JP. The training of the surgeon: Dr. Halsted's greatest legacy. *Am. Surg.* 1999; 65:1101–1102.

Kim VB, Chapman WH, Albrecht RJ, Bailey BM, Young JA, Nifong LW, Chitwood WR Jr. Early experience with telemanipulative robot-assisted laparoscopic cholecystectomy using Da Vinci. *Surg. Laparosc. Endosc. Percutan. Tech.* 2002; 12(1):34–40.

Korte C, Nair SS, Nistor V, Low TP, Doarn Cr, Schaffner G. Determining the threshold of time-delay for teleoperation accuracy and efficiency in relation to telesurgery. *Telemed. J. E. Health.* 2014; 20(12):1078–1086.

Krambeck AE, DiMarco DS, Rangel LJ, Bergstralh EJ, Myers RP, Blute ML, Gettman MT. Radical prostatectomy for prostatic adenocarcinoma: a matched comparison of open retropubic and robot-assisted techniques. *BJU Int.* 2009; 103(4):448–453.

Kwoh YS, Hou J, Jonckheere EA, Hayati S. A robot with improved absolute positioning accuracy for CT guided stereotactic brain surgery. *IEEE Trans. Biomed. Eng.* 1988; 35(2):153–161.

Lafranco AR, Castellanos AE, Desai JP, Meyers, WC. Robotics surgery: a current perspective. *Ann. Surg.* 2004; 239(1):14–21.

Le CQ, Lightner DJ, VanderLei L, Segura JW, Gettman MT. The current role of medical simulation in American urological residency training programs: an assessment by program directors. *J. Urol.* 2007; 177(1):288–291.

Lee J, Nah KY, Kim RM, Ahn YH, Soh EY, Chung WU. Differences in postoperative outcomes, function, and cosmesis: open versus robotic thyroidectomy. *Surg. Endosc.* 2010; 24(12):3186–3194.

Lee JY, O'Malley BW, Newman JG, Weinstein GS, Lega B, Diaz J, Grady MS. Transoral robotic surgery of craniocervical junction and atlantoaxial spine: a cadaveric study. *J. Neurosurg. Spine* 2010; 12(1):13–18.

Liu C, Peresic D, Samadi D, Nezhat F. Robotic assisted laparoscopic partial bladder resection for the treatment of infiltrating endometriosis. *J. Minim. Invasive Gynecol.* 2008; 15(6):145−148.

Lobe TE, Wright SK, Irish MS. Novel uses of surgical robotics in head and neck surgery. *J. Laparoendosc. Adv. Surg. Tech. A* 2005; 15(6):647−652.

Loulmet D, Carpentier A, D'Attellis N, Berrebi A, Cardon C, Ponzio O, Aupecle B, Relland JY. Endoscopic coronary artery bypass grafting with the aid of robotic assisted instruments. *J. Thorac. Cardiovasc. Surg.* 1999; 118(1):4−10.

Lum MJ, Rosen J, King H, Friedman DC, Donlin G, Sankaranarayanan G, Harnett B, Huffman L, Doarn C, Broderick T, Hannaford B. Telesurgery via Unmanned Aerial Vehicle (UAV) with a field deployable surgical robot. *Stud. Health Technol. Inform.* 2007; 125:313−315.

Maeso S, Reza M, Mayol JA, Blasco JA, Guerra M, Andradas E, Plana MN. Efficacy of the Da Vinci surgical system in abdominal surgery compared with that of laparoscopy. *Ann. Surg.* 2010; 252(2):254−262.

Magrina JF, Espada M, Munoz R, Noble BN, Kho RM. Robotic adnexectomy compared with laparoscopy for adnexal mass. *Obstet. Gynecol. Obstet. Gynecol.* 2009; 114(3):581−584.

Magrina JF, Zanagnolo V, Noble BN, Kho RM, Magtibay P. Robotic approach for ovarian cancer: perioperative and survival results and comparison with laparoscopy and laparotomy. *Gynecol. Oncol.* 2011; 121(1):100−105.

Marescaux J, Leroy J, Gagner M, Rubino F, Mutter D, Vix M, Butner SE, Smith ML. Transatlantic robot-assisted telesurgery. *Nature* 2001; 413(6854):379−380.

Masterson TA, Cheng L, Boris RS, Koch KO. Open vs. robotic-assisted radical prostatectomy: a single surgeon and pathologist comparison of pathologic and oncologic outcomes. *Urol. Oncol.* 2013; 31(7):1043−1048.

Matthews CA, Reid N, Ramakrishnan V, Hull K, Cohen S. Evaluation of the introduction of robotic technology on route of hysterectomy and complications in the first year of use. *Am. J. Obstet. Gynecol.* 2010; 203(5):499e1−499e5.

McCool RR, Warren FM, Wiggins RH 3rd, Hunt JP. Robotic surgery of the infratemporal fossa utilizing novel suprahyoid port. *Laryngoscope* 2010; 120(9):1738−1743.

McLeod IK, Melder PC. Da Vinci robot-assisted excision of a vallecular cyst: a case report. *Ear Nose Throat. J.* 2005; 84(3):170−172.

Mehrabi A, Yetimoglu CL, Nickkholgh A, Kashfi A, Kienle P, Kostan-tinides L et al. Development and evaluation of a training module for the clinical introduction of the da Vinci robotic system in visceral and vascular surgery. *Surg. Endosc.* 2006; 20:1376−1382.

Menon M, Tewari A, Baize B, Guillonneau B, Vallancien G. Prospective comparison of radical retropubic prostatectomy and robot-assisted anatomic prostatectomy: The Vattikuti urology institute experience. *J. Urol.* 2002; 60(5):864−868.

Mihaljevic T, Jarrett CM, Gillinov AM, Williams SJ, DeVilliers PA, Stewart WJ, Svensson LG, Sabik JF 3rd, Blackstone EH. Robotic repair of posterior mitral valve prolapse versus conventional approaches: potential realized. *J. Thorac. Cardiovasc. Surg.* 2011; 141(1):72−80.

Mohr FW, Falk V, Diegeler A, Autschback R. Computer-enhanced coronary artery bypass surgery. *J. Thorac. Cardiovasc. Surg.* 1999; 117(6):1212−1214.

Moore EJ, Olsen KD, Kasperbauer JL. Transoral robotic surgery for oropharyngeal squamous cell carcinoma: a prospective study of feasibility and functional outcomes. *Laryngoscope* 2009; 119(11):2156−2164.

Mottrie A, Wilson TG. Systemic review and meta-analysis of perioperative outcomes and complications after robot-assisted radical prostatectomy. *Eur. Urol.* 2012; 62(3):431–452.

Muhlmann G, Klaus A, Kirchmayr W, Wykypiel H, Unger A, Holler E, Nehoda H, Aigner F, Weiss HG. DaVinci robot-assisted laparoscopic bariatric surgery: is it justified in a routine setting? *Obes. Surg.* 2003; 13(6):848–854.

Nakamura N, Sugano N, Nishii T, Kakimoto A, Miki H. A comparison between robotic-assisted and manual implantation of cementless total hip arthroplasty. *Clin. Orthop. Relat. Res.* 2010; 468(4):1072–1081.

Nam EJ, Kim SW, Kim S, Kim JH, Jung YW, Paek JH, Lee SH, Kim JW, Kim YT. A case-control study of robotic radical hysterectomy and pelvic lymphadenectomy using 3 robotic arms compared with abdominal radical hysterectomy in cervical cancer. *Int. J. Gynecol. Cancer* 2010; 20(7):1284–1289.

Nathoo N, Cavusoglu MC, Vogelbaum MA, Barnett GH. In touch with robotics: neurosurgery for the future.*Neurosurgery* 2005; 56(3): 421–33.

Netravali NA, Shen F, Park Y, Bargar WL. A perspective on robot assistance for knee arthroplasty. *Adv. Orthop.* 2013; 970703.

Nguan CY, Kwan K, Al Omar M, Beasley KA, Luke PP. Robotic pyeloplasty: experience with three robotic platforms. *Can. J. Urol.* 2007; 14(3):3571–3576.

Nguan CY, Morady R, Wang C, Harrison D, Browning D, Rayman R, Luke PP. Robotic pyeloplasty using internet protocol and satellite network- based telesurgery. *Int. J. Med. Robot.* 2008; 4(1):10–14.

Nguan CY, Miller B, Patel R, Luke PP, Schlacha CM. Pre-clinical remote telesurgery trial of da Vinci telesurgery prototype. *Int. J. Med. Robot.* 2008; 4(4):304–309.

Nifong LW, Rodriquez E, Chitwood WR Jr. 540 consecutive robotic mitral valve repairs including concomitant atrial fibrillation cryoablation. *Ann. Thorac. Surg.* 2012; 94(1):38–42.

Nix J, Smith A, Kurpad R, Nielsen ME, Wallen EM, Pruthi RS. Prospective randomized controlled trial of robotic versus open radical cystectomy for bladder cancer: perioperative and pathologic results. *Eur. Urol.* 2010; 57(2):196–201.

Novara G, Ficarra V, Mocellin S, Ahlering TE, Carroll PR, Graefen M, Guazzoni G, Menon M, Patel VR, Shariat SF, Tewari AK, Van Poppel H, Zattoni F, Montorsi F, Mottrie A, Rosen RC, Wilson TG. Systemic review and meta-analysis of studies reporting oncologic outcome after robot-assisted radical prostatectomy. *Eur. Urol.* 2012; 62(3):382–404.

Novara G, Ficarra V, Rosen RC, Artibani W, Costello A, Eastham JA, Graefen M, Guazzoni G, Shariat SF, Stolzenburg JU, Van Poppel H, Zattoni F, Montorsi F, Mottrie A, Wilson TG. Systematic review and meta-analysis of perioperative outcomes and complications after robot assisted radical prostatectomy. *Eur. Urol.* 2012; 62(3): 431–52.

Oliveira CM, Nguyen HT, Ferraz AR, Watters K, Rosman B, Rahbar, R. Robotic surgery in Otolaryngology and head and neck surgery: a review. *Minim Invasive Surg.* 2012; 2012:286563.

O'Malley BW Jr, Weinstein GS, Snyder W, Hockstein NG. Transoral robotic surgery (TORS) for base of tongue neoplasms. *Laryngoscope* 2006; 116(8):1465–1472.

Paley PJ, Veljovich DS, Shah CA, Everett EN, Bondurant AE, Drescher CW, Peters WA 3rd. Surgical outcomes in gynecologic oncology in the era of robotics: analysis of first 1000 cases. *Am. J. Obstet. Gynecol.* 2011; 204(6):551e1–9.

Pandya S, Motkoski JW, Serrano-Almeida C, Greer AD, Latour I, Sutherland GR. Advancing neurosurgery with image-guided robotics. *J. Neurosurg.* 2009; 111(6):1141–1149.

Park SE and Lee CT. Comparison of robotic-assisted and conventional manual implantation of a primary total knee arthroplasty. *J. Arthroplasty* 2007; 22:1054–1059.

Partin AW, Adams JB, Moore RG, Kavoussi LR. Complete robot-assisted laparoscopic urologic surgery: a preliminary report. *J. Am. Coll. Surg.* 1995; 181(6):552–557.

Paul HA, Bargar WL, Mittlestadt B, Musits B, Taylor RH, Kazanzides P, Zuhars J, Williamson B, Hanson W. Development of a surgical robot for cementless total hip arthroplasty. *Clin. Orthop. Relat. Res.* 1992; 285:57–66.

Payne TN, Dauterive FR. A comparison of total laparoscopic hysterectomy to robotically assisted hysterectomy: surgical outcomes in a community practice. *J. Minim. Invasive Gynecol.* 2008; 15(3):286–291.

Pearle AD, O'Loughlin PF, Kendoff DO. Robot assisted unicompartmental knee arthroplasty. *J. Arthroplasty* 2010; 25:230–237.

Perez M, Xu S, Chauhan S, Tanaka A, Simpson K, Abdul-Muhsin H, Smith R. Impact of delay on telesurgical performance: study on the robotic simulator dV-Trainer. *Int. J. Comput. Assist. Radiol. Surg.* 2016; 11(4):581–587.

Perez-Cruet MJ, Welsh RJ, Hussain NS, Begun EM, Lin J, Park P. Use of the da Vinci minimally invasive robotic system for resection of a complicated paraspinal schwannoma with thoracic extension: case report. *J. Neurosurg.* 2012; 72(1):e209–214.

Plate JF, Mofidi A, Mannava S, Smith BP, Lang JE, Poehling GG, Conditt MA, Jinnah RH. Achieving accurate ligament balancing using robotic-assisted unicompartmental knee arthroplasty. *Adv. Orthop.* 2013; 2013:837167.

Prajapati PM, Solanki AS, Sen DJ. Robotic surgery: A new hope in medical science. *Int. J. Pharm.* 2012; 3(1):10–12.

Prasad SM, Ducko CT, Stephenson ER, Chambers CE, Damiano RJ Jr. Prospective clinical trial of robotically assisted endoscopic coronary grafting with 1-year follow up. *Ann. Surg.* 2001; 233(6):725–732.

Pruitt JC, Lazzara RR, Dworkin GH, Badhwar V, Kuma C, Ebra G. Totally endoscopic ablation of lone atrial fibrillation: initial clinical experience. *Ann. Thorac. Surg.* 2006; 81(4):1325–1331.

Pruthi RS, Nix J, McRackan D, Hickerson A, Nielsen ME, Raynor M, Wallen EM. Robotic-assisted laparoscopic intracorporeal urinary diversion. *Eur. Urol.* 2010; 57(6):1013–1021.

Rasmus M. Preliminary clinical results with the MRI-compatible guiding system INNOMITON. *Int. J. Cars. S.* 2007; 2(s1):138–145.

Rassweiler J, Henkel TO, Potempa DM, Coptocat MJ, Miller K, Preminger GM, Alken P. Transperitoneal laparoscopic nephrectomy: training, technique, and results. *J. Endourol.* 1993; 7(6):505–516.

Rassweiler JJ, Scheitlin W, Heidenreich A, Laguna MP, Janetschek G, Laparoscopic retroperitoneal lymph node dissection: Does it still have a role in the management of clinical stage I nonseminomatous testis cancer? A European perspective. *Eur. Urol.* 2008; 54(5):1004–1015.

Rininsland H. ARTEMIS. A telemanipulator for cardiac surgery. *Eur. J. Cardiothorac. Surg.* 1999; 16:S106–111.

Rininsland H. Basics of robotics and manipulators in endoscopic surgery. *Endosoc. Surg. Allied. Technol.* 1993; 1(3):154–159.

Royal College of Physicians and Surgeons of Canada. *Competence by Design (CBD): Moving towards competency-based medical education.* 2016. http://www.royalcollege.ca/portal/page/portal/rc/resources/cbme.

Satava RM. Surgical robotics: the early chronicles: a personal historical perspective. *Surg. Laparosc. Endosc. Percutan. Tech.* 2002; 12(1):6–16.

Schilling J, Engel AM, Hassan M, Smith JM. Robotic excision of atrial myxoma. *J. Card. Surg.* 2012; 27(4):423–426.

Schizas C, Thein E, Kwiatkowski B, Kulik G. Pedicle screw insertion: robotic assistance versus conventional C-arm fluoroscopy. *Acta. Orthop. Belg.* 2012; 78(2):240–245.

Schulz AP, Seide K, Queitsch C, von Haugwitz A, Meiners J, Kienast B, Tarabolsi M, Kammal M, Jugens C. Results of total hip replacement using the Robodoc surgical assistant system: clinical outcome and evaluation of complications for 97 procedures. *Int. J. Med. Robot.* 2007; 3(4):301–306.

Schurr MO, Buess G, Neisius B, Vogues U. Robotics and telemanipulation technologies for endoscopic surgery. A review of the ARTEMIS project. Advanced Robotic Telemanipulator for Minimally Invasive Surgery. *Surg. Endosc.* 2000; 14(4):375–381.

Scott DJ, Young WN, Tesfay ST, Frawley WH, Rege RV, Jones DB. Laparoscopic skills training. *Am. J. Surg.* 2001; 182(2):137–42.

Shiomi A, Kinugasa Y, et al. Robot-assisted versus laparoscopic surgery for lower rectal cancer: the impact of visceral obesity on surgical outcomes. *Int. J. colorectal Dis.* 2016; 31(10):1701–1710.

Skolarus TA, Zhang Y, Hollenbeck BK. Robotic surgery in urologic oncology: Gathering the evidence. *Expert. Rev. Pharmacoecon. Outcomes. Res.* 2010; 10(4):421–432.

Song EK, Seon JK, Park SJ, Jung WB, Park HW, Lee GW. Simultaneous bilateral total knee arthroplasty with robotic and conventional techniques: a prospective, randomized study. *Knee Surg. Sports Traumatol. Arthrosc.* 2011; 19(7):1069–1076.

Sterbis JR, Hanly EJ, Herman BC, Marohn MR, Broderick TJ, Shih SP, Harnett B, Doarn C, Schenkman NS. Transcontinental telesurgical nephrectomy using the da Vinci robot in a porcine model. *Urology* 2008; 71(5):971–973.

Sukovich W, Brink-Danan S, Hardenbrook M. Miniature robotic guidance for pedicle screw placement in posterior spinal fusion: early clinical experience with the SpineAssist. *Int. J. Med. Robot.* 2006; 2(2):114–122.

Sutherland GR, Lama S, Gan LS, Wolfsberger S, Zareinia K. Merging machines with microsurgery: clinical experience with neuroArm. *J. Neurosurg.* 2013; 118(3):521–529.

Tae K, Ji YB, Cho SH, Lee SH, Kim DS, Kim TW. Early surgical outcomes of robotic thyroidectomy by a gasless unilateral axillo-breast or axillary approach for papillary thyroid carcinoma: 2 years' experience. *Head Neck* 2012; 34(5):617–625.

Tae K, Ji YB, Jeong JH, Lee SH, Jeong MA, Park CW. Robotic thyroidectomy by a gasless unilateral axillo-breast or axillary approach: our early surgical experiences: *Surg. Endosc.* 2011; 25(1):221–228.

Tae K, Kim KY, Yun BR, Ji YB, Park CW, Kim DS, Kim TW. Functional voice and swallowing outcomes after robotic thyroidectomy by a gasless unilateral axillo-breast approach: comparison with open thyroidectomy. *Surg. Endosc.* 2012; 26(7):1871–1877.

Takasuna H, Goto T, Kakizawa Y, Miyahara T, Joyama J, Tanaka Y, Kawaii T, Hongo K. Use of a micromanipulator system (NeuRobot) in endoscopic neurosurgery. *J. Clin. Neurosci.* 2012; 19(11):1553–1557.

Tewari A, Srivasatava A, Menon M, Members of the VIP Team. A prospective comparison of radical retrpubic and robot-assisted prostatectomy: experience in one institution. *BJU Int.* 2003; 92(3): 205−210.

Titan Medical Inc [Internet]. Ontario; 2016 [cited 2016 Sept 26]. Available from: http://www.titanmedicalinc.com/technology/

Tolley N, Arora A, Palazzo F, Garas G, Dhawan R, Cox J, Darzi A. Robotic-assisted parathyroidectomy: a feasibility study. *Otolaryngol. Head Neck Surg.* 2011; 144(6):859−866.

Turchetti G, Palla I, Pierotti F, Cuschieri A. Economic evaluation of da Vinci-assisted robotic surgery: a systematic review. *Surg. Endosc.* 2012; 26(3):598−606.

Wang W, Li J, Wang S, Su H, Jiang X. System design and animal experiment study of a novel minimally invasive surgical robot. *Int. J.Med. Robot.* 2016; 12(1):73−84.

Weinberg L, Rao S, Escobar PF. Robotic surgery in Gynecology: An updated systemic review. *Int. J. Gynecol. Obstet.* 2011; 2011:852061.

Wiewiorski M, Valderrabano V, Kretzschmar M, Rasch H, Markus T, Dziergwa S, Kos S, Bilecen D, Jacob AL. CT-guided robotically-assisted infiltration of foot and ankle joints. *Minim. Invasive Ther. Allied Technol.* 2009; 18(5):291−296.

Woo Y and Nacke EA. Robotic minimally invasive mitral valve reconstruction yields less blood product transfusion and shorter length of stay. *Surgery* 2006; 140:263−267.

Wu Z, Li M, Liu B, Cai C, Ye H, Lv C, Yang Q, Sheng J, Song S, Qu L, Xiao L, Sun Y, Wang L. Robotic versus open partial nephrectomy: A systematic review and meta-analysis. *PLoS One* 2014; 9(4):e94878.

Yen PL and Davies BL. Active constraint control for image-guided robotic surgery. *Proc. Inst. Mech. Eng. H.* 2010; 224(5):623−631.

Yoshiki H, Tadano K, Ban D, Ohuchi K, Tanabe M, Kawashima K. Surgical energy device using steam jet for robotic assisted surgery. *Conf. Proc. IEEE Eng. Med. Biol. Soc.* 2015; 2015:6872−6875.

ABOUT THE EDITORS

Dr. Huifang Chen, MD., PhD.
Professor of Surgery
Laboratory of Experimental Surgery, Research Center, CHUM
10th floor, R10. 480, University of Montreal
900 rue Saint Denis, Montreal, Quebec, Canada H2X 0A9
E. Mail: hui.fang.chen@umontreal.ca

Dr. Paulo N. Martins, MD., PhD, FAST, FACS
Department of Surgery
Division of Transplantation ,UMass Memorial Medical Center,
University of Massachusetts, Worcester, MA, USA
E. Mail: Paulo.martins@umassmemorial.org

INDEX

#

2D (two-dimensional), 3, 6, 20, 28, 35, 184, 185, 187, 188, 189, 194, 209, 237
3D (three-dimensional), 3, 6, 22, 26, 28, 184, 187, 188, 189, 190, 195, 201, 202, 203, 204, 206, 207, 208, 209, 210, 230, 247, 248, 249, 250, 251, 252, 323, 338, 374, 376, 377, 381, 382
3D laparoscopy, 29

A

AAV (Adeno-Associated Vector), 359, 369
absorption spectra, 337
acetylcholine, 366
ACF (aorto-caval fistula), 81, 101, 102, 105
acidosis, 139, 271, 343
ACL, 232, 252
action potential, 239
active feedback, 390
active oxygen, 295, 315
activity level, 364
acute liver failure, 108, 120, 121, 123, 125, 129
acute lung injury, 55, 58, 59
acute rejection, 272
acute respiratory distress syndrome, 38
adenectomy, 380
adenine, 270, 277
adenocarcinoma, 149, 213, 214, 396
adenosine, 38, 274, 288, 290, 320
adenosine triphosphate, 38, 290
adipose, 236, 240
adipose tissue, 236
adjustable gastric banding, 74
adventitia, 263
adverse effects, 273, 294, 367

AESOP, 374, 375, 376
aflatoxin, 142, 143
agar, 51
aggregation, 44, 63, 68, 241, 320, 321, 323, 324, 325, 328, 340, 341, 342, 343, 344, 346, 347, 353, 357
aggregation process, 324
airway epithelial cells, 238
alanine, 133, 299, 305
alanine aminotransferase, 133, 299
albumin, 45, 47, 236, 237, 241, 244, 280, 324, 330, 343
alcohol consumption, 154
alkaline phosphatase, 133, 151
ALS (anti-lymphocyte serum), 160, 172
ALT (Auxiliary Liver Transplantation), 121, 131, 133, 299, 300, 301, 302, 303, 304, 359, 367
alveoli, 46
ambient air, 198
amino acids, 275, 297, 303
ammonia, 123
amniotic fluid, 259
ampulla, 136
amylase, 137, 274, 280
analgesic, 61, 217
anastomosis, 16, 18, 32, 34, 52, 64, 74, 103, 116, 134, 239, 255, 263, 270, 377, 378, 389, 390, 394
anatomy, 11, 12, 16, 21, 22, 25, 58, 107, 109, 112, 113, 114, 115, 117, 124, 127, 148, 150, 151, 152, 153, 374, 384, 389
anemia, 260, 327, 336
anesthesia, 18, 22, 25, 26, 50, 51, 60, 61, 62, 63, 83, 87, 88, 92, 95, 96, 101, 102, 212, 217, 221, 261, 262, 361, 362, 370
angina, 272
angiogenesis, 122, 259, 260, 265, 266, 267
angiography, 234, 338

animal husbandry, 222
animal models, v, vi, 3, 4, 11, 12, 16, 17, 18, 22, 23, 24, 25, 26, 30, 32, 34, 35, 37, 39, 40, 53, 63, 65, 66, 67, 68, 69, 81, 82, 104, 107, 122, 129, 138, 139, 140, 143, 144, 145, 147, 148, 152, 155, 156, 159, 160, 161, 162, 164, 165, 169, 172, 174, 176, 211, 212, 213, 221, 222, 224, 225, 237, 240, 261, 262, 264, 266, 267, 276, 277, 280, 298, 304, 313, 317, 326, 327, 344, 359, 369, 389
animal welfare, 345
anoxia, 350
antibiotic, 50, 70, 88
antibody, 65, 162, 167, 171, 173, 175, 176, 178, 242, 252, 282, 287, 363, 364, 371
anti-cancer, 145, 187
anticoagulant, 345
anticoagulation, 241, 280
antigen, 160, 162, 163, 165, 166, 167, 168, 170, 175, 179, 258, 363, 364, 367
antigenicity, 369
antioxidant, 277, 283
antitumor immunity, 363, 364
antrum, 75
anuria, 46
anus, 27
aorta, 87, 90, 95, 97, 98, 102, 103, 110, 112, 119, 132, 240, 305, 389
aortic, 81, 88, 89, 96, 97, 239, 249, 305, 353, 380
  banding, 81, 87, 88, 95, 96
    stenosis, 96
  valve, 249, 305
aortocaval fistula, 82
APC (Antigen Presenting Cell), 162, 360, 363
aplasia, 224
aplastic anemia, 175
apnea, 384
apoplexy, 47
apoptosis, 137, 156, 163, 203, 276, 282, 293, 296, 303, 305
appendectomy, 4, 5, 7, 16, 28, 31, 33, 67
appendicitis, 50, 67
ARDS (acute respiratory distress syndrome), 38, 58, 138
arginine, 63, 150
ARs, 163
ARTEMIS, 375, 399, 400
arterioles, 44, 59, 318, 319, 328, 350, 354
arteritis, 326, 329
artery, 52, 59, 60, 61, 81, 82, 83, 87, 92, 94, 109, 110, 112, 113, 114, 116, 117, 124, 128, 132, 137, 148, 152, 237, 240, 242, 282, 292, 299, 300, 301, 309, 312, 367, 369, 378, 384, 397
arthroplasty, 378, 382

arthroscopy, 393
articular cartilage, 251
ascending colon, 51
ascites, 130, 212, 218, 219, 222
ascitic cells, 214
aseptic, 93, 197
aspartate, 38, 272, 299
atelectasis, 46
atherosclerosis, 62
atomic force, 234
ATP, 38, 43, 152, 187, 235, 270, 273, 274, 276, 285, 290, 294, 296, 300, 301, 302, 304, 305, 308, 322, 342, 353
atraumatic technique, 255, 257, 264
atrial fibrillation, 46, 377, 398, 399
atrial myxoma, 394, 400
atrial septal defect, 377, 394
atrophy, 137, 272, 295, 366
attachment, 109, 242, 243
automation, 185
autopsy, 172, 214, 218, 219
Azathioprine, 172

B

bacteremia, 47, 68
bacteria, 44, 47, 48, 49, 50, 51, 52, 53, 54, 55, 56, 57, 59, 60, 147, 177, 259
bariatric experimental surgery, 17, 77
bariatric experimental surgery models, 73
bariatric surgery, 6, 17, 34, 74, 79, 80, 398
bariatric surgical methods, 73
barium, 51
basement membrane, 260
basic research, 148
B-catenin, 141
beryllium, 55
betadine, 83, 93
bicarbonate, 278, 304
bilateral, 380, 400
bile, 13, 74, 107, 114, 116, 127, 129, 130, 131, 133, 134, 135, 136, 137, 144, 147, 148, 149, 150, 151, 153, 155, 279, 291, 299, 300, 301, 302, 303, 304, 308, 309
bile acids, 133
bile duct, 13, 107, 114, 116, 127, 129, 130, 131, 134, 137, 144, 149, 150, 151, 153, 155, 279, 308
bile duct ligation, 107, 129, 130, 131, 134, 144, 150
biliary cirrhosis, 131, 149
biliary obstruction, 155
biliary stricture, 289, 313
biliary tract, 109, 114, 144, 152, 299
biliopancreatic diversion, 74, 75, 80

biliopancreatic diversion with duodenal switch, 74, 80
bilirubin, 41, 47, 133, 299, 302, 304
biocompatibility, 17, 34, 247
biological processes, 281
biological samples, 185, 187, 193
biomarkers, 64, 184, 207, 292
biopsy, 142, 171, 192, 196, 197, 198, 200, 216, 374, 378, 381
biopsy needle, 197
biosciences, 357
bladder cancer, 387, 398
bleeding, 85, 96, 124, 145, 148, 218, 239, 263, 264, 377, 384
blood, 26, 41, 43, 44, 45, 46, 51, 54, 58, 59, 60, 61, 63, 66, 67, 68, 69, 71, 75, 82, 103, 123, 135, 137, 138, 139, 154, 155, 156, 160, 165, 169, 170, 171, 174, 182, 229, 231, 234, 236, 237, 239, 240, 241, 243, 245, 246, 257, 258, 259, 262, 263, 264, 266, 276, 278, 280, 282, 287, 292, 293, 296, 297, 298, 299, 301, 302, 305, 307, 314, 318, 319, 320, 321, 322, 323, 324, 325, 326, 327, 328, 329, 330, 332, 333, 336, 337, 338, 339, 340, 341, 342, 343, 344, 345, 346, 347, 348, 349, 350, 351, 352, 353, 354, 355, 356, 357, 364, 366, 369, 377, 379, 380, 384, 385, 386, 387, 391, 401
blood circulation, 351
blood clot, 241, 243, 257, 258
blood flow, 26, 44, 45, 51, 59, 67, 71, 123, 135, 138, 154, 155, 237, 240, 276, 280, 296, 298, 314, 319, 326, 327, 329, 330, 336, 344, 347, 348, 349, 353, 354, 369
blood plasma, 350
blood pressure, 41, 45, 46
blood stream, 240
blood supply, 137, 259, 262, 299, 301, 337
blood transfusion, 377
blood urea nitrogen, 297
blood vessels, 156, 231, 234, 258, 259, 263, 264, 318, 366
blood viscosity, 320, 321, 323, 325, 339, 341, 342, 347, 351, 354, 357
bloodstream, 43, 143
body fat, 75
Body Mass Index (BMI), 74, 75, 373
body weight, 23, 83, 85, 102, 109, 130, 142, 223
bone, 159, 160, 161, 162, 165, 167, 168, 169, 170, 174, 175, 177, 178, 179, 180, 185, 210, 234, 236, 243, 264, 329, 334, 352, 382
bone growth, 382
bone marrow, 159, 160, 161, 162, 165, 167, 168, 169, 170, 174, 175, 177, 178, 179, 180, 236, 243, 329, 352

bone marrow transplant, 159, 160, 161, 162, 165, 169, 170, 177, 179, 180
bone marrow transplantation, 159, 160, 161, 162, 165, 179, 180
bone resorption, 210
bowel, 18, 26, 41, 47, 50, 52, 74, 159, 160, 169, 172, 173, 176, 179, 180, 263, 280, 335
bowel sounds, 41
box trainer, 12, 19, 20
  simulators, 12, 19
BPH (Benign Prostate Hyperplasia), 184
brain, 152, 185, 190, 286, 290, 291, 292, 306, 315, 327, 329, 356, 361, 374, 381, 388, 395, 396
brain stem, 395
brain tumor, 381
breast cancer, 149, 208, 209, 210
bronchus, 60, 239
bursa, 217
bypass graft, 378

C

C reactive protein, 41
Ca^{2+}, 83, 270, 285, 361, 372
cadaver, 11, 18, 19, 34
calcium, 83, 197, 239, 272, 273, 275, 342
caliber, 131, 343
cancer, 62, 122, 142, 145, 146, 184, 187, 188, 189, 193, 196, 198, 201, 204, 205, 206, 207, 208, 209, 212, 213, 217, 221, 225, 244, 282, 359, 363, 364, 372, 379, 380, 395, 399, 400
cancer cells, 142, 188, 193, 205
cancer progression, 187, 189
capillary, 41, 42, 43, 44, 45, 46, 185, 210, 234, 241, 242, 257, 259, 260, 318, 319, 322, 325, 328, 329, 330, 332, 336, 339, 340, 342, 343, 344, 349, 350, 352
capillary refill, 41
carbohydrate metabolism, 236
carbohydrates, 77, 297
carbon dioxide, 23, 213
carbon monoxide, 270, 273, 337
carbon tetrachloride, 49, 55, 108, 129, 148
carboxylic groups, 242
carcinogen, 142, 143, 144
carcinogenesis, 140, 142, 144, 149, 155
carcinoma, 107, 108, 122, 140, 146, 152, 155, 214, 215, 223, 224, 225, 226, 400
cardiac arrest, 278, 293
cardiac output, 51, 59, 101
cardiac surgery, 26, 278, 377, 393, 399
cardiogenic shock, 344, 348
cardioplegia, 278

cardiovascular disease(s), 79, 81, 104, 244
cardiovascular system, 46, 73, 318
carotid arteries, 90, 95, 97, 98
cartilage, 232, 233, 234, 236, 251, 256
casein, 140
CASP (colon ascendens stent peritonitis model), 38
castration, 203
CAT (Chloramphenicol acetyltransferase), 360, 361
catheter, 51, 60, 74, 111, 117, 217, 359, 367, 369, 371
CBD (common bile duct), 13, 31, 107, 108, 110, 113, 114, 116, 128, 130, 131, 144, 279, 314, 400
CBDL (common bile duct ligation), 108, 131
C-C, 256, 257
CCA, 144
CCC (cholangiocarcinoma), 107, 108, 144, 148, 151, 155, 156
CCL (C-C Motif Chemokine Ligand), 256
CCL4 (carbon tetrachloride), 49, 55, 108, 129, 148, 168
CD (Cluster of Differentiation), 67, 71, 181, 186, 212, 214, 218, 251, 253, 256, 292, 328
CD8+, 165, 167, 176, 179
CD95, 167
CDL (closed duodenal loop), 108, 135, 149, 153
cDNA, 364, 365, 367, 371, 372
cecum, 50, 51, 70, 213
cell biology, 138, 206
cell culture, 151, 185, 187, 188, 193, 198, 207, 208, 209, 210, 361
cell cycle, 365
cell death, 203, 205, 273, 305
cell invasion, 207
cell line, 142, 147, 155, 165, 185, 187, 189, 200, 208, 211, 213, 214, 218, 219, 221, 225, 239, 241, 261, 361
cell membranes, 232
cell organization, 242
cell size, 345
cell surface, 44, 241, 323, 324
cellular energy, 45, 300
cellular immunity, 181
cellular properties, 324
cellulitis, 387
cellulose, 140
central nervous system, 58
cerebral blood flow, 336
cervical cancer, 380, 398
cervix, 212
challenges, 6, 25, 28, 65, 70, 229, 242, 292, 355, 374, 381, 391
channel blocker, 273, 287
chemical reactions, 186

chemokines, 165, 261, 264
chemotaxis, 257
chemotherapeutic agent, 207
chemotherapy, 155, 164, 166, 183, 187, 190, 196, 200, 201, 203, 213, 214, 224, 383
CHF (chronic heart failure), 81, 82, 83
Chinese medicine, 274
cholangiocarcinoma, 107, 108, 144, 148, 151, 155, 156
cholangitis, 137, 148
cholecystectomy, 5, 16, 18, 27, 28, 30, 32, 34, 35, 144, 379, 389, 394
cholecystitis, 34, 47, 52
cholelithiasis, 5, 12, 148, 152
cholestasis, 67, 116, 125, 128, 133, 148, 150, 156
cholesterol, 140, 148, 153, 299
cholic acid, 140
choline, 129, 130, 131
cholinesterase, 138
chondroitin sulfate, 240, 250
chromatography, 185, 207
chronic diseases, 272, 326, 329
chronic heart failure, 81, 82, 83
chronic heart failure (CHF), 83
chronic rejection, 271
chyle, 384
circulation, 65, 68, 117, 128, 130, 131, 135, 151, 155, 156, 169, 200, 237, 240, 242, 260, 292, 322, 323, 328, 341, 342, 343, 350, 352, 357
cirrhosis, 62, 107, 108, 129, 130, 131, 134, 147, 148, 149, 150, 151, 152, 154
CL (caudate lobe), 30, 64, 67, 108, 109, 110, 111, 112, 113, 114, 115, 116, 121, 128, 144, 149, 180, 197, 198, 246, 250, 265, 311, 350, 372, 397
clinical application, 160, 194, 266, 277, 282, 291, 296, 301, 307, 367
clinical assessment, 349, 395
clinical diagnosis, 173
clinical examination, 214
clinical interventions, 318
clinical judgment, 9
clinical presentation, 173, 259
clinical problems, 166
clinical symptoms, 171, 318
clinical syndrome, 37, 82, 137
clinical trials, vii, 37, 53, 62, 70, 166, 176, 187, 207, 269, 279, 283, 298, 304, 355, 381, 388, 392, 396
clinical versus experimental sepsis, 37
CNS, 178, 209
CO_2, 198, 200, 212, 213, 216, 217, 223, 302, 337
coarctation, 87
cognitive abilities, 10, 11, 32
cognitive load, 28

cognitive psychology, 32
colectomy, 378
colic, 109, 213
collaboration, 373, 391
collagen, 133, 188, 232, 233, 237, 238, 245, 246, 258, 259, 262
collateral, 117, 149, 155
collisions, 322
colon, 16, 32, 38, 51, 56, 67, 71, 76, 107, 122, 145, 146, 190, 213, 371, 389
colon cancer, 122, 145, 146
colonization, 259, 264
colonoscopy, 33
colorectal cancer, 146, 207
coma, 46, 292
common bile duct, 13, 31, 107, 108, 110, 113, 114, 117, 130, 131, 144, 279, 314
common bile duct (CBD) stricture, 107
communication systems, 391
complementarity, 283
complexity, 6, 136, 185, 190, 261, 262, 297, 307, 322, 380, 387
comprehension, 187, 198
computed tomography, 317, 318, 338, 392
confocal microscopy, 183, 185, 192, 200, 201, 202, 204, 205, 326, 329, 331
confounding variables, 380
congestive heart failure, 83
congestive HF, 81, 104
conjugation, 242, 252
connective tissue, 127
control group, 167, 272, 274, 382
controlled studies, 35, 138
controlled trials, 4, 5, 33, 379
conversion rate, 27, 379, 380
copolymer, 49, 198
cornea, 232
coronary artery bypass graft, 377, 392, 397
coronary artery ligation, 82, 83
coronary ligation, 92
corticosteroids, 171, 174
cranial nerve, 384
creatinine, 46, 271, 274, 292, 295, 296, 297, 305, 306
cryopreservation, 272, 273, 277
CT scan, 22
CTA, 340
CTO, 184, 202, 204
cultivars, 361
cultivation, 248
culture, 53, 142, 188, 189, 190, 191, 192, 198, 202, 207, 208, 209, 210, 237, 239, 240, 241, 243, 244, 249, 280, 282, 297, 361

culture conditions, 237
culture medium, 198, 280, 361
current limit, 245
Cutan Section, 76
CVD, 81, 104
cyclophosphamide, 155, 164, 173
cyclosporine, 160, 166, 169, 172, 175, 177, 181
cyst, 378, 383, 397
cystectomy, 387, 395
cysteine, 272
cystic duct, 13, 144
cytochrome, 45, 140, 302, 319, 336
cytocompatibility, 239
cytokines, 42, 49, 162, 163, 165, 172, 235, 236, 257, 259, 260, 271, 293, 296, 315, 320, 352, 361, 363, 364
cytomegalovirus, 170
cytometry, 171, 183, 185, 201, 203, 204, 205, 340
cytoplasm, 281, 322
cytoskeleton, 258, 265
cytotoxicity, 163

D

data analysis, 331, 335
data set, 335
data transfer, 390, 391
daVinci, 373, 375, 376, 377, 379, 380, 381, 383, 384, 385, 386, 387, 388, 389, 390, 391, 392, 395
    skills simulator, 21
    surgical system, 375, 376, 377, 379, 381, 388, 395
death rate, 51
deaths, 38, 144, 173, 219
decellularization, 229, 230, 231, 232, 233, 234, 237, 238, 239, 240, 241, 243, 244, 245, 246, 247, 248, 249, 250, 252, 253
decontamination, 198
deep brain stimulation, 381
deformability, 43, 44, 68, 69, 320, 321, 322, 323, 328, 339, 340, 342, 343, 344, 346, 347, 350, 351, 352, 353, 357
dendritic cell, 245
dengue, 372
deoxyribonucleic acid, 148, 151, 260
depolarization, 156
depth perception, 7, 28, 387
dermis, 259
descending colon, 30
desiccation, 262, 264
detectable, 132, 171, 174, 175
detergents, 155, 231, 232, 238

diabetes, 34, 41, 62, 73, 79, 138, 150, 249, 262, 266, 326, 329
dialysis, 296, 307
diapedesis, 257
diaphragm, 13, 75, 109, 110, 112
diaphragmatic hernia, 18
diarrhea, 170, 173
DIC, 38, 43, 44, 56, 317, 344
didactic teaching, 7
diffusion time, 194
digestive enzymes, 74
dilated cardiomyopathy, 82
disaster area, 391
discrimination, 205
discs, 112
disease model, 23, 181, 282
diseases, ix, 73, 81, 107, 161, 165, 211, 236, 282, 317, 324, 363, 364, 372
disinfection, 83
disseminated intravascular coagulation, 38, 63, 317
dissolved oxygen, 273
diverticulitis, 50, 64
dizziness, 28
DNA, 122, 208, 210, 232, 233, 234, 244, 256, 260, 267, 281, 359, 360, 361, 362, 363, 364, 366, 367, 368, 369, 370, 371, 372
sequencing, 208
DNA vaccine(s), 359, 363, 364, 370, 371, 372
domain optical coherence tomography, 338
donors, 27, 149, 152, 175, 245, 279, 286, 287, 290, 291, 292, 293, 304, 308, 311, 313, 314, 315, 369
drug discovery, 207
drug metabolism, 236, 237
drug reactions, 170
drug resistance, 185, 187
drug testing, 198, 206
drug therapy, 206
drug treatment, 143
duodenum, 74, 76, 109, 110, 114, 117, 135, 137, 144
dynamic viscosity, 339
dysplasia, 144

E

E. coli, 51, 52, 56, 59, 60, 64, 65, 68, 70, 130, 353
ECG, 94
ECM, 184, 188, 189, 229, 230, 231, 232, 233, 238, 242, 250, 255, 258, 259, 260, 261
economics, 183, 184
ECs, 319, 320, 322, 342, 343
ectoderm, 236

edema, 41, 44, 45, 55, 135, 136, 137, 147, 152, 155, 239, 257, 259, 260, 275, 276, 278, 281, 282, 294, 297, 305, 306, 343, 344
EEG, 46
elastic deformation, 321, 322
elastin, 232, 233, 238, 239, 245, 246
electric field, 233
electrical properties, 244
electrocautery, 26, 263
electrodes, 337
electrolyte, 271
electron microscopy, 305
electrophoresis, 185, 208, 210
electroporation, 233, 248, 251, 359, 361, 369, 370, 371, 372
ELISA, 233
emboli, 152, 386
embolization, 152, 386
embryonic stem cells, 208, 236, 246
encephalopathy, 46, 71, 123
endocrine, 117, 138, 307
endoderm, 236
endometrial carcinoma, 225
endometriosis, 393, 397
endoscope, 27, 28, 375, 376
endoscopic-laparoscopic interdisciplinary training entity (ELITE), 22
endoscopy, 334, 381
endothelial cells, 123, 230, 231, 241, 242, 243, 245, 260, 317, 319, 350, 353, 357
endothelial dysfunction, 44, 348, 349
endothelium, 44, 241, 295, 319, 320, 322, 323, 325, 328, 342, 343, 346, 347, 356
endothelium-derived P-selectin, 320
EndoTower, 20
endotoxemia, 48, 49, 59, 65, 66, 68, 71, 348
endotracheal intubation, 96
end-stage renal disease, 284
energy, 25, 26, 45, 271, 276, 277, 289, 300, 301, 302, 305, 306, 307, 315, 321, 322, 324, 335, 337, 361, 389, 401
energy transfer, 337
environment control, 214
environmental contamination, 186
environmental factors, 59
enzyme(s), 45, 83, 133, 135, 136, 142, 147, 152, 190, 207, 232, 238, 258, 300 301, 372
enzyme inhibitors, 190, 207
EPC, 230, 243
epidermis, 262, 361
epinephrine, 42
epithelial cells, 133, 238, 239, 240, 242, 299
epithelial ovarian cancer, 211, 212, 222, 224, 225

epithelium, 76, 144, 151, 181, 241, 247, 279
epitopes, 245
ergonomics, 264, 374
Erythrocyte aggregation, 323
erythrocyte sedimentation rate, 318, 323, 340
erythrocytes, 44, 299, 323, 324, 333, 336, 342, 343, 344, 347, 349, 354
esophagus, 5, 18, 74, 76, 112, 113
ESR, 318, 323, 340
ethanol, 62, 83, 93, 130, 135, 136, 137, 138, 147, 152, 155, 198
ethical implications, 25
ethyl alcohol, 88
Eurotransplant, 285, 293
ex vivo, 16, 26, 32, 170, 183, 187, 188, 190, 192, 193, 206, 208, 222, 239, 251, 270, 282, 284, 292, 296, 297, 298, 299, 301, 302, 307, 308, 309, 310, 311, 313, 315, 316, 330, 341, 389
   patient-derived, 183, 192
excessive fat tissue, 73
excision, 16, 397, 400
experimental
   design, 81
   laparoscopy, 4
   models, 69, 153, 155, 211
   wound models, 255
exposure, 6, 51, 135, 142, 143, 168, 175, 233, 238, 257, 264, 279, 328, 329, 382, 383
external fixation, 381
extracellular matrix, 187, 229, 231, 247, 248, 249, 250, 258, 266, 267
extraction, 13
extravasation, 240
exudate, 46
ex-vivo
   machine perfusion, 289

fibrinogen, 44, 257, 266, 320, 322, 323, 324, 343, 344, 347
fibroblast growth factor, 266
fibroblast proliferation, 259
fibroblasts, 209, 238, 240, 257, 258
fibrogenesis, 133
fibrosis, 130, 131, 133, 134, 140, 148, 153, 155, 260, 272, 295, 315
fidelity, 19, 159, 176
FIGO, 214
filtration, 66, 339, 340, 376, 388
fistulas, 105
flexibility, 376, 384
flow cytometry, 171, 183, 185, 201, 203, 204, 205
FLS (Fundamentals of Laparoscopic Surgery), 4, 6, 36
fluid balance, 41
fluorescence, 27, 137, 171, 192, 202, 203, 326, 329, 330, 331, 332, 333, 348, 351, 352, 353, 354, 355, 356
Food and Drug Administration, 278
food intake, 17
Fourier, 335, 338
fractures, 382
free radicals, 260, 271, 274, 294, 343, 349, 352
friction, 323, 325
functional capillary density, 318, 328, 330
functional changes, 328
functional MRI, 338
functional organs, 245
functionalization, 242
fundamentals of laparoscopic surgery, 4, 6, 36
fungi, 49, 54, 142
furan, 144, 149, 155
future laparoscopy, 4
future of clinical liver machine perfusion, 302

F

fabrication, 156, 185, 186, 187, 193, 195, 246, 359
failing heart, 105
fascia, 53, 262
fasting, 50
fat, 16, 18, 73, 77, 97, 130, 131, 139, 153, 154, 243, 262, 379
feces, 52, 53, 56
Federal Drug and Administration (FDA), 278, 373, 374, 376, 381, 382, 383
femur, 374, 378
fiber optics, 334
fibrillation, 378
fibrin, 52, 56, 257, 266

G

gallbladder, 110, 111, 114, 128, 139, 144, 148
gallstones, 137, 139, 148, 154
gastrectomy, 17, 73, 74, 75, 78, 79, 80, 378, 396
gastric mucosa, 79
Gastric Plication, 73, 74, 75, 76, 78, 79
gastroenterostomy, 74
gastroesophageal reflux, 5
gastroschisis, 174
GB (Gallbladder), 108, 128
GCS (Glasgow Coma Scale), 38
gender differences, 344, 345
gene expression, 80, 105, 188, 208, 272, 282, 316, 352, 360, 365, 366, 368, 369, 371, 372

Gene Gun, 359, 360, 361, 362, 363, 364, 365, 366, 371, 372
gene silencing, 281, 282
gene therapy, vii, ix, 261, 269, 308, 359, 364, 365, 366, 368, 371, 372
gene transfer, 105, 359, 361, 363, 364, 366, 367, 369, 371
general anesthesia, 26, 361, 370
general surgeon, 12
general surgery, 3, 6, 17, 73, 378, 379
genes, 92, 104, 139, 235, 236, 261, 281, 282, 293, 359, 360, 361, 362, 365, 371
genetic factors, 138, 161, 163, 211
genetic mutations, 189
genetics, 281
genitals, 16
genomics, 185
geometry, 193, 328, 339, 341, 354
germ layer, 236
gestation, 261
Ghrelin, 17, 73, 74, 75, 76
ginseng, 274
glandular section, 76
glucocorticoids, 167
glucose, 41, 61, 123, 124, 194, 197, 200, 237, 244, 277, 278, 280, 300
glutamate, 278
glutamine, 198
glutathione, 274, 278, 303
glycol, 270, 273, 275, 279, 286, 294, 324
glycoproteins, 324
glycosaminoglycans, 233
goblet cells, 144
Gori, 342, 343, 344, 349
graft dysfunction, 270, 281
graft healing, 259
gravitational force, 28, 339
growth factor, 142, 148, 155, 163, 240, 257, 258, 267, 270, 271, 297
growth hormone, 79, 80
guiding principles, 263
gunpowder, 360, 361
GVH (graft-versus-host), 159
GVHR (Graft-versus-host responses), 159
gynecology, 211, 378, 379, 380, 401

H

hair cells, 361
haplotypes, 164, 167, 179
haptoglobin, 324
HBV, 142, 143
HCC, 107, 108, 140, 141, 142, 143

head and neck cancer, 395
healing, 138, 255, 256, 258, 259, 260, 261, 263, 264, 265, 266, 352
health, 35, 73, 82, 183, 184, 206, 350, 388, 393
health care, 206, 388, 393
health care costs, 393
health care system, 206, 393
heart disease, 350
heart failure, 67, 81, 82, 88, 92, 96, 101, 102
Heart Machine Preservation, 305
heart rate, 38, 83, 87, 88, 96, 102, 251
heart transplantation, 269, 275, 282, 288, 290, 305, 367
heart valves, 231, 232, 245, 246, 249, 252
heat shock protein, 296
heat transfer, 186
helium, 213, 361
hematocrit, 139, 318, 320, 321, 324, 325, 328, 341, 342
hematoma, 384, 386
hematuria, 387
hemoglobin, 52, 297, 303, 318, 322, 327, 330, 336, 337, 343
hemorheology, 317, 347, 349, 350, 357
hemorrhage, 44, 63, 64, 135, 136, 139, 170
hemorrhagic, 62, 136, 138, 149, 154, 156, 212, 218, 328, 349, 352, 356
hemostasis, 11, 134, 143, 257, 264, 266
hepatectomy, 13, 14, 15, 27, 31, 36, 107, 108, 120, 121, 122, 123, 124, 125, 127, 129, 140, 141, 147, 148, 149, 150, 151, 152, 153, 154, 156
  technique, 108
hepatic failure, 139, 149, 152, 154
hepatic fibrosis, 153, 155
hepatic stellate cells, 154
hepatitis, 108, 129, 142, 153, 363, 370, 372
hepatocellular carcinoma, 107, 149, 150, 153, 155
hepatocytes, 131, 133, 142, 143, 154, 208, 235, 236, 237, 238, 249, 250
hepatoma, 143
hepatomegaly, 142
hepatopancreatobiliary surgery, 108
  experimental models, v, 107
hernia, 17, 218, 219, 255
hernia repair, 17
heterogeneity, 40, 147, 151, 185, 187, 188, 189, 207, 319, 327, 331, 333
HF (heart failure), 36, 67, 81, 82, 88, 92, 96, 101, 102, 104, 177, 351
hiatal hernia, 18
hip arthroplasty, 378, 382, 398, 399
hip replacement, 382, 393, 395, 400
histidine, 275, 277, 278, 279, 293, 294

histocompatibility antigens, 160
histogram, 340
histological examination, 25
histology, 139, 172, 283, 299, 300, 301, 302, 303, 306
histone, 232
historical data, 380
HIV, 370, 371
HLA, 162, 166, 168, 169, 170, 178, 245
HLA antigens, 170
homeostasis, 230, 241, 270, 278, 282, 300
homogeneity, 242, 243
hormones, 17, 62, 74, 161
host-versus-graft (HVG), 159
HPB anatomy, 107
HPB models, 107
HPB research, 107
HPV, 235
HSCT, 160, 161, 162, 168, 170, 171
human body, 22
human diseases, 107, 165, 211, 317
human genome, 260
human skin, 265, 337
human subjects, 243
humidity, 334
hybrid, 19, 21, 28, 35
hydrodynamic method, 359, 367, 369
hydrogels, 188
hydrogen, 66, 273, 283
hydrogen gas, 283
hydrogen sulfide, 273
hydroxyl, 294
hygiene, 262
hypercalcemia, 136
hyperkalemia, 278
hyperplasia, 122
hypersensitivity, 65, 66
hypertension, 58, 62, 129, 131, 149, 153
hypertrophy, 82, 87, 88, 95, 101, 105
hypoglycemia, 49
hypotension, 40, 41, 59
hypotensive, 56
hypothermia, 49, 270, 272, 284, 297, 308, 315
hypothermic kidney perfusion, 292
hypothermic liver perfusion, 301
hypovolemia, 139, 343
hypovolemic shock, 355
hypoxemia, 41
hypoxia, 45, 66, 139, 189, 190, 191, 192, 260, 320, 343, 353, 354
hysterectomy, 380, 389, 394, 397, 398, 399

I

ICAM, 150, 296
icterus, 47
IFN, 55
IFN-β, 55
IL-8, 257, 260
ileostomy, 64
ileum, 52, 172, 331
IMA, 308
image analysis, 352, 354
imaging modalities, 193, 376
immune activation, 55, 168
immune function, 62, 328
immune reaction, 244
immune response, 63, 154, 165, 171, 174, 175, 213, 229, 244, 245, 246, 259, 364, 371, 372
immune system, 23, 54, 55, 65, 161, 163, 165, 166, 171, 174, 175, 190, 245, 259, 283
immunobiology, 162, 165
immunocompromised, 143, 161, 211
immunogenetics, 161
immunogenicity, 230, 231, 245, 275
immunoglobulin, 324, 343, 367
immunomodulation, 271
immunostimulatory, 286
immunosuppression, 54, 163, 166, 171, 174, 175, 177, 179, 229, 235, 244
immunosuppressive agent, 161
immunotherapy, 224, 363
implant placement, 382
implants, 212, 213, 222, 374, 382, 394
improvements, 4, 6, 17, 295, 318, 382, 384
in situ hybridization, 171
in utero, 160
inbreeding, 167
incisional hernia, 212, 221
incubation period, 201, 203, 280
incubator, 198
induction, 48, 54, 60, 61, 62, 83, 96, 122, 137, 139, 142, 146, 155, 162, 164, 169, 172, 217, 218, 235, 265, 283
induction methods, 60
induction time, 218
INF, 342
infection, 37, 40, 41, 48, 50, 54, 56, 57, 59, 62, 65, 71, 142, 151, 155, 170, 174, 264, 266, 267, 272
infectious agents, 257
inferior vena cava, 13, 109, 110, 111, 112, 113, 116, 117
inflammation, 49, 55, 64, 65, 66, 67, 71, 131, 135, 137, 139, 257, 258, 259, 264, 283, 286, 317, 318, 319, 320, 342, 346, 351

inflammatory disease, 267
inflammatory mediators, 342
inflammatory response, 25, 38, 40, 54, 55, 56, 57, 58, 64, 69, 245, 258, 259, 262, 272, 281, 283, 296, 320
influenza, 364, 369
influenza vaccine, 369
influenza virus, 364
infrared spectroscopy, 318, 327, 336, 348
infrastructure, 222, 391
infusion model, 49
inguinal hernia, 18, 31, 33, 391
injections, 53, 57, 212, 214, 218, 219, 221, 383
innate immune response, 283
innate immunity, 286
inner ear, 361
innominate, 90, 95, 97, 98
innovator, 309
inoculation, 51, 52, 53, 57, 61, 122, 142, 155, 364
insecticide, 138
insulin, 64, 79, 241, 244, 270, 271, 280
integrity, 45, 196, 231, 232, 233, 234, 237, 238, 240, 241, 244, 255, 256, 257, 279, 292
intensive care unit, 38, 306
intercourse, 386
interference, 124, 214, 221, 272, 281, 336, 368, 369, 372
interferon, 66, 71, 364
interleukin-8, 266
intervention strategies, 211
intestinal villi, 331
intestine, 23, 178, 236, 329, 331, 351, 389
intra-abdominal abscess, 68
intracellular calcium, 273
intragastric balloon, 74
intravenously, 48, 60, 68, 161, 353
investigative tools, 107
ion channels, 239
ionizing radiation, 259
IRI, 278, 279, 290, 293, 302, 306
iron, 66, 294, 302, 343
irradiation, 160, 161, 165, 166, 169, 170, 177, 262
irrigation, 274, 277
IRS, 336
ischemia, ix, 47, 52, 83, 92, 105, 123, 125, 129, 135, 137, 147, 148, 172, 179, 230, 235, 263, 272, 273, 274, 275, 276, 279, 280, 282, 283, 284, 285, 286, 287, 289, 290, 291, 292, 293, 295, 297, 299, 300, 301, 302, 303, 304, 305, 306, 309, 310, 313, 315, 316, 326, 327, 334, 342, 343, 346, 349, 350, 351, 352, 353, 355, 356

ischemia reperfusion injury, 272, 273, 274, 287, 289, 300, 302, 304, 313, 342, 346, 351, 352, 353, 355

J

jaundice, 137
jejunum, 74, 135
joints, 383, 401

K

K^+, 270, 278, 279, 320, 322, 353
keratinocyte, 258, 265
key findings, 317
kidney, 23, 46, 65, 83, 109, 110, 127, 132, 153, 169, 175, 185, 190, 229, 240, 246, 250, 252, 253, 269, 271, 272, 273, 274, 276, 277, 282, 283, 284, 285, 286, 287, 289, 290, 291, 292, 293, 294, 295, 296, 297, 298, 301, 307, 308, 310, 311, 312, 313, 314, 315, 316, 329, 335, 386, 389
kidney machine perfusion preservation, 291
kidney transplantation, 127, 153, 269, 273, 274, 277, 282, 283, 284, 285, 286, 290, 295, 296, 308, 311, 312, 313, 314
killer cells, 224
knee arthroplasty, 382, 398, 399, 400

L

labeling, 243, 326, 330, 331
lab-on-a-chip, 184, 185
laceration, 213, 386
lactate dehydrogenase, 290
lactate level, 41, 123, 305
lactose, 276
laparoscope, 14
laparoscopic cholecystectomy, 5, 13, 20, 26, 27, 212, 379, 391, 396
laparoscopic hepatobiliary surgery, 12
laparoscopic nephrectomy, 16, 22, 399
laparoscopic simulator, 3, 4, 10, 11, 19, 31, 32, 33, 35
laparoscopic surgery, 3, 4, 5, 6, 9, 10, 12, 19, 21, 22, 26, 27, 28, 29, 30, 32, 33, 34, 35, 212, 216, 223, 224, 225, 374, 379, 380, 391, 392, 393, 400
learning curve, 6
laparoscopic suturing, 7, 8, 19, 30
laparoscopic table, 214
laparoscopic training, 4, 5, 17, 18, 19, 22, 25, 30, 32, 34, 35

laparoscopy, 3, 4, 5, 6, 9, 10, 11, 12, 16, 17, 21, 23,
    26, 27, 28, 29, 30, 32, 33, 35, 212, 213, 216, 217,
    218, 219, 221, 222, 223, 224, 225, 226, 334, 374,
    380, 387, 394, 395, 397
laparotomy, 61, 211, 212, 213, 214, 217, 218, 219,
    221, 222, 223, 224, 280, 380, 397
LapMentor II, 20
LapMentor/, 20
LapSim, 20
L-arginine, 65, 135, 139
larynx, 84, 233
Laser Doppler perfusion imaging technology, 335
Laser Doppler tissue flowmetry, 334
Laser Speckle Imaging, 336
Leahy, 327, 330, 333, 334, 335, 337, 347, 349, 350,
    351, 353, 354, 355, 356
LED, 349
Left Anterior Descending (LAD) ArteryLigation, 81
left atrium, 82
left coronary artery ligation, 82, 83, 92
left ventricle, 81, 83, 86, 87
legislation, 25
leptin(s), 73, 74, 75, 79, 80
lesions, 137, 139, 147, 278, 290, 291, 384, 395
leucocyte, 134
leukemia, 165, 175, 180
leukocytes, 44, 68, 170, 318, 319, 325, 330, 331,
    344, 353, 355
leukocytosis, 49
leukopenia, 49
ligament, 74, 108, 109, 110, 111, 116, 126, 128, 399
ligand, 79
light cycle, 214
light scattering, 338, 355
light transmission, 341
linear function, 321
lipases, 232
lipid metabolism, 236
lipid peroxidation, 343
liposomes, 356
liquid chromatography, 185
lithography, 187, 193
Liver,
    anatomy, 108, 109, 114
    engineering, 234
    transplantation, 116, 123, 149, 153, 154, 155,
        156, 169, 170, 173, 176, 177, 178, 181, 269,
        290, 298, 299, 301, 303, 304, 310, 311, 312,
        313, 314, 315, 363, 367
liver cancer, 149, 156
liver cirrhosis, 147, 148
liver damage, 154
liver disease, 13, 133, 143, 153

liver failure, 107, 108, 120, 121, 123, 125, 129, 153,
    155
liver function tests, 123
liver metastases, 122, 146, 148, 153, 154
liver transplant, 116, 121, 123, 149, 153, 154, 155,
    156, 169, 170, 171, 173, 176, 177, 178, 181, 269,
    290, 298, 299, 301, 303, 304, 310, 311, 312, 313,
    314, 315, 363, 367
local anesthesia, 88
local anesthetic, 364
loci, 170
logistics, 18, 390
longevity, 304, 305
(LOS) Length of Stay, 373, 377, 379, 382, 401
low fat diet, 155
LTx, 281
luciferase, 362, 364, 366, 367
lumen, 16, 28, 51, 76, 134, 343
lung cancer, 207, 209, 210, 238
lung function, 306
lung machine preservation, 306
lung transplantation, 23, 269, 284, 285, 290, 309
lymph node, 110, 167, 172, 329, 356, 380, 385, 387,
    399
lymphadenopathy, 173
lymphocytes, 133, 167, 170, 171, 180, 364
lymphoid, 161, 172, 173, 224
lymphoid tissue, 172, 173
lysine, 197

M

machine organ preservation, vi, 289
machine perfusion, 289, 290, 291, 292, 295, 296,
    298, 299, 300, 302, 303, 304, 305, 306, 307, 308,
    309, 310, 311, 312, 313, 314, 315, 316
macro-hemorheological changes, 343
macromolecules, 275, 294, 322, 323, 324, 346
macrophages, 43, 59, 156, 257, 258, 260, 342, 363
magnesium, 197, 276, 277
magnetic resonance, 318, 338, 392
magnetic resonance imaging, 318, 338, 392
major histocompatibility complex, 160, 179, 181
malabsorption, 17
malaria, 364
mammalian cells, 281
mannitol, 275, 277, 278, 294
mapping, 337
marker genes, 361, 362, 366
marrow, 160, 161, 165, 166, 167, 168, 175, 179,
    180, 181, 182, 243, 259
marsupialization, 383
mast cells, 342, 351

matrix metalloproteinase, 154, 258
mean arterial pressure, 38, 41
mechanical properties, 200, 232, 236, 238
mechanical ventilation, 45, 60, 67, 282
medical, 7, 22, 23, 25, 26, 35, 53, 74, 160, 166, 183, 184, 206, 302, 306, 375, 396, 399, 400
medical care, 166, 183, 184
medical science, 302, 399
medicine, vii, 31, 34, 35, 183, 184, 196, 207, 209, 274, 304, 318, 345, 347, 351, 373, 392
melanoma, 363, 372
mellitus, 62, 73
MEMS, 184
meningitis, 48, 53, 68, 70
mercury, 331
mesenchymal stem cells, 169, 248
mesentery, 280, 319
mesoderm, 236
messenger ribonucleic acid, 260
meta-analysis, 19, 27, 30, 33, 35, 279, 293, 311, 379, 384, 386, 398, 401
metabolic acidosis, 172
metabolic change, 342
metabolic responses, 65
metabolic syndrome, 73
metabolism, 17, 64, 190, 191, 209, 270, 275, 278, 291, 294, 296, 297, 299, 305
metabolites, 135, 138, 190, 319, 320, 343, 350
metabolizing, 82
metastasis, 108, 120, 122, 143, 223, 224, 225, 363
methodology, 185, 211, 298, 304, 317, 318, 326, 328, 329, 345, 369
methyl methacrylate, 195
methylprednisolone, 53, 173, 281
MFI, 318, 331, 332, 333
MHC, 160, 162, 163, 164, 165, 167, 168, 172, 174, 175, 177, 178, 179, 247, 371
microcirculation, 43, 66, 68, 70, 71, 135, 137, 138, 274, 287, 294, 317, 318, 319, 320, 322, 323, 325, 327, 328, 329, 331, 334, 335, 336, 337, 341, 342, 343, 344, 345, 346, 348, 349, 350, 351, 352, 353, 354, 355, 356, 357
microcirculatory inflammation, 317
microcirculatory perfusion, 70, 317, 328, 336, 356
micro-dissected tissue, v, 183, 184, 185, 192, 196, 199, 200, 203
microenvironments, 210
microfluidic device, 183, 185, 186, 187, 189, 190, 192, 193, 195, 196, 198, 201, 207
microfluidics, 184, 185, 186, 187, 190, 209
micro-hemodynamic features, 328
micrometer, 186
microorganism(s), 62, 259

micro-rheology, 318, 345
microRNA, 265, 266, 301, 311
microscope, 87, 96, 125, 197, 202, 328, 329, 331
microscopy, 137, 183, 185, 192, 200, 201, 202, 204, 205, 234, 318, 324, 326, 329, 331, 337, 338, 340, 341, 347, 348, 351, 352, 354, 355, 356, 357
microspheres, 152
microstructure, 240
micro-ultrasound devices, 338
microvasculature, 319
migration, 5, 17, 243, 258, 260, 325, 341, 342
mini gastric bypass, 74
miniaturization, 375, 387
Minimally Invasive Surgery (MIS), 3, 5, 9, 10, 18, 21, 27, 30, 225, 374, 375, 381, 386, 388, 395
Minimally Invasive Surgical Trainer – Virtual Reality (MIST-VR), 19, 20
MISTELS/FLS trainer, 21
mitochondria, 310, 319
mitochondrial damage, 272, 300
mitogen, 272
mitral valve, 377, 393, 397, 398, 401
mitral valve prolapse, 397
MMP, 256, 258, 282, 287
MMP-2, 282, 287
MMPs, 282
model of hepatic metastases of colon carcinoma, 107
models of acute liver failure, 107, 123
models of cirrhosis, 107
models of hepatocellular carcinoma, 107
Models of Liver Resection, 120
modifications, 58, 82, 176, 278, 361
modules, 389
modulus, 322
mold, 193, 195, 197
molecular biology, 144, 281
molecular weight, 278, 324
molecules, 165, 186, 194, 236, 269, 270, 273, 276, 281, 283, 315, 319, 337, 342, 343
momentum, 322
monoclonal antibody, 149, 163, 168
monocyte chemoattractant protein, 257
monolayer, 185, 188, 200, 361
morbidity, 37, 59, 82, 125, 139, 161, 255, 256, 279, 290, 387, 390, 392
morphine, 60
morphological abnormalities, 326, 329
morphology, 13, 44, 135, 146, 188, 205, 280, 320, 326, 341
mortality, 5, 37, 41, 47, 50, 51, 52, 55, 59, 68, 69, 70, 71, 82, 95, 107, 123, 124, 125, 134, 136, 137,

138, 139, 152, 161, 162, 170, 171, 174, 201, 205, 290
mortality rate, 50, 52, 55, 82, 123, 125, 134, 136, 137, 138, 162, 171
mouse, 48, 49, 55, 57, 58, 63, 68, 71, 81, 92, 93, 95, 96, 101, 107, 109, 111, 114, 120, 121, 124, 125, 126, 127, 128, 140, 142, 143, 144, 150, 151, 153, 156, 159, 160, 161, 164, 165, 167, 189, 190, 212, 213, 218, 221, 222, 223, 239, 252, 267, 347, 354, 362, 364
MRI, 318, 338, 381, 383, 399
mRNA, 83, 88, 281, 283, 296, 361, 364
mucin, 52, 53
mucosa, 334, 363, 364, 372
multiple factors, 6, 9, 165
multiple myeloma, 208
multiple sclerosis, 166
multivariate analysis, 279
muscle atrophy, 365, 372
muscles, 334, 335, 359, 366
musculoskeletal, 22, 73
mutation(s), 139, 140, 141
myelomeningocele, 381
myocardial infarction, 82, 95, 348, 377, 387
myocardial ischemia, 82, 352
myocardium, 46, 82, 88, 94, 250
myocyte, 105
myofibroblasts, 258
myoglobin, 336
myosin, 88

N

Na$^+$, 101, 270, 278, 279, 322, 352
NAD, 302
NADH, 330
naked DNA, vi, 359, 360, 366, 367, 368, 371, 372
NAS, 279
National Aeronautics and Space Administration (NASA), 374, 375, 390
National Institutes of Health, 74, 79, 80
natural evolution, 122
natural killer cell, 180
natural orifice translumenal endoscopic surgery (NOTES), 3, 4, 16, 17, 22, 26, 27, 28, 29, 30, 31, 35, 395
Near-infrared spectroscopy, 336
necrosis, 46, 69, 123, 129, 130, 135, 136, 137, 139, 147, 153, 155, 257, 299, 300, 303
negative effects, 277
neonates, 18, 62, 71, 356
neoplasm, 384
neovascularization, 146, 259

nephrectomy, 16, 18, 22, 26, 31, 32, 33, 34, 237, 385, 386, 389, 393, 394, 396, 399, 400, 401
nephron, 286, 394
nephropathy, 282
nerve, 75, 120, 245, 257, 270, 271, 366, 372, 382, 384
nerve growth factor, 257, 270, 271
nervous system, 42
neurons, 361
neurosurgery, 350, 381, 394, 398, 399, 400
neutropenia, 170
neutrophils, 44, 168, 257, 342, 350
NFκB (nuclear factor kappa B), 38, 342
NGF (nerve growth factor), 257, 270, 271
nicotine, 355
NIRS (near-infrared spectroscopy), 318, 327, 336, 348
Nissen fundoplication, 5
nitric oxide, 38, 65, 68, 70, 71, 105, 147, 241, 265, 273, 318, 319, 347, 352, 355, 356
nitric oxide synthase, 71, 105, 147, 352
nitrite, 45
nitrogen, 45, 320, 350
nitrous oxide, 213
NK cells, 170
NMP (Normothermic Machine Perfusion), 290, 291, 295, 296, 297, 298, 299, 300, 301, 302, 303, 304, 305, 306, 307, 310
NMR, 338
Nobel Prize, ix, 160
NOD (nucleotide-binding oligomerization domain-like (*receptor*)), 38, 42
nodules, 143
nonhuman primate, vii, 58, 159, 178, 180
non-neoplastic diseases, 161
norepinephrine, 42
normal distribution, 200
normothermic liver perfusion, 299
NOTES technique, 16, 17, 28
Nuclear Magnetic Resonance, 351
nucleic acid, 202, 232, 283, 360
nucleotides, 260
nutrition, 291, 384

O

obesity, 17, 31, 73, 74, 77, 79, 80, 379, 400
obstructive sleep apnea, 384
olfactory nerve, 53
oligomerization, 38, 42
omentum, 22, 75, 114, 280, 335
oncogenes, 142, 144, 235
one dimension, 190

open heart surgery, 393
Open-source Heidelberg laparoscopy phantom (OpenHELP), 21
operating table, 212, 222, 376, 381
operations, 3, 12, 17, 19, 26, 75, 376, 379, 381, 385, 387, 388, 389, 392
optical fiber, 334
optical properties, 327, 334
optical systems, 216
optimization, 196, 206, 238
oral cavity, 331, 363, 378, 383
orbit, 347
organ engineering, 230, 231, 235, 236, 242, 244, 247, 250, 252
organ preservation, ix, 230, 269, 270, 271, 272, 273, 274, 276, 277, 278, 281, 283, 284, 285, 291, 292, 294, 297, 307, 308, 314
organelles, 194
organotypic tissue, 184, 190
Orthopedics, 381
osmolality, 278, 354
osmotic pressure, 276, 277
Otolaryngology, 378, 383, 384, 398
ovarian cancer, 209, 211, 212, 213, 222, 223, 224, 225, 226, 380, 397
ovarian tumor, 212, 213, 225
ovaries, 160
ox, 284, 290, 292, 294, 295, 296, 297, 298, 300, 302, 304, 309, 311, 312, 313, 330
oxidative damage, 296
oxidative stress, 23, 131, 278, 343
oxygen, 41, 43, 45, 59, 70, 71, 138, 187, 189, 190, 192, 193, 194, 195, 237, 241, 260, 266, 271, 272, 273, 274, 276, 278, 284, 292, 294, 296, 297, 299, 300, 301, 306, 309, 310, 314, 315, 318, 320, 321, 327, 336, 337, 343, 344, 348, 349, 350, 353, 356, 384
  tensions, 337
oxygen consumption, 59, 260, 296, 300, 301, 337, 348
oxygen plasma, 193, 195
oxygenation, 43, 46, 68, 69, 240, 259, 264, 273, 282, 291, 294, 295, 296, 297, 299, 300, 301, 306, 310, 314, 315, 318, 322, 327, 337, 345, 355, 356
oxyhemoglobin, 319, 336, 338

P

pacemaker, 378
pain, 5, 27, 28, 87, 217, 259, 267, 318, 383, 386
pancreas, 23, 47, 109, 110, 113, 114, 116, 117, 118, 119, 120, 135, 137, 147, 148, 150, 151, 152, 156, 169, 241, 244, 247, 253, 273, 274, 276, 277, 280, 290, 306, 307, 313, 329, 335, 351
pancreas anatomy, 117
pancreas transplant, 273, 307
pancreatic acinar cell, 139
pancreatic machine preservation, 306
pancreatic transplantation, 117, 269, 290
pancreatitis, 107, 117, 135, 136, 137, 138, 139, 147, 148, 149, 150, 152, 153, 154, 155, 156, 351, 356
paracentesis, 212, 224
paradigm shift, 4
parasites, 54, 137, 364
parathyroidectomy, 401
parenchyma, 25, 121, 124, 126, 170
parenchymal cell, 231, 241, 242, 243, 245, 319
partial portal vein ligation, 131
partial thromboplastin time, 41
participants, 7, 12, 283, 284, 390
particle bombardment, 361
pathogenesis, 72, 102, 138, 147, 149, 155, 258, 342
pathogens, 42, 45, 67, 245, 262, 283
pathologist, 196, 197, 397
pathology, 138, 164, 209, 356, 384
pathophysiological, 42, 46, 48, 63, 142, 165, 334, 344, 347
pathophysiology, 37, 38, 39, 40, 50, 53, 54, 58, 62, 63, 64, 68, 81, 82, 101, 104, 107, 129, 131, 135, 136, 139, 140, 153, 162, 318, 344, 348, 349, 353
patient care, 9, 207, 388, 392
pattern recognition, 270, 283
PCR, 151, 171
pediatric surgery training, 18, 23
pelvic floor, 16
pelvis, 388
pepsin, 76
peptide(s), 17, 162, 165, 166, 267, 270, 271
peptides
perforation, 5, 50
perfusion, 25, 41, 44, 45, 70, 135, 136, 156, 190, 191, 192, 193, 208, 231, 233, 234, 235, 237, 238, 239, 240, 241, 242, 243, 244, 246, 247, 251, 252, 270, 275, 279, 281, 282, 284, 285, 286, 287, 289, 290, 291, 292, 294, 295, 296, 297, 298, 299, 300, 301, 302, 303,304, 305, 306, 307, 308, 309, 310, 311, 312, 313, 314, 315, 316, 317, 327, 328, 333, 334, 335, 336, 338, 341, 342, 344, 348, 351, 354, 356, 372, 377
pericardium, 86, 93
pericytes, 257
periodicity, 335
peripheral blood, 165, 167, 171, 175, 243
peripheral blood mononuclear cell, 175
peristalsis, 334

Index

peritoneal carcinomatosis, 212, 224
peritoneal cavity, 16, 50, 52, 61, 280
peritoneum, 16, 23, 109, 112, 125, 134, 334
peritonitis, 38, 45, 48, 50, 51, 52, 55, 56, 57, 61, 64, 65, 66, 67, 71
permeability, 44, 59, 66, 105, 149, 152, 156, 193, 242, 319, 320, 326, 330, 339, 342, 343, 344, 348, 356
permit, 104, 107, 125, 164
peroxidation, 300
peroxynitrite, 343
personalized approach, 183, 184
PET, 338
PGD, 270, 281
pH, 43, 139, 197, 214, 240, 275, 302, 307, 342, 350
phagocyte, 258
pharmacokinetics, 65
pharmacological agents, 53
pharmacology, 206
phenol, 198
phenotype, 139, 167, 234, 235, 242, 265
phosphate, 49, 55, 197, 214, 271, 277, 278, 294, 367
Phosphate-Buffered Saline (PBS), 184
Phosphate-buffered sucrose (PBS), 270, 271
phospholipids, 302
phosphorescence, 337
phosphorylation, 272, 273
photoacoustic tomography, 338
photobleaching, 326
photolithography, 193
photons, 330, 333
phototoxicity, 355
physical characteristics, 234
physiology, 25, 58, 63, 185, 187, 255, 278, 298, 299, 305, 318, 351
PI3K, 208
pig(s), 3, 4, 11, 13, 14, 16, 17, 18, 22, 23, 24, 26, 32, 33, 34, 35, 40, 45, 48, 49, 52, 55, 56, 57, 58, 59, 60, 63, 64, 66, 68, 70, 114, 116, 159, 160, 165, 168, 176, 225, 262, 265, 267, 272, 276, 279, 286, 287, 296, 303, 308, 309, 310, 312, 313, 314, 315, 316, 350, 359, 366, 369, 370, 372
pigmentation, 334
pilot study, 222, 223, 246
plasma levels, 48
plasma proteins, 320, 324, 330, 351
plasma viscosity, 44, 320, 322, 339, 342, 343, 344, 357
plasmid, 144, 361, 363, 364, 366, 369, 370, 372
plasmid DNA, 369, 370, 372
platelet aggregation, 241
platelet count, 41, 343
platelets, 68, 257, 260, 302, 324, 329, 344, 353
platform, 102, 167, 185, 191, 194, 195, 203, 206, 209, 250, 375, 376, 386, 387, 389, 391
pleural effusion, 377
plexus, 299, 313
PMMA, 184, 195
PNA, 153
pneumonectomy, 239
pneumonia, 48
polarity, 188
polarization, 235, 260, 318, 327, 330, 350
polycarbonate, 340
polymer, 195, 323
polymerase, 88
polymerase chain reaction, 88
polymers, 187, 323, 324
polypeptide, 271
polypropylene, 17, 34, 49, 79
polysaccharide, 49
polystyrene, 193
population, 16, 18, 23, 167, 176, 203, 242, 312, 379, 385
Porcine model(s), 11, 12, 16, 17, 18, 25, 32, 44, 45, 65, 68, 284, 286, 295, 302, 304, 353, 371, 389, 390, 394, 395, 400
portability, 299
portal hypertension, 129, 130, 131, 147, 150, 151, 152, 154, 155, 156
portal systemic shunt, 107
portal vein, 14, 25, 45, 108, 109, 110, 112, 113, 114, 116, 117, 122, 124, 127, 128, 129, 131, 132, 134, 146, 148, 152, 237, 243, 280, 299, 300, 301, 302, 308, 314, 369
positive correlation, 324
positive feedback, 343
positron, 225
positron emission tomography, 225
postoperative complications, 221, 382, 384
postoperative outcome, 27, 396
post-transplant, 162, 283, 295, 297, 304, 314
potassium, 270, 271, 274, 276, 277, 278, 279, 280, 281, 294
pregnancy, 162
preservation, ix, 179, 180, 197, 229, 230, 232, 233, 234, 235, 238, 269, 270, 271, 272, 273, 274, 275, 276, 277, 278, 279, 280, 281, 282, 283, 284, 285, 286, 287, 288, 289, 290, 291, 292, 293, 294, 295, 296, 297, 298, 299, 300, 301, 303, 304, 305, 306, 307, 308, 309, 310, 311, 312, 313, 314, 315, 316
primary cells, 230, 235, 242
primary tumor, 145, 196
probability, 184, 197
probe, 45, 185, 186, 333, 334, 335
procurement, 183, 196, 279, 281, 292, 293, 305

progenitor cell, 174, 182, 230, 235, 238, 240, 243, 257, 352
prognosis, 68, 170, 353
pro-inflammatory, 48, 49, 54, 257, 320
proliferation, 122, 131, 133, 134, 141, 142, 144, 148, 150, 151, 155, 168, 176, 179, 188, 209, 235, 240, 242, 244, 257, 258, 264, 293
proline, 86, 87, 100, 101, 103
propagation, 239, 320
prophylactic, 131
prophylaxis, 166, 179
prostaglandin(s), 156, 281, 319, 320, 353
prostate, v, 183, 184, 196, 197, 198, 201, 203, 204, 393
　cancer, 183, 184, 196, 198, 201, 203, 393
prostatectomy, 16, 26, 183, 196, 378, 385, 386, 393, 394, 396, 397, 398, 401
prostheses, 249
protein kinases, 42
protein-protein interactions, 231
proteins, 58, 143, 162, 194, 231, 232, 233, 272, 320, 323, 324, 326, 363, 364
proteinuria, 295
prothrombin, 257
proto-oncogene, 140, 142, 144
prototype, 28, 377, 398
Pseudomonas aeruginosa, 49, 52, 53, 71
psychomotor ability, 7
pulmonary artery, 60, 61, 82, 239, 240, 281
pulmonary embolism, 383
pulmonary hypertension, 59
pulmonary vascular resistance, 306
pulp, 323
PUMA, 374, 381
PVP, 299, 324
pylorus, 78, 114
pyogenic, 258

Q

quality of life, 82, 183, 184, 383
quantitative technique, 205

R

rabbit model, 18, 23, 33
radiation, 161, 164, 166, 178, 180, 213, 256, 260
radiation therapy, 213
radical cystectomy, 387, 395, 398
radical hysterectomy, 380, 398
radical reactions, 343
radicals, 342, 343, 349, 352

radio, 166
radiotherapy, 209, 214
radius, 324, 339
Ramadan, 310
Raman spectroscopy, 356
RANTES, 265
rash, 170, 173
Rat,
　models, 16, 144, 169, 240
　stomach, 76, 78
reactions, 49, 54, 217, 338, 342, 343, 344
reactive oxygen, 43, 260, 270, 272, 278, 320
reactive sites, 319
reagents, 58, 96, 163, 186, 193, 238
recellularization, 229, 230, 231, 237, 239, 240, 241, 243, 244, 245, 251, 252
receptor(s), 38, 42, 65, 67, 69, 79, 105, 148, 149, 163, 166, 261, 267, 270, 283, 320, 324, 347, 366
reconstruction, 16, 248, 338, 382, 383, 386, 387, 401
recovery, 3, 4, 5, 27, 28, 51, 83, 92, 122, 149, 178, 200, 201, 272, 273, 295, 296, 301, 303, 314, 315, 377, 379, 383, 386, 387
rectal prolapse, 395
red blood cell count, 320, 341
red blood cell deformability, 43, 68, 322, 346, 353
red blood cells, 297, 319, 320, 321, 322, 323, 324, 325, 329, 330, 331, 332, 333, 336, 338, 340, 341, 342, 343
regeneration, ix, 13, 108, 117, 120, 121, 122, 123, 124, 129, 135, 137, 138, 149, 150, 152, 153, 156, 237, 248, 250, 255, 256, 259, 312
regenerative capacity, 122
regenerative medicine, 235, 256
remission, 218
renal cell carcinoma, 386, 394
renin, 87
resection, 15, 30, 64, 74, 75, 108, 116, 120, 121, 122, 123, 124, 125, 126, 128, 129, 153, 155, 213, 223, 378, 383, 384, 386, 391, 393, 397, 399
resistance, 46, 48, 51, 59, 183, 187, 188, 196, 208, 259, 260, 272, 276, 295, 297, 301, 306, 307, 319, 325, 342, 344
respiratory failure, 217
respiratory rate, 83, 87, 88
response, 25, 37, 38, 40, 41, 48, 49, 51, 54, 55, 56, 57, 58, 59, 64, 65, 66, 69, 71, 83, 120, 131, 145, 150, 151, 156, 164, 165, 171, 173, 174, 175, 179, 183, 184, 185, 188, 190, 192, 201, 205, 206, 207, 208, 245, 256, 257, 258, 259, 262, 266, 272, 296, 319, 320, 327, 336, 338, 348, 355, 363, 391
responsiveness, 153, 343
restoration, 259, 306, 382

reticulum, 83
rheology, 44, 63, 64, 68, 69, 317, 318, 328, 342, 344, 345, 346, 349, 351, 352, 354
right ventricle, 290, 305
risk factors, 170
risk management, 5
RNA, 180, 232, 256, 260, 269, 270, 272, 281, 282, 283, 285, 286, 287, 288, 361, 368, 369, 372
RNA Interference, 269
RNAi, 281, 283
RNAs, 260
robotic surgery, vii, ix, 3, 21, 26, 30, 373, 374, 375, 378, 380, 388, 391, 392, 393, 395, 396, 397, 398, 399, 400, 401
robotics, 374, 375, 377, 379, 381, 383, 387, 388, 389, 392, 394, 395, 397, 398, 399, 400
rodent models, 105, 107, 129, 211, 212, 213
rodents, 38, 40, 48, 49, 52, 54, 55, 56, 57, 59, 62, 82, 107, 114, 120, 122, 124, 125, 127, 129, 131, 137, 148, 159, 160, 161, 162, 176, 213, 214, 221, 262
rotating camera, 20
Roux-en-Y gastric bypass, 17, 74
rubber, 96, 193, 389
ruthenium, 285

S

safety, 5, 16, 19, 80, 273, 298, 305, 327, 374, 377, 380, 381, 390
Salmonella, 59
salpingo-oophorectomy, 380
salts, 136
saturation, 41, 273, 327, 336, 337, 384
scaling, 376, 388
scanning electron microscopy, 234
scar tissue, 214, 215, 218, 258
scarring, ix, 255, 258, 265, 267, 386
scatter, 203
scavengers, 274, 278, 306, 310
schistosomiasis, 129, 130
SDS, 230, 232, 238, 239, 240, 241
secretin, 138
sensitivity, 48, 49, 55, 63, 164, 187, 188, 189, 196, 204, 205, 206, 210, 303, 307, 345, 350
sensitization, 135, 138, 163, 175, 176, 177, 178
sepsis, 37, 38, 39, 40, 41, 42, 43, 44, 45, 46, 47, 48, 49, 50, 52, 53, 54, 56, 57, 58, 59, 60, 61, 62, 63, 64, 65, 66, 67, 68, 69, 70, 71, 72, 171, 172, 327, 334, 337, 343, 344, 346, 350, 352, 353, 355, 356
septic shock, 41, 44, 46, 63, 64, 65, 66, 67, 68, 69, 70, 71, 327, 328, 336, 353, 355, 356
serine, 232
serotonin, 152

serum, 41, 46, 129, 130, 133, 137, 151, 160, 172, 180, 197, 271, 274, 292, 295, 297, 330, 354, 367, 369
serum albumin, 330
sex differences, 171
sex hormones, 62
shear rates, 339
sheep, 16, 40, 48, 49, 55, 56, 58, 59, 65, 66, 69, 70, 237, 356
sheep models, 16
signal transduction, 296
signaling pathway, 282
signs of dehydration, 101
silicon, 22, 193, 208, 209
silk, 90, 97, 131, 134, 144
SIMENDO VR, 21
simulation-based training, 18, 30
Single Incision Laparoscopic Surgery (SILS), 3, 26, 27
siRNA, 256, 270, 272, 281, 282, 283, 286, 287, 288, 361, 369
skeletal muscle, 327, 351, 353
skills training, 4, 6, 34, 395, 400
sleep apnea, 378
sleeve gastrectomy, 17, 73, 74, 75, 78, 79, 80
small animal models, 22, 63, 81, 159
small bowel transplantation, 159, 172, 176, 180
small intestine, 74, 76, 177, 233, 250, 276, 354, 355, 389
small-for-size syndrome, 123
smooth muscle cells, 257, 266, 319
Society of American Gastrointestinal and Endoscopic Surgeons (SAGES), 6
sodium dodecyl sulfate (SDS), 231
soft lithography, 187, 193
solid tumors, 197, 213
somatic cell, 236
somnolence, 46
spatial ability, 9, 10, 33, 35
spatial memory, 10, 11
spectroscopy, 324, 327, 336, 337, 355
sphincter, 74, 137
spinal fusion, 400
spine, 329, 388, 392, 396
spleen, 76, 119, 120, 159, 164, 167, 174, 177, 323, 364
splint, 116
Sprague-Dawley rats, 102, 331
squamous cell, 208, 397
squamous cell carcinoma, 397
starch, 270, 274, 278, 294
stasis, 45, 323, 341, 342
stem cell differentiation, 236

stem cells, 175, 181, 189, 209, 230, 235, 236, 238, 239, 240, 245, 247, 248, 250, 259
stenosis, 124, 125, 131, 152, 304
stent, 35, 38, 51, 52, 56, 67, 71, 386
stereomicroscope, 198
sterile, 55, 60, 78, 88, 93, 96, 101, 197, 198, 214, 217, 222
sternum, 88, 89, 96
steroids, 171, 173
stimulation, 122, 136, 240, 248, 292, 319, 347
stimulus, 48
stomach, 74, 75, 76, 77, 78, 109, 110, 112, 117, 119, 236, 364
stress, 27, 31, 88, 120, 123, 129, 150, 194, 212, 234, 237, 238, 239, 319, 320, 322, 323, 340, 342, 344, 349, 352, 374
strictures, 137, 299
stroke, 55, 305, 354, 386
stroke volume, 55
stroma, 207
stromal cells, 163, 189, 203
structural protein, 143, 343
subcutaneous injection, 51, 53, 221
subcutaneous tissue, 53
submucosa, 280
subnormothermic and rewarming liver perfusion, 300
substrate(s), 236, 256, 271, 274, 277, 281
sucrose, 140, 270, 271, 294
sulfate, 51, 230, 238, 277
superior vena cava, 240
surface structure, 323
surface treatment, 195
surgical intervention, 345
surgical removal, 150
surgical resection, 183
surgical technique, vii, 3, 5, 17, 31, 143, 156, 374, 377, 394
surgical tissue handling, 255
survival, 45, 50, 51, 66, 70, 71, 104, 107, 123, 125, 131, 135, 139, 147, 166, 168, 169, 172, 174, 179, 180, 198, 200, 201, 203, 205, 206, 212, 222, 224, 225, 229, 230, 237, 240, 241, 242, 244, 245, 272, 275, 279, 280, 285, 293, 298, 302, 303, 304, 305, 345, 356, 364, 367, 371, 382, 386, 393, 397
survival rate, 51, 66, 123, 125, 212, 222, 272, 303, 364
suture, 51, 53, 57, 86, 87, 88, 90, 94, 95, 97, 100, 101, 103, 126, 217, 221, 263
swelling, 218, 271, 318, 343, 352
syndrome, 38, 40, 65, 71, 105, 123, 150, 161, 172, 303, 346, 378, 384
synergistic effect, 166

synthesis, 65, 133, 151, 258, 259, 280, 353
systolic blood pressure, 41
systolic pressure, 88, 295

T

T cell, 133, 162, 163, 164, 165, 166, 168, 169, 170, 171, 172, 173, 175, 176, 179, 180, 245
T cell receptor (TCR), 162, 164
T lymphocytes, 364
T regulatory cells, 165, 169
target organs, 147, 162, 167, 177, 282, 366
Task Trainer, 20
TBI, 160, 161, 164, 166, 167, 168, 175, 180
techniques of liver resection, 124
telesurgery, 373, 376, 390, 391, 393, 396, 397, 398
tendinitis, 258
tendon, 234, 263, 264
tensile strength, 234, 238, 258, 259, 261
testis, 399
TGF, 256, 257, 258, 260, 266
the liver regeneration model, 122
therapeutic agents, 53, 136, 183, 185, 187, 188, 192, 196, 200, 292
therapeutic approaches, 37, 102, 171
therapeutic benefits, 318
therapeutic response, 183, 184, 190, 192, 206, 207, 208
thermal energy, 25
third dimension, 209
thoracoscopy, 395
thoracotomy, 82, 93, 94, 95, 96, 97, 377
thorax, 82, 84
three-dimensional laparoscopy, 26
three-dimensional model, 22
three-dimensional space, 3, 6
thrombin, 241, 257, 265, 266, 272, 286
thrombocyte, 257
thrombocytopenia, 170
thrombomodulin, 302
thrombosis, 263, 266, 280, 299, 306, 312, 316, 344, 383
thrombus, 320
thymus, 89, 97, 167, 174, 214
thyroid, 383, 384, 400
thyroid gland, 383
time constraints, 305
time frame, 196, 201, 206
time periods, 7
TIMP, 287
TIMP-1, 287
tissue engineering, vii, ix, 235, 239, 246, 248, 249, 250, 251, 252, 253

tissue perfusion, 25, 45, 51, 59, 322, 356, 376
tissue regeneration, 255, 259
tissue viability imaging, 337
titanium, 14, 124
TLR, 38, 48, 55, 283
TLR2, 261
TLR3, 283
TNF, 38, 48, 49, 55, 56, 57, 59, 152, 163, 257, 261, 302, 342
TNF-alpha, 152
TNF-α, 38, 48, 49, 55, 56, 57, 59, 163, 302
Togo, 151, 152
total costs, 379
total parenteral nutrition, 172
toxicity, 175, 283, 326, 369
toxicology, 191, 209
toxicology studies, 209
toxin, 62, 129, 138, 366, 372
trachea, 57, 88, 93, 231, 233, 242, 248
tracheostomy, 60
training programs, 12, 19, 388, 396
transaminases, 296
transcription factors, 156, 320, 342
transduction, 144
transection, 74
transfection, 144, 361, 364, 365, 371
transferrin, 324
transfusion, 182, 384, 385, 386, 401
transgene, 105, 273
transition metal, 273
translocation, 163
transplant, 29, 161, 162, 163, 165, 166, 167, 169, 170, 171, 172, 173, 174, 175, 177, 180, 208, 229, 239, 269, 277, 283, 287, 292, 293, 294, 295, 298, 359
transplant recipients, 173
transplantation, vii, ix, 33, 108, 117, 122, 123, 129, 151, 153, 154, 159, 160, 161, 166, 167, 169, 170, 172, 173, 174, 175, 176, 177, 178, 179, 180, 181, 182, 229, 230, 235, 237, 240, 245, 247, 249, 250, 251, 255, 269, 270, 271, 274, 275, 276, 277, 279, 281, 282, 283, 284, 285, 286, 287, 289, 290, 291, 292, 293, 294, 295, 296, 297, 298, 299, 301, 302, 303, 304, 305, 306, 307, 308, 309, 310, 313, 314, 362, 366, 367, 368, 369, 372, 403
transurethral resection, 183, 196
transverse aortic constriction, 82, 95
transverse colon, 117
trauma, 3, 4, 27, 28, 40, 43, 62, 63, 65, 66, 68, 120, 263, 264, 292, 343, 351, 396
tremor, 26, 374, 376, 388
trypsin, 135, 147, 153, 232
tryptophan, 269, 270, 271, 275, 277, 278, 294

tumor, 32, 38, 65, 68, 70, 120, 122, 140, 142, 143, 144, 145, 146, 148, 156, 183, 185, 187, 189, 190, 192, 196, 197, 198, 200, 201, 206, 207, 208, 212, 213, 214, 217, 218, 219, 221, 222, 223, 224, 225, 226, 259, 318, 363, 364, 377, 378, 380, 383, 386, 389
tumor cells, 122, 142, 143, 145, 187, 197, 214, 223
tumor development, 221
tumor growth, 122, 148, 187, 212, 214, 222, 223, 224, 225, 226
tumor necrosis factor, 38, 65, 68, 70
tumoral injection, 218
tumorigenesis, 222
tungsten, 361
turnover, 152, 235, 236, 262, 293
TURP (Transurethral Resection of the Prostate), 183, 184, 196, 203
type 1 diabetes, 282
type 2 diabetes, 17
typhoid fever, 59
tyrosine, 144, 260, 267

U

ultrastructure, 147, 265, 305
umbilical cord, 236
unconjugated bilirubin, 133
underlying mechanisms, 365
urea, 237, 296
ureter, 16, 241, 389
urinary bladder, 60
urinary tract, 54
urine, 41, 46, 143, 298, 386
URO Mentor, 21
urologic laparoscopic training, 16
urology, 16, 32, 34, 35, 269, 378, 385, 389, 395, 400

V

vaccine, 359, 363, 364, 370, 371, 372
variations, 17, 47, 112, 114, 116, 117, 300
vascular cell adhesion molecule, 352
vascular surgery, vii, 397
vascular wall, 325, 344
vascularization, 109, 231, 241, 260
vasculature, 21, 112, 127, 153, 240, 241, 242, 245, 249, 250, 292, 338
vasculitis, 326, 329
vasoconstriction, 257, 274, 281, 338, 343
vasodilation, 44, 319, 320, 334, 343, 353
vasomotor, 320
vasopressin, 63, 150

vasopressor, 44
vasospasm, 271
VCAM, 296
VEGF (Vascular Endothelial Growth Factor), 147, 149, 212, 213, 256, 257, 258, 260, 266
VEGFR, 260
vein, 13, 60, 61, 110, 112, 113, 114, 116, 117, 124, 125, 126, 128, 130, 131, 132, 134, 152, 156, 230, 237, 239, 242, 251, 280, 298, 299, 325, 341, 366, 367, 369, 383, 384
velocity, 321, 325, 326, 327, 330, 332, 333, 336, 339, 350, 360, 371
ventilation, 60, 62, 85
venules, 44, 319, 325, 328, 354
vessels, 44, 45, 69, 102, 104, 112, 117, 124, 137, 237, 241, 259, 263, 306, 318, 319, 321, 322, 325, 328, 330, 331, 332, 337, 343, 350
video microscopy, 353
video trainers, 16, 19
villus, 189, 209
viral gene, 142, 366, 367
viral vectors, 235, 361, 366, 371
viscera, 119, 132, 382
viscoelastic properties, 322
viscosity, 44, 239, 274, 275, 276, 278, 279, 294, 320, 321, 322, 323, 325, 328, 339, 340, 341, 342, 343, 344, 345, 347, 349, 350, 351, 354, 357
visual field, 11, 221
visualization, 23, 26, 93, 117, 248, 328, 330, 331, 345, 349, 354, 376, 385, 387
vitamin K, 47, 131
vitamins, 140, 275, 294

VR (Virtual Reality), 11, 12, 19, 21, 28, 30, 31, 33, 35, 389, 390
   models, 11
   trainer, 9

W

water, 38, 46, 60, 88, 92, 96, 144, 194, 195, 197, 213, 214, 232, 233, 261, 319, 322, 331
water vapor, 213
weight loss, 17, 73, 74, 75, 80
white blood cell count, 41
white blood cells, 302, 325
World War I, 161
wound dehiscence, 263
wound healing, ix, 80, 255, 256, 257, 258, 259, 260, 261, 262, 263, 264, 265, 266, 267, 326, 327, 336
wound infection, 5, 260, 374
wound physiology, 255
wounding, 255, 256, 257, 261, 262

X

xenograft(s), 140, 142, 143, 144, 188, 200, 206, 207, 208, 209, 210, 211, 212, 213, 214, 218, 221, 222, 223, 225
   models, 140, 142, 143, 200, 210, 211, 213, 221

Z

Zeus, 373, 374, 376, 390, 391, 396